HEMATOLOGY

principles and procedures

BARBARA A. BROWN B.A., M.T. (ASCP), M.S.

Supervisor, Hematology Section, Clinical Pathology Department,
Tufts New England Medical Center Hospital
Boston, Massachusetts

HEMATOLOGY

principles and procedures

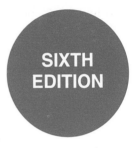

SIXTH
EDITION

Lea & Febiger ● 1993 ● Philadelphia, London

Williams & Wilkins
Rose Tree Corporate Center, Building II
1400 North Providence Road, Suite 5025
Media, PA 19063-2043 USA

Executive Editor—R. Kenneth Bussy
Development Editor—Tanya Lazar
Project Editor—Lisa Stead
Manuscript Editor—Denise Wilson
Production Manager—Samuel A. Rondinelli

Library of Congress Cataloging-in-Publication Data

Brown, Barbara A.
    Hematology : principles and procedures / Barbara A. Brown ; [contributors, chapters 2, 6, and color plates, Rouette C. Hunter, chapter 7, Alison O'Hare, chapters 5 and 6, Gloriana Erim]. — 6th ed.
        p.   cm.
    Includes bibliographical references and index.
    ISBN 0-8121-1643-7
    1. Blood—Examination. 2. Hematology—Technique. I. Title. [DNLM: 1. Hematologic Diseases—diagnosis—laboratory manuals. 2. Hematology—instrumentation—laboratory manuals. WH 25 B877h]
    RB45.B76   1993
    616. 1'5—dc20
    DNLM/DLC
    for Library of Congress   92-49057
                                                                                              CIP

First Edition, 1973
  Reprinted, 1974
Second Edition, 1976
  Reprinted, 1977, 1978, 1979
Third Edition, 1980
  Reprinted, 1981, 1982 (Twice)
Fourth Edition, 1984
  Reprinted, 1985 (Twice)
Fifth Edition, 1988
Sixth Edition, 1993

NOTE: Although the author(s) and the publisher have taken reasonable steps to ensure the accuracy of the drug information included in this text before publication, drug information may change without notice and readers are advised to consult the manufacturer's packaging inserts before prescribing medications.

Cover art courtesy of: D. Zucker-Franklin, M. F. Greaves, C. E. Grossi, A. M. Marmount: Atlas of Blood Cells, Function and Pathology. Second Ed. Philadelphia, Lea & Febiger, 1988.

Print number: 5   4   3   2

*A dedication and thank you
to Bettina G. Martin, M.S., M.B.A.,
without whose direction and support
the first (and all subsequent) editions
of this book would never have been written.*

PREFACE

In the sixth edition of *Hematology: Principles and Procedures* the scope and purpose of the book remain the same: to give the new student a basic knowledge of hematology, coagulation, and instrumentation in preparation for understanding more advanced texts. This book may also be an aid to technologists requiring a review of theory and procedures after having been away from the field for a period of time. Supervisors and technologists in hematology and coagulation may find the book useful in the preparation of procedure manuals and for troubleshooting technical problems. Other workers in the allied health professions may find the text helpful to them in the areas of hematology and coagulation.

A review of universal precautions has been added to Chapter 1, and statistical analysis of laboratory testing has been increased. Chapter 2 has been updated, and the color plates have been reorganized and expanded. Routine hematology procedures (Chapter 3) have been updated in regard to universal precautions, the ESR procedure expanded, and a new test for hemoglobin S added. In Chapter 4, additions have been made to the sections on blood parasites and quantitation of hemoglobin F, and a red cell zinc protoporphyrin test has been added. Coagulation theory has been updated in Chapter 5 and several new procedures added. The chapter on diseases has been reorganized and updated. Because of the increased variety of hematology and coagulation instrumentation, the format of the Automation chapter has been changed slightly. With space constraints it is not possible to describe all related instruments currently manufactured. The principles and operation of the most widely used instruments are described. This includes the addition of 14 new instruments/models, including an automated reticulocyte analyzer and an automated ESR instrument.

I appreciate the information and assistance that I received from Rose Mikulski (Bio/Data Corp.), Alan Burton (Coulter Corp.), Jeff Williams, Steve Gauthier, and Judith Burns (Baxter Diagnostics Inc.), Beth Peterson-Shedd (TOA Medical Electronics Co., Ltd.), Diann Thurston (Ortho Diagnostics Systems, Inc.), Carolyn Steinberg (Instrumentation Laboratory), John Perini (Organon Teknika), C. Scott Palubiak (Isolab, Inc.), International Technidyne Corp., Brent L. Riley (Miles, Inc.), Richard Minnihan (Medical Laboratory Automation), Don Pepin (Miles, Inc.), Karen Civetti (Vega Biomedical), and John Dean (Abbott Diagnostics).

I am most appreciative of the help of the contributors, listed previously. I am indebted to Elizabeth Golden, M.T. (ASCP), Chief Technologist: Special Coagulation (Medical Center Hospital of Vermont) for her review and suggestions in the coagulation section of the book. In addition, a thank you to Marcie LaFountain for the art work, Rouette Hunter, M.T. (ASCP) for taking additional photomicrographs for the color plates, Mary R. Donahoe, M.T. (ASCP) for proofreading assistance, and a special thanks to Theresa Kuszaj for her proofreading help on all editions of this book.

For this and all previous editions I am most grateful to the staff at Lea & Febiger for their valuable assistance and for helping to make this book successful.

Randolph, MA   Barbara A. Brown

CONTRIBUTORS

Chapters 2, 6, and Color Plates
Rouette C. Hunter, M.T. (ASCP)
Assistant Supervisor, Hematology
Tufts New England Medical Center Hospital
Boston, Massachusetts

Chapter 7
Alison O'Hare, M.T. (ASCP)
Section Leader, Hematology
Tufts New England Medical Center Hospital
Boston, Massachusetts

Chapters 5 and 6
Gloriana Erim, M.T. (ASCP)
Medical Technologist III, Hematology
Special Coagulation Coordinator
Tufts New England Medical Center Hospital
Boston, Massachusetts

CONTENTS

3. • Routine Hematology Procedures

4. • Special Hematology Procedures

5. • Coagulation

6. • Diseases

7. • Automation

BASIC LABORATORY TECHNIQUES

Hematology is defined as the study of blood. This textbook deals primarily with the cellular elements of the peripheral blood and bone marrow, and with those components of the plasma that function in the process of blood coagulation and fibrinolysis.

To perform laboratory testing various tools are used; those common to most hematology procedures are described in this chapter. It is important to understand the principles of operation for the microscope, the centrifuge, and the spectrophotometer. A procedure for collection of blood specimens is also included, as is a brief description of universal precautions for working with blood and other body fluids. Quality control of patient test results, methods for evaluation of new laboratory procedures, and the determination of normal testing ranges should also be understood by the medical technologist.

COMPOSITION OF BLOOD

The total blood volume in an adult is 5 to 6 liters, or 7 to 8% of the body weight. Approximately 45% of the blood is composed of formed elements: *red blood cells, white blood cells,* and *platelets.* The red cells contain hemoglobin, which binds oxygen; the white blood cells defend the body against foreign substances, such as infections; and the platelets primarily function in the stoppage of bleeding. The remaining 55% of the blood is the fluid portion, of which approximately 90% is water and 10% is composed of proteins (albumin, globulin, and fibrinogen), carbohydrates, vitamins, hormones, enzymes, lipids, and salts.

When coagulation is prevented by the use of an anticoagulant, the liquid portion of the blood is termed *plasma* and contains the protein fibrinogen. If a blood specimen is allowed to clot, the liquid portion released from the clot is called *serum* and does not contain any fibrinogen due to the fact that the fibrinogen was utilized to form the fibrin threads of the blood clot.

As the blood circulates throughout the body, oxygen is transported from the lungs to the tissues, products of digestion are absorbed in the intestine and carried to the various tissues of the body, and substances produced in various organs are transferred to other tissues for use. Cellular elements of the blood may also be transported to fight infection or aid in blood coagulation. At the same time, waste products from the tissues are picked up by the blood to be excreted through the skin, kidneys and lungs.

UNIVERSAL PRECAUTIONS

Universal precautions may be defined as a method for controlling infection in which all blood and certain body fluids are treated as if infected with hepatitis B, human immunodeficiency virus (HIV), or other disease-producing blood-borne pathogens. The *reason* for universal precautions is that all patients infected with blood-borne pathogens cannot be readily identified. Therefore, certain precaution techniques are used for all patients.

Under universal precautions the following policies are applicable to laboratory personnel.

1. Skin and mucous membrane exposure to

1

blood and other body fluids must be prevented.

2. Gloves must be worn when there is any possibility of coming in contact with blood or other body fluids. When removing gloves they must be disposed of in biohazardous waste. Gloves must never be reused.

3. Masks and protective eyewear (goggles) or face shields are to be worn if there is a possibility of droplets or spattering of the blood or body fluid. Use of plexiglas shields in the work area is an alternative.

4. Gowns or laboratory coats should be worn when working with blood or body fluids. These coverings must be removed before leaving the laboratory and may not be taken home for washing.

5. Any skin surfaces that become contaminated with blood or body fluids should be washed immediately. Hands must be washed upon removal of gloves.

6. It is of utmost importance that any cuts or scratches be well protected from contamination with blood or body fluids.

7. During phlebotomy, used needles should not be recapped, bent, or broken by the technologist. The unsheathed needle should be placed directly into an appropriately labeled puncture-resistant biohazard container for disposal.

8. All specimens for centrifugation must be centrifuged in a closed tube (a top must be on every tube).

9. Special care must be taken to avoid leaking of specimen tubes or containers.

10. All pipetting must be carried out using mechanical pipet devices.

11. All laboratory work benches must be decontaminated with the appropriate germicide (10% Clorox, for example) when work has been completed (at least once per shift).

12. Instrumentation must be decontaminated prior to servicing. If this is not possible, a warning should be placed on the equipment.

13. All materials coming in contact with blood or body fluids must be placed in biohazardous waste containers when finished with and disposed of according to the institution's infective waste disposal policy.

14. No precaution labels are used on any patient specimens because of the fact that *all* specimens are considered infectious and handled accordingly.

COLLECTION OF BLOOD

The medical technologist most often comes in contact with a patient during the process of blood collection. The patient in a hospital is anxious, fearful, and in ill health. He is anxious about his physical condition; he fears because he does not know what will happen next; his disease may or may not be life threatening; and he is physically uncomfortable as a result of his illness or injury. He is also separated from his known surroundings and family. For these reasons, a person's mental attitude is often at its worst when he is in the hospital as a patient. It is important, therefore, for the medical technologist to show the patient, at all times, the kindness and understanding that can mean so much.

When the technologist is dealing with a child, his approach is doubly important. This may be the first time the child has had a blood test. If it turns out to be a horrendous experience, it will be remembered and feared by the child for many years. Therefore, it is important to gain the child's confidence before proceeding with blood collection. The child should be informed of what is going to happen. If the child is told that the puncture will not hurt, the child's confidence will be lost because this statement is generally not true. A routine venipuncture may be compared to a bee sting, while the fingerstick may be described as a mother pricking her finger with a needle or pin while sewing.

The techniques used in obtaining blood are not learned overnight. They are an art that must be developed by study, observation, and practice, until the technologist has the necessary skill and self confidence. Skill, patience, understanding—these are the qualities of a good phlebotomist.

Blood specimens are commonly obtained from a patient's vein. Under some circumstances, as outlined below under Microsample Technique, a skin puncture will be used for this purpose. Irrespective of the method used certain techniques are common to all phlebotomy procedures:

1. The *correct patient identification* is critical.

For hospital patients this is accomplished by checking the identification wrist band for the correct name and hospital identification number. The procedure for outpatients is not as easy. The phlebotomist should ask the patient for his or her full name and any other information specific for that patient that can be verified by the requisition slip. (Misidentification of a patient is a serious error and can have disastrous implications for the patient.)

2. The *correct specimen identification* is equally as important as patient identification. Each blood specimen obtained should be labeled with the patient's first and last name, the hospital identification number, patient location, time, date, and the phlebotomist's initials.

3. To be consistent with laboratory safety guidelines and universal precautions, gloves must be worn at all times while performing phlebotomy techniques to protect the technologist from acquiring blood-borne infections such as hepatitis B or HIV. In addition, the phlebotomist's hands should be washed between each patient when removing gloves.

4. The puncture site should be cleaned by rubbing vigorously with a pad thoroughly moistened with 70% isopropanol (v/v). The area is then dried using sterile gauze. Once the phlebotomy site has been cleaned the decontaminated area should not be touched. Betadine should not be routinely used to clean the phlebotomy area because contamination with this substance will cause some erroneous test results (falsely elevates potassium, uric acid, and phosphorus results).

5. All sharp objects such as lancets and needles must be disposed of in special puncture-resistant disposable needle containers labeled as biohazardous. Needles should not be bent, broken, or resheathed before disposal. All other objects such as gauze and alcohol prep swabs should be placed in biohazardous waste containers.

Microsample Technique

Microsampling refers to blood collection by skin puncture and is frequently used on the following types of patients:

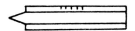

FIG. 1–1. Blood lancet.

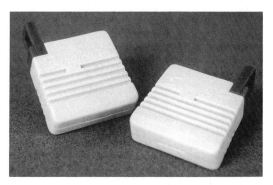

FIG. 1–2. Tenderfoot® disposable heel incision device. (Courtesy of International Technidyne Corp., Edison, NJ.)

1. *Infants less than 6 months* of age generally do not have a large blood supply, and it is dangerous to remove the volume of blood involved in venipuncture.

2. In *young children,* if only a small amount of blood is needed, a skin puncture is performed on the finger.

3. When an *adult* has poor veins, when the veins cannot be used because of intravenous (I.V.) infusions, or in the case of a severely burned patient, the finger may be used as the phlebotomy site.

Reagents and Equipment

1. Isopropyl alcohol, 70% (v/v), or prepared alcohol prep pads.
2. Sterile gauze pads.
3. Skin puncture device.
   a. Sterile blood lancet (Fig. 1–1).
   b. Tenderfoot® heel incision device (Fig. 1–2) (manufactured by International Technidyne Corp., Edison, NJ) is a semiautomated, disposable instrument which makes a standardized incision 1 mm deep and 2.5 mm in length. (The wound depth of 1 mm is sufficient to reach the vascular bed in an infant's heel.) To use this device:
      1) When the phlebotomy area has been cleaned and dried, remove

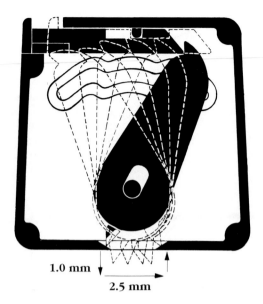

1.0 mm

2.5 mm

FIG. 1–3. Tenderfoot® disposable heel incision device (inside mechanism). (Courtesy of International Technidyne Corp., Edison, NJ.)

the Tenderfoot from its wrapper, being careful not to touch the blade-slot end on any nonsterile surface.

2) Remove the safety clip.

3) Select the phlebotomy site and place the blade-slot surface against the area. The instrument surface should be flush with the skin surface.

4) Press trigger. The tip of the blade ejects through the blade-slot while moving horizontally from one side of the slot to the other side and completely retracts into the opposite end of the blade-slot (Fig. 1–3).

c. Tenderfoot® Preemi is similar to the Tenderfoot described above and is for use on very small babies (3 to 4 pounds) or for collection of smaller amounts of blood. The incision is 0.85 mm deep and 1.75 mm in length.

d. Tenderlett™ (International Technidyne Corp.) (Fig. 1–4) is an automated, disposable incision device for obtaining blood samples from the fingertip. It is specially shaped to place on the fingertip, thus minimizing skin indentation. When the trigger is pressed, a

surgical blade quickly protrudes from the device at a 30° angle and then automatically retracts. The action of the blade is so fast it cannot be seen by the naked eye, while the angle of the blade is set for maximum blood flow. There are three sizes of Tenderlett for use with different age groups (size of finger). The Tenderlett Toddler will make an incision depth of 0.85 mm × 0.46 mm long and may be used on infants as young as 6 months old. For children up to 7 or 8 years of age the Tenderlett Junior (1.25 mm deep × 0.67 mm long) may be used. The Tenderlett is used for the older child and adult and has an incision size of 1.75 mm deep × 0.94 mm long.

4. Appropriate capillary tubes (Figs. 1–5, 1–6, and 1–7), Microtainers (Fig. 1–8), Unopette (Fig. 1–9), and/or pipets and diluting fluids.

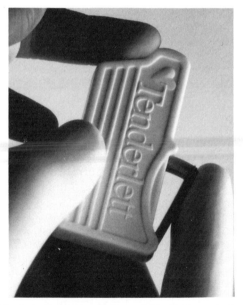

FIG. 1–4. Tenderlett™ disposable incision device. (Courtesy of International Technidyne Corp., Edison, NJ.)

FIG. 1–5. Caraway pipet.

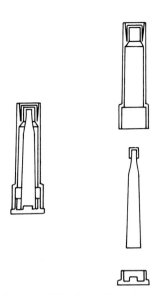

FIG. 1–6. Sarstedt 300 μL capillary blood collection system.

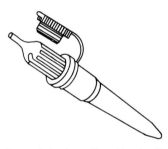

FIG. 1–7. Sarstedt 1 mL capillary blood collection system.

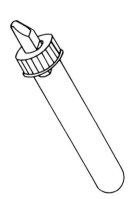

FIG. 1–8. Becton Dickinson Microtainer.

Procedure

1. *Location of phlebotomy site.* When obtaining blood from infants less than 1 year of age, blood is generally obtained from the heel of the foot. The site chosen should be on the inside (medial) or outside (lateral) portion of the bottom (plantar surface) of the foot. An imaginary line may be drawn from the middle of the large toe to the heel, and a line from between the fourth and fifth toes to the heel. The area outside of these two lines is considered acceptable as a phlebotomy site. Either side of the bottom surface of the heel, however, is the recommended and most commonly used area (Fig. 1–10). At no time should the back or sides of the heel be used. The depth of the puncture must be no greater than 2.4 mm in order to avoid damage to the bone. Because the blood vessels of an infant's heel are located between 0.35 and 1.6 mm below the surface of the skin, the puncture need not be any deeper than 1.6 mm. The third or fourth finger should be used when the patient is older than 1 year. The middle finger is most often used. The puncture should be made perpendicular to the fingerprint, on the palmar surface of the end portion of the finger, slightly off-center, but not on the side or tip of the finger (Fig. 1–11). The puncture should be

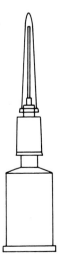

FIG. 1–9. Unopette.

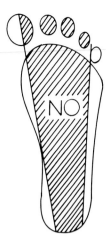

FIG. 1–10. Acceptable/unacceptable puncture sites on the foot.

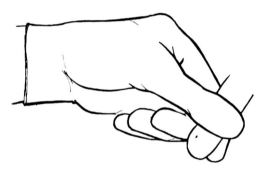

FIG. 1–11. Site of fingertip puncture.

no deeper than 3.1 mm because the distance between the skin surface and bone will vary from 3.1 to 10.9 mm. The distance to the bone is only 1.5 to 2.4 mm in infants 6 months old, so the finger is not used on this age group of children unless special devices are used. The puncture site should contain no swelling, and previous puncture sites should not be repunctured.

2. *Preparation of the puncture site.*
   a. Make certain the puncture site is warm. If it is not, use a *warm* moist cloth (not to exceed 42°C) and cover the site for 3 to 10 minutes.
   b. Clean the site with 70% isopropanol (v/v) and thoroughly dry with a sterile gauze. (Any alcohol left on the puncture site may cause the blood to hemolyze.)

3. Holding the finger (or foot), firmly puncture the site. If a lancet is used, insert it through the skin as far as it will go, but do not depress the surface of the skin because this will force the lancet to penetrate to an unsafe depth. With a good single puncture, 0.5 mL of blood may be obtained.

4. Using sterile dry gauze, wipe away the first drop of blood.

5. Apply moderate pressure, approximately 1 cm behind the site of the puncture to obtain a drop of blood.

6. Release this pressure immediately to allow recirculation of the blood.

7. Hold the collection tube (or pipet) in a horizontal to slightly downward position. When the tube comes in contact with the drop of blood, it should flow freely into the collection tube. If multiple tubes are to be collected, EDTA specimens should be filled first, followed by any other anticoagulated tests. Containers with no additives should be filled last.

8. Repeat steps 5, 6, and 7 until enough blood has been collected.

9. When blood collection is complete, the foot may be elevated above the body (the finger may be held in an upward position) and a sterile gauze pad pressed against the puncture site until bleeding stops. Application of an adhesive bandage is questionable on children less than 2 years of age because of resultant skin irritation, whereas slightly older children may remove the adhesive bandage and chew or aspirate it.

Discussion

1. Blood from a skin puncture is a mixture of venous, arterial, and capillary blood. The concentration of some constituents in the blood will differ between skin puncture blood and an arterial or venous specimen. Because of this, test reports should indicate if the blood sample was obtained from a skin puncture.

2. Excessive massaging or squeezing of the finger or foot will cause tissue juice to mix

with and dilute the blood. This will result in erroneous test results and increased clotting of the blood.

3. Excess crying will affect some test results (most notably, the white blood cell count may increase considerably). It is advisable to wait 30 minutes to 1 hour following a crying episode before obtaining the blood specimen.
4. The thumb, big toe, and ear lobe should not be used as a skin-puncture site for phlebotomy.
5. When collecting blood for hematology tests, the finger must be wiped dry after each test. (Platelets clump immediately in the blood at the puncture site.) Because of platelet adhesiveness and aggregation at the site of puncture, it is advisable to collect the platelet count and blood smears (if requested) first when samples for a number of tests are to be obtained.

Venipuncture

A venipuncture must be performed with care. The veins of a patient are the main source of blood for testing and the entry point for medications, intravenous solutions, and blood transfusions. Because there are only a limited number of easily accessible veins in a patient, it is important that everything be done to preserve their good condition and availability. Part of this responsibility lies with the medical technologist.

The ideal procedure is to have the patient lie down. If this is not possible, the patient should sit in a sturdy, comfortable chair with his or her arm firmly supported on a table or chair arm and easily accessible to the technologist. A patient should never stand or sit on a high stool during any process of blood collection. The technologist must be ready for the occasional patient who faints during this procedure; however, this rarely occurs with hospital inpatients who are lying flat in bed. There should be nothing in the patient's mouth at the time of phlebotomy, such as a thermometer or food.

Reagents and Equipment

1. Isopropyl alcohol, 70% (v/v), or prepared 70% alcohol prep pads.
2. Sterile gauze pads.
3. Tourniquet.
4. Appropriate test tubes for tests ordered.
5. Vacutainer holder (Fig. 1–12) or syringe (Fig. 1–13). The vacutainer system is the most widely used since it allows the blood to pass directly from the vein into the test tube.
6. Sterile, disposable needle. The choice of needle depends on the size of the vein. The most commonly used needles are 20-, 21-, and 22-gauge. The higher the gauge number, the smaller the inner diameter (bore) of the needle. For small veins, the 21- or 22-gauge needle is recommended. The length of needle used is chosen by the individual technologist. The two most widely used needle lengths are one inch and 1½ inches. Blood may be obtained from most deep veins with a one inch needle. If the vacutainer system is used, a special vacutainer needle (Fig. 1–12) is used. The hypodermic needle (Fig. 1–14) is employed with use of the syringe technique.
7. Band-aid.

Procedure

1. Prepare the vacutainer assembly: Insert the shorter end of the vacutainer needle into the holder. (The end of the needle is generally covered by a rubber like sleeve to prevent blood leaking from the needle when collecting more than one tube of blood.) Insert the first tube into the vacutainer holder until the top is even with the line on the holder. Do *not* puncture the top of the tube with the inside needle. Each tube contains a vacuum that draws the appropriate amount of blood into the tube. Puncturing the top causes loss of this vacuum.
2. When using a syringe to draw blood, move the plunger up and down in the barrel once or twice to make certain it does not stick. Expel all air from the syringe. Place the needle on the syringe (while keeping the cap on the shaft of the needle) and twist it to make certain it fits securely.
3. Apply the tourniquet several inches above the bend of the elbow, as shown in Figures 1–15 and 1–16, just tightly

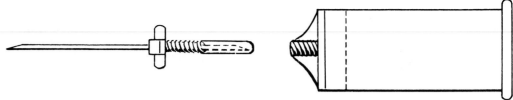

FIG. 1–12. Vacutainer holder and multisample needle.

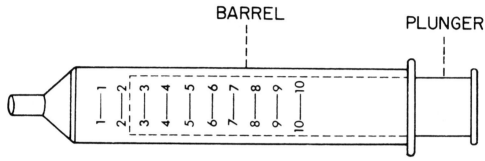

BARREL   PLUNGER

FIG. 1–13. Syringe.

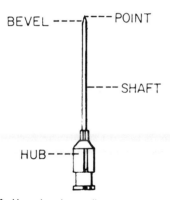

FIG. 1–14. Hypodermic needle.

enough to be uncomfortable. The patient's arm should be in a slightly downward position so that when blood enters the vacutainer tube it will go directly to the bottom of the tube and not remain at the top where it might flow back into the patient's vein.

4. Ask the patient to make a tight fist. This makes the vein more easily palpable.

5. Select a suitable vein for puncture (Fig. 1–17). The veins of the arm, which are the site of the majority of venipunctures, are the cephalic, median cephalic, and median basilic. The median cephalic vein is well anchored in tissue and does not roll when punctured. The median basilic vein, at the inner portion of the arm, tends to roll in many patients, whereas the cephalic vein is located on the edge of the outer part of the arm where the outside skin tends to be a little tougher.

6. Using the index finger of the left hand, palpate the arm until the best vein has been found. It should feel similar to an elastic tube. (A frequent error is failure to find the best vein because of carelessness or haste.) If the vein is not readily palpable, one of several techniques may be used to help locate the vein: (1) Force blood into the veins by massaging the arm from the wrist to the elbow, (2) tap sharply on the vein site with the index and third finger to cause the vein to dilate, (3) apply a warm, moist cloth (about 40°C) to the vein site, or, (4) allow the arm to hang in a vertical position so that the veins will fill to capacity with blood.

7. When the vein has been chosen, cleanse the puncture site with 70% alcohol. Dry the area with sterile gauze.

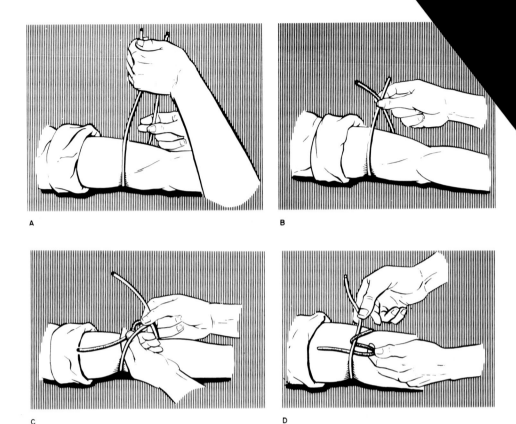

FIG. 1–15. Method of tourniquet application. A. Stretch the tourniquet to obtain the correct amount of tension. B. Grasp both sides of the tourniquet with the right hand while continuing to maintain the proper tension. C. With the left hand, reach through the loop and grasp the left side of the tourniquet. D. With the left hand, pull the tourniquet halfway through the loop. Release hands carefully.

8. Grasp the patient's arm 1 to 2 inches below the puncture site, pulling the skin tight with your thumb.

9. Hold the vacutainer assembly, or syringe, with the opposite hand, between the thumb and last three fingers. Rest the index finger against the hub of the needle to serve as a guide.

10. The needle should be in the bevel up position (needle opening facing upward), pointing in the same direction as the vein, and should make an approximate 15° angle with the arm.

11. The vein should be entered slightly below the area where it can be seen. In this way, there is tissue available to serve as an anchor for the needle.

12. A prominent vein may be entered quickly with a one-step puncture of the skin and vein. When the veins are

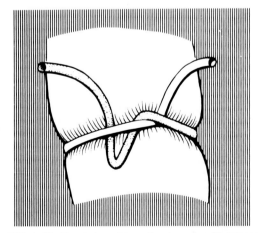

FIG. 1–16. Front view of tourniquet on arm. To release the tourniquet, carefully pull the end of the tourniquet on the left (shaded end).

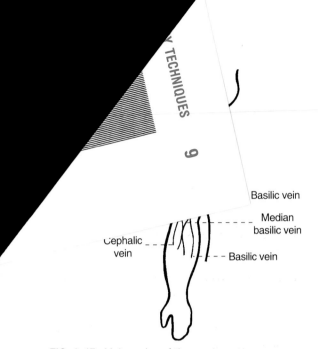

FIG. 1–17. Major veins of the arm.

deeper or the entry more difficult, a two-step procedure may be followed. First, the skin is punctured, and then, if need be, the free index finger is used to palpate above the puncture site to confirm the exact location of the vein. The second step is to puncture the vein.

13. As the needle enters the vein slightly less resistance will be felt.

14. If the vacutainer assembly is being used, as soon as the needle is in the vein, push the tube firmly but carefully into the holder as far as it will go, ensuring that the needle in the arm is kept in position. Maintain slight pressure on the bottom of each tube until it is filled.

15. If a syringe is used, a small amount of blood will flow into the neck of the syringe as the needle enters the vein. Care should be taken when pulling back on the plunger. Do not pull back with too much force since this may cause the blood to hemolyze, the force may pull the wall of the vein down on top of the bevel of the needle causing the blood flow to stop, or, the needle may inadvertently be pulled out of the vein.

16. The tourniquet should be loosened as soon as the blood enters the tube or syringe. The tourniquet should not be left on longer than 1 minute. If it remains on for longer periods, the blood in the

area will have an increased concentration of cells (hemoconcentration). (If desired, the patient may open his fist as soon as the blood begins to flow.)

17. The tourniquet must be released before the needle is removed from the vein.

18. Apply a sterile, dry gauze to the puncture site and quickly and smoothly withdraw the needle from the patient's arm.

19. Have the patient apply gentle pressure to the site of puncture for several minutes until the bleeding has stopped. Apply a bandaid if desired. The patient may also keep his arm raised in a vertical position for several minutes to decrease pressure in the blood vessel.

20. If a syringe is employed, the tubes to be filled should be placed in a test tube rack. As soon as the syringe is filled, the stopper(s) should be punctured with the needle and the tube(s) allowed to fill with blood until the blood flow stops. This process should be accomplished quickly before the blood begins to clot. The syringe should be disposed of with the unsheathed needle attached, as described previously.

Discussion

1. When the vacutainer system is being used to obtain several tubes of blood, collect a non-anticoagulated tube first. Coagulation specimens should be collected next, followed by tubes containing heparin, EDTA, and oxalate/fluoride (in the order listed). If a coagulation specimen is to be drawn first, a "discard" tube should be filled with several mL of blood first and then discarded. This prevents contamination of the specimen with tissue fluid from the venipuncture site. As soon as a tube containing anticoagulant is filled, mix the tube by inversion about 10 times while the next tube is filling with blood.

2. In the event that you have been unable to puncture the vein immediately, use your free index finger to locate the vein. It may be that the needle has not gone deeply enough, or perhaps it is slightly to the left or right of the vein. Do not attempt to puncture the vein from that

location. This is painful to the patient and may cause tissue damage. Withdraw the needle until the point is almost to the surface of the skin and then redirect the needle. This procedure is acceptable if the needle is close to the vein, but care should be taken that the patient is not caused too much pain. Sometimes a second venipuncture is necessary.

3. If the patient is receiving intravenous therapy in both arms, it is acceptable to puncture a vein below the intravenous site if the therapy is stopped for a minimum of 2 minutes, or if a different vein from the intravenous location is used.

4. A technologist or student should not stick a patient more than two times. If the blood sample has not been obtained after the second attempt, it is usually advisable to call another technologist. By this time, both you and the patient have lost confidence.

5. It is important that pressure be applied to the site of the venipuncture. Failure to follow this procedure leads to a hematoma (bleeding into the tissues).

6. If the area surrounding the puncture site begins to swell while blood is being withdrawn, this usually indicates that the needle has gone through the vein or the bevel of the needle is halfway out of the vein and blood is leaking into the tissues. The tourniquet should be released and the needle withdrawn immediately, with pressure applied to the site.

7. In some instances, it is almost impossible to locate a vein in the arm. In such cases, the veins of the lower arm, wrist, or hand may be used. The student should gain a reasonable amount of skill and confidence before attempting a venipuncture in these areas. The technologist should not perform a venipuncture on the veins in the ankle or foot.

8. When a venipuncture must be carried out on a small child, it is very important to release the tourniquet when the blood starts to enter the syringe. Children's veins are small and collapse quickly because blood is removed from the vein faster than it enters it.

9. When performing a venipuncture in the lower arm or hand, on small children, or on a patient with poor or small veins, a syringe or pediatric (small) vacutainer assembly and tubes is generally used. The use of standard sized vacutainer tubes tends to collapse these veins.

10. At all times be careful not to stick yourself with the needle. If this happens, report it to the supervisor immediately.

Isolation Techniques

Isolation techniques are used (1) to prevent the spread of infection from a patient to hospital personnel or to other patients, and (2) to shield or protect an infection-prone patient from pathogens. Five types of isolation have been described and are outlined below.

1. Strict isolation is used in cases of contagious diseases that can be transmitted by direct contact via the air. Examples are meningococcal meningitis, rabies, diphtheria, viral encephalitis, polio, measles, smallpox, and mumps. A gown, mask, and gloves are generally worn by the technologist. All articles in the room are considered contaminated, and handwashing is critical.

2. Enteric isolation techniques are used when coming in contact with patients who have dysentary and other disorders that spread through direct contact, such as Salmonella, Escherichia coli, and parasitic infections. The technologist is generally required to wear a gown and gloves.

3. In respiratory isolation, the patient has infections that are transmitted via droplets or by an airborne route. Examples are tuberculosis and whooping cough. In these cases the technologist should always wear a mask. Gloves are required as part of universal precautions.

4. Wound and skin isolation is used in cases of skin infection that may be transmitted directly or indirectly. The technologist will usually be required to wear gown and gloves.

5. Protective isolation requires the technologist to protect the patient from infection. These are patients with leukemia, severe burns, body radiation, kidney transplants, and plastic surgery. The technologist is usually required to wear a gown, mask, gloves, and sometimes shoe coverings.

Articles may be removed from the room because the patient does not have an infection but has a lowered resistance to infection.

When drawing blood from a patient in isolation, there are several general guidelines the technologist should adhere to:

1. Before entering the patient room, check the door for the type of isolation and review the directions indicated.
2. Leave the phlebotomy basket outside and carry in to the room only those supplies necessary.
3. Put on the necessary clothing as indicated (except gloves).
4. Once in the patient room place a clean paper towel on the table. All supplies should be kept on this towel.
5. Wash hands and put on gloves.
6. Perform phlebotomy.
7. Wash tourniquet in soap and water or 70% isopropanol. (In protective isolation this step should be performed prior to phlebotomy.)
8. Discard all needles, gauze, and like materials in the appropriate receptacles in the room (except in protective isolation).
9. Remove gown, gloves, mask, etc.
10. Wash hands.
11. Clean outside of specimen tubes with 70% isopropanol. (This step is not necessary in protective isolation.)
12. Discard paper towel.

ANTICOAGULANTS

Most hematology and coagulation procedures must be performed on whole blood or plasma. Therefore, as soon as the blood is withdrawn from the patient, it is mixed with an anticoagulant to prevent coagulation. The three most commonly used anticoagulants in the hematology laboratory are discussed below.

1. **EDTA** (sequestrene or versene) is generally available as the disodium, dipotassium, or tripotassium salt of ethylenediaminetetraacetic acid. It is the most widely used anticoagulant for hematologic procedures. The dipotassium salt is more soluble than the disodium salt and

is used in concentrations of 1.5 ($\pm$0.25) mg/mL. Tripotassium EDTA is normally used in the liquid form. This mixes more easily with the blood specimen and therefore results in fewer clotted specimens. EDTA prevents coagulation by binding the calcium in the blood. (Calcium is required for blood coagulation.) This anticoagulant also prevents formation of artifacts and may be used for the preparation of blood films up to 2 to 3 hours following blood collection. EDTA will, on rare occasions, cause platelet clumping or aggregation of the white blood cells. Excessive concentrations of EDTA cause shrinkage of the red blood cells leading to a decreased spun hematocrit, an increased MCHC, and a falsely low erythrocyte sedimentation rate. The hemoglobin, however, will not be affected. Increased concentrations also cause degenerative changes in the white cells and the platelets will swell and break up, causing a falsely increased platelet count (due to the broken fragments). After approximately 3 hours at room temperature, degenerative cellular changes will begin to occur and will become evident on a stained blood smear. The white blood cells may show vacuolation of the cytoplasm, more homogeneous nuclei, irregular or poorly defined cytoplasmic borders, and development of irregularly shaped nuclei. The platelets will increase in size and then disintegrate. After about 6 hours the red blood cells will begin to swell, causing an increased MCV, a decreased erythrocyte sedimentation rate, and an increase in the osmotic fragility. Generally, the older the blood specimen the more morphologic changes will occur. The hemoglobin is stable for several days. Refrigeration of the blood at 4°C will slow down the degenerative process, and there will be little evidence of change in the hematocrit, white blood count, or red blood count after 24 hours.

2. **Sodium citrate** (buffered or nonbuffered) is used for coagulation studies in a concentration of 1 part 0.109 M sodium citrate (trisodium citrate dihydrate) to 9 parts whole blood. (Concentrations of 0.109 M and 0.129 M have been used. The International Committee for Standardization in Hematology has recommended 0.109 M

[3.2%].) Sodium citrate prevents coagulation by binding the calcium of the blood in a soluble complex and also helps the platelets retain their functional capabilities. Buffered sodium citrate 0.109 M (trisodium citrate dihydrate and citric acid) may increase the stability of factors V and VIII.

3. **Heparin** may be used in a concentration of 15 to 30 units/mL of whole blood. Coagulation is prevented by its interaction with antithrombin III and subsequent inhibition of thrombin. The use of heparin as an anticoagulant does not alter the size of the red blood cells, but may cause clumping of the white cells and platelets. It is, therefore, of limited use in hematology and is the anticoagulant of choice for only a few special hematology procedures (e.g., osmotic fragility test) because the addition of salts to the blood affect some test results. When a blood smear is prepared from a heparinized specimen and Wright-stained, a blue colored background may be obtained. This is especially noticeable in the presence of abnormal proteins.

THE MICROSCOPE

Microscopes are basically classified by the type of light source used. The microscope used in the routine hematology laboratory is, in simple terms, a magnifying glass. It is termed a **compound light** (bright light or bright field) **microscope** because it contains two separate lens systems, the objective and the ocular (eyepiece). This microscope consists of an **eyepiece, objective,** a **mechanical stage,** a **substage condenser** system with an **iris diaphragm,** and a **light source** (Fig. 1–18).

1. The conventional **eyepiece lens,** or ocular, has a magnification of 10 ×. (× is used to designate the units of magnification, known as diameters. If a lens has a magnification of 10 ×, this does not mean that it magnifies an object to 10 times its original area, but rather that the diameter of the object is magnified 10 times its original size.) A monocular microscope consists of one eyepiece; a binocular microscope, the most commonly used today, contains two eyepieces.

2. Most light microscopes contain three **objectives lenses,** each with different powers of magnification. The most commonly employed objectives in hematology are 10 × (low power), 40 × (high dry), and 100 × (oil immersion). A fourth lens, 50 × (low oil immersion), may be utilized by experienced technologists for performing a differential cell count. These lenses are mounted on a disc, which is rotated to the desired position.

3. The **optical tube length** is the distance between the eyepiece and objective lenses and is generally 160 mm.

4. The specimen slide to be studied is placed on the **stage,** which contains a moveable assembly to facilitate the study of different parts of the slide.

5. The most commonly used **substage condenser** is the Abbe condenser which directs the beam of light from the source onto the specimen. It consists of two lenses (Fig. 1–18). The light is focused on the slide (specimen) by raising or lowering the condenser system. Lack of a substage condenser will cause fuzzy rings and haloes around the object being studied.

6. The **iris diaphragm** contains a number of leaves that the operator may open or close to increase or decrease the amount of light illuminating the object (Fig. 1–19).

7. Microscopes contain a built-in light source at their base, which usually contains a transformer for adjusting the light intensity. There may also be a neutral density filter present in the light source. Centering screws (in the light source or condenser) enable the viewer to center the light passing up through the condenser. A **field iris diaphragm** may also be present in the light source. It may be opened or closed and is used in focusing the light which passes up through the condenser.

The **image** seen by the eye through a compound microscope is termed the *virtual image* and is upside down and reversed. The right side is seen as the left side and vice-versa; therefore, movement of the slide on the stage will also appear reversed when looking through the microscope.

The total **magnification** of the microscope is equal to the magnification of the eyepiece times the magnification of the objective lens. For example, using a 10 × eyepiece and the 40 × objective lens, the total magnification is 400 ×. The magnification of each system is printed on each of the appropriate parts.

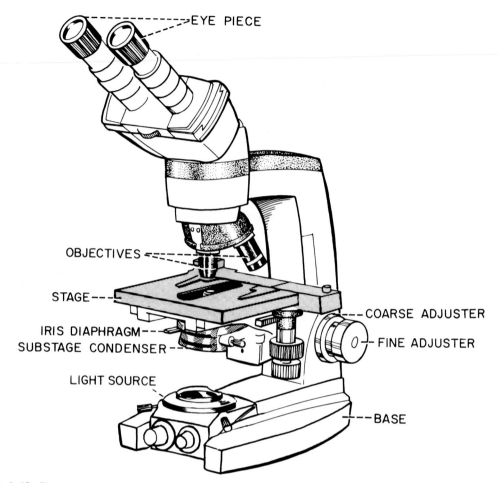

FIG. 1–18. Binocular microscope.

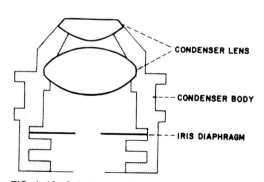

FIG. 1–19. Substage condenser and iris diaphragm.

The **numerical aperture** is a designation of the amount of light entering the objective from the microscopic field (or, as in the condenser, the amount of light entering the substage condenser from the light source). It may be thought of as a method for expressing the fraction of the wave front admitted by a lens (Fig. 1–20). The numerical aperture is constant for any single lens and is dependent on the radius of the lens (AC) and the focal length of the lens (PC).

$$\text{Numerical aperture} = R \times \sin \mu$$

μ = The angle made by the one ray passing through the edge of the lens, with the other ray passing through the center of the lens

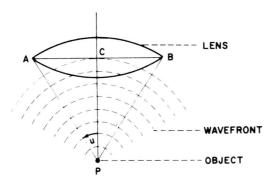

FIG. 1-20. Numerical aperture.

R = The refractive index of the medium between the object and the objective lens

The numerical aperture of the objective should be the same as the numerical aperture of the substage condenser. If these numerical apertures are not similar, interference effects occur.

The **refractive index** of a substance is calculated as the speed with which light travels in air divided by the speed with which light travels through the substance. (Since light travels more slowly through immersion oil, the numerical aperture is increased by placing oil between the oil immersion objective and the object.)

Resolving power is the useful limit of magnification. It is the ability of the microscope, at a specific magnification, to distinguish two separate objects situated close to one another and the ability of the lens to reveal fine detail. The smaller the distance between the two specific objects that can be distinguished apart, the greater the resolving power of the microscope.

$$\text{Minimal distance between two objects (resolvable distance)} = \frac{0.612 \times \lambda}{\text{Numerical aperture}}$$

λ = The wavelength of the light

The resolving power is, therefore, dependent on the wavelength of light and the numerical aperture. The light source remains constant and so, in routine work, may be ignored. The larger the numerical aperture, the smaller the resolvable distance, and hence, the more efficient the resolving power.

Depth of field is the capacity of the objective lens to focus in different planes at the same time. This is largely dependent on the numerical aperture. The greater the numerical aperture, the smaller the depth of field. It is possible to increase the depth of field slightly by closing the iris diaphragm (thus decreasing the numerical aperture).

Different wavelengths of light are not bent in the same way as they pass through the lens and, therefore, are not brought to the same focus. These are called **chromatic aberrations** (Fig. 1-21).

With **spherical aberrations,** the light waves, as they travel through the lens, are bent differently, depending on which part of the lens they pass through. Rays passing through the peripheral portions of the lens are brought to a shorter focal point than those rays passing through the thicker part of the lens (Fig. 1-22). To compensate for aberrations, **achromatic** and **apochromatic lenses** are employed. The achromatic lens is the most commonly used lens for color correction. It brings rays of two colors to a common focus and obtains a reasonable compromise for the remaining colors. Apochromatic lenses are the finest lenses produced and correct for chromatic and spherical aberrations. This lens brings three colors (blue, yellow, and red) to a common focus.

A factor that must be taken into consideration for the most effective use of the microscope lens is the **medium** between the objective and the object being studied. The low power (10 ×) and high dry objective lenses (40 ×) use air. When oil immersion lenses are employed, a drop of oil should be used; otherwise, bending of the light waves occurs (Fig. 1-23).

Operating Procedures

1. With the 10× objective in position, place the object to be studied (slide or counting chamber) on the microscope stage.
2. Adjust the distance between the eyepieces as necessary.
3. Focus the object, using the coarse adjustment knob. Bring the object into sharp focus with the fine adjustment knob.
4. While looking through the microscope, close the field diaphragm on the light source so that the image of the leaves of the diaphragm may be seen in the field of view.

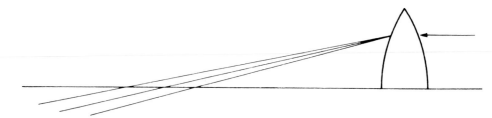

FIG. 1–21. Chromatic aberration.

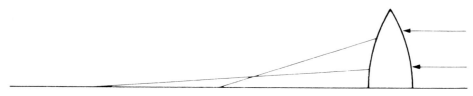

FIG. 1–22. Spherical aberration.

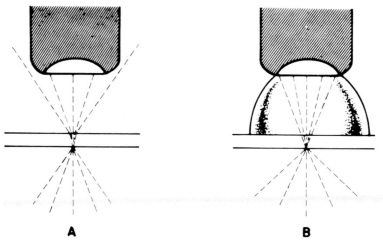

FIG. 1–23. Light path through the high dry objective lens (A) and oil immersion objective lens (B).

5. Focus the condenser by raising or lowering it until the leaves of the iris diaphragm are in sharp focus. The condenser should now be left in this position for use with all like objects.

6. Center the light source by using the two centering screws (these will be located on the light source or the condenser) so that the image of the field diaphragm in the field of view is in the center. Open the field diaphragm until the iris leaves just disappear from view.

7. Remove one eyepiece and, while looking into the microscope (without the eyepiece), close the condenser diaphragm. Reopen the diaphragm until the diaphragm leaves just disappear from view. (Further closing of the condenser diaphragm may increase contrast and depth of focus, depending on the specimen.) This procedure allows you to obtain the best resolving power for the microscope. Replace the eyepiece.

8. Generally, as you increase the magnifi-

cation of the microscope (change objectives), the condenser diaphragm must be opened while the field diaphragm (light source) is further closed. The condenser and field diaphragms should not be used to control light intensity. This is generally done by adjusting the transformer setting on the light source or by using filters.

Discussion

1. When employing the high-dry or oil immersion objectives, a suitable field for study should be found and focused using the low power objective ($10\times$). A drop of oil may then be placed on the slide and the oil immersion objective swung into place. Never use oil with the high-dry objective.
2. To clean the lenses, only lens paper should be used. The paper is designed for this purpose and will not scratch the lenses, which other, more harsh paper or material might do.
3. The oil must be removed from the oil immersion lens (with lens paper) whenever it is not in use in order to prevent oil seepage to the inside of the lens.
4. If a solvent is used to clean the lenses, the structures holding the objective lenses may loosen in time because of the dissolving qualities of these solutions.
5. If the field of study is dirty, the cause may be dirt on the eyepiece. Revolve the eyepiece as you are looking through the microscope. If the dirt also revolves, the eyepiece needs cleaning.

Phase Microscopy

Phase microscopy is employed in hematology for counting platelets. Performing this procedure on a light microscope is tedious and more prone to error because the platelets are unstained and are very small. Phase microscopy enables the viewer to see unstained platelets and structures in larger cells due to differences in the refractive index, shape, and absorption characteristics of the cells and cellular components.

Light travels in waves. If two sets of light

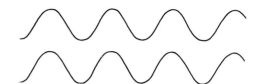

FIG. 1–24. Light waves in phase.

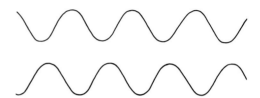

FIG. 1–25. Light waves out of phase.

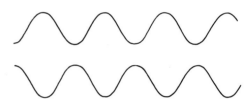

FIG. 1–26. Light waves out of phase.

waves in phase are allowed to travel through the same medium, they remain in phase (Fig. 1–24), and the brightness of the light is the sum of the two amplitudes (height of the peaks). If only one of these two light waves passes through an object, it is slowed down; the two waves are then out of phase (Fig. 1–25), and the light is diminished. If the two light waves are out of phase by one-half of a wavelength, there will be no light because the peak of one wave is cancelled by the trough of the other light wave (Fig. 1–26).

When rays of light pass through a slide containing unstained cells, platelets, or tissues, those rays which pass through the cells may be retarded or slowed down but not diffracted from their pathway. These are termed direct rays. Other light waves may be retarded and, at the same time, diffracted. The amount of retardation of the light wave is dependent on the optical density, refractive index, and shape of the cell or cellular component.

For maximum contrast between the cell and its surroundings, the light wave should be retarded by one-quarter of a wavelength. Unstained cells and tissues, however, are not able to retard the wavelength to this great a degree. Therefore, two additional parts are added to the light microscope to increase the small wave changes by approximately one-quarter of a wavelength. This then becomes the phase microscope. An **annular diaphragm** is placed below, or in the substage condenser, and a **phase shifting element** is situated in the rear focal plane of the objective. The light passes up from its source, through the clear circular area of the annular diaphragm (Fig. 1–27), and through the specimen. The phase shifting element is constructed so that light waves pass quickly through the clear areas (Fig. 1–27) but are retarded by one-quarter of a wavelength when going through the shaded circular area. These two components are so situated that the diffracted rays pass directly through the clear area of the phase shifting element. All light waves that are undiffracted pass through the treated (shaded) areas of the phase shifting element and are, therefore, slowed by an additional one-quarter of a wavelength. These alterations in the phases of the light waves increase the contrast and enable the viewer to get a more highly visible picture of the cells and their components.

Electron Microscopy

Magnifications greater than 1500× to 2000× are not practical with the light microscope due to a decreased efficiency in resolving power. For this reason, the electron microscope has come into use, where magnifications of 50,000× may be obtained with a high degree of resolving power. There are two types of electron microscope in common use today. The **transmission electron microscope (TEM)** employs a beam of electrons in place of the beam of light (in the bright light microscope). This beam of electrons, invisible to the eye, passes through the specimen being studied and is then focused onto a fluorescent screen or photographic plate to make the image visible to the human eye. The **scanning electron microscope (SEM)** was more recently developed. It looks at the surface of the tissue or cell and gives the viewer a three-dimensional image by striking the surface of the tissue with a focused beam of electrons. The deflected electrons, in addition to electrons emitted from the surface of the tissue or cells, are focused onto a photographic film or cathode ray tube to form a visible three-dimensional image. The specimen examined with the SEM is thicker than that used with the TEM, and the beam of electrons does not pass through the specimen as occurs with the TEM.

PHOTOMETER/SPECTROPHOTOMETER

If a substance can be converted to a soluble, colored material, its concentration may be determined by the amount of color present in the solution. The filter photometer and spectrophotometer are instruments used for this type of measurement in which a photocell or photomultiplier tube is used to detect the amount of light that passes through a colored solution from a light source. To obtain the greatest sensitivity, the light permitted to pass through the solution is of a particular wavelength (that wavelength which shows maximum absorbance for the color of the solution). If a filter is used to determine the wavelength, the instrument is termed a **filter photometer** or **colorimeter.** In the **spectrophotometer,** the wavelength is selected by a prism, or diffraction grating.

As shown in Figure 1–28, the *light source* (1) passes through a *monochromator* (filter, prism, or diffraction grating) (2). Only light of the present wavelength can pass from the monochromator through the *cuvet* (3) containing the material to be measured. The amount of light passing through the solution (those light waves not absorbed by the material) comes in contact with the photocell or photomultiplier tube (4), where the light energy is converted into electrical energy, which is then measured by the *galvanometer* (5). A scale located on the galvanometer is generally calibrated to read **optical density (O.D.)** or **percent transmittance (%T).** Optical density, or absorbance, measures the

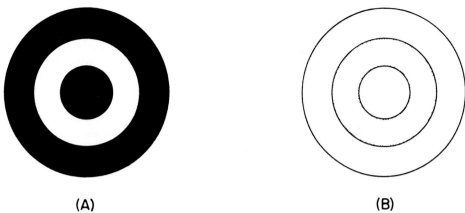

(A) **(B)**

FIG. 1–27. Annular diaphragm (A) and phase-shifting element (B).

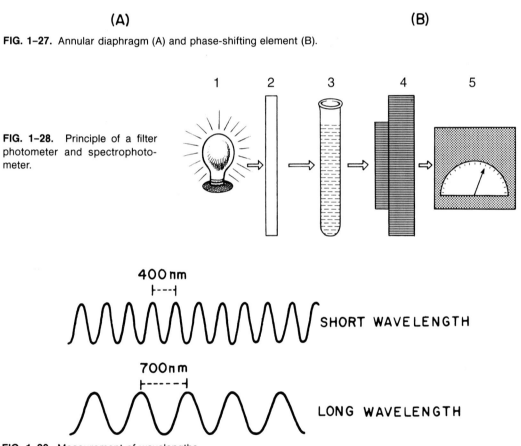

FIG. 1–28. Principle of a filter photometer and spectrophotometer.

FIG. 1–29. Measurement of wavelengths.

amount of light absorbed by the solution. The percent transmittance measures the amount of light allowed to pass through the solution. All colors which make up light have a wavelength of a specific length measured in **nanometers (nm)** (Fig. 1–29). A blue solution is blue because all colors except blue have been absorbed by the solution. In other words, the blue color (that particular wavelength) passes through the solution.

The principle of photometry is based on the Lambert-Bouger-Bunsen-Roscoe-Beer laws, which have been combined to give what is commonly known as **Beer's law.** According to this law, the absorbance (optical density) of a solution is directly proportional to the concentration of the solute (material in solution being tested for) and the length of the light path through this solution. Since the predetermined wavelength is the same and cuvets with a given, constant diameter are employed, the length of the light path through the solution is set, and the optical density is, therefore, directly proportional to the concentration of the solute. If the optical density and concentration of a standard are known, the unknown concentration may be calculated if its optical density is known.

$$\frac{\text{Concentration of unknown}}{\text{Concentration of standard}} = \frac{\text{Optical density of unknown}}{\text{Optical density of standard}}$$

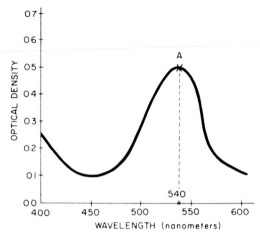

FIG. 1–30. Determination of wavelength.

Optical Density vs. % Transmittance

If L represents the light energy entering the solute and Lo is the light energy leaving the solute (that light hitting the photocell), then $\frac{Lo}{L}$ equals the transmittance (T) of the solute. If the energy leaving the solute is the same as the energy entering the solute, then $\frac{Lo}{L} = 1$ and, $1 \times 100 = 100\%$ transmittance, and the solution does not contain any of the material for which it is being tested. Optical density and % transmittance are related logarithmically to each other:

$$\text{O.D.} = -\log T \; or \; \text{O.D.} = 2 - \log\%T$$

When plotting a curve using optical density, regular graph paper is used. In plotting percent transmittance, semilog paper is employed. If solutions of varying concentrations are used, a straight line curve will be obtained if the test follows Beer's law. There are several conditions under which Beer's law will not hold true, in which case a straight line curve will not be obtained.

Determination of the Wavelength

To determine the optimal wavelength to be used for a specific test, an absorbance curve, reading optical density, should be plotted against the wavelength, as shown in Figure

1–30. Using a single concentration of the solution and the appropriate blank, take optical density readings at a series of different wavelengths. Plot the results on graph paper. Where the absorbance is at a maximum (point A), there should be maximum sensitivity, and this will, therefore, be the wavelength (540 nm) chosen for this test. Care should be taken that (1) the solution follows Beer's law in the wavelength chosen, (2) the sensitivity is not so great as to give too many readings at the extreme ends of the scale (for the greatest accuracy, readings should be taken between 20% transmittance and 90% transmittance), and (3) interfering substances are not picked up at this wavelength.

Preparation of a Curve

To construct a curve for a specific test, various known concentrations of the substance must be used. A graph is made, plotting the concentration of the substance (on the X axis, or abscissa) against the optical density or % transmittance readings (on the Y axis, or ordinate). All unknown readings from this curve should then fall in between the highest and lowest standards used in setting up the curve. The graph should be checked daily, using known controls. When new reagents are used or changes made to the photometer/spectrophotometer, a new curve should be made up. Graphs and tables supplied with a new instrument by the manufacturer should not be used, for the obvious reason that reagents and conditions in your laboratory are not the same as those found in the manufacturer's laboratory.

Discussion

1. Reagent blanks should generally be used with all tests and must contain all the reagents used in the unknown, with the exception of the unknown specimen.
2. Care must be taken to ensure that the cuvets used are not scratched. It is advisable to use the same cuvet for each sample. Rinsing the cuvet between samples is unnecessary if drainage is efficient, except in cases where the unknown is more diluted or concentrated than the previous sample. In this instance, rinse the cuvet with a small amount of the mixture to be read next.
3. The cuvet should be placed in the spectrophotometer facing in exactly the same direction for each reading. If the cuvet is turned slightly, there may be a significant difference in the reading.
4. It may be necessary to allow the instrument to warm-up for a time when first turned on. See manufacturer's directions.
5. Any turbidity present in the sample will cause erroneous results unless the procedure is being used to measure turbidity.
6. When taking readings on more than one sample, it may be necessary to recheck the reagent blank between specimen unknowns. This will depend on the stability of the instrument. It may be possible to read numerous samples without resetting the reagent blank.
7. Instrument quality control procedures should be performed at regular intervals according to manufacturer's directions: stray light check, wavelength calibration, and linearity checks at various wavelengths.

CENTRIFUGATION

A centrifuge is used to sediment particles suspended in a liquid or to separate different densities of a mixture. Centrifuges may vary from small table-top models to the much larger floor types. Refrigerated centrifuges are also available for maintaining the specimens at a lower temperature during the centrifugation process.

Centrifuges generally contain an *on/off switch* for turning the electrical power on and off, a *timer* that automatically turns the centrifuge off after a preset time, and a *tachometer* or *dial* for setting the speed (RPM) of the centrifuge (a few centrifuges will not contain this dial and can only be used at maximum speed). A *braking device* for rapidly stopping (de-accelerating) the centrifuge may also be present. The centrifuge *head* contains the *cups* (*shields* or *carriers*) that hold the specimens during the process of centrifugation. There are two types of heads that may be used interchangeably in most centrifuges: (1) the *horizontal head* and (2) the *angle head.* The specimen cups in the *horizontal centrifuge heads* are in a vertical position when the centrifuge is at rest. During centrifugation, the cups move to a horizontal position. As the specimen is centrifuged, the particles being sedimented travel down through the liquid to the bottom of the tube. When the centrifuge stops and the tubes swing to a vertical position there may be some remixing of the sediment with the supernatant liquid. These centrifuge heads are capable of speeds up to about 3000 RPM. Higher speeds than this will generally cause excessive heat buildup as a result of air friction. *Angle centrifuge heads* are capable of higher speeds and contain drilled holes that hold the tubes at a fixed angle (approximately 52° angle with the center shaft around which they rotate). There is much less heat developed during centrifugation because of very low air friction. During centrifugation, the particles travel across the column of liquid to the side of the tube where they clump together and then rapidly move to the bottom of the tube.

Specimens must be centrifuged for a specific time and at a certain speed, depending on the type and purpose of the specimen. This information should be included in all laboratory procedures, and may be critical for accurate test results.

The force generated by a centrifuge is termed the **relative centrifugal force (RCF)** × gravity and is calculated from the RPM (of the centrifuge head), the radius (distance, in centimeters, from the center shaft to the middle of the specimen tube), and a constant factor (1.118×10^{-5}), according to the following formula:

RCF = Constant $\times$ r $\times$ RPM^2
RCF = $1.118 \times 10^{-5} \times$ r $\times$ RPM^2
where r = radius

Most centrifuge instruction manuals will contain a *nomogram*, which is a chart for automatically determining the RCF when the radius and RPM are known.

When operating the centrifuge it is important that the tubes and cups on opposite sides of the head weigh the same (i.e., are balanced). The carriers and tubes must also be placed in the centrifuge in a geometrically symmetrical arrangement with each cup and its contents being of the same weight. If the centrifuge vibrates excessively during operation, it should be stopped and the load rebalanced. When centrifuging body fluid specimens, tubes should be covered. The centrifuge cover must be closed and locked into place at all times during operation.

The **ultracentrifuge** is an extremely high-speed centrifuge able to reach very high RCF values.

Centrifuges require regular maintenance. The brushes and timer should be checked and the RPM measured. A strobe light or a mechanical or electronic tachometer (available from most laboratory distributors) may be used to check the routinely used speeds on the centrifuge. The temperature of refrigerated centrifuges should also be closely monitored.

STATISTICAL TOOLS USED TO EVALUATE LABORATORY TESTING

In hematology, as in other areas of the laboratory, various statistical tools are used to help control the quality of test results, evaluate new test procedures, and define reference intervals (normal ranges) for test methods.

Quality Control of Test Results

The Quality Control Specimen

Quality control (Q.C.) specimens are used in the laboratory to ensure that patient testing is performed within acceptable limits of variation. In hematology, both commercially prepared and within-laboratory-prepared specimens may be used.

Generally, commercially prepared specimens are assayed (test results provided by the manufacturer). Controls that are prepared within the laboratory are tested multiple times to obtain a range of values. The Q.C. specimen should resemble the patient specimen as closely as possible and should show assay values within the same ranges as the patient results. This normally necessitates using three levels of control: abnormal high, abnormal low, and normal. If only two levels of control are used, abnormal high and normal are preferred. The frequency of testing quality control specimens will vary according to the particular procedure and the testing patterns within each laboratory. In a large, busy laboratory, a Q.C. specimen may be run every hour, whereas in a smaller operation quality control testing may be performed once each 8-hour shift. However, any time a change has occurred in a procedure that may affect test results (e.g., new reagents or change of instrument tubing or lamp), a Q.C. specimen should be run.

Assay of Control Specimens

Before a Q.C. specimen may be used as a control, an acceptable range of values must be determined. When using a commercial control the manufacturer will generally include the acceptable range for each lot of control. However, this range will differ from one laboratory to another, and the precision of the method should be determined for each testing center. If possible, the control should be tested over a period of at least 3 to 4 weeks by different technologists, that is, under conditions similar to that of patient testing. In these circumstances the results will not be exactly the same each time the test is performed because of random errors inherent in all procedures (this does not include use of malfunctioning equipment, expired reagents, etc.). **Precision** is defined as the variation of results when numerous tests are performed on the same sample. It is also referred to as **random error** (error with no set pattern) and may be measured using standard deviation, coefficient of variation, and variance.

Standard deviation (S.D.) is used to determine the acceptable range of values for a control using the following formula:

$$S.D. = \sqrt{\frac{\Sigma(\overline{X} - X)^2}{N - 1}}$$

Σ = sum of   X = individual values
$\overline{X}$ = mean   N = number of values

Using the WBC control values in Table 1–1 above, the S.D. may be calculated as shown below.

1. Determine the mean for the white blood cell count (WBC):

$$\overline{X} = \frac{\Sigma X}{N}$$

$$\overline{X} = \frac{204.4}{31} = 6.59 \times 10^3/\mu L \text{ or } 6590/\mu L$$

2. Calculate the difference from the mean for each individual control result $(\overline{X} - X)$. Square this difference for each result $(\overline{X} - X)^2$ (see Table 1–1).
3. Add all of the squared differences (Table 1–1).
4. Calculate the S.D. (results are expressed in the same units as the substance being tested):

$$S.D. = \sqrt{\frac{\Sigma(\overline{X} - X)^2}{N - 1}} = \frac{0.60}{31 - 1} = 0.14 \times 10^3 \text{ WBC}/\mu L \text{ or}$$

or

$$140 \text{ WBC}/\mu L$$

$$S.D. = \sqrt{\frac{\Sigma X^2 - \frac{(\Sigma X)^2}{N}}{N - 1}}$$

This formula is much easier to use with a non-programmed calculator

5. 1 S.D. = 140 WBC/μL (0.14 × 10³ WBC/μL)
   2 S.D. = 280 WBC/μL (0.28 × 10³ WBC/μL)
   3 S.D. = 420 WBC/μL (0.42 × 10³ WBC/μL)

The acceptable range for a Q.C. specimen is considered ±2 S.D. Therefore, using the previous figures for the WBC control and rounding off the numbers to the closest hundred, the acceptable value obtained each time it is run should be 6.6 × 10³/μL ±0.30 × 10³/μL, or 6300 to 6900/μL.

Before calculating the final S.D., results considered outliers should be eliminated from the calculations. (An outlier is considered any value that exceeds the mean by 3.0 to 3.5 S.D., depending on the number of test values. The larger the number of values, the

TABLE 1–1. WBC CONTROL VALUES FOR OCTOBER

Date	WBC × 10³ /μL	$(\overline{X} - X)$	$(\overline{X} - X)^2$
Oct 1	6.4	0.2	.04
2	6.7	−0.1	.01
3	6.8	−0.2	.04
4	6.7	−0.1	.01
5	6.7	−0.1	.01
6	6.6	0.0	.00
7	6.4	0.2	.04
8	6.6	0.0	.00
9	6.8	−0.2	.04
10	6.7	−0.1	.01
11	6.6	0.0	.00
12	6.7	−0.1	.01
13	6.5	0.1	.01
14	6.5	0.1	.01
15	6.4	0.2	.04
16	6.6	0.0	.00
17	6.7	−0.1	.01
18	6.3	0.3	.09
19	6.6	0.0	.00
20	6.7	−0.1	.01
21	6.5	0.1	.01
22	6.5	0.1	.01
23	6.5	0.1	.01
24	6.4	0.2	.04
25	6.6	0.0	.00
26	6.8	−0.2	.04
27	6.5	0.1	.01
28	6.5	0.1	.01
29	6.6	0.0	.00
30	6.6	0.0	.00
31	6.9	−0.3	.09
Total	204.4		0.60

greater the deviation allowed. For example, with 20 values a 3.0 S.D. is acceptable, whereas with 100 values an S.D. of 3.47 is allowable. Each outlier should be documented and a note made as to the action taken. There should be no more than two outliers per 100 test values. If there are three or more a serious problem may exist, and the method and materials should be examined.) After calculating the S.D. review all control values obtained. Identify and delete the outliers and then recalculate the S.D.

The **coefficient of variation (C.V.)** is the S.D. expressed as a percentage of the mean (average):

$$C.V. = \frac{S.D.}{\overline{X}} \times 100$$

Using the previous figures from the WBC control, the C.V. for this control would be

$$C.V. = \frac{140/\mu L}{6590/\mu L} \times 100 = 2.12\%$$

Because the C.V. is always expressed as a percentage it can be used to compare the precision of methods expressed in different units of measure.

Variance is also an indicator of precision and is defined as the standard deviation squared:

$$Variance = S.D.^2 = \frac{\Sigma(\overline{X} - X)^2}{N - 1} \text{ test unit}^2$$

The variance for the WBC control would therefore be:

$$Variance = (0.14)^2 = 0.0196/\mu L^2$$

It does not give as clear a picture of precision as S.D. and C.V. and is rarely used.

Normal Frequency (Gaussian) Distribution

When the average value of a group of Q.C. specimens is calculated, most of the values will be found to be close to the average, with approximately half being lower than the average and the remainder being higher than the average. The closer the value to the average the more frequent these values will occur, whereas the most infrequently occurring values will show a larger deviation from the average. If the control values are graphed plotting the concentration on the X-axis against the number of results on the Y-axis, a bell-shaped curve known as a normal frequency distribution curve will result (Fig. 1–31). This normal distribution curve is also termed the **Gaussian distribution curve.** The central point of the curve represents the mean value for the series of tests. When Gaussian distribution is present the **mean** (average value), the **mode** (most frequently occurring value), and the **median** (middle value within the range) will be the same or nearly the same value. This curve may be described in terms of distances from the mean, using standard deviation as the unit to measure this distance (Fig. 1–32). (Standard deviation is based on the assumption that the distribution of a set of values will follow the Gaussian distribution curve.) The central area of the curve from −1 S.D. to +1 S.D. contains 68% of the values obtained. Within ±2 S.D., 95% of the values are found, and 99.7% of the test values are contained within ±3 S.D. There will be 0.3% of the values outside of ±3 S.D. Therefore, one might expect to receive a control value outside the 2 S.D. limit 5% of the time or 1 out of every 20 samples.

Quality Control Graphs

Once a control specimen has been assayed (a mean value and range of acceptability), a quality control graph should be prepared and the Q.C. values charted each time the control is tested. Use of these charts simplifies the evaluation of control data. Three quality control graphs will be described briefly here: Levey-Jennings control chart, twin-plot graph, and the cumulative sum (CUSUM) graph.

The **Levey-Jennings graph** is the most widely used quality control chart. As seen in Figure 1–33 the date is plotted along the X-axis and the control value is represented on the Y-axis. A horizontal line is drawn through the mean, at +2 S.D., and at −2 S.D. (Lines indicating ±1 S.D. are optional.) Each time the control is tested the result is plotted on the chart.

When two control samples (normal and abnormal) are run, the **twin plot graph of Youden,** modified by D. B. Tonks, may be used (see Fig. 1–34). This same graph may also be employed using two control values by the same method or one control value from each of two separate methods. The graph is prepared by drawing on the vertical axis the mean +2 S.D. and the mean −2 S.D. limits for the abnormal control, or control No. 2. On the horizontal axis, mark off the mean +2 S.D. and the mean −2 S.D. limits for the normal control, or control No. 1. Draw a square field in the middle of the graph connecting the 2 S.D. limits. The cross in the middle of the square denotes the mean for both control samples. The line drawn connecting the bottom left corner with the top right corner denotes the line of normal distribution.

The **CUSUM graph** is a third method for charting control results. In this method, after the mean for the control is determined, this result is subtracted from each control result as it is obtained. The resulting value is added to the total of the previous days to give a

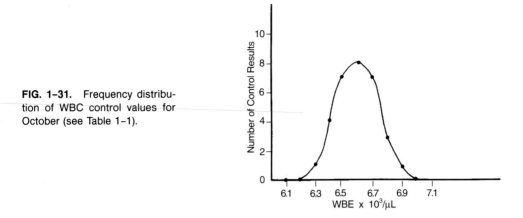

FIG. 1–31. Frequency distribution of WBC control values for October (see Table 1–1).

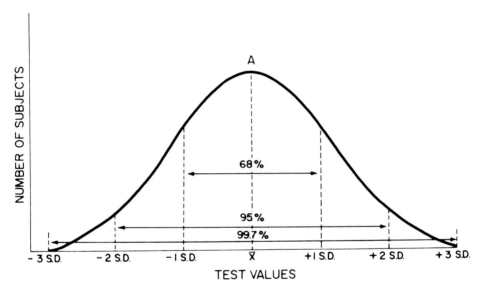

FIG. 1–32. Gaussian curve (normal frequency distribution curve).

cumulative difference from the mean. Each day the control is run, the cumulative difference is plotted on the graph. The CUSUM graph consists of a single line representing the mean. Negative cumulative differences fall below the mean line, and positive differences are plotted above the line (Fig. 1–35).

Acceptability of Patient Testing

Recalling the normal distribution (Gaussian) curve, 5% (5/100) of the control test values will fall between 2 and 3 S.D. This may or may not indicate a problem. Therefore, when this does occur the control should be repeated, preferrably using a new bottle or, if applicable, a new lot number. If two levels of control are used and if

(1) *Both control values are within ±2 S.D.*, accept all data.
(2) *One control is within ±2 S.D. and the second control falls between 2 and 3 S.D.*, re-run the out of range control. If this control is now acceptable the patient data are accepted as valid. If the repeat control is still not acceptable, the sample results from that run must be rejected. Troubleshoot the

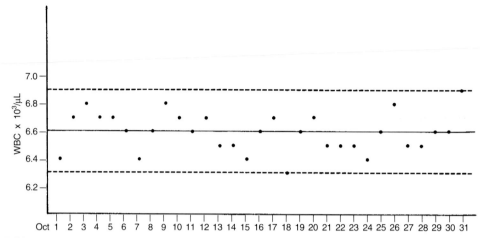

FIG. 1–33. Levey-Jennings graph of WBC control values for October (see Table 1–1).

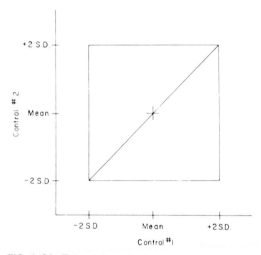

FIG. 1–34. Twin-plot graph.

test procedure and re-run controls and patient samples.

(3) *Both controls are out of range,* reject all results, troubleshoot the problem(s) and re-run controls and patient samples.

Control values should be plotted on the Q.C. graphs as soon as possible after they are obtained. A control value must not only be examined for its accuracy (should fall within ±2 S.D.) but must also be compared with previous values. Shifts and trends are systematic errors in a test procedure and can be detected easily by examination of the Levey-Jennings chart. Generally, a **shift** is thought to occur when the control value is on one side of the mean for approximately 6 consecutive days or is beyond 1 S.D. (on the same side of the mean) for at least 4 consecutive days. A **trend** is said to occur when the control value moves in the same direction (increases or decreases) for 6 consecutive days. The control graph should also be examined for an increased scatter of results—that is, the plotted points fall further above and below the mean. This indicates poor precision and will therefore cause increased S.D. and C.V. values.

James O. Westgard has described a multirule system for identifying out-of-control Q.C. results based on control procedures initially described by W.A. Shewhart and later by Levey-Jennings. **Westgard's multirule** may be used with the Levey-Jennings Q.C. chart to decide if a run of tests is to be accepted or rejected. If one control exceeds the mean by 2 S.D. (±2 S.D.) or more this is considered a "warning" and all control data must be further inspected in order to determine acceptance or rejection of the run. This is termed rule 1_{2s}. (Each rule has been given a symbol in the form of A_{Ls}, where A = number of control values in question, L = limit of the control, and s = S.D.) If rule 1_{2s} (above) has been broken, all control results must be examined and the following rules applied to determine whether or not the test run is to be rejected. Therefore, if rule 1_{2s} is broken, reject the run if any one of the following rules is true.

1. 1_{3s} = One control exceeds the mean by ±3 S.D.

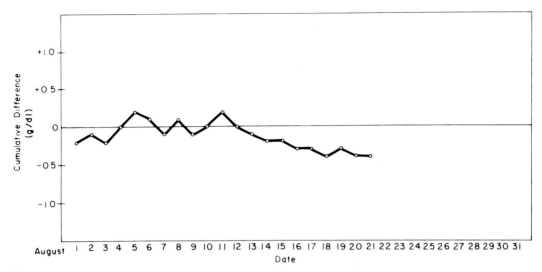

FIG. 1–35. Cumulative difference graph for hemoglobin (August).

2. 2_{2s} = One control exceeds the mean by 2 S.D. in the same direction (+ or −) two consecutive times (or two controls in the same run).

3. R_{4s} = Two controls in the same run differ by 4 S.D. (for example, one control of +2 S.D. and the other control −2 S.D.).

4. 4_{1s} = Four consecutive controls exceed the mean by 1 S.D. or more in the same direction.

5. $10_{\bar{x}}$ = Ten consecutive control values fall on the same side of the mean (10 consecutive runs or, for example, two controls in five consecutive runs).

The specific rule violated will give an indication of the type of problem. Rejection of test results by rules 1_{3s} and R_{4s} indicates a random error, whereas systematic errors cause test rejection by rules 2_{2s}, 4_{1s}, and $10_{\bar{x}}$.

When using the twin-plot graph, the control values should be plotted each day (Fig. 1–36). Several details should be noted when interpreting this graph: (1) Under normal conditions, when the test procedure is in control, the plotted control values should fall along the diagonal line of normal distribution, as seen in Figure 1–36 for July 1 through July 7. (2) If one of the controls is high and the other control is low, something is probably wrong. Both control samples were not affected in the same manner in the procedure, and patient values may be erratic. This condition shows up in the chart by the

appearance of the plotted point in the lower right or upper left corner of the square, as shown in Figure 1–36 for July 8. (3) The plotted values should fall along the diagonal line from the lower left corner to the top right corner. An uneven distribution in one of the two corners indicates an upward or downward shift, and, therefore, an out-of-control situation. Note that beginning with July 9, all values are in the upper right corner, indicating an upward trend (Fig. 1–36). (4) If, at any time, both control values fall outside the ±2 S.D. limit, something is wrong with

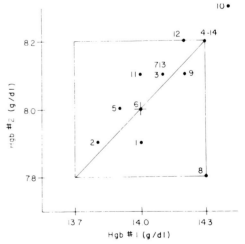

FIG. 1–36. Twin-plot chart for normal and abnormal hemoglobin results (July).

the procedure and the cause for these results should be found. In Figure 1–36, the control values for July 10 were both outside of normal limits.

When using the CUSUM graph, the plotted chart should show a line moving back and forth close to and above and below the 0 line (Fig. 1–35, Aug. 1 though Aug. 12). If the graph begins to show a trend upward or downward, this indicates a trend toward high or low control results, respectively. Beginning on Aug. 12 there is a downward trend of the control. Any time five or six successive plots go down or up on this graph, it is an indication that the test is out of control.

Internal/External Quality Control

Quality control programs may be divided into internal and external programs—both are an important component of the total quality control program.

Internal quality control consists of running assayed control specimens along with patient testing. The S.D., C.V., monthly mean, and cumulative mean should be calculated for each control at the end of every month. When calculating these parameters, delete (and document problems and actions) all outliers. Also, when there is a shift or trend noted, this data should not be included in the monthly statistics but, again, should be documented with appropriate action described. When using the same lot number of control the new results should agree closely with the previous month's results. If there is any question as to the agreement of the values, the t test (see later in this section) may be used to decide if the differences are significant. The C.V. for most tests in hematology should be less than 5%. Complete records must be kept of all quality control results. When values fall outside of acceptable limits, written explanations (documentation) must be maintained describing the problem(s) and the action(s) taken.

The **external quality control** program is performed similarly in the laboratory except that control results are generally compared with other laboratories within the city, state, or country. Numerous commercial Q.C. programs are available for certain test procedures. At the end of a month's testing the laboratory submits its results to the manufacturer or organization directing the program, who in turn sends the laboratory a report containing monthly and cumulative means, S.D.s, and C.V.s for the individual laboratory and for the group. Also included will be the standard deviation index (S.D.I.) (see below) for the laboratory. External Q.C. may not always be performed daily, may not always be pre-assayed, and should not be used as a substitute for internal Q.C.

A unit of measure used in the external Q.C. program is the **standard deviation index (S.D.I.)** (also termed **Z score**). The S.D.I. measures both systematic and random error and basically denotes how many standard deviations a particular number is from the mean. It is commonly used to relate the performance of your laboratory to other laboratories participating in the same external quality control program. It is calculated for each test procedure as follows:

$$\text{S.D.I.} = \frac{\text{Mean (your lab)} - \text{Mean (all labs)}}{\text{S.D. (all laboratories)}}$$

The perfect S.D.I. is 0 (zero) but should always be less than 1.0. If the S.D.I. exceeds 1.5 a problem may exist with your procedure, and if it exceeds 2.0 this indicates that you should take immediate action to determine and correct the problem.

Evaluation of Test Procedures

When a new test method or instrument is introduced into the laboratory a plan should be developed for evaluating this new procedure. Following is an outline of some studies that may be performed prior to acceptance of a new instrument or procedure for patient testing.

1. A preliminary procedure should be written.
2. A linearity study should be performed using dilutions and/or high and low standards to determine how high or low test results may be considered valid before diluting and/or double-checking results.
3. The precision (reproducibility) of the method should be determined using standard deviation and coefficient of variation (variance may be used if desired) as described previously.

4. The **accuracy** (agreement with the true value) of the test should be studied. The method(s) used here will depend on the specific test or procedure and will consist of testing standards and controls, determining interfering substances, and detecting any other problems that may interfere with test results.
5. A comparison study should be performed in which test values using the new method are compared with test results obtained by the reference or current method. This may also be termed a parallel study.
6. The normal range for the new procedure must be determined.
7. A final procedure should be written.
8. All technologists will need to be trained.

When performing a comparison study between the two procedures (new and current or reference), a minimum of 30 to 50 patient samples should be tested by both methods over a period of 3 to 5 days. The patient samples should represent values over the entire range of the test. Each sample should be tested by both methods at approximately the same time so that age of specimen and/or laboratory conditions do not differ for either test. After performing the two procedures as described above, several statistical studies of these results may be used to determine if there is a significant difference between the two methods. Several studies will be described here: the determination of the slope and Y intercept and the t test. Both of these tests are based on Gaussian distribution and may be used with small groups of about 30 samples. In addition, the correlation graph with the line of linear regression will be described. The F test is also included, which compares the precision of two methods and determines if there is a significant difference in the S.D., C.V., and variance between the two methods.

Slope and Y-intercept

Determination of the slope and Y-intercept is one of the most useful ways of comparing methods. Slope represents proportional systematic error using the following formula:

$$\text{Slope} = s = \frac{\Sigma XY - \dfrac{(\Sigma X)(\Sigma Y)}{N}}{\Sigma X^2 - \dfrac{(\Sigma X)^2}{N}}$$

Where X = current or reference method values
Y = new method values
Σ = sum of
N = number of values

If both procedures are in complete agreement the slope will be 1.0. However, a slope of 0.95 to 1.05 is considered acceptable for the agreement of two procedures.

Comparing hemoglobin results from a new instrument (B) with those results from the currently used instrument (A) (Table 1–2), the slope may be calculated:

$$s = \frac{\Sigma XY - \dfrac{(\Sigma X)(\Sigma Y)}{N}}{\Sigma X^2 - \dfrac{(\Sigma X)^2}{N}}$$

$$= \frac{7030.02 - \dfrac{(513.4)(527.1)}{40}}{6839.28 - \dfrac{(513.4)^2}{40}}$$

$$= \frac{7030.02 - 6765.33}{6839.28 - 6589.49}$$

$$= \frac{264.69}{249.79}$$

$$= 1.06$$

The Y-intercept represents constant systematic error and may be calculated:

$$\text{Y-intercept} = \overline{Y} - s\overline{X}$$

Where $\overline{Y}$ = mean of values by new method
$\overline{X}$ = mean of values by reference or current method
s = slope

The value obtained for the Y-intercept is more difficult to interpret and depends on the substance being measured. Perfect correlation between the two procedures will give a Y-intercept value of 0. The lower the number the better the correlation of the two methods.

Using the test results in Table 1–2 the Y-intercept is calculated:

$$\overline{Y} = \frac{Y}{N} = \frac{527.1}{40} = 13.18$$

$$\overline{X} = \frac{X}{N} = \frac{513.4}{40} = 12.84$$

$$\begin{aligned}
\text{Y-intercept} &= \overline{Y} - s\overline{X} \\
&= 13.18 - (1.06)(12.84) \\
&= 13.18 - 13.61 \\
&= -0.43
\end{aligned}$$

TABLE 1–2.   RESULTS OF HEMOGLOBIN TESTS USING INSTRUMENTS A AND B

Test No.	Inst. A (X)	X²	Inst. B (Y)	Y²	D (A − B)	D²	XY
1	9.3	86.49	9.3	86.49	0.0	0.00	86.49
2	14.7	216.09	15.4	237.16	−0.7	0.49	226.38
3	13.2	174.24	13.6	184.96	−0.4	0.16	179.52
4	13.9	193.21	14.1	198.81	−0.2	0.04	195.99
5	12.1	146.41	12.2	148.84	−0.1	0.01	147.62
6	15.2	231.04	15.5	240.25	−0.3	0.09	235.60
7	8.3	68.89	8.6	73.96	−0.3	0.09	71.38
8	11.3	127.69	11.5	132.25	−0.2	0.04	129.95
9	15.6	243.36	16.2	262.44	−0.6	0.36	252.72
10	12.3	151.29	12.5	156.25	−0.2	0.04	153.75
11	14.1	198.81	14.4	207.36	−0.3	0.09	203.04
12	12.0	144.00	12.2	148.84	−0.2	0.04	146.40
13	16.5	272.25	17.4	302.76	−0.9	0.81	287.10
14	10.3	106.09	10.3	106.09	0.0	0.00	106.09
15	14.6	213.16	15.1	228.01	−0.5	0.25	220.46
16	10.6	112.36	10.7	114.49	−0.1	0.01	113.42
17	12.6	158.76	12.8	163.84	−0.2	0.04	161.28
18	9.2	84.64	9.5	90.25	−0.3	0.09	87.40
19	10.4	108.16	10.6	112.36	−0.2	0.04	110.24
20	14.7	216.09	15.4	237.16	−0.7	0.49	226.38
21	15.6	243.36	16.2	262.44	−0.6	0.36	252.72
22	12.5	156.25	12.6	158.76	−0.1	0.01	157.50
23	18.7	349.69	19.1	364.81	−0.4	0.16	357.17
24	10.4	108.16	10.7	114.49	−0.3	0.09	111.28
25	15.7	246.49	16.3	265.69	−0.6	0.36	255.91
26	16.3	265.69	17.0	289.00	−0.7	0.49	277.10
27	11.6	134.56	11.7	136.89	−0.1	0.01	135.72
28	14.3	204.49	14.8	219.04	−0.5	0.25	211.64
29	15.3	234.09	16.1	259.21	−0.8	0.64	246.33
30	14.7	216.09	15.1	228.01	−0.4	0.16	221.97
31	12.9	166.41	13.6	184.96	−0.7	0.49	175.44
32	6.1	37.21	6.2	38.44	−0.1	0.01	37.82
33	12.1	146.41	12.4	153.76	−0.3	0.09	150.04
34	11.8	139.24	12.1	146.41	−0.3	0.09	142.78
35	10.2	104.04	10.7	114.49	−0.5	0.25	109.14
36	13.5	182.25	13.6	184.96	−0.1	0.01	183.60
37	11.1	123.21	11.3	127.69	−0.2	0.04	125.43
38	12.4	153.76	12.4	153.76	0.0	0.00	153.76
39	12.6	158.76	12.7	161.29	−0.1	0.01	160.02
40	14.7	216.09	15.2	231.04	−0.5	0.25	223.44
Total	513.4	6839.28	527.1	7227.71	−13.7	6.95	7030.02

Correlation Graph

The slope and Y-intercept may be visually seen by constructing a correlation graph. The results obtained by the reference method are plotted on the X-axis, whereas the new method results are plotted along the Y-axis. (If the two methods give identical results all points will fall along a line that makes a 45° angle with the X and Y axes [**line of perfect correlation**] and also passes through 0. The Y intercept will be 0.) When all points have been plotted, draw a line that best fits all of the points. This is termed the regression line (Fig. 1–37).

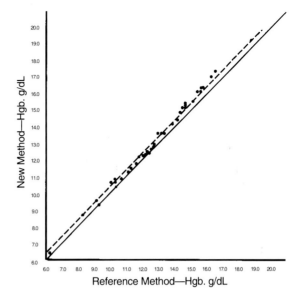

FIG. 1–37. Correlation graph and line of correlation for hemoglobin results using two different procedures (see Table 1–2).

t Test

The t test, also called the paired t test or the student t test, compares the accuracy of two methods in that it tests the difference between the mean value of each procedure. The reference or current method is considered to reflect the true value. The t test is based on a **null hypothesis,** which assumes that there is no difference between the two methods. The t value is calculated as follows:

$$t = \frac{\overline{D}}{SD_D} \sqrt{N}$$

D = difference between the two results
$\overline{D}$ = mean of the differences
SD_D = S.D. of the differences
N = number of paired results (number of samples analyzed)

$$SD_D = \sqrt{\frac{\Sigma D^2 - \frac{(\Sigma D)^2}{N}}{N - 1}}$$

When the t value has been obtained the null hypothesis is either accepted or rejected by comparing the t value with the critical value of t, as shown in Table 1–3. (Degrees of freedom = the number of paired results minus 1, or N − 1.) If the calculated t value is equal to or larger than the t value in Table 1–3 the null hypothesis is rejected and the difference between the two procedures is assumed to be

significant. If the calculated t value is less than the value in the t table the null hypothesis is accepted and it is assumed there is no significant difference between the two methods. (The table of t values shown here in Table 1–3 gives t values at a 95% probability or confidence level. This may be written as p = 0.05 and means that there are only 5 chances in 100 that these data appear only by chance. The critical t value is located at the ±2 S.D. point of the normal distribution curve at this level of confidence. Remember, with normal frequency distribution 95% of the values will fall within ±2 S.D.)

Using the values in Table 1–2 the t value for the comparison of the two hemoglobin methods may be calculated as follows:

$$S.D._D = \sqrt{\frac{\Sigma D^2 - \frac{(\Sigma D)^2}{N}}{N - 1}}$$

$$= \sqrt{\frac{6.95 - \frac{(13.7)^2}{40}}{39}}$$

$$= \sqrt{\frac{6.95 - 4.69}{39}}$$

$$= \sqrt{0.0579}$$

$$= 0.24$$

$$\overline{D} = \frac{\Sigma D}{N} = \frac{13.7}{40} = 0.34$$

$$t = \frac{\overline{D}}{S.D.} \sqrt{N}$$

$$= \frac{0.34}{0.24} \sqrt{40}$$

$$= 1.42 \times 6.32$$

$$= 8.97$$

It can be seen that the calculated t value exceeds the critical value of t, indicating a significant difference between the two hemoglobin methods.

F Test

The F test is used to compare the precision of two procedures and is calculated using the following formula:

$$F = \frac{S.D.^2 \text{ (method showing larger variance)}}{S.D.^2 \text{ (method showing smaller variance)}}$$

If both methods have the same precision the F value will be 1.0. As the difference in precision between the two methods increases, the F value will increase. To determine whether the F value shows a significant difference, refer to the Critical Values of F table (95% confidence level) (Table 1–4). Using the degrees of freedom (number of test values minus 1) for each procedure, look up the appropriate critical F value. If the calculated F value is smaller than the critical F value the differences in precision are not significant. However, if the calculated F value is the same as or higher than the critical F value, the smaller S.D. is considered to have significantly more precision than the test with the larger S.D. For example, if hemoglobin method A has a standard deviation of 0.13 g/dL based on 31 control results, and method B shows a standard deviation of 0.26 g/dL as calculated from 25 sets of results, the F value would be calculated as

$$F = \frac{S.D.^2 \text{ (larger S.D.)}}{S.D.^2 \text{ (smaller S.D.)}}$$

$$= \frac{(0.26)^2}{(0.13)^2}$$

$$= \frac{0.068}{0.017}$$

$$= 4.0$$

TABLE 1–3. CRITICAL VALUES OF t (95% CONFIDENCE LEVEL)

Degrees of Freedom	Critical Value of t	Degrees of Freedom	Critical Value of t
1	12.706	31	2.040
2	4.303	32	2.037
3	3.182	33	2.035
4	2.776	34	2.032
5	2.571	35	2.030
6	2.447	36	2.028
7	2.365	37	2.026
8	2.306	38	2.024
9	2.262	39	2.023
10	2.228	40	2.021
11	2.201	41	2.020
12	2.179	42	2.018
13	2.160	43	2.017
14	2.145	44	2.015
15	2.131	45	2.014
16	2.120	46	2.013
17	2.110	47	2.012
18	2.101	48	2.011
19	2.093	49	2.010
20	2.086	50	2.009
21	2.080	60	2.000
22	2.074	70	1.994
23	2.069	80	1.990
24	2.064	90	1.987
25	2.060	100	1.984
26	2.056	200	1.972
27	2.052	300	1.968
28	2.048	400	1.966
29	2.045	500	1.965
30	2.042	600	1.964

Referring to Table 1–4 (the larger S.D. has 24 degrees of freedom [number of results minus 1] and the smaller S.D. has 30 degrees of freedom), the critical value of F at 95% confidence is 1.89. Therefore, there is a significant difference in precision between the two methods, with the new method (B) showing a significant increase in precision over the current method (A).

Determination of Normal Range (Reference Interval)

The purpose of laboratory testing is to identify the abnormal patient. To determine this, a normal range (or reference interval) must

TABLE 1–4.   CRITICAL VALUES OF F (95% CONFIDENCE LEVEL)

		Degrees of Freedom (larger number)										
		2	4	6	8	10	12	14	16	20	24	30
D	2	19.00	19.25	19.33	19.37	19.39	19.41	19.42	19.43	19.44	19.45	19.46
E G	4	6.94	6.39	6.16	6.04	5.96	5.91	5.87	5.84	5.80	5.77	5.74
R E	6	5.14	4.53	4.28	4.15	4.06	4.00	3.96	3.92	3.87	3.84	3.81
E S	8	4.46	3.84	3.58	3.44	3.34	3.28	3.23	3.20	3.15	3.12	3.08
O	10	4.10	3.48	3.22	3.07	2.97	2.91	2.86	2.82	2.77	2.74	2.70
F	12	3.88	3.26	3.00	2.85	2.76	2.69	2.64	2.60	2.54	2.50	2.46
F R	14	3.74	3.11	2.85	2.70	2.60	2.53	2.48	2.44	2.39	2.35	2.31
E E	16	3.63	3.01	2.74	2.59	2.49	2.42	2.37	2.33	2.28	2.24	2.20
D O	20	3.49	2.87	2.60	2.45	2.35	2.28	2.23	2.18	2.12	2.08	2.04
M	24	3.40	2.78	2.51	2.36	2.26	2.18	2.13	2.09	2.02	1.98	1.94
	30	3.32	2.69	2.42	2.27	2.16	2.09	2.04	1.99	1.93	1.89	1.84

be determined for each procedure. The normal or reference range for a test will depend on a number of factors such as the particular test method, geographical location, interfering substances, age, and sex, to name a few.

Procedure

1. Select a large number (100 to 300) of normal, healthy individuals.
2. Perform the test and record the results for each individual.
3. Determine if the normal population of test results has Gaussian distribution by constructing a frequency distribution graph (described previously in this section). If the resultant curve is Gaussian, calculation of the mean, mode, and median will show these three numbers to be almost the same.
4. To determine the normal range if the frequency distribution curve is normal (Gaussian), calculate the standard deviation. The normal range will be ±2 S.D.

and will contain 95% of the normal population.

When interpreting patient results, a test value that falls outside of the ±3 S.D. limit is said to be abnormal. If the test value falls between the second and third standard deviation limit, this may or may not be considered abnormal or may be classified as borderline.

To check or verify a previously run normal range or to confirm published data, testing may be limited to 25 to 50 normal individuals. In these circumstances 95% of the values obtained should fall within the normal range.

If the normal study data does not show normal Gaussian distribution, the resulting curve will be skewed. The test values may show log normal distribution and would then need to be logarithmically transformed. In this circumstance calculation of the coefficient of variation would generally show a value greater than 15 to 20%. For dealing with non-Gaussian data the reader is referred to more sophisticated texts on statistical analysis.

HEMATOPOIESIS

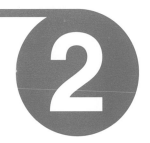

There are three types of cellular elements present in the blood: red blood cells (erythrocytes), white blood cells (leukocytes), and platelets (thrombocytes) (Fig. 2–1). (The platelet is not considered a true cell in that it does not contain a nucleus.) Each of these cells has its own function, differs morphologically from the others, and has a life span characteristic for that particular cell type. In health, the destruction and production of cells is balanced, and, therefore, the number of cells present in the blood at any particular time is relatively constant. *Hematopoiesis* is a term used to signify the production of blood cells.

In the same way that a person goes through various stages until he becomes an adult, the blood cells must also go through certain stages before they mature and are able to carry out their intended functions. In a healthy person, only the mature adult cells are found in the blood, whereas in many diseases, immature and abnormal forms of the cells may be present. For this reason, it is imperative that the student of medical technology be able to identify the immature and abnormal cell forms.

In the fetus, hematopoiesis takes place at various intervals in the liver, spleen, thymus, bone marrow, and lymph nodes (Fig. 2–2). Within 2 weeks of embryonic life, primitive red blood cells are produced in the yolk sac. By the second month, granulocytes and megakaryocytes begin to appear and the liver and spleen become the primary sites of cell development. Lymphocyte production starts at approximately the fourth month, and monocytes are produced by the fifth month; at this time, the bone marrow has assumed its primary role in hematopoiesis.

At birth, and continuing into adulthood, major blood cell production is confined to the bone marrow and is known as *medullary hematopoiesis.*

In the child, hematopoietic bone marrow (red marrow) is located in the flat bones of the skull, clavicle, sternum, ribs, vertebrae, and pelvis and also in the long bones of the arms and legs. By 18 years of age and for the remainder of the adult life, the red marrow is normally confined to the flat bones only (skull, clavicle, sternum, ribs, vertebrae, pelvis, and the proximal ends of the long bones [femur and humerus]). The remaining marrow space is occupied by fat cells (yellow marrow), which can be replaced by hematopoietic cells under certain situations of intensive stimulation.

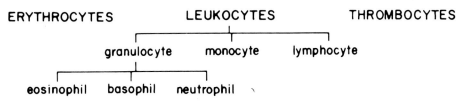

FIG. 2–1. Cellular elements in the peripheral blood.

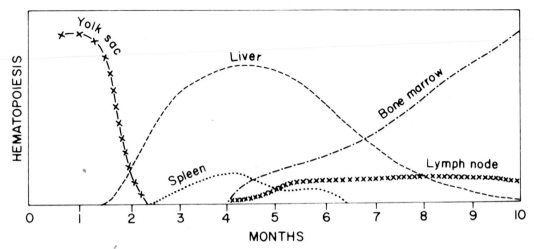

FIG. 2–2. Hematopoiesis in the fetus. (Modified from Wintrobe, M.M: *Clinical Hematology*, 8th Ed., Lea & Febiger, Philadelphia, 1981.)

In certain disease states, the bone marrow is unable to produce sufficient numbers of hematopoietic cells, and the liver and spleen may then become the sites of *extramedullary hematopoiesis*. This can occur in hemolytic anemias, where there is increased demand placed on the bone marrow. However, in cases of aplastic anemia and the leukemias, blood cells are not produced because of the fibrotic nature of the bone marrow or infiltration with malignant cells.

ORIGIN AND INTERRELATIONSHIP OF BLOOD CELLS

One of the more perplexing and controversial problems in hematology has concerned the origin of the blood cells and their relationship to one another. Today, as shown in Figure 2–3, it is believed that an uncommitted pluripotential stem cell in the bone marrow gives rise to (1) the lymphoid stem cell, and, (2) the myeloid or hematopoietic stem cell. (Stem cells have the ability to reproduce themselves and to differentiate. They can repopulate the bone marrow after injury or lethal irradiation, which is the essence of bone marrow transplantation. They are not morphologically identifiable and are thought to look very similar to the small or intermediate sized lymphocyte.) Stem cells are present in small numbers in the bone marrow and account for less than 1% of the population. The

hematopoietic or multipotential stem cell is thought to be the common precursor for red cells, granulocytes, monocytes, and megakaryocytes (platelets) and gives rise to the committed or unipotential stem cells through stimulation by various environmental factors within the body.

Existence of the stem cells has been shown by various culture techniques. The uncommitted stem cell has been given the designation CFU-S (colony forming unit-spleen), while those stem cells committed to forming blood cells are termed CFU-C (colony forming unit-culture) and require CSF (colony stimulating factor) to proliferate (multiply) and differentiate.

The lymphocyte precursor (CFU-L) and CFU-S have a more primitive pleuripotential stem cell in common that gives rise to both the CFU-S and the lymphocyte. The lymphoid stem cell leaves the bone marrow for differentiation into B lymphocytes in the lymph nodes and T lymphocytes in the thymus. (T and B lymphocytes will be described later in this chapter.)

The primitive red blood cells have been termed burst forming units—erythroid (BFU-E), which, in turn, give rise to colony forming units—erythroid (CFU-E) in response to erythropoietin. The primitive eosinophils (colony forming unit—eosinophil [CFU-Eo]) give rise to eosinophils in response to a substance (Eo-CSF) produced by stimulated lymphocytes. CFU-Meg is the primitive megakaryocytic line which gives rise to the

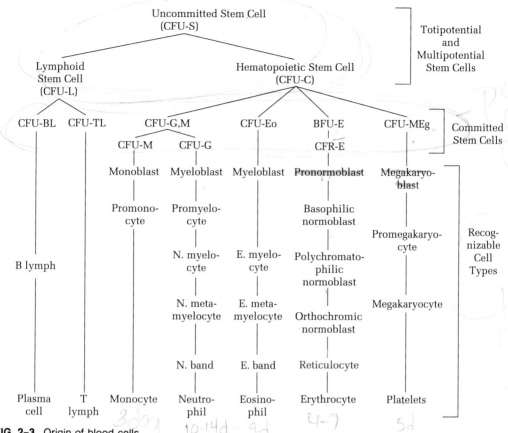

FIG. 2–3. Origin of blood cells.

megakaryocyte and ultimately the platelets, in response to Meg-CSF and thrombopoietin. CFU-G,M gives rise to the monocytes and neutrophils in response to GM-CSF. Colony forming units for basophils (CFU-Baso) also exist. Because of their limited number little research has been done in this area.

CELL STRUCTURE

As an aid in identifying cells, it is important to know their basic structure and composition. One should also have an understanding of the function of the cellular components.

The *plasma* or *cellular membrane* surrounds the outer limits of the cell and maintains the integrity of the interior of the cell. It is composed of three distinct layers: a middle lipid layer located between two layers of protein (Fig. 2–4). These proteins—actin, myosin,

and tubulin—form microfilaments and microtubules to maintain the shape (cytoskeleton) and structure of the plasma membrane. The "head" of the phospholipid molecules (adjacent to each protein layer) is the water-soluble portion and is positively charged. The inner ends of the lipids, or "feet," repel water (are water-insoluble). Also present in the cell membrane are small pores through which

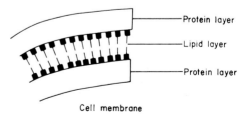

FIG. 2–4. Schematic diagram of a portion of a cell membrane.

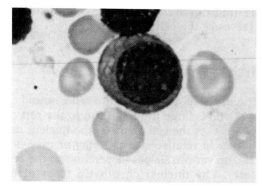

FIG. 2–6. Pronormoblast (center).

a. Granular or nongranular; specific or nonspecific granules.
b. Color (staining properties).
c. Relative amount.

When attempting to identify a cell, it is important to note the degree to which the cells take up the stain. For example, if all cells seem bluer than normal, the staining technique may be poor, and cell identification must be made accordingly.

Unless otherwise stated, all cells in this text are described as they appear in Wright-stained smears.

RED BLOOD CELLS

The red blood cells are produced in the bone marrow.

Pronormoblast (Rubriblast) (Fig. 2–6).

Size: 14 to 20 μm in diameter.

Cytoplasm: Deeply basophilic.
Relatively small amount, appearing as a band around the nucleus.
May show a lighter staining area around the nucleus (perinuclear halo).
Non-granular.

Nucleus: Relatively large. N/C ratio is about 8:1.
Round or slightly oval.
Reddish purple in color.
Fine chromatin pattern.
Usually 1 to 2 nucleoli.

Nucleoli are larger than those found in the myeloblast and may stain with a slightly bluish tint.

Basophilic Normoblast (Prorubricyte) (Fig. 2–7).

Size: 12 to 17 μm in diameter.

Cytoplasm: Intensely basophilic.
Relative amount of cytoplasm increased over previous stage (pronormoblast).
Non-granular.

Nucleus: Relatively large. N/C ratio is about 6:1.
Round or slightly oval.
Centrally located.
Chromatin pattern is slightly coarser than in the previous stage.
Nucleoli are usually not visible if present.

Polychromatophilic Normoblast (Rubricyte) (Fig. 2–8).

Size: 10 to 15 μm in diameter.

Cytoplasm: Blue-gray to pink-gray (shows a large range in color) due to the start of hemoglobin production in the cell.
A slight increase in relative amount.
Non-granular.

Nucleus: Round.
Smaller than previous stage. N/C ratio is approximately 4:1.

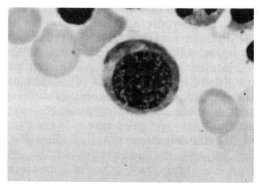

FIG. 2–7. Basophilic normoblast (center).

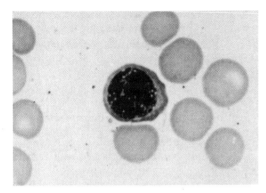

FIG. 2–8. Polychromatophilic normoblast.

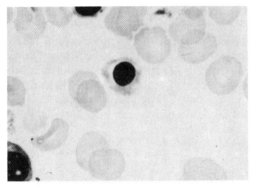

FIG. 2–9. Orthochromic normoblast (small cell in center).

More condensed. The chromatin pattern is coarse and clumped. Stains a deeper blue-purple. Parachromatin is distinct.

Orthochromic Normoblast (Metarubricyte) (Fig. 2–9).

Size: 7 to 12 μm in diameter.

Cytoplasm: Pinker than previous stage because of increased hemoglobin production.
Increased in amount compared to previous stage.
Non-granular.

Nucleus: N/C ratio is about 1:2. Small, pyknotic nucleus (a homogeneous blue-black mass with no structure). This is a primary difference between the rubricyte and the metarubricyte. Nucleus may be bizarre in form and partially extruded from the cell.

Reticulocyte.

Size: 7 to 10 μm in diameter. (Approximately the same size or slightly larger than the mature red blood cell.)

Cytoplasm: Pink to a slight pinkish gray.
Contains a fine basophilic reticulum of RNA, which only stains with supravital stain (see Reticulocyte Count in Chapter 3).

Nucleus: None present.

Mature Red Blood Cell.

Size: 6 to 8 μm in diameter.

Cytoplasm: Pink in color.
The mature red blood cell is a non-nucleated, round, biconcave cell (Fig. 2–10).

Erythropoiesis

Normally, the rate of production of red blood cells determines the hemoglobin level (and red blood cell count) in the peripheral blood and shows little variation among normal individuals. The packed red cell volume (hematocrit) is fairly consistent at 40 to 45%, and is optimal for the delivery of oxygen to the tissues.

Red blood cells exist and develop in the bone marrow as *erythroblastic islands* consisting of a macrophage surrounded by concentric rings of maturing normoblasts. The macrophage serves to supply the developing red cells with iron for hemoglobin synthesis. They also phagocytize extruded nuclei and dying red cells. During maturation of the erythroid cell, three to four mitotic divisions occur between the pronormoblast and the polychromatophilic normoblast stages. Thus, up to sixteen erythrocytes may be produced

FIG. 2–10. Cross section of the mature red blood cell.

from each pronormoblast. It takes approximately 3 days for the pronormoblast to develop into the orthochromic normoblast. When the cell reaches the orthochromic normoblast stage, the nucleus is extremely condensed and the cell is incapable of further mitosis. After approximately 1 more day, the nucleus is extruded. The resultant reticulocyte is slightly larger than the normal mature red blood cell and is slightly adhesive (sticky), appearing to be coated with a globulin, part of which may be transferrin. This characteristic may be responsible for keeping it in the bone marrow for an additional 2 to 3 days before it is released into the peripheral blood as a more mature reticulocyte. There are fewer reticulocytes in the peripheral blood than in the bone marrow. The red blood cells of the circulating blood have a life span of approximately 120 days, ± 20 days.

Production of red blood cells (erythropoiesis) is initiated by a hormone, called erythropoietin, which is produced mainly by the kidney and found in the plasma. Erythropoietin, in conjunction with interleukin-3, produced by T cell lymphocytes, is responsible for the formation of erythrocyte colony-forming units (CFU-E) from burst-forming units (BFU-E). When a person's hemoglobin level is below normal, the oxygen content of the blood drops and the oxygen tension in the kidneys is reduced (*hypoxia*). This condition stimulates the kidneys to increase their production of erythropoietin, which activates the CFU-E of the bone marrow to differentiate into pronormoblasts. An increased number of red blood cells are then produced. In addition, the rate of mitosis is increased and the maturation process of the red blood cells in the bone marrow is shortened. Hemoglobin is manufactured more quickly, and the reticulocytes are not delayed as long before they are released into the peripheral blood. As a result, the immature reticulocytes prematurely released may appear somewhat larger than the normal circulating red blood cells (generally 20 to 25% larger) and are polychromatophilic (staining gray to blue-gray in color). These cells are frequently termed *shift cells* and may be indicative of increased red blood cell production. In more severe conditions wherein the marrow is seriously stressed, as in hemolytic anemias, even larger macroreticulocytes or *stress reticulocytes* may appear in the circulation.

Various substances are required for the production of new red cells and hemoglobin. Iron is needed for both the proliferation and maturation of the red blood cell. Folic acid and vitamin B_{12} are necessary for normal DNA replication and cell division. Manganese, cobalt, zinc, and vitamins C, E, B_6, thiamine, riboflavin, and pantothenic acid are also needed for normal erythropoiesis, along with the hormones, erythropoietin, thyroxine, and androgens.

Hemoglobin Structure and Synthesis

The primary function of the red blood cell is to manufacture hemoglobin, which, in turn, transports oxygen to the tissues and carbon dioxide from the tissues to the lungs. The hemoglobin molecule is composed of four subunits, each containing heme and the protein, globin. Every heme group is capable of carrying 1 mole of oxygen, and therefore each hemoglobin molecule is able to transport 4 moles of oxygen. The synthesis of heme begins in the mitochondria with the formation of delta-aminolevulinic acid from glycine and succinyl-coenzyme A in the presence of pyridoxal phosphate (vitamin B_6) and delta-aminolevulinic acid synthetase (Fig. 2–11). The process then continues in the cytoplasm of the cell, where two molecules of delta-aminolevulinic acid condense in the presence of delta-aminolevulinic acid dehydrase to form porphobilinogen. Four molecules of porphobilinogen combine to form urophyrinogen III in the presence of uroporphyrinogen I synthetase and uroporphyrinogen III cosynthetase. Coproporphyrinogen III is then formed by the action of uroporphyrinogen decarboxylase, which removes four carboxyl groups from the acetic acid side chains. Heme is then produced in the mitochondria, where protoporphyrinogen IX is formed by the action of coproporphyrinogen oxidase. Protoporphyrin IX is formed in the presence of protoporphyrinogen oxidase, and ferrous iron is incorporated into the molecule in the presence of the enzyme ferrochelatase (heme synthetase) to form the heme molecule (Fig. 2–12). The atom of iron is located in the center of the structure and, in the ferrous state (Fe^{++}), binds oxygen.

Iron is delivered to the maturing red blood

Succinyl coenzyme A + Glycine

Pyridoxal phosphate | delta-Aminolevulinic acid synthetase

delta-Aminolevulinic acid

delta-Aminolevulinic acid dehydrase

Porphobilinogen

Uroporphyrinogen III cosynthetase

Uroporphyrinogen III

Uroporphyrinogen decarboxylase

Coproporphyrinogen III

Coproporphyrinogen oxidase

Protoporphyrinogen IX

Protoporphyrinogen oxidase

Protoporphyrin IX

Ferrochelatase | Fe^{++}

Heme molecule

FIG. 2–11. Biosynthesis of heme.

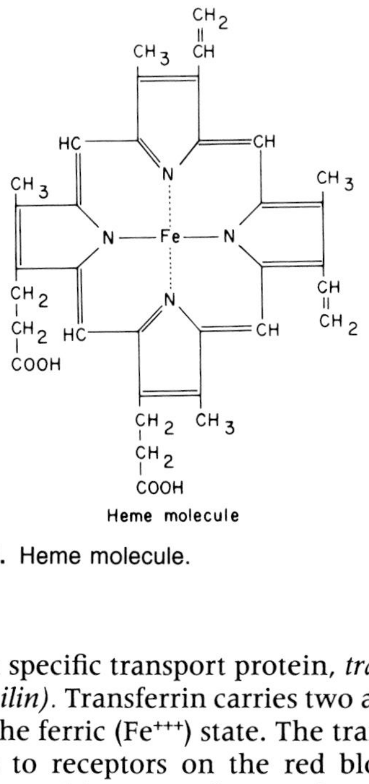

FIG. 2–12. Heme molecule.

cell by a specific transport protein, *transferrin (siderophilin)*. Transferrin carries two atoms of iron in the ferric (Fe^{+++}) state. The transferrin attaches to receptors on the red blood cell membrane. This causes the membrane to invaginate, forming an intracellular vacuole. The iron is then released into the cytoplasm as the vacuole fuses with a lysosome. The transferrin-receptor complex then returns to the cell membrane, and the transferrin molecule is released back into the plasma to repeat the cycle. The major portion of this iron is used in heme synthesis. Upon insertion into the red blood cell, the iron is reduced from the ferric (Fe^{+++}) to the ferrous (Fe^{++}) state; it proceeds to the mitochondria, where it enters the protoporphyrin molecule. Some of the iron not used for heme production may accumulate in the cytoplasm of the red blood cell as ferritin aggregates. (This may be demonstrated by the Prussian blue stain.) Cells containing these aggregates are called *sideroblasts*, and are found in the normal bone marrow.

While the heme molecule is being synthesized, the globin portion of hemoglobin is produced on specific ribosomes in the cytoplasm of the red blood cells. The globin in each hemoglobin molecule consists of four polypeptide chains which determine the type of hemoglobin formed. (In the normal adult, three hemoglobin types are present: hemoglobins A, F, and A_2, with hemoglobin A having a concentration of approximately 96 to 97%.) The polypeptide chains are composed of amino acids arranged in a specific sequence. Each chain is bent and coiled and forms a three-dimensional structure. The type and number of amino acids and their sequence are dependent on the type of chain being formed and are determined by the DNA molecules in the nucleus of the cell. This information in the nucleus of the cell is transferred to the cytoplasmic ribosomes by messenger RNA. Once the ribosome receives this information, it can function, without further messages from the nucleus, to synthesize the polypeptide chains from amino acids delivered by transfer RNA. Hemoglobin A is composed of four polypeptide chains, two alpha (α) and two beta (β) chains. Hemoglobin F is made up of two α and two gamma (γ) chains, whereas hemoglobin A_2 is composed of two α and two delta (δ) chains. (The amounts of hemoglobin A and F are significant in that they will show increased levels in certain disorders of globin synthesis.) α Chain synthesis is controlled by two pairs of genes on chromosome 16, and the genes for γ, δ, and β chain synthesis are on chromosome 11.

Using hemoglobin A as an example, when the individual α and β chains are produced, one α and one β chain combine to form a *dimer*. These dimers are then free in the cytoplasm of the cell, where $\alpha\beta$ dimers combine with the heme molecule and form the tetrad hemoglobin molecule consisting of two α chains, two β chains, and four heme groups (Fig. 2–13). This tetrahedral structure gives the hemoglobin molecule its nearly spherical shape. One heme group is attached to each polypeptide chain by a linkage from the iron in the heme group, to a specific amino acid (histidine) in each α and β chain. When globin production is decreased (as is found in certain disorders of impaired synthesis of protoporphyrin III or porphyrin), there is no corresponding decrease in iron uptake by the red blood cell. As a result, the excess iron may accumulate in the cytoplasm of the red blood cell as ferritin aggregates or may build up in the mitochondria and may be seen around the nucleus of the immature red blood cell *(ringed sideroblast)*.

The production of heme and globin begins in the polychromatophilic normoblast stage and ends in the reticulocyte, which is able to synthesize hemoglobin for approximately 2 days after the cell has lost its nucleus. No hemoglobin synthesis takes place in the mature red blood cell.

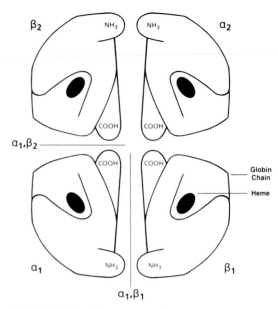

FIG. 2–13. Graphic representation of the hemoglobin A molecule. (From McKenzie, S.B.: *Textbook of Hematology*, Lea & Febiger, Philadelphia, 1988.)

Function of Hemoglobin

The red blood cell functions primarily to supply oxygen to the tissues and remove carbon dioxide. It is the hemoglobin molecule within the red blood cell that is responsible for supplying the tissues with oxygen. The normal hemoglobin molecule has an attraction (affinity) for oxygen (which binds to the iron). As soon as one atom of iron binds oxygen, because of a shift in the configuration of the hemoglobin molecule, the remaining three atoms of iron more readily bind oxygen. In other words, the affinity of hemoglobin for oxygen increases as the molecule binds more oxygen. This characteristic has been termed *heme-heme interaction.*

The amount of oxygen which the hemoglobin molecule binds varies in relationship to the amount of oxygen in the blood. For example, when the oxygen tension in arterial blood is high (about 95 mm Hg), the hemoglobin molecule is about 95% saturated with oxygen. This conformation of the hemoglobin molecule in the oxygenated form is termed the *relaxed (R) state.* In this condition the faces of the hemoglobin dimers have moved apart to bind oxygen. However, in the veins and tissues, the oxygen tension is

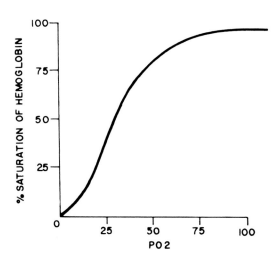

FIG. 2–14. Oxygen dissociation curve of hemoglobin.

lower. The hemoglobin molecule picks up and binds oxygen while in the capillary system of the lungs. As this hemoglobin travels through the tissue capillaries, in which the oxygen concentration is decreased, it releases this oxygen to the tissues. The deoxygenated form of hemoglobin is called the *tense (T) state.* Here, the $\alpha_1\beta_2$ faces of the hemoglobin molecule fit closely together.

The affinity of hemoglobin for oxygen is represented graphically by the *oxygen dissociation curve* (Fig. 2–14), in which pO_2 represents the partial pressure or tension of oxygen in the tissues plotted against percent hemoglobin saturation. P_{50} represents hemoglobin's affinity for oxygen and is used to designate the partial pressure of oxygen at which the hemoglobin molecule is 50% saturated with oxygen. (Normally, the partial pressure of oxygen is 26.6 mm Hg when the hemoglobin is half saturated with oxygen.) The normal oxygen dissociation curve is sigmoidal in shape and shows its steepest slope at the pO_2 levels that are generally found in the tissues. In this area of the curve, hemoglobin gives up and binds oxygen with relatively small changes in pO_2. A decreased affinity of the hemoglobin molecule for oxygen shifts this curve to the right, and hemoglobin then gives up oxygen readily. If this curve shifts to the left, hemoglobin has an increased affinity for oxygen (it binds oxygen readily but does not release it to the tissues easily). The P_{50} therefore, increases as the curve shifts to the right

and decreases with a shift to the left. The normal position of the oxygen dissociation curve is dependent on carbon dioxide, hydrogen ions (pH), 2,3 DPG, temperature, and on the structure of the hemoglobin molecule.

Hemoglobin's affinity for oxygen as influenced by the pH has been termed the *Bohr effect.* As the pH becomes more acid, hemoglobin's affinity for oxygen decreases. In the tissues, due to the presence of lactic acid and carbon dioxide, the pH is more acid, and hemoglobin is further influenced to release oxygen to the tissues. In the lungs, the pH rises (becomes more basic), which favors the uptake of oxygen by the red cells. The organic phosphate 2,3 DPG also affects hemoglobin's affinity for oxygen. When the hemoglobin molecule releases oxygen, the beta chains move apart allowing 2,3 DPG to enter. The 2,3 DPG binds with the deoxygenated hemoglobin, thereby having an inhibitory effect on hemoglobin binding with oxygen. Hemoglobin gives up more oxygen to the tissues with increased concentrations of 2,3 DPG in the blood, and the oxygen dissociation curve is shifted to the right.

The type of hemoglobin present also influences the oxygen dissociation curve. Hemoglobin F (fetal hemoglobin) has a higher affinity for oxygen than hemoglobin A because of the fact that the γ chains of hemoglobin F bind 2,3 DPG less strongly than the β chains of hemoglobin A. Therefore, a higher saturation level of oxygen occurs with hemoglobin F because of the inhibitory nature of 2,3 DPG (in binding oxygen to the hemoglobin A molecule).

The major portion of carbon dioxide is transported from the tissues by the red blood cell. Carbon dioxide diffuses into the red cell and reacts with water to form carbonic acid (H_2CO_3). Hydrogen ions, liberated from the H_2CO_3 (leaving free bicarbonate or $H_2CO_3^-$), are free to combine with deoxygenated hemoglobin, further decreasing the affinity of the hemoglobin molecule for oxygen. (Deoxygenated hemoglobin has more affinity for hydrogen ions because oxygenated hemoglobin is the stronger acid.) (The enzyme, carbonic anhydrase catalyzes the conversion of carbon dioxide to bicarbonate in the red cell, and then also catalyzes the release of carbon dioxide from the bicarbonate when the red cell is in the capillaries of the lungs.) Some of the carbon dioxide remaining in the tissues combines with the amino acid groups of deoxygenated hemoglobin to form *carbaminohemoglobin*. Also, a small amount of carbon dioxide is removed from the tissues by the plasma in solution.

Erythrocyte Membrane

The normal, mature red blood cell may be described as a 'biconcave disk'. This distinctive shape allows the red cell to have maximum membrane surface area for its size, which facilitates the transfer of gases in and out of the cell. In addition, it enables the red blood cell to easily undergo the changes in shape necessary for its travel through such areas as the microvasculature.

The red blood cell membrane is composed of protein (50%), lipid (40%), and a small amount of carbohydrate (10%) and can be penetrated by most solutes. The membrane is two molecules thick and contains tightly packed phospholipids. The polar surfaces of the phospholipids face the inside and the outside of the cell, with the nonpolar groups at the center of the membrane. The external surface of the membrane is rich in the phospholipids phosphatidylcholine, glycolipid, and sphingomyelin, while the internal surface contains phosphatidylethanolamine, phosphatidylinositol, and phosphatidylserine. The cholesterol content of the membrane depends upon the concentration of the plasma cholesterol, bile acids, and the activity of the enzyme, lecithin:cholesterol acyltransferase (LCAT).

There are two classes of proteins in the membrane: integral and peripheral (Fig. 2–15). The integral proteins, primarily glycophorin A and component a, are in contact with both the inner and outer surfaces of the membrane. Glycophorin A is probably responsible for the negative charge of the red blood cell surface. Spectrin and actin are *peripheral proteins* which are present on the inner portion of the membrane and create the framework or cytoskeleton for the cell and thus determine the shape of the red blood cell. They are attached to the inner ends of the integral proteins. Actin is a contractile protein that contributes to the deformability of the red cell. The spectrin molecule consists of an α and a β chain in a helix (circular pattern like a spring).

The integral membrane proteins carry various antigens on the membrane surface, while some antigens are also attached to the glycolipid portions of the membrane surface. Over 300 red blood cell antigens have been identified of which most are intrinsic components appearing on the membrane during early development of the red cell.

Changes in the shape of the red blood cell may result from alterations in the plasma lipids. Increases in cholesterol and phospholipid may be one cause of target cells. With increased concentrations of membrane cholesterol, the red cell has excess membrane or surface area which then makes the red cell appear as a target or spiculated red blood cell. *Acanthocytes* (in patients who lack beta lipoprotein) result from abnormalities in the ratios of membrane lecithins and sphingomyelins. An abnormality in the peripheral proteins may be responsible for the shape of the red blood cell in hereditary elliptocytosis and spherocytosis. Cells which lack the Rh antigens are termed Rh null cells, appear as stomatocytes on the peripheral smear, and have a shortened life span.

Metabolism of the Red Blood Cell

The mature red blood cell consists primarily of hemoglobin (about 90% of the dry weight). The membrane is composed of lipids and proteins. In addition, there are numerous enzymes present which are necessary for oxygen transport and cell viability. The red blood cell derives its energy from the breakdown of glucose. About 90% of the glycolysis in the red blood cell follows the anaerobic *Embden-Meyerhof* pathway (Fig. 2–16). In this way, two moles of adenosine triphosphate (ATP) are generated for every glucose molecule broken down to lactic acid. ATP is used to control the flow of sodium and potassium into and out of the red blood cell (for osmotic equilibrium via the cation pump), maintain the biconcave shape of the cell, and protect the membrane lipids.

The *methemoglobin reductase pathway* (Fig 2–16) maintains the iron present in the hemoglobin molecule in a functional reduced state (Fe^{++}) for oxygen transport.

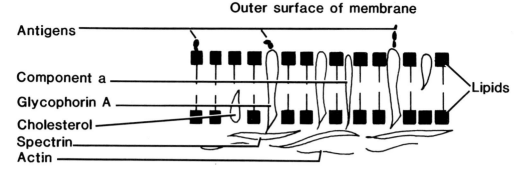

Outer surface of membrane

Antigens

Component a

Glycophorin A

Cholesterol

Spectrin

Actin

Lipids

Inner surface of membrane

FIG. 2–15. Diagrammatic illustration of the red blood cell membrane.

The *Rapoport-Leubering pathway* allows for the production of 2,3 diphosphoglycerate (2,3 DPG), which regulates the affinity of the hemoglobin molecule for oxygen. The 2,3 DPG combines reversibly with the deoxygenated hemoglobin, decreasing the affinity of hemoglobin for oxygen.

The remaining 10% of the glucose molecules follow the aerobic *hexose monophosphate shunt* (pentose phosphate pathway) (Fig. 2–16), where reduced glutathione is made available to prevent oxidative denaturation of hemoglobin. When the red blood cell is exposed to an oxidant drug, the activity of the hexose monophosphate shunt increases in order to maintain the hemoglobin molecule in its reduced state. Decreased activity of an enzyme in this pathway, results in oxidized hemoglobin, which denatures and precipitates as *Heinz bodies.* (Heinz bodies and pieces of the red cell membrane are removed by the spleen macrophages.)

DNA and RNA present in the early stages of the maturing red blood cell are absent in the mature cell.

Breakdown of the Red Blood Cell

As a red blood cell ages, there is a decrease in its enzymes, a decrease in ATP, a decrease in size, and an increase in density. As a result, the red cell membrane loses deformability and undergoes membrane damage. Approximately 1% of the red blood cells leave the circulation each day and are broken down by the mononuclear phagocytic system (MPS) (see p. 68). This may be termed extravascular

destruction and most commonly occurs in the spleen. About 90% of aged red cell destruction is extravascular. (Severely damaged red cells may be removed by the liver, while some completely damaged red cells will be destroyed as they circulate through the vascular system [intravascular destruction].)

When the red cell has been removed from the circulation, the membrane is disrupted and the hemoglobin is broken down within the macrophages of the MPS by the action of the enzyme, heme oxygenase. The iron returns to the plasma transferrin and is carried back to the erythroid bone marrow for reuse by new red blood cells, or, the iron may be stored within the MPS as ferritin and hemosiderin. The amino acids from the globin are returned to the amino acid pool. The protoporphyrin ring is broken at the α methene bridge, yielding biliverdin and carbon monoxide. The biliverdin is reduced to bilirubin in the MPS and is then carried by the plasma albumin as unconjugated bilirubin to the liver for eventual excretion (Fig. 2–17). Bilirubin is conjugated in the liver with glucuronic acid to bilirubin glucuronide and is excreted in the bile to the intestinal tract. Bacterial flora converts bilirubin glucuronide to urobilinogen, which is excreted in the feces as urobilin. The carbon monoxide appears in the blood attached to hemoglobin as carboxyhemoglobin and is exhaled in the lungs.

Ten percent of aged red cell destruction occurs intravascularly, and when hemoglobin is released directly into the blood, it dissociates into $\alpha\beta$ dimers and becomes attached

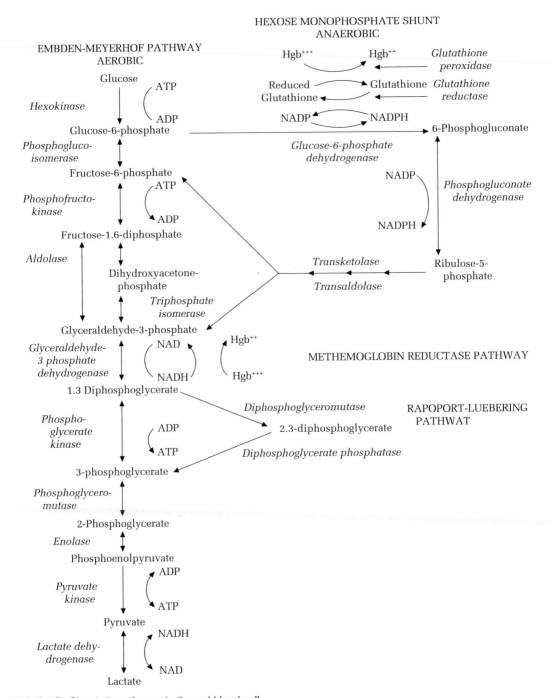

FIG. 2–16. Glycolytic pathways in the red blood cell.

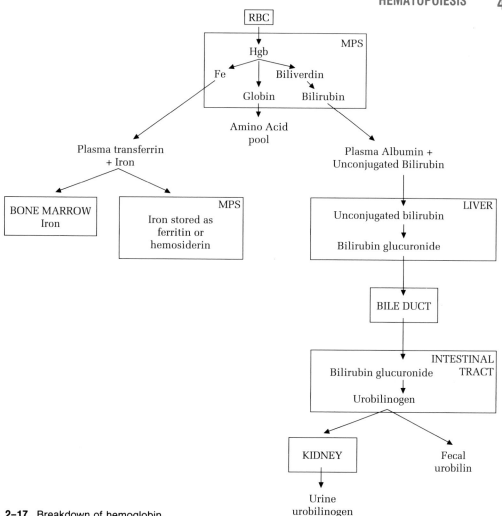

FIG. 2–17. Breakdown of hemoglobin.

to *haptoglobin* (a plasma globulin). The hemoglobin-haptoglobin complex is taken to the MPS and processed in the normal way, because it is too large a complex to be filtered by the kidneys. If the plasma haptoglobin becomes depleted, the hemoglobin (dimers) are converted to *hemosiderin,* are excreted as free hemoglobin, or oxidized to methemoglobin in the urine. If free hemoglobin is present in the blood, it may be oxidized to *methemoglobin.* If this occurs, the heme groups dissociate and are bound to another transport protein, *hemopexin,* leave the circulation via the liver, and are catabolized. If all hemopexin is used up, the excess heme groups will combine with albumin to form *methemalbumin* until hemopexin becomes available for transfer to the liver.

Megaloblastic Erythropoiesis

A nuclear maturation defect occurs in vitamin B_{12} and folic acid deficiencies. As a result, the red blood cell and its precursors are much larger in sizer than normal. Thus, the term *megaloblast* is used, 'megalo' meaning large. The maturation of the megaloblast proceeds through the same stages of development as the normal red blood cell. Because of the defect in nuclear development (abnormal or inhibited DNA synthesis due to a depletion of the DNA precursor thymidine triphosphate), maturation of the nucleus takes longer than the cytoplasm, which matures at a more normal rate. Cell division is delayed because of the nuclear defect, resulting in a red cell that is larger than normal because of prolonged

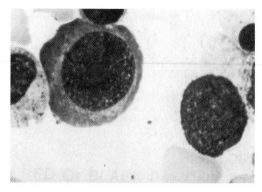

FIG. 2–18. Promegaloblast (large cell in center).

mitotic phases of cell division. However, RNA synthesis proceeds at a normal rate; therefore, development of the cytoplasm continues. As a result, the cytoplasm appears to have matured to one stage, whereas the nucleus appears larger than normal and much more immature *(asynchronism)*. The nuclear chromatin in these cells shows a much more open pattern with increased or prominent parachromatin.

Promegaloblast (Fig. 2–18).

Size: 19 to 28 μm in diameter.

Cytoplasm: More abundant than in the pronormoblast.
Deeply basophilic.
Non-granular.

Nucleus: Fine chromatin pattern.
Chromatin pattern is more open than in the pronormoblast.
3 to 8 nucleoli.
N/C ratio 5:1.

Basophilic Megaloblast (Fig. 2–19).

Size: 17 to 24 μm in diameter.

Cytoplasm: Deeply basophilic.
Non-granular.

Nucleus: No nucleoli visible.
Chromatin pattern is coarser than in the basophilic normoblast.
N/C ratio is 4:1.

Polychromatophilic Megaloblast (Fig. 2–20).

Size: 15 to 20 μm in diameter.

Cytoplasm: Blue-gray to pinkish-gray.
May contain *Howell-Jolly bodies* (nuclear fragments).

Nucleus: Chromatin pattern is coarser and more open than in the poly-chromatophilic normoblast.
There may be a breaking up of the nucleus *(karyorrhexis)*.
N/C ratio is 2:1.

Orthochromic Megaloblast (Fig. 2–21).

Size: 10 to 15 μm in diameter.

Cytoplasm: Pink in color.
More abundant than is found in the orthochromic normoblast.

Nucleus: Chromatin may be clumped but is much less condensed than the normal orthochromic normoblast.
N/C ratio is about 1:1.

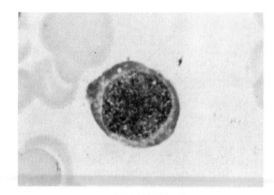

FIG. 2–19. Basophilic megaloblast.

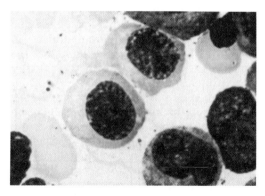

FIG. 2–20. Polychromatophilic megaloblast (large cell in center).

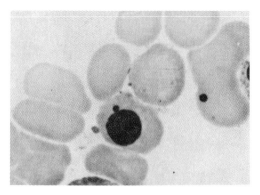

FIG. 2–21. Orthochromic megaloblast (center).

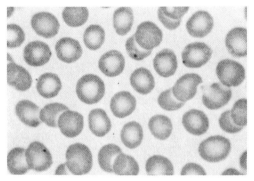

FIG. 2–22. Normal red blood cells. (Magnification × 1000)

Macrocyte.

Size: 9 to 12 μm in diameter.

The macrocyte may appear oval on the stained blood smear.

Red Blood Cell Morphology

In anemias and other disease states, the mature red blood cells of the peripheral blood may show certain significant changes. The terms applied to each of these abnormalities are defined and illustrated on the following pages.

Normal red blood cells (discocytes), Figure 2–22 (see also Fig. 2–28) are round, have a small area of central pallor, and show only a slight variation in size. (As the relative amount of hemoglobin in the red cell decreases [or increases], the area of central pallor will increase [or decrease] accordingly.)

Microcytic red blood cells, Figure 2–23,

show a decrease in size and are found in thalassemia and a variety of anemias such as iron deficiency and hemolytic anemia.

Macrocytic red blood cells, Figure 2–24, are increased in size and may be found in liver disease and the megaloblastic anemias. When associated with vitamin B_{12} or folic acid deficiency, the macrocytes may appear slightly oval in shape.

Anisocytosis, Figure 2–25, indicates a variation in the size of the red blood cells.

Hypochromia, Figure 2–26, denotes red blood cells with a large area of central pallor and is due to a decreased concentration of hemoglobin in the cell. Hypochromia is characteristically present in iron deficiency anemia but is also present in other forms of anemia.

Polychromatophilia indicates young red blood cells which contain residual RNA. These cells are generally larger than normal

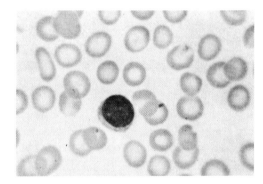

FIG. 2–23. Microcytes (compare red blood cell size with the size of the lymphocyte nucleus). (Magnification ×1000)

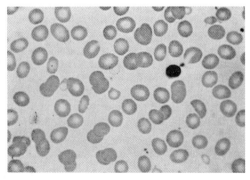

FIG. 2–24. Macrocytes, oval. (Compare red blood cell size with the size of the lymphocyte nucleus.) (Magnification ×500)

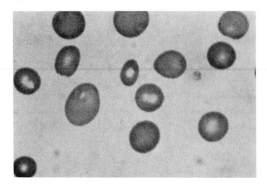

FIG. 2–25. Red blood cells showing anisocytosis. (Magnification ×1000)

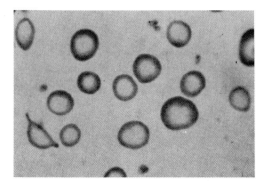

FIG. 2–26. Hypochromic red blood cells. (Magnification ×1000)

and stain a pinkish gray to pinkish blue color (Plate V). When stained supravitally with brilliant cresyl blue they show up as reticulocytes.

Spherocytic red blood cells, Figures 2–27 and 2–28, are almost spherical in shape. They are not biconcave like a normal red blood cell and do not have the central area of pallor which a normal red cell shows. The spherocyte, therefore, has less surface area for its size. These cells are associated with hemolytic anemia, ABO hemolytic disease of the newborn, and hereditary spherocytosis. In some hereditary red cell enzyme deficiencies, the spherocytes may have many fine needle-like projections on the surface of the cell.

Spheroidocytes, Figures 2–29 and 2–28, are thicker than normal red blood cells (more spherical than the normal red cell, but less spherical than the spherocyte), have a higher than normal concentration of hemoglobin,

and show a small area of pallor that is usually off-center.

Target cells (leptocytes), Figure 2–30 (see also Fig. 2–28), show a centrally stained area with a thin outer rim of hemoglobin and are associated with liver disease and certain hemoglobinopathies (abnormal hemoglobins): sickle cell anemia and hemoglobin CC, E, and SC diseases.

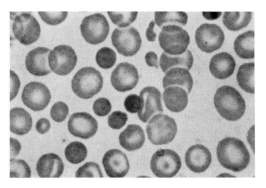

FIG. 2–27. Spherocytes. (Note the group of three spherocytes in the center of the illustration that show no area of central pallor. There are several more spherocytes also present.) (Magnification ×1000)

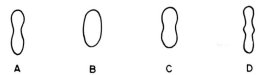

A **B** **C** **D**

FIG. 2–28. Cross section of A, the normal red blood cell; B, the spherocyte; C, the spheroidocyte; and D, the target cell.

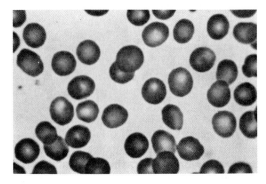

FIG. 2–29. Spheroidocytes. (Note the red blood cells showing only a small off-center area of pallor.) (Magnification ×1000)

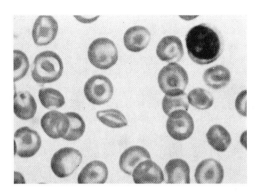

FIG. 2–30. Target cells. Note the *pocketbook-shaped* red blood cell located near the center of the illustration. (Magnification ×1000)

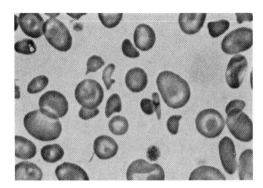

FIG. 2–32. Poikilocytosis of the red blood cells. Small red blood cell fragments, or schistocytes, are also present. (Magnification ×1000)

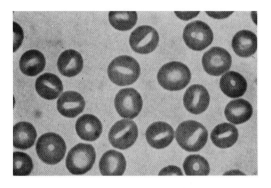

FIG. 2–31. Stomatocytes. (Note the oval-shaped area of central pallor in the red blood cells as compared to the round area in normal red blood cells. (Magnification ×1000)

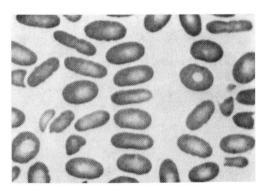

FIG. 2–33. Numerous ovalocytes and elliptocytes. (Magnification × 1000)

Stomatocytes, Figure 2–31, show a slit-like (rectangular) area of central pallor. These red blood cells have lost the indentation on one side and may be found in liver disease, alcoholism, electrolyte imbalance, and hereditary stomatocytosis.

Poikilocytosis, Figure 2–32, indicates a variation in the shape of the red blood cells.

Ovalocytes, Figures 2–33 and 2–34, are oval-shaped red blood cells. *Elliptocytes,* more oval than ovalocytes, are cigar-shaped. Both of these cells are found in hereditary elliptocytosis in large numbers. They are also present in various anemias but at a much lower concentration, no more than 6 to 10% of the mature red blood cell population. (These cells show normal shape in the nucleated and reticulocyte stages.)

Teardrop shaped red blood cells, Figure

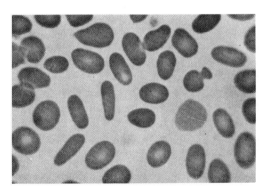

FIG. 2–34. Ovalocytes and elliptocytes. Note the *pincer cell* (red blood cell, shown in the upper right, which appears as if it has been pinched). (Magnification × 1000)

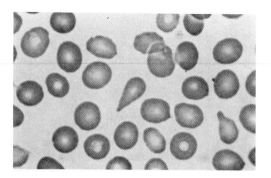

FIG. 2–35. Teardrop-shaped red blood cell (center of illustration). (Magnification ×1000)

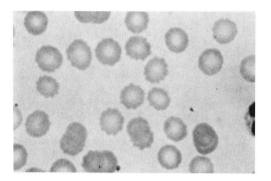

FIG. 2–36. Crenated red blood cells. (Note that the projections on the surface of the red blood cells are rounded, not pointed as in the burr cell.) (Magnification ×1000)

2–35, are found most notably in myelofibrosis, pernicious anemia, myeloid metaplasia, thalassemia, and some hemolytic anemias.

Crenated red blood cells (echinocytes), Figure 2–36, have blunt spicules evenly distributed over the surface of the red blood cell and are usually artifactual due to faulty drying of the blood smear, or, may be a result of hyperosmolarity.

Burr cells, Figures 2–37 and 2–38, are red blood cells with uniformly spaced, pointed projections on their outer edges. These cells occur in uremia, acute blood loss, cancer of the stomach, and pyruvate kinase deficiency.

Schistocytes, Figure 2–32, are red blood cell fragments and may occur in microangiopathic hemolytic anemia, uremia, severe burns, and hemolytic anemias caused by physical agents, as in disseminated intravascular coagulation (DIC).

Acanthocytes, Figure 2–39, are red blood cells with irregularly spaced projections. These spicules vary in width but usually contain a bulbous, rounded end. These cells have a decreased survival time and are found in abetalipoproteinemia and certain liver and lipid metabolism disorders.

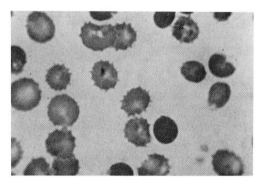

FIG. 2–37. Burr cells. (Magnification ×1000)

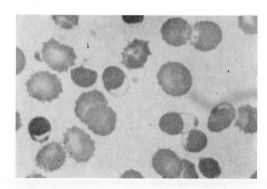

FIG. 2–38. *Blister cells* and burr cells. (Magnification ×1000)

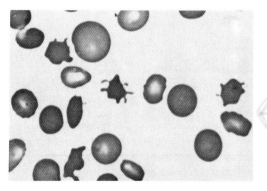

FIG. 2–39. Acanthocyte (center). (Magnification × 1000)

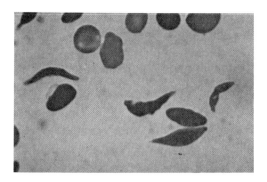

FIG. 2–40. Sickled red blood cells. (Magnification × 1000)

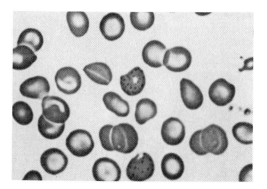

FIG. 2–41. Basophilic stippling (note the stippling in the red blood cell having a flattened side). (Magnification ×1000)

Sickle cells (drepanocytes), Figure 2–40, are red blood cells in the shape of a sickle or crescent due to the formation of rod-like polymers of hemoglobin S within the cell. To be considered sickle cells, they must come to a point at one end. These cells are associated with hemoglobin S and are found in sickle cell anemia, hemoglobin SC disease, and hemoglobin Sβ thalassemia.

Basophilic stippling, Figure 2–41, is present as many coarse or fine, purple-staining granules in the red blood cell. The granules result from aggregation of ribosomes and are found in lead poisoning, anemias with impaired hemoglobin synthesis, refractory anemias, alcoholism, and megaloblastic anemias.

Siderocytes are deposits of iron in the red blood cell. They are generally seen near the periphery of the cell and may appear as a single granule or as multiple granules. When

present on a Wright-stained smear, the granules appear less vividly stained than Howell-Jolly bodies and are termed *Pappenheimer bodies* (Fig. 2–42.) In contrast, when the iron deposits are stained only by iron stains, as in the Prussian blue reaction, the cells are termed *siderocytes*. In the bone marrow, siderocytes may appear in a ring formation around the nucleus of a sideroblast and are called *ringed sideroblasts*. These iron-staining granules are present in sideroblastic and megaloblastic anemias, alcoholism, following splenectomy, and in some hemoglobinopathies.

Howell-Jolly bodies, Figure 2–43, are round, purple staining nuclear fragments (DNA) in the red blood cell. They generally appear singly in hemolytic anemia, following splenectomy, and in cases of splenic atrophy

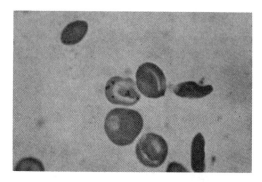

FIG. 2–42. Pappenheimer bodies (present in the red blood cell located in the middle of the illustration). (Magnification ×1000)

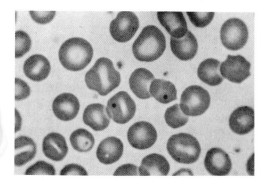

FIG. 2–43. Howell-Jolly bodies (one Howell-Jolly body is located in each of the two red blood cells shown in the center of the illustration). (Magnification ×1000)

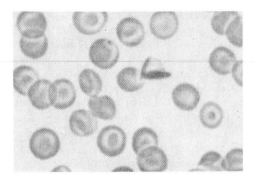

FIG. 2–44. Hemoglobin C crystal. Target cells are also present. (Magnification ×1000)

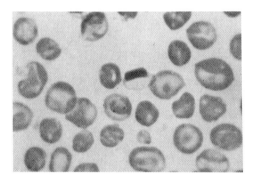

FIG. 2–45. Hemoglobin C crystal. Target cells are also present. (Magnification ×1000)

as in sickle cell anemia. Multiple Howell-Jolly bodies in a red blood cell occur in megaloblastic anemia and in other forms of nuclear maturation defects.

Hemoglobin C crystals, Figures 2–44 and 2–45, are tetragonal in shape and may be found in patients with homozygous hemoglobin C disease and characteristically in patients with hemoglobin SC disease.

Cabot rings, Figure 2–46, are purple staining threadlike filaments in the shape of a ring or figure 8 in the red blood cell. They are thought to be microtubules from a mitotic spindle and are seen rarely in pernicious anemia and lead poisoning. They probably indicate abnormal erythropoiesis.

Platelets on top of red blood cells, Figure 2–47, should not be confused with a red blood cell inclusion body. Compare the platelet with those in the surrounding field. Also, there is generally a nonstaining halo surrounding the platelet when it is positioned on top of the red blood cell.

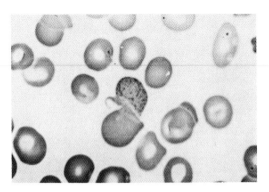

FIG. 2–46. Cabot ring. (Note the red blood cell in the center containing basophilic stippling and partially covered by another red blood cell. The cabot ring appears as a faintly stained circle within the red blood cell.) (Magnification ×1000)

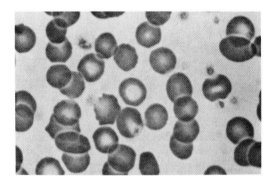

FIG. 2–47. Note the platelet on top of the red blood cell. When seen, there is generally a halo or clear-staining area in the red blood cell surrounding the platelet. (Magnification ×1000)

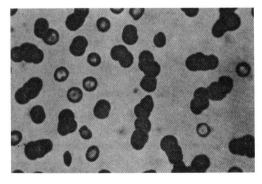

FIG. 2–48. Rouleaux formation of the red blood cells. (Magnification ×500)

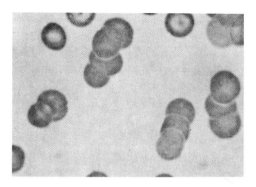

FIG. 2–49. Rouleaux formation of the red blood cells. (Magnification ×1000)

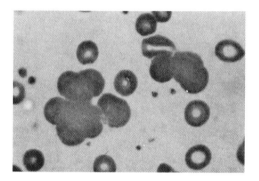

FIG. 2–50. Agglutination of the red blood cells. (Magnification ×1000)

Rouleaux formation, Figures 2–48 and 2–49, represents erythrocytes arranged in rolls or stacks. This may be due to an artifact (as a result of delay in smearing the blood once the drop has been placed on the slide) or, may be due to the presence of high concentrations of abnormal globulins or fibrinogen. This formation of red cells is found in multiple myeloma and macroglobulinemia.

Agglutination of the red blood cells, Figure 2–50, is found in patients who have a cold agglutinin (antibody), or autoimmune hemolytic anemia. Note the clumping of the red blood cells rather than the stacking as found in rouleaux formation. When agglutination of the red blood cells is seen on a blood smear, routine automated methods of red blood cell counting and sizing should not be utilized.

Crescent bodies are faintly staining bodies in the shape of a quarter moon. They are probably ruptured red blood cells.

When examining a blood smear, any of the preceding red blood cell morphology or inclusions should be noted. An occasional crescent body, however, may be ignored. Whenever possible, a red blood cell abnormality should be described in as much detail as possible. For example, when poikilocytosis is present, the type(s) of irregularly shaped cells should be noted. The generally accepted methods of reporting red blood cell irregularities include commenting on the degree of variability present (slight, moderate, marked, or 1+, 2+, 3+). Regardless of the method chosen, it should be used consistently. The reporting of red blood cell morphology varies widely between technologists. It is, therefore, helpful for each laboratory to have a uniform grading system. Also, the significance of different types of abnormal morphology will vary and, therefore the degree of grading may depend on the abnormality present. Refer to Table 2–1 for an example of a grading system for red blood cell morphology. In addition, it is important to select the proper area of the smear when determining morphology. The recommended areas on wedge or coverslip smears are those fields in which some red blood cells begin to overlap.

WHITE BLOOD CELLS AND PLATELETS

Granulocytes

There are three types of mature granulocytes: the neutrophil, eosinophil, and basophil. These three cell lines are distinguishable from each other by the presence of specific granules that appear in the myelocyte stage.

The committed stem cell for the neutrophils (and monocytes), CFU-G,M, gives rise to the myeloblast. The eosinophil, however, is thought to have its own committed stem cell, CFU-Eo, which gives rise to the myeloblast for further maturation to the eosinophil. The committed stem cell from which the basophil ultimately develops has not yet been identified. Because the maturation of the neutrophil, eosinophil, and basophil are very similar, and because these three cell types are granulocytic, their development is described simultaneously on the following pages.

In general, as the granulocytes mature, the nuclear chromatin becomes more condensed, nucleoli disappear, and abundant basophilic

TABLE 2-1. RED BLOOD CELL MORPHOLOGY GRADING CHART

Morphology	Grade As:
Polychromatophilia Helmet Cells Tear drop RBC Acanthocytes Schistocytes Spherocytes	1+ = 1 to 5/field 2+ = 6 to 10/field 3+ = >10/field
Poikilocytosis Ovalocytes Elliptocytes Burr Cells Bizarre-shaped RBC Target Cells Stomatocytes	1+ = 3 to 10/field 2+ = 11 to 20/field 3+ = >20/field
Rouleaux	1+ = aggregates of 3 to 4 RBC 2+ = aggregates of 5 to 10 RBC 3+ = numerous aggregates with only a few free RBC
Sickle cells Basophilic stippling Pappenheimer bodies Howell-Jolly bodies	Grade as Positive only

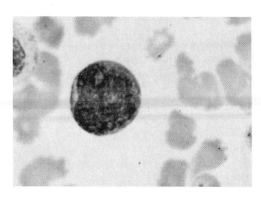

FIG. 2-51. Myeloblast (center).

cytoplasm with nonspecific granulation progresses to more scant cytoplasm containing granulation specific for the eosinophil, basophil, or neutrophil. The nucleus indents and becomes segmented, and overall cell size decreases.

Myeloblast (Figs. 2–51 and 2–52).

Size: 15 to 20 μm in diameter.

Cytoplasm: Small amount in relation to the rest of the cell.
Usually a moderate blue in color.
Texture is smooth and usually nongranular.

Nucleus: Round or slightly oval.
Occupies about four-fifths of the cell. N/C ratio of 4:1.
Extremely fine chromatin pattern.
Reddish purple in color.
Contains two to five nucleoli.

Promyelocyte (Figs. 2–52 and 2–53).

Size: 15 to 21 μm in diameter. This cell is normally slightly larger than the myeloblast.

Cytoplasm: Pale blue to basophilic.
Contains a few to many, large blue to reddish purple staining nonspecific (primary) granules.

Nucleus: Occupies half or more of the cell. N/C ratio of 3:1 to 2:1.
Oval or round.

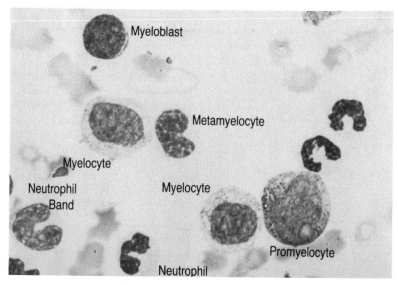

FIG. 2-52. Myeloblast, promyelocyte, myelocytes (two), metamyelocyte, neutrophilic band, neutrophils. Note the coarsening of the nuclear chromatin as the cell matures.

Chromatin pattern may become a little coarser, although it will still be relatively fine.

Two or three nucleoli present.

Myelocyte (Figs. 2-52 and 2-54). This is the last stage capable of cell division.

Size: 12 to 18 μm in diameter.

Cytoplasm: Moderate amount.

May contain a few patches of blue.

Few to moderate number of non-specific granules.

Small, specific (secondary) granules begin to appear in this stage.

Neutrophil myelocyte: the pink specific granules may be seen as pinkish or lighter staining areas in the cytoplasm, usually appearing near the nucleus first.

Eosinophil myelocyte: the specific granules first appear as dirty orange to blue. These granules are larger than the specific and nonspecific granules of the neutrophil.

Basophil myelocyte: the specific granules are few, large, and stain a dark blue-purple.

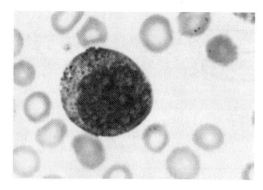

FIG. 2-53. Promyelocyte (center).

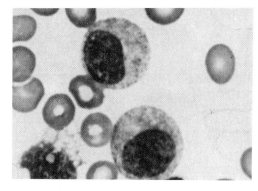

FIG. 2-54. Myelocytes, two.

2 types of Neutro
① segmental
② Band

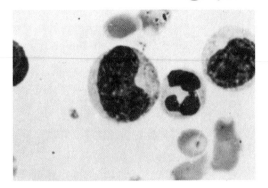

FIG. 2–55. Metamyelocyte and neutrophil.

Nucleus: Oval or round.
Chromatin pattern becomes coarser and more condensed.
Generally shows no nucleoli.
Nucleus may be centrally located or eccentric.
N/C ratio is 1:1.

Metamyelocyte (Figs. 2–52 and 2–55).

Size: 10 to 15 μm in diameter.

Cytoplasm: Moderate to abundant amount giving a decreased N/C ratio.
A few nonspecific granules. Full complement of specific granules.
Neutrophil metamyelocyte: the granules are pinker and more numerous.
Eosinophil metamyelocyte: the granules are a brighter orange-red and more numerous.
Basophil metamyelocyte: the dark purple to black granules are more numerous.

Nucleus: Indented or kidney-shaped.
Chromatin pattern is coarse and clumped and stains dark purple.

Neutrophil

Band (Figs. 2–52 and 2–56).

Size: 9 to 15 μm in diameter.

Cytoplasm: Same as the metamyelocyte.

Nucleus: Elongated or band-shaped.
Deeply indented from the metamyelocyte stage.
Chromatin pattern is coarse and clumped.

Segmented Neutrophil (Figs. 2–52, 2–55, and 2–57).

Size: 9 to 15 μm in diameter.

Cytoplasm: Full complement of pink to rose-violet specific granules.
Abundant amount.
Few nonspecific granules are present.

Nucleus: Normally two to five lobes connected by thin nuclear filaments.
Coarse, clumped chromatin pattern.

Eosinophil (Fig. 2–58).

Size: 9 to 15 μm in diameter.

Cytoplasm: Contains the full complement of large, reddish-orange granules.

Nucleus: Usually has two lobes.
Coarse, clumped chromatin pattern.

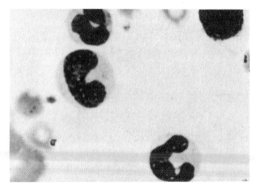

FIG. 2–56. Neutrophilic band.

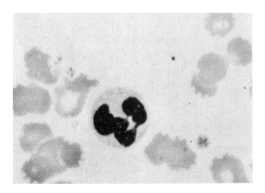

FIG. 2–57. Neutrophil (center).

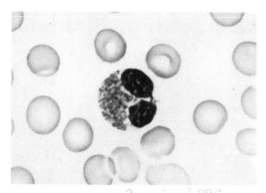

FIG. 2–58. Eosinophil. *3x size of RBC*

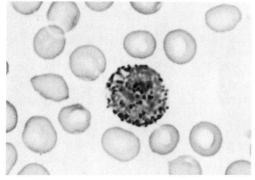

FIG. 2–59. Basophil. *2x size RBC*

Basophil (Fig. 2–59).

Size: 10 to 16 μm in diameter.

Cytoplasm: Stains slightly pink to colorless. Contains specific dark purple to blue-black granules.
There are fewer granules present than found in the eosinophil. The granules are water-soluble and tend to wash out when stained (probably because of improper fixation).

Nucleus: Does not appear as coarse as in the neutrophil or eosinophil.
Generally unsegmented or bi-lobed, rarely has three or four lobes.

When routinely differentiating white blood cells, it should be noted that, except in unusual circumstances, the different stages of the eosinophil or basophil are not identified. The cells are denoted merely as eosinophils or basophils. The neutrophil stages are always differentiated. Identification of the neutrophil band varies from one laboratory to another. In this text, a neutrophil is considered to be mature if the nucleus is indented by greater than one half of its diameter.

With present staining techniques, it is often impossible to differentiate the various types of blast cells. Many times, the cell is merely termed a 'blast' cell. Otherwise, the cell is identified by the company it keeps, that is, by placing it in the same family as the identifiable cells in the immediately surrounding area.

Neutrophilic Granulocytes

Neutrophil production and maturation occur in the bone marrow. The mature neutrophil moves into the lungs, spleen, and liver from the peripheral blood and then into the tissues where it carries out its major functions of ingesting and killing invading microorganisms.

Neutrophil Kinetics

As the myeloblast develops into the mature segmented neutrophil, the myeloblast, promyelocyte, and myelocyte undergo cell division. These cells constitute the mitotic pool (or proliferative compartment) where both cell division and maturation occur (Fig. 2–60), and will generally undergo a total of three to five cell divisions over a period of 6 to 7 days. During the promyelocyte stage the cell produces primary (azurophilic) granules. The number of granules per cell will decrease with each cell division. At the myelocyte stage the cell produces secondary (specific) granules. (Synthesis of primary granules stops when the cell begins secondary granule production.)

Once the cell reaches the metamyelocyte stage it is no longer capable of mitosis. It spends the next 6 to 14 days in the maturation and storage pools, during which time it develops into the segmented neutrophil. The number of bands and segmented neutrophils in the storage pool is about 15 times the number in the peripheral blood and the mitotic pool is approximately one-third the size of the storage pool.

When the neutrophilic cells are mature,

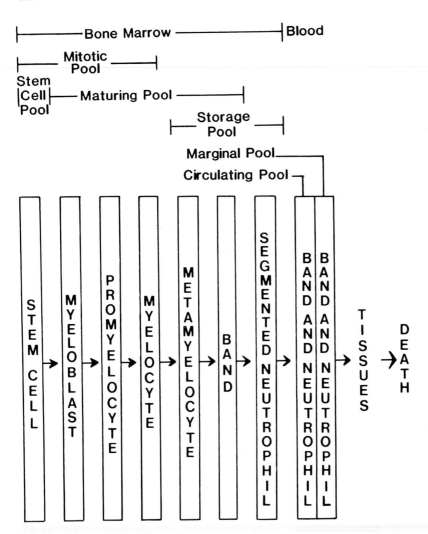

FIG. 2–60. Neutrophil kinetics.

they are ready for release into the peripheral blood. The release of marrow cells into the blood is only partially understood and is most probably based on a selective type of release of mature cells rather than a random release. It has been determined that a granulocytic CSF (colony stimulating factor) produced by macrophages and endothelial cells regulates granulocyte production and maturation and controls the movement of granulocytes through the sinusoid wall of the bone marrow to the blood. Granulocyte-CSF also enhances the function of the neutrophil during phagocytosis, oxidation, degranulation, and chemotaxis. The exact mechanisms and controls are still unknown.

When the mature neutrophils leave the storage pool they enter the peripheral blood, where approximately 50% of the neutrophils circulate freely and make up the *circulating pool*. The remaining 50% adhere to the walls of the blood vessels or are sequestered in the capillaries and constitute the *marginal pool*. (The cells in the marginal pool are not included in the white blood cell count. Therefore, in a blood sample, the number of neutrophils counted in a white blood cell count and differential represents only half the number actually present in the peripheral blood.) The cells are continually changing back and forth between the marginal and circulating pools. A small percentage of bands are also normally released to the peripheral blood along with mature neutrophils. The segmented neutrophil is generally released to the peripheral blood first, before the band. When the demand for neutrophils in the peripheral blood increases, as soon as the numbers of segmented neutrophils in the storage pool has become depleted, the number of bands entering the peripheral blood from the storage pool increases. This is reflected by an increased percentage of bands in the white blood cell differential count. The average time the neutrophil spends in the peripheral blood is considered to be about 10 hours. According to this figure, the neutrophils in the peripheral blood are completely replaced by neutrophils from the bone marrow almost 2.5 times every 24 hours. The neutrophils do not return to the bone marrow once they enter the peripheral blood. They have a lifespan of about 5 days.

From the marginal pool, the neutrophils randomly enter the tissues and body cavities where they carry out their major functions. The cells leave the peripheral blood randomly, regardless of the age of the cell or the length of time it has been in the marginal or circulating pool. Normally, the neutrophils enter the tissues at the same rate as other neutrophils leave the storage pool and enter the peripheral blood. Once the neutrophil has entered the tissues, it is utilized to fight infection, or it leaves the body via excretions from the intestinal tract, the urinary tract, the lungs, or the salivary glands. It may also be destroyed by the mononuclear phagocytic system within 4 or 5 days.

Physiology and Function of the Neutrophil

Neutrophils are metabolically active. They are capable of both aerobic and anaerobic glycolysis for their source of energy. Their major function is to stop or retard the action of foreign material or infectious agents by means of: (1) moving into the area of inflammation or infection, (2) phagocytosis of the foreign material, and (3) killing and digestion of the offending material.

The primary (nonspecific) and secondary (specific) granules of the neutrophil are packaged and released from the Golgi apparatus. In the mature neutrophil, the ratio of specific granules to nonspecific granules is about 2 or 3:1. The primary granules are membrane-bound lysosomes and contain acid phosphatase, peroxidase, esterase, sulfated mucosubstance, β-galactosidase, arylsulfatase, lysozyme, and other basic proteins. The secondary granules contain aminopeptidase, collagenase, muramidase, lactoferrin, lysozyme, and a number of basic proteins. Alkaline phosphatase is no longer thought to be contained in the granules but may reside on the neutrophil plasma membrane.

The neutrophil is capable of both random locomotion (*chemokinesis*) and directed locomotion (*chemotaxis*). This locomotion is possible only if the neutrophil is attached to a surface. The neutrophil is normally spherical in shape but becomes bipolar or ameboid when in contact with a surface. The tail end, or *uropod*, is blunt and adhesive; the front end, or *protopod*, extends pseudopods, which results in the creeping movement of the neutrophil along a surface. This locomotion is made possible by actin and myosin contractile filaments. The cells in the marginal pool move by locomotion through the unruptured walls of the blood vessels (*diapedesis*) and travel to the tissues and body cavities. Neutrophil granules release the enzyme collagenase, which aids in its movement through the tissues. In the presence of infection, inflammation, or a foreign substance, the neutrophils in the area of the foreign matter quickly move, within minutes, by diapedesis to the damaged or infected area. This directed locomotion is brought about by *chemotactic factors,* such as secretions from transformed lymphocytes and macrophages, endotoxins and other products from bacteria, and activated complement. The neutrophils are able to distinguish foreign particles and damaged cells. This is of utmost importance to its function of phagocytosis. *Opsonins* (specific antibodies, complement, etc.) enhance phagocytosis and increase chemotaxis. They act on the foreign particles by coating them. The surface of the neutrophil membrane contains receptors for complement (C3b) and for the Fc portion of IgG. The neutrophil is able to bind the coated matter and phagocytose it.

When the neutrophil phagocytizes foreign particles, the cell membrane moves inward and encloses the material by the process of *endocytosis,* forming a phagocytic vacuole (*phagosome*), the walls of which had been the

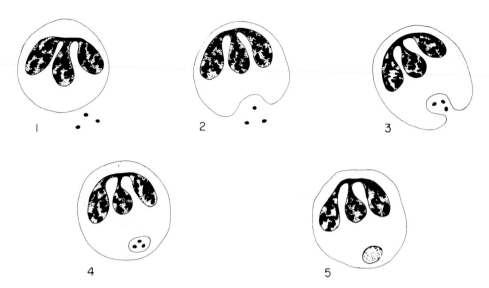

FIG. 2–61. Phagocytosis of bacteria by the neutrophil.

cell's outer membrane (Fig. 2–61). During phagocytosis, a number of metabolic changes take place: increased glycolysis and lipid synthesis, increased monophosphate shunt activity, a decrease in pH within the phagosome, and increased oxygen consumption. There is also the formation of oxidants such as superoxide (O_2^-) from oxygen (catalyzed by the enzyme NADPH oxidase), and hydrogen peroxide from superoxide, all of which are highly active oxygen radicals.

Once the phagocytic vacuole is formed, the specific neutrophil granules will first fuse with the phagosome membrane (forming a *phagolysosome*), emptying their contents into the phagosome. (This process is known as *degranulation.*) Following this, the nonspecific granules release their contents into the phagosome. Myeloperoxidase from the primary granules in combination with the hydrogen peroxide generated form a highly reactive peroxide halide, which is an effective way for the neutrophil to kill bacteria, viruses, and fungi. This process is referred to as the *respiratory burst* and is essential for the destruction of phagocytized material. When the bacteria have been killed, the phagosome is known as a *secondary lysosome.* The cell may then expel the digested residue (*exocytosis*). The neutrophil is also capable of *pinocytosis* (ingestion of small amounts of liquid). The combination of phagocytosis and pinocytosis

is termed *endocytosis.* Once the neutrophil has lost its granules, the cell dies and is removed by the macrophages.

In the presence of an inflammatory process, the neutrophils continually move into the infected area, phagocytize, die, and are, in turn, phagocytized by macrophages. The neutrophils are generally the first phagocytic cell to reach infected areas and are followed by the monocyte. These two cell types continue their migration to the area until all of the foreign material has been phagocytized. Under normal conditions, the neutrophil will spend 4 to 5 days in the tissues before senescence (growing old) and destruction.

Neutrophilia

(1) Extreme exercise and also the administration of certain drugs cause a decrease in the proportion of neutrophils in the marginal pool. These cells become part of the circulating pool and are reflected by an increased white blood cell count and an increased percentage of neutrophils in the differential count. (2) In the presence of infection, an increased number of neutrophils are present in the marginal pool. These cells then enter the tissues at a faster rate. The influx of neutrophils from the storage pool increases until the rate of outflow to the tissues is exceeded by the rate of inflow from the storage pool

in the bone marrow. (3) In chronic infection, the high rate of influx of neutrophils into the peripheral blood and the corresponding increased outflow may remain unchanged and a steady state of neutrophilia is maintained.

Neutropenia

When the absolute neutrophil count is less than 1000/μL, the patient is prone to recurrent infections. However, when the count drops to less than 500/μL the patient is seriously open to infection from bacteria or fungi.

(1) Certain drugs cause an increased number of neutrophils to enter the marginal pool, resulting in a lower percentage of neutrophils in the circulating pool. (2) In a severe infection, the outflow of cells to the tissues may exceed the input from the bone marrow storage pool. (3) Decreased production in the bone marrow from congenital causes, cytotoxic drugs, or aplastic anemia gives rise to decreased numbers of neutrophils available to the peripheral blood. (4) An increased loss of white blood cells (as might occur with splenomegaly), whereby the spleen sequesters (removes from the blood and holds) and destroys the cells, may also lead to neutropenia.

The Eosinophil

The majority of eosinophils are produced in the bone marrow. They most likely originate from their own committed stem cell and not the same committed stem cell as the neutrophils. The maturation process of the eosinophil, however, closely parallels that of the neutrophil. They are slightly larger than neutrophils and the nuclei of the cells average fewer lobes than found in the mature neutrophil. The eosinophils will average 2.1 lobes in the normal person.

The colony stimulating factor (CSF) which stimulates the production of eosinophils from the committed stem cell (CFU-Eo) is produced by T lymphocytes, and is termed the Eo-CSF. It also plays an important role in the prolonged in vitro survival of eosinophils, as well as increasing their tonicity against parasites.

The eosinophil is primarily a tissue cell. Once it is released into the peripheral blood from the bone marrow, it will be randomly removed from the blood independently of its age. Its half-life in the blood is about 8 hours; there is a diurnal variation in eosinophil counts, with the highest counts occurring at night. From the blood it moves into the tissues where it localizes in areas exposed to the external environment, most notably in the skin, nasal membranes, lungs, and gastrointestinal tract. Steroid compounds act by inhibiting the release of the eosinophil from the bone marrow and enhance their movement into the tissues. For each eosinophil in the peripheral blood there are 300 to 500 eosinophils in the tissues where their life span is probably several days. Once they migrate to the tissues they are still able to return to the peripheral circulation. The eosinophils are motile and capable of locomotion in a manner similar to the neutrophils.

The eosinophil is metabolically more active than the neutrophil. The mitochondria are larger and more numerous, and the Golgi zones are more developed. Although the eosinophil membranes have receptors for complement and IgG, they are present on fewer of the cells than found in the neutrophils.

The mature eosinophil contains two types of granules. The larger granules are the more numerous and contain a very dense elliptical crystalloid core, which primarily consists of what is termed *major basic protein* (MBP), which is toxic to helminth parasites and may also become toxic to the body's own tissues. Production of these granules stops when the eosinophil becomes mature. The second type of granule present is smaller than the first and may not appear in the cell until after the myelocyte stage. The eosinophilic granules contain peroxidase, β-glucuronidase, acid β-glycerophosphatase, arylsulfatase (contained in small granules), phospholipase, acid phosphatase, ribonuclease, and cathepsin. The peroxidase is a different form than that found in the neutrophil. In addition, the eosinophil granules differ from those in the neutrophil in that they lack lysozyme, phagocytin, and neutrophil bactericidal cationic proteins.

The functions of the eosinophil are not completely understood. They are capable of phagocytizing foreign material and antigen-antibody complexes in a limited way. However, these are probably not their primary functions. One proposed function describes the eosinophil as an *anti-inflammatory cell* in that they may modulate reactions in which basophils and mast cells are active. Basophils contain eosinophil chemotactic factors. In addition, eosinophils: (1) are thought to prevent basophil and mast cell degranulation, (2) contain histaminase which can inactivate the histamine from mast cells, (3) contain aryl-sulfatase B which inactivates leukotrienes released by the mast cell, (4) contains phospholipase D to inactivate platelet-activating factor, and (5) are capable of neutralizing the heparin released by mast cells by the action of the major basic protein (present in the large eosinophil granule). The eosinophils also appear to function by providing some defense against helminth parasites by first moving to the site of parasite infection. The cells then attach to the surface of the parasites where they release hydrolytic enzymes from their granules that damage and degrade the larval wall of the parasitic invaders.

Basophils and Mast Cells

It is thought that basophils develop from a cell similar to the myeloblast. The stem cell from which it originates has not yet been identified and it may or may not be a separate stem cell from that of the neutrophil and monocyte, or eosinophil. The cell matures in a manner similar to the eosinophil and is produced in the bone marrow. Once released from the bone marrow to the peripheral blood, the basophil remains in the circulation for approximately the same amount of time as the neutrophil before it moves into the tissues. Tissue mast cells are widely distributed throughout the body including the skin, lung tissue, thymus, spleen, and bone marrow, where they are long-lived and are of mesenchymal origin. They are normally not present in the peripheral blood.

The granules of the basophil are larger than the azurophilic granules found in the promyelocyte, and may be slightly irregular in shape. They are water soluble and stain a deep purple with Wright stain. During maturation, the nucleus does not segment as completely as the neutrophil and the nuclear chromatin in the mature basophil has a condensed and somewhat smudged appearance. The mast cells are slightly larger than the basophil, have a round or oval nucleus, and contain abundant purple staining (Wright stain) granules that are slightly smaller and less soluble than the basophil granules. The mast cell granules are sufficiently abundant to obscure the nucleus.

The basophil exhibits chemotaxis and some phagocytic activity. It is also capable of a sluggish motility. The basophil granules contain serotonin, peroxidase, a vasoconstrictive histamine compound, and the anticoagulant heparin. They synthesize an eosinophil chemotactic factor, a slow reacting substance of anaphylaxis, and platelet activating factor (PAF) to promote platelet aggregation and adhesion. The biochemical make up of the mast cell is similar and, in addition, it contains serotonin and some proteolytic enzymes.

Basophils and mast cells appear to function similarly in inflammatory processes. They appear to participate in immediate hypersensitivity immune reactions and are also involved in some delayed hypersensitivity reactions. Their membranes readily bind immunoglobulin E and when specific antigens react with the membrane-bound IgE, rapid degranulation occurs and the contents of the basophil/mast cell granules are released to the surrounding area, producing an anaphylactic shock reaction that can be severe. Hyperimmune responses to toxins and wasp or bee stings can result in vasoconstriction and bronchioconstriction. This, in turn, will lead to the accumulation of eosinophils in the area (due to the eosinophil chemotactic factor released from the cells).

Monocytes

The monocyte is produced in the bone marrow.

Monoblast (Fig. 2–62).

Size: 12 to 20 μm in diameter.

Cytoplasm: Moderately basophilic to blue-gray.
Nongranular.

Nucleus: Ovoid or round in shape.
Light blue-purple in color.
Fine, lacey chromatin.
One to two nucleoli.
N/C ratio is 4:1 to 3:1.

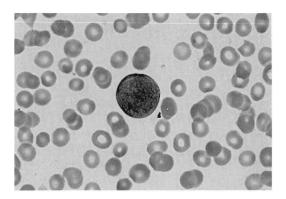

FIG. 2–62. Monoblast.

Promonocyte (immature monocyte) (Fig. 2–63).

Size: 14 to 18 μm in diameter.

Cytoplasm: Blue-gray.
May contain fine dustlike azurophilic granules.
Ground glass appearance.
Moderate amount.

Nucleus: Oval, may have a single fold or fissure.
One to five nucleoli.
Fine chromatin pattern.
N/C ratio is 3:1 to 2:1.

Monocyte (Fig. 2–64).

Size: 14 to 20 μm in diameter.

Cytoplasm: Abundant.
Blue-gray.
Outline may be irregular because of the presence of pseudopods.
Many fine azurophilic granules, giving a ground glass appearance.
Vacuoles may sometimes be present.

Nucleus: Round, kidney shaped, or may show slight lobulation. It may be folded over on top of itself, thus showing brainlike convolutions.
No nucleoli are visible.
Chromatin is fine and lacey (not clumped), arranged in skein-like strands.

Physiology and Biology of the Monocyte

The monocyte arises from the same bipotential stem cell as the neutrophil, the CFU-G, M (colony forming unit granulocyte, monocyte). From this stem cell arises the CFU-M (monocyte), the stem cell committed to forming monocytes. The precursor to the monocyte is the monoblast and is morphologically indistinguishable from the myeloblast. Cytochemical stains may be used to differentiate the two cell lines. Monoblasts are positive for nonspecific esterase, which is inhibited by sodium fluoride, and negative for peroxidase and Sudan black stains. Myeloblasts are positive for both peroxidase and Sudan black and contain both nonspecific and specific (α naphthyl chloroacetate esterase) esterases. Unlike the other white blood cells in the peripheral blood, the monocyte is considered to be an immature cell. When it leaves the blood, it travels to the tissues, where the cell line spends most of its time, maturing and differentiating into specific types of macrophages

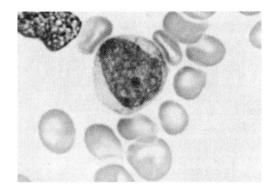

FIG. 2–63. Promonocyte (immature monocyte).

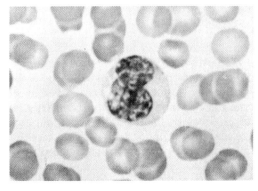

FIG. 2–64. Monocyte.

depending on the site of maturation in the various tissues.

The immature monocyte, or promonocyte, is less phagocytic and less motile than the monocyte. Once the promonocyte is formed it will undergo two mitotic divisions within a period of 2 to 2½ days under normal conditions. Mature monocytes are released into the peripheral blood 12 to 24 hours after their last mitotic division. The mature monocyte in the peripheral blood has a well-developed Golgi apparatus, rough endoplasmic reticulum, numerous mitochondria, and variable amounts of ribosomes and polyribosomes. There are nucleoli present in the nucleus in about 50% of the monocytes, as seen by electron microscopy. The granules in the cytoplasm of the monocyte are packaged by the Golgi apparatus, represent primary lysosomes, and contain acid phosphatase and arylsulfatase, and esterase activity. These lysosomes become numerous in the macrophage. The monocyte and macrophage are actively motile cells which are capable of chemotaxis, are able to move through blood vessel walls and migrate to areas of inflammation, and may extend multiple pseudopods. They respond to such substances as chemotactic inhibitors and MIF (migration inhibition factor), which is produced by the T lymphocytes to immobilize and restrict the macrophage to areas of inflammation. The monocyte and macrophage are capable of phagocytosis and pinocytosis, the energy for which is generated by glycolysis. When there are areas of inflammation present in the body, the production of monocytes is increased and their numbers increase in the peripheral blood.

Life Span of the Monocyte

The bone marrow contains the developing monocyte precursors and supplies monocytes to the peripheral blood. The proliferation of monocytes in the bone marrow takes about 55 hours. They undergo no maturation in the bone marrow and leave there randomly, in no specific order. The marginal pool of monocytes in the peripheral blood is about 3.5 times the size of the circulating pool. The mature monocyte spends about 12 hours in the peripheral blood before going to the tissues.

Development of the Monocyte into the Macrophage

The monocyte moves via diapedesis through the blood vessel walls into the various tissues and transforms into the macrophage, at the same time becoming actively phagocytic. It is also thought that some macrophages are produced by cell division of existing macrophages. As the macrophage develops from the monocyte, the cell increases in size as a result of increased cytoplasmic content. One or more nucleoli develop and there is an increase in the hydrolytic enzymes. In addition, the Golgi apparatus and the number of mitochondria increase. There is also an increased number of secondary lysosomes as a result of increased phagocytosis. Once the monocyte leaves the circulation it is pleuripotential, capable of differentiating into specific types of macrophage depending on the location in the tissues to which it has migrated. Monocytes and differentiated macrophages constitute the *mononuclear phagocytic system (MPS)*, a term that has replaced the outdated reticuloendothelial system (RES). They may become the Kupffer cells of the liver sinusoids, osteoclasts in bone, macrophages of inflammatory areas, connective tissue macrophages (histiocytes), pulmonary alveolar macrophages, or microglial cells of the nervous system. Overall, the macrophage is more active than the monocyte and has a much richer supply of acid hydrolases. Once the monocyte leaves the blood it may spend several months, or longer, in the tissues where it will eventually die. Macrophages generally do not re-enter the peripheral blood for recirculation, although an occasional macrophage may enter the blood via the lymphatic system.

The Macrophage

The macrophage is a large cell, ranging in size from 15 to 80 μm in diameter. It has an eccentric nucleus that may be egg-shaped, indented, or elongated. The chromatin appears spongy, and there are generally one to two nucleoli. The cell has abundant sky blue cytoplasm which contains many coarse azure granules. It is usually vacuolated, and may contain ingested material. The cytoplasmic outline may be irregular because of the presence of pseudopods. There is large variation in the appearance of the macrophage, depending on the site from which the cell has been derived. Some macrophages may develop epithelioid characteristics and may fuse to form giant multinucleated cells. Macrophages have been divided into two categories: (1) *fixed macrophages* and (2) *unfixed (wandering) macrophages*. When stimulated, some of the fixed macrophages may become actively motile, phagocytic, wandering macrophages. The fixed, nonphagocytic macrophage has also been termed a *histiocyte*. Examples are the fixed dendritic cells of the thymus and spleen. Macrophages are found scattered throughout the body. There are macrophages lining the sinusoids of the spleen and bone marrow, and alveolar macrophages in the lungs; they are present in the skin as Langerhans cells; there are freely migrating macrophages in the pleural cells; and they are also found at sites of inflammation and in peritoneal, pleural, and synovial fluids. The macrophage lives much longer in the tissues than does the neutrophil. It is capable of cell division and can be stimulated to synthesize a number of enzymes and other substances, depending on the body's needs.

Properties and Functions of the Monocyte and Macrophage

As the monocyte transforms into an activated macrophage, the cell surface becomes sticky and develops numerous fan-like folds for optimal phagocytosis. Both the monocyte and macrophage show active chemotaxis and *necrotaxis* (attraction to dead or dying cells); however, compared to neutrophils, monocytes are much slower to appear at inflammatory sites. Pinocytosis and micropinocytosis increase as the cell matures into the macrophage. Phagocytosis of antigens by the monocyte and macrophage requires that certain antigens be coated with an antibody *(opsonization)*. The monocytes and macrophages are also capable of *necrophagocytosis* (ingestion of dying cells and cellular debris) that, along with pinocytosis, does not require antibody coating of the material being ingested. The primary functions of the monocyte and macrophage are:

1. *Defense mechanism against microorganisms (including fungi) and tumor cells.* They primarily control microbial infections such as mycobacteria, brucella, listeria, and salmonella. When an antibody coated antigen is present, the monocyte or macrophage travels to the site by the use of chemotaxis. It then attaches to the antigen and extends pseudopods around the material, forming a phagosome. *Primary lysosomes* in the cytoplasm of the monocyte or macrophage fuse with the phagosome; acid hydrolases enter the area to digest or degrade the antigen and they become *secondary lysosomes*. Particle ingestion is also accompanied by the release of powerful microbiocidal substances such as superoxide (O_2^-) and hydrogen peroxide (H_2O_2). The digested material may then be released from the cell *(exocytosis)*. The macrophage contains Fc receptor sites for the IgG and IgM immunoglobulins on their surface, which greatly enhances their recognition and ingestion of foreign particles. Also, ingestion of particles by these cells is enhanced by certain factors present in the plasma such as antibodies and complement (C3b). The macrophage is able to phagocytize more quickly and has a greater capacity for phagocytosis than either the neutrophil or the monocyte. The cell is also capable of anaerobic phagocytosis, functioning in the center of wounds where oxygen is decreased. Unlike the neutrophil, both the monocyte and macrophage are able to synthesize new enzymes and regenerate lysosomes. Macrophages also are capable of destroying a variety of other cells, such as fungi, protozoa, and tumor cells. Activated macrophages produce substances such as cachectin that destroy some tumor cells coated with specific antibodies. The macrophage attaches to the Fc portion of the immunoglobulin and exerts a direct cytolytic effect on the tumor cell.

2. *Removal of damaged and old cells, plasma proteins, and plasma lipids.* They play an important part in the removal of old and damaged red blood cells (as in the spleen) and also in wound debridement through phagocytosis. Splenic macrophages also remove red cells sensitized with autoantibody (in autoimmune hemolytic anemia), and platelets (in autoimmune thrombocytopenia). The plasma proteins and lipids are removed by the macrophage

via pinocytosis. The process by which the macrophage identifies the cells and proteins to be removed is largely unknown. One factor may be the less negative charge of cell membranes (due to a decrease in their sialic acid content upon aging).

3. *Participation in iron metabolism.* Some tissue macrophages contain heme oxidase activity which enables them to break down the hemoglobin present in red blood cells. Macrophages of the spleen are involved in erythrophagocytosis of abnormal red cells, as are the macrophages of the bone marrow (nurse cells of erythroblastic islands). The iron, from the hemoglobin, remains in the macrophage, binding with apoferritin (in the macrophage) to form aggregates of ferritin. It may subsequently form hemosiderin. The ferritin will later leave the macrophage, bind to transferrin, and be available for use in hemoglobin production.

4. *Processes antigen information for lymphocytes.* Macrophages serve an important role in the immune response as antigen presenting cells. They interact with antigens by membrane attachment, ingestion, and by subsequent modification of the antigen, and will secrete a lymphocyte activating factor, *interleukin-1 (IL-1).* (Three forms of IL-1 are known: αIL-1, which activates B lymphocytes; βIL-1, which activates T helper cells; and IL-1, which stimulates cytotoxic T cells. In turn, activated T cells produce interleukin-2 [IL-2], which regulates macrophage function.) The processed antigen is presented to the lymphocyte on specific cytoplasmic surface sites. The T lymphocyte may then undergo blast transformation, and the B lymphocytes may produce antibody. The macrophage can interact with both B and T lymphocytes and is, therefore, also active in cell mediated immunity.

5. *Production and secretion of various substances.* The macrophages release lysosomal enzymes into the surrounding area which decompose tissue components and contribute to the inflammatory response. These enzymes include acid phosphatase, lipase, nucleases, proteinase, collagenase, elastase, various glycosidases, and plasminogen activator for lysing fibrin clots. They are an important source of colony stimulating factor (CSF) with a monopoietic hormone-like effect, which is felt to be an important ingredient for the control of leukopoiesis and the development of CFU-M from CFU-G, M. They secrete an erythropoietic factor, substances concerned with the stimulation and differentiation of T and B lymphocytes, materials which suppress lymphocyte function, chemotactic factors, and chemotactic factor inhibitors. The macrophage produces and secretes high levels of pyrogen upon stimulation (causes fever), and prostaglandins that inhibit the function of activated lymphocytes. They also secrete such miscellaneous substances as thromboplastin, platelet activating factors, transferrin, protease inhibitors (α2-macroglobulin and α1-antitrypsin), and transcobalamin II (vitamin B_{12} transport protein), as well as a stimulatory factor for hepatocytes of the liver to secrete fibrinogen. Complement factors, interferons (antiviral compounds), lysozymes, hydrogen peroxide, and superoxide are also secreted by the macrophages for use in the body's defense system.

Lymphocytes

Lymphocytes are produced by the lymph nodes, spleen, thymus, and bone marrow.

Lymphoblast (nonleukemic lymphoblast) (Fig. 2–65).

Size: 10 to 18 μm in diameter.

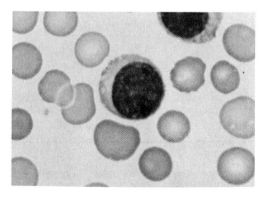

FIG. 2–65. Immature lymphocyte (center).

Cytoplasm: No granules present.

Appears smooth.

Moderate to dark blue. May stain deep blue at the periphery and a lighter blue near the nucleus.

More abundant than in the myeloblast.

Nucleus: Chromatin pattern is somewhat coarse.

Round or oval in shape.

Generally contains one to two distinct nucleoli.

N/C ratio is 4:1.

Prolymphocyte.

Size: May be the same size as the lymphoblast or smaller.

Cytoplasm: Moderate to dark blue.

Usually nongranular, but may contain occasional azurophilic granules.

More abundant than in the lymphoblast.

Nucleus: Round, oval, or slightly indented.

Chromatin pattern is more clumped than in the lymphoblast.

May contain one to two nucleoli.

Mature Lymphocyte

The lymphocytes found in the peripheral blood occur in varying sizes. For purposes of description, they are divided into three categories: small, medium, and large, with a size variation of 8 to 16 μm in diameter. In addition to differing in size, the relative amount of cytoplasm varies. Generally, the larger the lymphocyte, the more abundant the cytoplasm.

Small Lymphocyte (Fig. 2–66).

Size: 8 to 10 μm in diameter. (Approximately the size of a normal red blood cell.)

Cytoplasm: Usually forms a thin rim around the nucleus.

Moderate to dark blue.

Nucleus: Chromatin pattern is dense and clumped.

Round or oval in shape and may be slightly indented.

No nucleoli are visible.

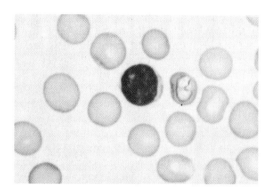

FIG. 2–66. Small mature lymphocyte.

Medium Lymphocyte.

Size: 10 to 12 μm in diameter.

Cytoplasm: More abundant than in the small lymphocyte.

Pale to moderately blue.

May or may not contain a few nonspecific azurophilic granules.

Nucleus: Round or oval in shape and may be slightly indented.

Chromatin pattern is clumped but not as dense looking as in the small lymphocyte.

No nucleoli are visible.

Large Lymphocyte.

Size: 12 to 16 μm in diameter.

Cytoplasm: Abundant.

Clear, very pale blue.

May or may not contain a few nonspecific azurophilic granules.

Nucleus: Round or oval in shape and may be slightly indented.

Chromatin pattern is coarse.

No nucleoli are visible.

May be eccentrically located.

Biology and Physiology of the Lymphocyte

The lymphocytes are vital to the immune system. They function in the production of circulating antibodies and in the expression of cellular immunity. The mature lymphocyte has little or no endoplasmic reticulum, only a small Golgi apparatus, possesses only a few mitochondria, and the ribosomes are free and in clusters. Depending upon the functional state of the lymphocyte (whether it is active or resting), it may have microvilli projections on its outer surface, or, it may have a relatively smooth outside surface. The nucleus of the lymphocyte usually contains a nucleolus, which, because of the denseness of the nucleus, is generally not visible under light microscopy.

Using special staining procedures, the lymphocyte is negative for chloroacetate esterase, alkaline phosphatase, and peroxidase and is positive for acid phosphatase. Lymphocytes show variable staining for the periodic acid Schiff (PAS) stain, and the cytoplasm may illustrate a block pattern of staining (the stain is aggregated).

The lymphocyte is actively motile and, during locomotion, has the appearance of a hand mirror. Locomotion occurs as the lymphocyte crawls over or around other cell surfaces. When moving, the nucleus is at the leading end of the cell with the cytoplasm trailing behind, appearing as the handle of the mirror. Lymphocytes also extend a trailing uropod studded with microvillae for attachment to "target" cells.

The Lymphocytic System

The lymphocytic system in the adult is comprised of the primary lymphopoietic organs, made up of the bone marrow and thymus, and the secondary, or peripheral, lymphatic system, which includes the lymph nodes, spleen, gut-associated lymphoid tissues (lymph nodules of the intestines, which are also termed *Peyer's patches,* and the *Waldeyer's ring* of lymphoid tissue in the tonsils), and the blood. The lymph tissue is composed of lymphatic vessels that form a dense network in most of the tissues of the body. The smaller vessels unite with each other to form larger vessels until all of the lymphatic vessels come together and form two main trunks: the right lymphatic duct and the thoracic duct. These two main vessels open into the veins of the neck. Lymph nodes are located along these lymphatic vessels to drain and filter lymphatic fluid from the tissue spaces. The contents of the vessels pass through the lymph nodes on their way to the thoracic and lymphatic ducts. Lymphatic fluid enters the lymph node via the afferent lymph vessel, passes through the sinuses, and exits via the efferent lymph vessel. The sinuses are lined with macrophages, which remove foreign antigens. B lymphocytes proliferate in the region of the outer cortex, and the paracortical area consists mainly of T helper lymphocytes. The central medulla of the lymph node contains both T and B cells (Fig. 2–67).

The bone marrow is the body's largest lymphopoietic mass. The source of lymphocyte replacement is the stem cell compartment in the bone marrow. Production of lymphocytes in the bone marrow and thymus is independent of antigenic stimulation and events occurring in other areas of the lymphoid system.

These two organs (bone marrow and thymus) provide the peripheral lymph system with a supply of lymphocytes that can become immunocompetent when stimulated by an antigen. The fate of the lymphocytes produced in the bone marrow varies; some of these cells may serve as lymphocyte stem cells, while some lymphocytes may migrate to the peripheral lymphatic system. Most of the marrow lymphocytes, however, probably die randomly in the bone marrow and serve as building blocks for future generations of lymphocytes. In the thymus, most of the lymphocytes are replaced every 3 to 4 days. A few of these lymphocytes will migrate to thymus-dependent areas of the spleen and lymph nodes, whereas the remainder will die in the thymus or migrate out of the thymus and die elsewhere.

Lymphocyte Subpopulations

There are two main functional classes of lymphocytes: B lymphocytes and T lymphocytes. These cells are morphologically similar and cannot be distinguished from each other on a Wright-stained smear.

The B lymphocyte is derived from the bone marrow and was so named because it was originally discovered in birds, where it was programmed by an organ called the bursa of Fabricius. (The equivalent organ in the human is thought to be the bone marrow.) The B lymphocyte accounts for 10 to 20% of normal blood lymphocytes in the adult. The B lymphocyte migrates from the bone marrow to the peripheral lymphatic tissues (including

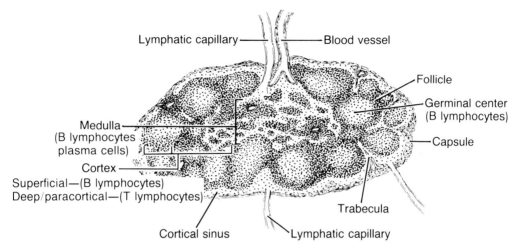

Lymphatic capillary — Blood vessel

Follicle

Germinal center (B lymphocytes)

Medulla (B lymphocytes plasma cells)

Capsule

Cortex

Superficial—(B lymphocytes)
Deep/paracortical—(T lymphocytes)

Cortical sinus

Trabecula

Lymphatic capillary

FIG. 2–67. Schematic drawing of a lymph node. (From McKenzie, S.B.: *Textbook of Hematology*, Lea & Febiger, Philadelphia, 1988.)

the primary follicles and red pulp of the spleen, and follicular and medullary regions of the lymph nodes) where it interacts with antigens and differentiates into a plasma cell that secretes immunoglobulins (IgG, IgM, and IgA) for defense against infections (this is termed *humoral immunity*). The plasma cell is the final stage of maturation for the B cell.

T lymphocytes mature in the thymus and then travel to the peripheral tissues (including the paracortical regions of the lymph nodes) where they interact with antigens to form specific *effector cells* which act in delayed hypersensitivity reactions, suppression of tumors, graft rejection, and against some intracellular organisms. This is termed *cellular immunity*. The T lymphocytes may also assist in regulating both humoral and cellular immune responses. T lymphocytes make up 60 to 80% of the lymphoid cells in the adult blood lymphocyte pool.

A third population of lymphocytes appears to exist which lack the characteristics of the mature T and B lymphocytes, and are termed *null* lymphocytes. Less than 10% of adult lymphocytes are in this category.

Life Span, Circulation and Recirculation of Lymphocytes

The majority of lymphocytes are long-lived, with a life span of about 4 years. Some lymphocytes, however, may live as long as 10 years. The remaining lymphocytes, about 15%, are short-lived, lasting 3 to 4 days.

Those lymphocytes present in the peripheral blood are generally in transit from one lymphoid tissue to another or to sites of inflammation. The lymphocytes have two basic patterns of circulation: (1) There is a recirculation of the mature, differentiated lymphocytes continually moving from one area of the lymphatic system to another. (2) Immature lymphocytes will travel from the bone marrow to the thymus and from there to the peripheral or secondary lymphoid organs. These cells then migrate via the lymphatic vessels to thymus-dependent areas in the peripheral lymphatic system and most probably become the long-lived T lymphocytes. They make up most of the recirculating pool of lymphocytes, although both the B and T lymphocytes are able to recirculate and will travel back and forth between the blood, bone marrow, and peripheral lymphoid tissue. They will enter the thymus, however, only from the bone marrow. It is thought that T lymphocytes have their own patterns of recirculation in that some T lymphocytes travel only to the lymph nodes, whereas other T lymphocytes only recirculate to the gut area. T cells do not appear to migrate back to the thymus. Antigenic stimulation will transform short-lived, noncirculating lymphocytes into long-lived, recirculating cells, and during an immune response, the rate of blood flow

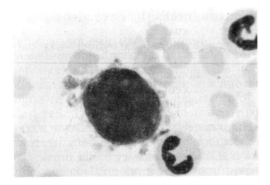

FIG. 2-69. Megakaryoblast. (Magnification ×1000).

Megakaryoblast (stage I) (Fig. 2-69).

Size: 20 to 50 μm in diameter.

Cytoplasm: Varying shades of blue.
Usually darker than the myeloblast.
May have small, blunt pseudopods.
Small to moderate amount. Usually a narrow band around the nucleus. As the cell matures, the amount of cytoplasm increases.
Usually nongranular.

Nucleus: Round, oval, or may be kidney shaped.
Fine chromatin pattern.
Multiple nucleoli that generally stain blue.
N/C ratio is about 10:1.

Promegakaryocyte (stage II).

Size: 20 to 60 μm in diameter.

Cytoplasm: More abundant than previous stage.
Less basophilic than in the blast.
Granules begin to form in the Golgi region.

Nucleus: Chromatin becomes more coarse.
Multiple nucleoli are visible.
Irregular in shape; may even show slight lobulation.
N/C ratio is 4:1 to 7:1 depending on the ploidy.

Granular megakaryocyte (stage III) (Fig. 2-70).

Size: 30 to 90 μm in diameter.

Cytoplasm: Abundant.
Pinkish blue in color.
Very fine and diffusely granular.
Usually has an irregular peripheral border.

Nucleus: Small in comparison to cell size.
Multiple nuclei may be visible or the nucleus may show multilobulation.
Chromatin is coarser than in the previous stage.
No nucleoli are visible.
N/C ratio is 2:1 to 1:1.

Mature megakaryocyte (stage IV).

Size: 40 to 120 μm in diameter.

Cytoplasm: Contains coarse clumps of granules aggregating into little bundles, which bud off from the periphery to become platelets.

Nucleus: Multiple nuclei are present, or the nucleus is multilobulated.
No nucleoli visible.
N/C ratio is less than 1:1.

Platelet (thrombocyte)

Size: 1 to 4 μm in diameter.

Cytoplasm: Light blue to purple.
Very granular.
Consists of two parts: (1) the *chromomere*, which is granular and located centrally, and (2) the *hyalomere*, which surrounds the chromomere and is nongranular and clear to light blue.

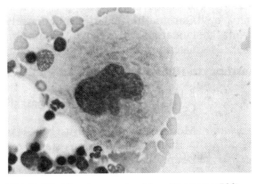

FIG. 2-70. Megakaryocyte. (Magnification ×500).

Nucleus: None present.

Maturation of the Megakaryocyte

The committed stem cell for the megakaryoblast (CFU-Meg) arises from the same uncommitted hematopoietic stem cell (CFU-C) as the erythroid and myeloid cell lines. *Megakaryocyte colony stimulating factor* (CSF-Meg) causes the committed stem cells to proliferate and differentiate into the megakaryoblast, whereas *thrombopoietin* stimulates differentiation and maturation of the megakaryocytes and also influences their size and thus the number of platelets produced.

The maturation of the megakaryoblast is unique. It is unable to undergo cell division, and, as it matures, the nucleus becomes lobulated and the cytoplasm increases in amount and becomes more granular. Nuclear and cytoplasmic maturation do not occur together or on parallel levels; nuclear maturation occurs first before cytoplasmic maturation begins. Initially, the nucleus contains a paired set of chromosomes (termed *diploid*). As the cell begins to mature, DNA synthesis takes place, and the nuclear material duplicates itself, resulting in a two-lobed nucleus in which each nuclear lobe contains a paired set of chromosomes (this process is termed *endomitosis*) whereby the DNA content of the cell doubles but cell division does not occur. The entire nucleus now contains two-paired sets of chromosomes and may be termed 4 N, in which 4 represents the *ploidy value* of 4 single sets of chromosomes and N stands for nuclear number. The nuclear number generally undergoes further divisions, yielding 4 sets of paired chromosomes (4-lobed nucleus) and is termed 8 N. Further nuclear divisions give rise to 8 sets of paired chromosomes (8-lobed nucleus, or 16 N), then 16 sets of paired chromosomes (16-lobed nucleus, or 32 N), and so on. Another term used to describe the increased numbers of chromosomes over the diploid number is *polyploid*. The majority of mature megakaryocytes in the bone marrow are 8 and 16 N, with a few being 32 N. When the cell has acquired all of its nuclear lobes, the cytoplasm begins to mature, becoming larger in size and more granular. During the entire process of nuclear and cytoplasmic maturation, there is no division of the cytoplasm.

Physiology and Biology of the Megakaryocyte

The maturing megakaryocyte contains a Golgi region around the nucleus where specific granules are packed to be distributed throughout the cytoplasm, except at the peripheral borders of the cell, which remain free of granules until platelets begin to form. Polyribosomes and rough endoplasmic reticulum are present at the beginning of cytoplasmic maturation. It takes 4 to 5 days for the megakaryocyte to mature in the bone marrow.

Megakaryocytes, or megakaryocyte fragments, frequently escape from the bone marrow and appear in the peripheral blood. They may occasionally be seen on a routine peripheral blood smear, but will more often be found if buffy coat smears are prepared. Megakaryocyte fragments may be seen more frequently in the blood in chronic myelogenous leukemia, various forms of cancer, myelofibrosis, polycythemia vera, Hodgkin's disease, leukocytosis due to infection, and following surgery. The presence of *dwarf* or *micro megakaryocytes* indicate an abnormal production and are found in myeloproliferative disorders and myelodysplastic syndromes. These cells have a single lobed nucleus and are about the size of a lymphocyte. The nuclear chromatin may be densely clumped or fine and loose, but generally has a smudged appearance. The cytoplasm is pale blue and foamy, which may be granular or agranular.

Platelet Production

Platelets are produced directly from the megakaryocyte cytoplasm. As the megakaryocyte matures, the granules in the cytoplasm cluster into small groups, and a network of tubules develops (by the invagination of the megakaryocyte cell membrane), many of which open to the outside of the cell. This membrane system is called the *demarcation membrane system* (*DMS*). These tubules fuse to form fissures, which ultimately form the margins and plasma membranes of individual platelets. The megakaryocytes in the bone marrow lie adjacent to the sinus walls. The cytoplasm fragments into individual platelets which are released into the peripheral blood over a period of several hours. The entire megakaryocyte cytoplasm is thus broken away, and the nucleus is left to degenerate and be processed by the monocyte-macrophage system. Each megakaryocyte generally produces between 2,000 to 4,000 platelets in this manner. Thus, the platelet is a portion of the megakaryocyte cytoplasm and, as such, contains no nucleus. As a general rule, the more nuclear lobes the megakaryocyte possesses, the larger the cytoplasmic mass, and, therefore, the more platelets produced. Conversely, megakaryocytes with lower ploidy values produce larger platelets that are denser and more functionally active. Increased production of platelets may be accomplished by means of three possible mechanisms: the number of megakaryocytes in the bone marrow may increase, the size of the megakaryocytes may increase, and there may be a decrease in the maturation time of the megakaryocyte. Major platelet production takes place in the bone marrow, where the megakaryocytes make up less than 1% of the nucleated cells of the marrow.

Platelet Life Span

Once the platelet is released into the peripheral blood, it has a life span of 9 to 12 days. The young platelets are larger and less dense than older platelets, and are associated with accelerated platelet production in the bone marrow. Also, they are metabolically more active and more effective in hemostasis. At any one time, approximately two thirds of the platelets are in the blood, whereas the remaining one third are in the spleen, which constitutes the splenic platelet pool. The platelets in the spleen are interchangeable with those in the blood. A high percentage of the platelets in the spleen are young platelets. Damaged and nonfunctioning platelets are generally removed from the blood, principally by the macrophages in the spleen. The platelet turnover rate is approximately 35,000 platelets ($\pm 4,300$) per μL each day.

Platelet Structure

The circulating platelet is circular to ellipsoidal in shape, 1 to 4 μm in diameter, and has a volume of approximately 6 to 7.5 fL

(Fig. 2–71). It may be divided anatomically into four areas: peripheral zone, sol-gel zone, organelle zone, and the membranous system.

The *peripheral zone* is basically composed of the membranes and is responsible for platelet adhesion (attachment of the platelet to blood vessel surfaces) and aggregation (attachment of the platelets to each other). The platelet membrane originates from the plasma membrane of the megakaryocyte. The peripheral zone may be divided into three areas. The external surface of the platelet has a fuzzy coating, termed the *glycocalyx* (1), and is primarily composed of glycoproteins including coagulation factors V, VIII, and fibrinogen. It is important in platelet reactions with thrombin, von Willebrand factor, and fibrinogen. The *plasma membrane* (2) lies directly beneath the glycocalyx and is composed of a bilayer of asymmetrically distributed phospholipids imbedded with integral proteins, of which arachidonic acid is a major component. Glycoprotein Ib functions as a receptor for the von Willebrand factor, and glycoproteins IIb and IIIa are receptors for fibrinogen as well as the von Willebrand factor. The third portion of this zone is a sub-membranous area where messages from the external membrane are translated into chemical signals causing activation and a physical change in the platelet. A number of platelet membrane receptor sites have been identified for ADP, collagen, serotonin, epinephrine, thrombin, von Willebrand factor, and factors V and Xa.

The *sol-gel zone* lies directly beneath the platelet membrane and is composed of *microfilaments* (3) and *microtubules* (4). They provide a cytoskeleton to maintain platelet shape, and a contractile system. Microfilaments contain the proteins actin and myosin which, upon stimulation of the platelet, will interact to form actomyosin *(thrombosthenin)*, a contractile protein, important in clot retraction. The microtubules are composed of the protein *tubulin*, which maintains the platelet's disc shape.

The *organelle zone* is composed of the mitochondria, alpha granules, dense bodies, and a lysosomal type granule. The *alpha granules* (5) are the most numerous and contain a number of substances including platelet factor 4, β thromboglobulin, platelet derived growth factor (PDGF), thrombospodin, von Willebrand factor, fibrinogen, fibronectin,

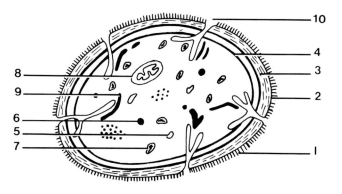

FIG. 2-71. Normal platelet structure.

and factor V. The *dense bodies* (6) contain ADP, ATP, calcium, serotonin, and pyrophosphate, and play an important role in platelet aggregation. The *mitochondria* (8) are important for ATP synthesis for platelet metabolism. The *lysosomal granules* (7) contain acid phosphatase and hydrolytic enzymes.

The *membranous system* is composed of the *dense tubular system* (9) and the *surface connecting system* (*open canicular system*) (10). The dense tubular system is derived from smooth endoplasmic reticulum and sequesters (holds) calcium for platelet activation processes. It also synthesizes prostaglandin. The surface connecting system, as an invagination of the plasma membrane, acts as a canal for the release of the granule constituents and cytoplasm to the exterior of the platelet. (This system is also involved in platelet phagocytosis.)

The platelet is composed of about 60% protein, 30% lipid, 8% carbohydrate, various minerals, water, and nucleotides. It contains over ninety different enzymes. Other proteins present include glycoproteins and coagulation factors. Fibrinogen, along with most of the other coagulation factors, has been demonstrated in association with the platelet. In addition, the platelet is able to synthesize amino acids, proteins, fatty acids, and phospholipids, and glycogen is the main carbohydrate present. The platelet has an active energy metabolism, using glucose as its main energy source.

Platelet Function

Platelets function in primary hemostasis (the stoppage of bleeding) and in maintaining capillary integrity. (This is discussed in greater detail in Chapter 5.)

White Blood Cell and Platelet Morphology

Toxic granulation (Plate IVa) consists of dark blue-black cytoplasmic granules in the neutrophil. They are thought to be primary granules, show increased alkaline phosphatase activity, and are found in acute infections, drug poisoning, and burns.

Döhle bodies (Plate IVb) appear as single or multiple light blue or grayish staining areas in the cytoplasm of the neutrophil. They are rough endoplasmic reticulum containing RNA and may represent localized failure of the cytoplasm to mature. They are found in infections, poisoning, burns, and following chemotherapy.

Hypersegmented neutrophils (Plate IVc) are neutrophils with a six- or more, lobed nucleus. This represents an abnormality in the maturation of the neutrophil and may be acquired (as in megaloblastic erythropoiesis) or inherited (*Undritz anomaly*). Normally, approximately 50 to 60% of the neutrophils contain three lobes, no more than 20% have four lobes, and there may be an occasional five-lobed neutrophil. Any time there is an increased percentage of four- and/or five-lobed neutrophils present, hypersegmentation should be reported. In cases of pernicious anemia and folic acid deficiency, neutrophils with more than five lobes are commonly found. Hypersegmented neutrophils are also found in chronic infections. The **Barr** (sex chromatin) **body** (Plate IVd) represents the second X chromosome in females and may be seen in 2 to 3% of the neutrophils in females. It is a small, well-defined, round projection of nuclear chromatin that is connected to the nucleus of the neutrophil by a single, fine strand of chromatin. The Barr body can be differentiated from small, non-specific nodules of chromatin in that these latter projections are not attached to the nucleus with as fine a strand of chromatin. The number of Barr bodies in a cell is one less than the number of X chromosomes present in a cell. Another term used to describe the Barr body is a *drumstick.* These chromatin bodies are not found in normal males.

Degenerated neutrophil with pyknotic nucleus (Plate IVe) results from the condensing of nuclear chromatin into a solid, structureless mass with no pattern. These cells are not counted in a differential cell count.

A **vacuolated neutrophil** (Plate IIIr) results when the degenerating cytoplasm begins to acquire holes or as the result of active phagocytosis (may reflect increased lysosomal activity). This condition may be found in septicemia and severe infection.

Giant neutrophils may be seen occasionally in a normal peripheral blood smear. These cells are much larger than normal neutrophils and are generally hyperlobulated. They may be found normally in a frequency of about 1 in every 20,000 neutrophils but may increase somewhat in frequency in disease states.

Pelger-Huët anomaly (Plate V e, f, g) indicates a failure of the neutrophil nucleus to segment properly. All of the neutrophils have no more than a bi-lobed nucleus. The nuclear chromatin is coarsely clumped. This benign anomaly may be inherited or acquired, as in certain leukemias. A person heterozygous for this characteristic shows numerous bi-lobed (dumbbell-shaped) nuclei, whereas the homozygous person has round neutrophil nuclei. The neutrophils in this anomaly appear to function normally.

Chédiak-Higashi syndrome (Plate V a, b) is a rare, fatal disorder found in children. It is inherited as an autosomal recessive characteristic. The granulocytes usually contain several very large, reddish-purple or greenish-gray staining granules in the cytoplasm. In the monocytes and lymphocytes they stain bluish purple and may be present singly, or there may be several in one cell. These granules represent abnormal lysosomes. Anemia,

neutropenia, and thrombocytopenia generally develop, and patients will show increased susceptibility to infection.

Alder-Reilly anomaly (Plate IVf) shows heavy, coarse blue-black granulation of the neutrophils, eosinophils, basophils, and sometimes, the lymphocytes and monocytes. This is an inherited condition and is commonly associated with Hurler's syndrome and Hunter's syndrome.

May-Hegglin anomaly is an inherited anomaly affecting the neutrophils and platelets. Larger than usual Döhle-like inclusion bodies are present in the neutrophils. Giant, bizarre platelets are present, and the platelets may be decreased in number. Some patients are asymptomatic, whereas others may exhibit bleeding tendencies. Platelet function may be abnormal.

Auer rods (Plate Vh) are rod-like bodies representing aggregated primary granules that stain a reddish purple. They are found in the cytoplasm of myeloblasts, monoblasts, and promyelocytes in acute monocytic or acute myelogenous leukemia and erythroleukemia.

Smudge or **basket cell** (Plate IV j, k) is the disintegrating nucleus of a ruptured white blood cell.

Atypical platelets (Plate III o, p), abnormal in appearance, occur in some diseased states. In such cases, the platelet may have one or more of the following characteristics:

1. Large size (4 to 7 μm), seen in conditions associated with thrombocytopenia and thrombocytosis. Giant platelets are 7 to 8 μm or larger and are seen in myeloproliferative disorders.
2. Increased amount of hyalomere.
3. Granules decreased or absent (platelet appears gray in color). They stain very pale blue and are difficult to see on Wright-stained smears.
4. Zoned appearance.
5. Bizarre or irregular shapes.

Platelet satellitosis (platelets encircling the peripheral borders of neutrophils) is seen in a rare patient whose blood is anticoagulated with EDTA. This phenomenon is thought to be due to a serum factor which reacts in the presence of EDTA.

ROUTINE HEMATOLOGY PROCEDURES

3

COMPLETE BLOOD COUNT

The complete blood count (CBC) consists of the white blood cell count, red blood cell count, hemoglobin, hematocrit, and white blood cell differential. Also included are the red blood cell indices, which indicate the relative and absolute hemoglobin content and size of the average red blood cell. When performing the differential, the white blood cells are identified and categorized, all cells are examined for abnormalities, and the platelets are reviewed for number and morphologic features. The importance of the CBC cannot be underestimated. It is a screening procedure that is helpful in the diagnosis of many diseases, it is one indicator of the body's ability to fight disease, it is used to monitor the effects of drug and radiation therapy, and it may be employed as an indicator of the patient's progress in certain diseased states such as infection or anemia.

HEMOGLOBIN

The measurement of hemoglobin is one of several tests used to diagnose and follow the treatment of anemia. The normal range for the hemoglobin will vary with the age and sex of the individual. At birth, the hemoglobin concentration is normally in the range of 15 to 20 g/dL. This value decreases to about 9 to 14 g/dL at 2 months. By 10 years of age, the normal hemoglobin is between 12 and 15 g/dL. Normal adult values range from 12 to 16 g/dL for women and from 13 to 18 g/dL for men. There is a slight decrease in the hemoglobin level after 50 years of age. It

should be noted that there may be some fluctuations in the hemoglobin during a 24-hour period, with the hemoglobin being higher in the morning and lower in the evening. The hemoglobin may also show slightly lower values when the patient is lying down, whereas strenuous muscular activity will tend to increase it. Smokers will have a tendency toward slightly higher hemoglobin levels. Altitude has the effect of raising the hemoglobin. The higher the altitude the greater will be the hemoglobin increase.

Cyanmethemoglobin Method

Reagents and Equipment

1. Cyanmethemoglobin (hemiglobincyanide) (HiCN) reagent contains potassium cyanide (50 mg), potassium ferricyanide (200 mg), dihydrogen potassium phosphate (KH_2PO_4) (140 mg), and a nonionic detergent (1 mL) in 1 L of distilled water (may be obtained commercially). This reagent should be pale yellow in color and must have an O.D. reading of 0.0 when measured in a spectrophotometer at a wavelength of 540 nm against a water blank. Store reagent in a brown bottle at room temperature where it is stable for several months. Discard if reagent becomes cloudy.
2. Test tubes, 13 × 100 mm.
3. Pipets, 0.02 mL.
4. Controls, normal, and abnormal.
5. Spectrophotometer (540 nm).

Specimen

Whole blood, using EDTA as the anticoagulant. Capillary blood may also be used.

Principle

Whole blood is added to cyanmethemoglobin (HiCN) reagent. The potassium ferricyanide in the reagent converts the hemoglobin iron from the ferrous state (Fe^{++}) to the ferric state (Fe^{+++}) to form methemoglobin (Hi) which then combines with potassium cyanide to form the stable pigment, cyanmethemoglobin (HiCN). (Hi = hemiglobin = hemoglobin in which the iron has been oxidized to the ferric state. HiCN = hemiglobin cyanide = Hi which has been banded to the cyanide ions.) The nonionic detergent present in the reagent improves the lysis of the red blood cells and decreases the amount of turbidity resulting from abnormal proteins, such as lipoprotein. The color intensity of this mixture is measured in a spectrophotometer at a wavelength of 540 nm. The optical density of the solution is proportional to the concentration of hemoglobin. All forms of hemoglobin are measured with this method except sulfhemoglobin.

Procedure

1. For each patient and control to be tested, place exactly 5.0 mL of HiCN reagent into an appropriately labeled test tube. Place 5.0 mL of the reagent into a test tube to be used as the blank.
2. Add 0.02 mL of well-mixed whole blood or control blood to the appropriately labeled tube. Rinse the pipet 3 to 5 times with the HiCN reagent until all blood is removed from the pipet.
3. Mix the preceding solutions well and allow to stand at room temperature for at least 3 minutes (see #1 under Discussion) to allow adequate time for the formation of HiCN.
4. Transfer the mixture to a cuvette and read in a spectrophotometer at a wavelength of 540 nm using the HiCN reagent in the blank tube to set the optical density (O.D.) at 0.0. Record the readings for the patient and control samples from the O.D. scale and refer to the prepared chart for the actual value of the hemoglobin in g/dL.

Discussion

1. The dihydrogen potassium phosphate used in the reagent in place of sodium bicarbonate (in the original Drabkin's [HiCN] reagent) allows the test to be read at the end of 3 minutes instead of waiting for the original 15 minute reaction time that was necessary with the sodium bicarbonate.
2. Before the unknown sample is read, the solution must be crystal clear. If any turbidity is present, a falsely elevated result will be obtained. Clouding may be due to:
   a. An exceptionally high white blood cell count. (In such cases, centrifuge the mixture and use the supernatant as the test sample.)
   b. Hemoglobin S and hemoglobin C. (Dilute the mixture 1:1 with distilled water, read on the spectrophotometer, and multiply the result by 2.)
   c. Lipemic blood. (Add 0.01 mL of the patient's plasma to 5.0 mL of HiCN reagent and use this mixture as the patient blank.)
3. Over-anticoagulation of the blood does not affect the hemoglobin results.

Preparation of a Standard Hemoglobin Curve

Using the HiCN calibrator (must be approved by the International Committee for Standardization in Hematology), set up at least four dilutions according to the directions received with the reagent, or as shown in Table 3–1. Plot the hemoglobin in g/dL (on graph paper) on the abscissa (horizontal axis) against O.D. on the ordinate (vertical axis)— this is a straightline curve. (If percentage of transmittance is read, use semilogrithmic graph paper and plot as described for O.D. This will also be a straight line curve.) A chart may then be made to facilitate the reading of the test results.

Abnormal Hemoglobin Pigments

If hemoglobin is converted to an abnormal hemoglobin pigment, it is no longer capable of oxygen transport and, if this impairment is severe enough, a condition of hypoxia or cyanosis occurs. The three abnormal hemoglobin pigments of most significance are discussed briefly below.

1. **Carboxyhemoglobin** is formed by the

TABLE 3–1. DILUTIONS FOR A HEMOGLOBIN CURVE

Tube	HiCN Reagent	Stock Standard	Concentration of Hemoglobin
1	0.0 mL	5.0 mL	100% of assay value of hgb standard
2	1.0 mL	4.0 mL	80% of assay value of hgb standard
3	2.0 mL	3.0 mL	60% of assay value of hgb standard
4	3.0 mL	2.0 mL	40% of assay value of hgb standard

combination of hemoglobin with carbon monoxide, which is not capable of binding with or transporting oxygen. The hemoglobin molecule's affinity for carbon monoxide is more than 200 times greater than for oxygen, and therefore it readily combines with carbon monoxide even when it is present in low concentrations. The formation of carboxyhemoglobin is reversible. It is found in the blood of tobacco smokers in concentrations of 1 to 10%. Symptoms of headache, nausea, dizziness, and muscular weakness will occur at levels of 20 to 30%.

2. **Methemoglobin** is a type of hemoglobin in which the ferrous ion has been oxidized to the ferric state and is, therefore, incapable of combining with or transporting the oxygen molecule which is replaced by a hydroxyl radical. Methemoglobinemia may be acquired or inherited. Most cases are acquired and are primarily due to exposure to certain drugs and chemicals such as nitrates, nitrites, quinones, and chlorates. Inherited methemoglobinemia may be a result of a structural abnormality of the globin chains, or it may occur as a result of a red blood cell enzyme defect in which the methemoglobin formed cannot be converted back to the reduced form of hemoglobin. Methemoglobin formation is reversible and is normally present in the blood in concentrations of 1 to 2%.

3. **Sulfhemoglobin** is not normally found in the blood. When it is present, its formation is irreversible, and it remains for the life of the carrier red blood cell. Its exact nature is unknown, but it is thought to be formed by the action of certain drugs and chemicals such as sulfonamides and aromatic amines. It is incapable of transporting oxygen but can combine with carbon monoxide to form carboxysulfhemoglobin. The normal concentration in blood is less than 1%.

HEMATOCRIT

When anticoagulated whole blood is centrifuged the red blood cells, white blood cells, and platelets will sediment out, with the heaviest particles (red blood cells) falling to the bottom of the tube. (See Fig. 3–1.) The white blood cells are heavier than the platelets and will therefore settle on top of the red cells. The platelets, being the lightest formed elements in the blood, will form a layer on top of the white blood cells. The fluid portion of the blood (plasma) is the top portion of the centrifuged specimen. The volume of the red blood cells represents the **packed red cell volume (PCV)** and is expressed as a percentage of the total whole blood volume. The white blood cell and platelet portions of the centrifuged specimen are termed the **buffy coat.** The subcommittee of the National Committee for Clinical Laboratory Standards has recommended that the term packed cell volume (PCV) be used to describe the red

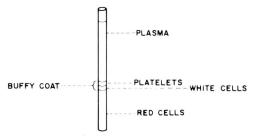

FIG. 3–1. Cell layers in centrifuged whole blood.

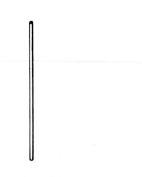

FIG. 3–2. Capillary hematocrit tube.

blood cell measurement and the term **hematocrit** be used to describe the method (materials) used. (The test name, hematocrit, however, is still widely used, and will be used in this text.)

The normal values for the hematocrit, like the hemoglobin, will vary with the age and sex of the individual. At birth, the normal range for the hematocrit is 45 to 60%. This range decreases to 27 to 44% by 1 year of age and then gradually increases to the adult levels of 36 to 48% for women and 40 to 55% for men. There is a slight decrease in the hematocrit level after 50 years of age. The hematocrit is decreased in anemia and increased in the various forms of polycythemia. The hematocrit reading closely parallels the hemoglobin values in an individual, so that those fluctuations seen in the hemoglobin will also be reflected in the hematocrit.

Microhematocrit Method

Reagents and Equipment

1. Microhematocrit tube, approximately 75 mm long with an inner bore of approximately 1.2 mm (Fig. 3–2). Two types of microhematocrit tubes may be purchased: (1) those which contain heparin (color coded with a red band) as the anticoagulant, for use with non-anticoagulated whole blood, and (2) plain tubes (color coded with a blue band) for use with anticoagulated whole blood. The microhematocrit tubes hold approximately 0.05 mL of whole blood.
2. Clay-like sealing compound.
3. Microhematocrit centrifuge capable of

producing an RCF of 10,000 to 15,000 g. The centrifuge should be able to reach maximum speed within 30 seconds.
4. Microhematocrit tube reader.

Specimen

Whole blood using dipotassium ethylene-diaminetetraacetic acid (EDTA) as the anticoagulant. (The liquid tripotassium salt of EDTA is thought to cause a 2 to 3% decrease in the hematocrit due to slight shrinkage of the red blood cells.)

Principle

Whole blood is centrifuged for maximum red blood cell packing. The space occupied by the red blood cells is measured and expressed as a percentage of the whole blood volume.

Procedure

1. Allow the capillary or well-mixed anticoagulated whole blood to enter two microhematocrit tubes until they are approximately two-third's filled with blood. (Air bubbles denote poor technique but do not affect the results of the test.)
2. Seal one end of the microhematocrit tube with the clay material by placing the dry end of the tube into the clay in a vertical position (the microhematocrit tube forms a 90° angle with the tray of clay). The plug should be 4 to 6 mm long. Make certain blood is not forced out the top of the microhematocrit tube during this process.
3. Place the two microhematocrit tubes in the radial grooves of the centrifuge head exactly opposite each other, with the sealed end away from the center of the centrifuge.
4. Centrifuge for 5 minutes.
5. Remove the hematocrit tubes as soon as the centrifuge has stopped spinning. Determine the results for both microhematocrits, using the microhematocrit tube reading device. Duplicate results should agree within 1 unit (%). If they do not, repeat the procedure. (When reading the hematocrit, it is important that the buffy coat not be included in the result. It is also important that reading errors due to parallax not occur. [Parallax is defined as an

object being seen in a different position by changing the position of the head, or as seen by one eye versus the other eye.]) The hematocrit may be expressed in either of two ways: (1) as a percentage, e.g., 42%, or, (2) as a decimal fraction, e.g., 0.42.

Discussion

1. Incomplete sealing of the microhematocrit tubes generally give falsely low results because, as the tubes spin, there is a greater loss of red blood cells than of plasma. To detect this problem, place a piece of white tape on the inner side surface of the centrifuge top. If the hematocrit tube leaks during centrifugation there will be a line of blood on the tape.
2. Inadequate centrifugation of the microhematocrit tubes or allowing the tubes to stand longer than several minutes after centrifugation, yields falsely elevated values.
3. The time and speed of centrifugation are extremely important to obtain maximum red blood cell packing. To determine the maximum packing time of the microhematocrit centrifuge, perform the microhematocrit procedure on two different blood samples, centrifuging them for 2 minutes. Read and record results. Prepare two more microhematocrits from the same blood samples and centrifuge for 2½ minutes. Read and record results. Repeat this procedure, increasing the centrifugation time by ½ minute until the hematocrit reading remains the same for two consecutive time periods. One of the two samples should have a hematocrit of >50%. Two sets of consistent readings should be obtained at 3 to 5 minutes of centrifugation. The longest of these centrifugation times should be used for routine testing. When maximum red blood cell packing has been achieved, the red cell layer will generally appear translucent.
4. If blood is overanticoagulated, the hematocrit reading will be falsely low due to shrinkage of the red blood cells.
5. When the microhematocrit is spun for the correct time period and at the proper speed, a small amount of plasma still remains in the red blood cell portion. This is termed *trapped plasma* and is usually expressed as a percentage of the red blood cell column. When comparing spun microhematocrit results with hematocrit results obtained on an electronic cell counter, the spun hematocrit results may vary from 1 to 3% higher because of this trapped plasma (unless the cell counter has been calibrated against spun microhematocrits uncorrected for trapped plasma). An increased amount of trapped plasma is found in macrocytic anemias, spherocytosis, thalassemia, hypochromic anemias, and sickle cell anemia (the amount of trapped plasma increases as the % of affected sickle shaped red blood cells increases).
6. For accurate results, anticoagulated blood samples should be centrifuged within 6 hours of collection when the blood is stored at room temperature.
7. It is recommended that heat sealing of the microhematocrit tubes not be used since it is difficult to obtain a flat sealing of the tube and the heat may cause damage to the red blood cells.
8. A **macrohematocrit** method for determining the packed red blood cell volume has been used in the past, but this method is rarely used today since it is more time consuming, requires larger amounts of blood, and generally contains a higher percentage of trapped plasma. In this method, a Wintrobe tube, calibrated from 0 to 100, is filled with anticoagulated whole blood and centrifuged at 2000 to 2300 g for 30 minutes. The ratio of the volume of the red blood cells to the total volume of blood is then determined and reported as the hematocrit reading.

BLOOD CELL COUNTS

Units of Reporting

The International Committee for Standardization in Hematology has recommended the liter (L) as the unit of volume. Cell counts are, therefore, expressed as the number of cells or formed elements (e.g., platelets, white blood cells, red blood cells) per liter of blood. The previous, traditional unit of reporting was cubic millimeters (cu mm, or, mm^3).

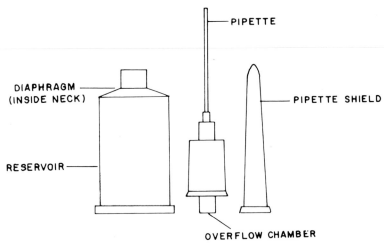

FIG. 3-3. Unopette.

Since the difference between 1 cu mm and 1 microliter (μL) (1 cu mm = 1.00003 μL) is felt to be insignificant, 1 μL is considered equivalent to 1 cu mm. Therefore:

1 cu mm = 1 μL = 10^{-6} liters

1×10^6 μL = 1 liter

A white blood count of 6,500 $\times$ 10^6/liter =

6.5 $\times$ 10^9/L

6.5 $\times$ 10^3/μL (or, 6,500/μL)

6.5 $\times$ 10^3/cu mm (or, 6,500/cu mm)

THE UNOPETTE SYSTEM

With a spotlight on technologist safety, the Unopette system has become a valuable method for standardizing the pipetting and diluting of blood or other body fluids for increased safety, accuracy, and precision. The Unopette is manufactured by Becton Dickinson Vacutainer Systems, Rutherford, N.J., and is available from most laboratory distributors.

The standard Unopette (Fig. 3-3) is made up of the following parts:

1. The *reservoir* contains a premeasured volume of diluting fluid and is sealed by a thin covering of plastic *(diaphragm)* located in the neck.
2. The *pipet* is self-filling and is available in various sizes (3 μL, 3.3 μL, 10 μL, 20 μL, 25 μL, 44.7 μL), depending on the procedure to be performed. Each pipet is color coded according to size. The end opposite the pipet tip is termed the *overflow chamber.*
3. The *pipet shield* protects the pipet and is also utilized to puncture the reservoir diaphragm just prior to use.

Procedure

1. Immediately before use, remove the pipet shield from the pipet. Using the pointed end of the shield, pierce the reservoir diaphragm firmly, inserting the shield as far as possible to obtain an opening large enough for the pipet tip.
2. Holding the pipet almost horizontally (about a 15° angle above the horizontal), touch the tip of the pipet to the blood sample. The pipet will automatically fill by capillary action. When the sample reaches the neck of the pipet, no more blood will enter. (If the pipet is tilted excessively, it may overfill.) Carefully wipe excess blood from the outside of the pipet without removing any blood from inside the tip. Place index finger firmly over the top of the pipet's overflow chamber.
3. Squeeze the reservoir slightly (do not lose any liquid) with other hand. With the pipet in a vertical position (finger covering the overflow chamber), carefully place the pipet into the reservoir and seat it firmly in the neck of the reservoir.
4. Remove index finger from the overflow

chamber and release the pressure on the reservoir. The sample will be drawn from the pipet into the diluting fluid. Squeeze and release the reservoir several times in order to rinse all blood from the pipet. (This must be done carefully to prevent the diluted sample from escaping through the top of the overflow chamber.)

5. Place index finger over the overflow chamber and invert the reservoir 10 to 15 times in order to completely mix the dilution.
6. Immediately prior to performing the test, carefully mix the dilution by inverting the reservoir 10 to 20 times. While mixing, rinse the pipet several times (carefully squeeze the reservoir) in case any sample entered the pipet while standing.
7. Any one of several methods may be used to remove the diluted sample from the reservoir. This will depend on the test being performed.
   a. For cell counting, as soon as the sample is well mixed, squeeze the reservoir, forcing the diluted sample up into (but not out of) the overflow chamber. Place index finger on the top of the overflow chamber and remove the pipet from the reservoir. The sample will drain from the pipet upon partial removal of the index finger from the top of the overflow chamber.
   b. The reservoir may be converted into a dropper assembly by removing the pipet and replacing it in the reservoir in a reverse position, with the overflow chamber seated firmly in the neck of the reservoir. The diluted sample may then be completely expelled from the reservoir by squeezing. This method may also be used to fill a hemocytometer, in which case the first three or four drops would be expelled from the reservoir and the counting chamber filled by gentle squeezing of the reservoir.
   c. If the entire diluted sample is to be removed from the reservoir, the pipet may be removed and the reservoir inverted and squeezed to expel the entire contents through the neck of the reservoir.
8. To store a diluted sample, the pipet shield may be installed on the top of the overflow

chamber (of the pipet), or the pipet may be removed from the reservoir, and the tip of the pipet shield inserted firmly into the reservoir opening.

Discussion

1. Specific Unopettes are available for a number of procedures, among which are red blood cell count, white blood cell count, platelet count, hemoglobin, reticulocyte count, eosinophil count, and the red blood cell fragility test. Unopettes are also available for dilution of blood for testing on the major hematology cell counters; there are also collection systems for a few chemistry procedures.

WHITE BLOOD CELL COUNT

The white blood cell count (WBC) denotes the number of white blood cells in 1 liter (L) of whole blood. In a normal, healthy individual, the WBC falls in the range of 4000 to 11,000 $\times 10^6$/L (or 4.0 to 11.0 $\times 10^9$/L). This count varies with age. The WBC of a newborn baby is 10.0 to 30.0 $\times 10^9$/L at birth. It decreases to a range of 6.0 to 17.0 $\times 10^9$/L at 1 year of age and drops to normal levels by age 21.

The WBC is a useful measurement to the physician. It is utilized to indicate infection and may also be employed to follow the progress of certain diseases and therapies. The WBC may be elevated in bacterial infections, appendicitis, leukemia, pregnancy, hemolytic disease of the newborn, uremia, and ulcers. The WBC may drop below normal values in viral diseases (such as measles), brucellosis, typhoid fever, infectious hepatitis, rheumatoid arthritis, cirrhosis of the liver, and lupus erythematosus. Radiation and certain drug therapy tends to lower the WBC. Patients will have white counts performed while receiving this treatment to ensure that the WBC does not become too low. A white count above 11.0 $\times 10^9$/L is termed **leukocytosis;** a white count below normal is known as **leukopenia.** The white count in children usually shows a greater variation in disease. For example, during infection, a child's WBC reaches much higher elevations than does an adult's white count in response to a corresponding infection. An individual's

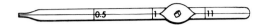

FIG. 3–4. Thoma white count pipet.

normal WBC is subject to variations, being slightly higher in the afternoon than in the morning. There is also an increase in the WBC following strenuous exercise, emotional stress, and anxiety.

In most laboratories an electronic method of counting white cells is used. This is discussed in chapter 7, Automation. The procedure for performing manual white blood cell counts is outlined in detail in this section because the manual WBC is still performed under various circumstances. The techniques outlined here are the same as those employed for the manual red blood cell count, platelet count, and direct eosinophil count. This detailed method is presented only once. Familiarize yourself with this procedure before progressing to the other manual counts outlined later in this chapter.

Manual White Blood Cell Count

Reagents and Equipment

1. Pipets, one of the following:
   a. WBC Unopette (1:20 dilution) is recommended because of ease of use and technologist safety.
   b. 20 μL pipet (also 10 × 75 mm test tubes with caps, and plain microhematocrit tube if this pipet is used).
   c. Thoma white count pipet (Fig. 3–4).
2. White count diluting fluid. Any one of the following diluting fluids may be used:
   a. Acetic acid, 2% v/v, in distilled water.
   b. Hydrochloric acid, 1% v/v, in distilled water.
   c. Turk's diluting fluid.
Glacial acetic acid	3 mL
Aqueous gentian violet, 1% w/v	1 mL
Distilled water	100 mL

   Note: If the WBC Unopette is used, diluting fluid is unnecessary since it is contained in the Unopette.
3. Microscope.
4. Clean gauze or Kimwipes.
5. Improved Neubauer hemocytometer (counting chamber) (Fig. 3–5) with coverglass.
   a. The hemocytometer with Neubauer ruling consists of two identically ruled platforms with a raised ridge on both sides of the two platforms on which a cover glass is placed. The space between the top of the platform and the cover glass over it is 0.1 mm (Fig. 3–6).
   b. Each of the two platforms contains a ruled area composed of nine large squares of equal size (Fig. 3–7). Each large square is 1 mm wide and 1 mm long. Therefore, the entire ruled area is 9 square mm (mm²) (3 mm wide and 3 mm long).
   c. The volume of the entire ruled area on one platform is 0.9 μL (width × length × depth, or, 3 mm × 3 mm × 0.1 mm). The volume of one large square is 0.1 μL.
   d. The four large corner squares, each of which is subdivided into 16 smaller squares, are labelled "W" and are the four squares used for counting white blood cells.

All hemocytometers used in the clinical laboratory must meet the specifications of the National Bureau of Standards (NBS) and are identified by those initials.

Specimen

Ethylene diamine tetra Acetic Acid

Whole blood, using EDTA as the anticoagulant. Capillary blood may also be used.

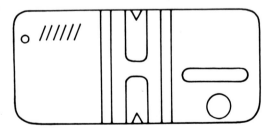

FIG. 3–5. Improved Neubauer hemocytometer.

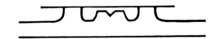

FIG. 3–6. Improved Neubauer hemocytometer (side view).

FIG. 3–7. Improved Neubauer hemocytometer, counting area.

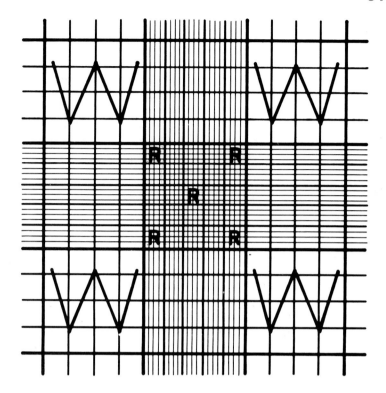

Principle

Whole blood is mixed with a weak acid solution to dilute the blood and hemolyze the red blood cells.

Procedure

1. Dilution of blood. Mix the specimen of whole blood for approximately 1 minute. Proceed with testing according to the blood dilution method used. Prepare duplicate dilutions on each specimen to be tested.
   a. WBC Unopette. Follow the procedure outlined in the Unopette section.
   b. 20 μL pipet (1:20 dilution).
      1) Place exactly 0.4 mL of diluting fluid into a 10 × 75 mm test tube. Remove exactly 0.02 mL (20 μL) of diluting fluid from the tube so that 0.38 mL remains.
      2) Add 0.02 mL of well-mixed whole blood to the tube. Cap tube and mix.
      3) A 1:21 dilution of blood may be used by adding 0.02 mL whole blood to 0.4 mL diluting fluid. (Final calculations of the WBC will need to be changed accordingly.)
   c. Thoma white count pipet.
      1) Draw the blood up to the 0.5 mark in the Thoma pipet. It is permissible for the blood to go slightly beyond the 0.5 mark. (If the blood is drawn up too far beyond this mark, however, the dilution is inaccurate because a small amount of blood continues to adhere to the inside of the stem when the excess blood is withdrawn from the pipet.)
      2) Remove the blood from the outside of the pipet with a clean gauze or Kimwipe. Be careful that the material does not withdraw any blood from the stem of the pipet. Place a nonabsorbent material to the end of the pipet, bringing the blood down to exactly the 0.5 mark. (If an absorbent material is used to remove the excess blood from the stem, the material tends to absorb the liquid portion of the blood and,

therefore the blood will have a higher concentration of cells.)

3) Holding the pipet almost vertical, place the tip into the fluid. Draw the diluting fluid into the pipet slowly, until the mixture reaches the 11 mark, while gently rotating the pipet to ensure a proper amount of mixing. (If the level of blood falls below the 0.5 mark at any time during this step, repeat the entire procedure, beginning with a clean pipet. Use fresh diluting fluid if any blood has entered the bottle. If the pipet has not been held in a vertical position while diluting the blood, air bubbles may form in the bulb. If this occurs, the dilution is inaccurate, and the procedure must be repeated, using a clean pipet. It is permissible for the level of the mixture to go slightly above or below the 11 mark.)

4) Place the pipet in a horizontal position and firmly hold the index finger of either hand over the opening in the tip of the pipet. Detach the aspirator from the other end of the pipet.

5) The dilution of blood is now complete. The white cell pipet is divided into units or volumes: 0.5, 1.0, and 11 (refer to the diagram of the white cell pipet, if necessary). The stem contains 1.0 unit and the bulb holds 10 units. The blood is drawn up into the pipet first. As the diluting fluid is aspirated, all of the blood is drawn up into the bulb. Therefore, if the blood is drawn up to the 0.5 mark and diluted to the 11 mark, there is 0.5 volume of blood and 9.5 volumes of diluting fluid in the bulb of the pipet, for a total of 10 volumes. The stem contains the last 1.0 volume of diluting fluid and contains no blood. The dilution of blood is, therefore, 0.5 in 10, or, 1:20.

2. Clean the counting chamber and cover glass with a lint free cloth. The use of 95% (v/v) ethanol also facilitates the cleaning

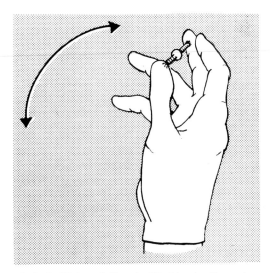

FIG. 3–8. Mixing of diluted white blood cell count.

process. Carefully place the cover glass on top of the ruled area of the counting chamber.

3. Mix the diluted white blood cell counts.
    a. If the WBC Unopette is used, follow the instructions outlined in that section for mixing the Unopette dilution.
    b. If 0.02 mL of blood was diluted in a test tube, cap the tube and mix well for 2 minutes.
    c. Mix the Thoma pipet for approximately 3 minutes to ensure hemolysis of the red blood cells and adequate mixing. This may be done with a mechanical shaker, or mix by hand: place the thumb over the tip of the pipet and the middle finger over the other end of the pipet. Mix the pipet in the direction shown in Figure 3–8.

4. Fill the counting chamber.
    a. If the WBC Unopette is used, refer to the corresponding section of the Unopette procedure and proceed as outlined below.
        1) Place the tip of the pipet on the edge of the ruled area of the counting chamber. Allow the mixture to seep under the coverglass gradually and exactly fill this area. (If the pipet is removed just before the area looks filled, the platform will fill without becoming flooded.) Care should be taken not to move

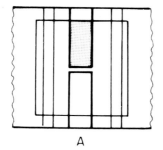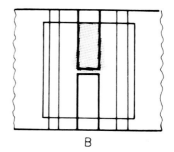

FIG. 3–9. Properly (A) and improperly (B) filled counting chamber.

the cover glass. (All steps should be done quickly so that the white blood cells in the mixture do not begin to settle out. Figure 3–9 illustrates proper and improper filling of the counting chamber. If it is filled improperly, reclean the counting chamber and cover glass. If there is enough diluted blood remaining repeat the above procedure and refill the counting chamber. Otherwise, repeat the entire procedure, preparing new dilutions.)

2) Fill the opposite side of the counting chamber with the second white count dilution.

3) When the counting chamber is filled, care should be taken that it is not jarred or the cover glass moved. The filled counting chamber should be allowed to stand for approximately 1 minute prior to performing the count to give the white blood cells time to settle.

b. If the 0.02 mL pipet was used and the diluted blood is in a test tube:

1) Half-fill a plain microhematocrit tube with the well-mixed dilution.

2) Hold the microhematocrit in a vertical position with the index finger covering the top of the microhematocrit tube.

3) Remove any excess liquid from the outside of the hematocrit tube with a piece of gauze.

4) Use the index finger to control the rate of flow. Follow the procedure as described above, steps 4 a 1, 2, 3.

c. Using the Thoma WBC pipet:

1) Hold the pipet in a vertical position with the right index finger covering the top of the pipet. Discard the first four drops of the mixture onto a piece of gauze. Remove any excess liquid from the outside of the pipet with a piece of gauze. Using the index finger to control the rate of flow, follow the procedure as described above, steps 4 a 1, 2, 3.)

5. Count the white blood cells.

a. Carefully, keeping the counting chamber horizontal at all times, place the hemocytometer on the stage of the microscope.

b. Using the low power (10×) objective, make certain the microscope light is adjusted correctly. In proper focus, the white blood cells should look like small dark or black dots.

c. Scan the four large corner squares marked 'W' (Fig. 3–7). For accurate white counts, there should be an even distribution of cells in all four large squares, with no more than a ten-cell variation between the four squares.

d. Beginning with the upper left square, count all white blood cells in the four large corner squares and add the results together to obtain the total number of cells. In counting the cells that touch the outside lines of the large square, count only those that touch the left (or right) and upper (or lower) outside lines (in counting chambers with double lines), disregarding those that touch the right (or left) and lower (or upper) outside margin. If the chamber has triple lines, count those cells that touch the middle of the three outside lines on two sides and disregard those touching the corresponding lines on the other two sides. (That is, count the cells touching either the right margin or the left margin and the cells on the upper margin or lower margin. It is irrelevant which sides are chosen, but it is important to be consistent and count the cells touching the same two lines every time.)

e. Count the cells on the opposite side of the counting chamber and record the number of cells counted in these four large squares. The total number of cells counted on each side of the counting chamber should agree within 10% of each other. If the counts do not agree the procedure should be repeated.

6. Calculation of the WBC.

a. For each of the two white counts performed, calculate the number of WBCs/μL, as shown below:

$$
\begin{array}{c}
\text{Number} \\
\text{of white} \\
\text{blood cells} \\
\text{counted}
\end{array}
\times
\begin{array}{c}
\text{Correction} \\
\text{for volume}
\end{array}
\times
\begin{array}{c}
\text{Correction} \\
\text{for dilution}
\end{array}
$$

Number of white blood cells counted. Add the total number of WBC counted in the four large squares of the counting chamber. For example:

Square 1	25 white cells	25
Square 2	34 white cells	34
Square 3	32 white cells	32
Square 4	31 white cells	31
Number of cells counted	=	122

Correction for volume. Obtain the WBC as the number of white blood cells in 1 μL of blood. Therefore, if the cells are counted in four large squares, the total volume counted is 4 (1.0 × 1.0 × 0.1) μL, or 0.4 μL. To obtain a volume of 1.0 μL, 0.4 is multiplied by 2.5 (1.0 ÷ 0.4). The correction factor for volume is then 2.5.

Correction for dilution. Since the blood was initially diluted 1:20, the correction factor for dilution is 20 (21 if using a 1:21 dilution).

b. Therefore:
WBC/μL = 122 × 2.5 × 20 = 6,100 WBC/μL.

c. WBC/L = 6,100 × 10^6 = 6.1 × 10^9/L.

d. Calculate the WBC for the second white count and average the two numbers for the final result.

Discussion

1. In certain conditions, such as leukemia, the WBC may be extremely high. If the white count is above 30.0 × 10^9/L, it is advisable to employ a larger dilution of blood. A platelet Unopette may be used or the blood may be diluted 1:101 (0.02 mL whole blood + 2.0 mL diluting fluid). Alternatively a Thoma red cell pipet may be used (see the section entitled Red Blood Cell Count), the blood drawn up to the 1.0 mark and diluted to the 101 mark with the white count diluting fluid (1:100 dilution). If the white count is markedly elevated, as in some leukemias, in which it may be as high as 100 to 300 × 10^9/L, a 1:200 dilution is used. This is accomplished by adding 0.02 mL of whole blood to 4.0 mL of diluting fluid (1:201 dilution), or by drawing the blood up to the 0.5 mark in the Thoma red cell pipet and diluting to the 101 mark with white count diluting fluid. The procedure for the WBC then proceeds as previously described. The correction factor for the dilution, however, changes accordingly.

2. Whenever the WBC drops below 3.0 × 10^9/L, a smaller dilution of the blood should be used to achieve a more accurate count. In this situation, the blood may be diluted 1:11 (0.02 mL whole blood + 0.2 mL diluting fluid) or drawn up to the 1.0 mark in a Thoma white cell pipet and diluted to the 11 mark with the white count diluting fluid for a dilution of 1:10. The white count then proceeds as previously outlined, with the appropriate correction factor used for the dilution.

3. It is important that the diluting fluid remain free from contamination. Often, small amounts of blood collect in the diluting fluid, causing inaccuracies and difficulties in distinguishing and counting the white blood cells.

4. It is imperative that the counting chamber and cover glass be free from dirt and lint. Again, contamination may cause inaccuracies and difficulties in counting white blood cells. (The counting chamber and

cover glass should be cleaned off immediately after completion of the count.)

5. Pipets must be free of dirt and dried blood. Never leave undiluted blood in a Thoma pipet. It quickly hardens and plugs up the pipet. Draw water or diluting fluid into the pipet and place it in a container of 10% aqueous Clorox solution.

6. There is an approximate 15% error for a manual WBC that falls within the normal range. It is advisable to count at least 100 WBC on each side of the counting chamber. Generally, the more cells counted, the lower the percentage of error.

7. The diluting fluids used for the white cell count destroy or hemolyze all non-nucleated red blood cells. In certain disease states, nucleated red blood cells (NRBC) are present in the peripheral blood. These cells, because they contain a nucleus, cannot be distinguished from the white blood cells. Therefore, any time there are five or more nucleated red blood cells per 100 white blood cells in a differential, the white blood cell count should be corrected as follows:

Corrected WBC

$$= \frac{\text{Uncorrected WBC}}{100 + \text{\# of NRBC/100 WBC}} \times 100$$

The white count is then reported as the 'Corrected' WBC.

8. Once the hemocytometer is filled, the counting of cells must proceed without delay. If too much time elapses, the fluid in the chamber begins to evaporate, causing inaccuracies in the count.

RED BLOOD CELL COUNT

The red blood cell count (RBC) is expressed as the number of red blood cells/liter (L) of whole blood. The normal RBC is 3.6 to 5.6 $\times 10^{12}$/L for females and 4.2 to 6.0 $\times 10^{12}$/L for males. The newborn shows an RBC of 5.0 to 6.5 $\times 10^{12}$/L at birth, which gradually decreases to 3.5 to 5.1 $\times 10^{12}$/L at 1 year of age. During childhood and adolescence, the normal values for the RBC are slightly below the normal adult values. There is also a slight decrease in the RBC after 50 years of age. In addition, strenuous physical activity tends to increase the red count, and there may also

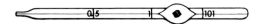

FIG. 3–10. Thoma red count pipet.

be daily fluctuations with the red count being highest in the morning and at its lowest in the evening. An increased red cell count is found in polycythemia vera and secondary polycythemia due to other causes, such as dehydration and the effect of altitude. The red count is below normal in anemia and secondarily in numerous other disorders.

As in the WBC, there are two basic methods used for counting red blood cells: the manual method and the procedure employing an electronic cell counter. The manual method for the RBC is similar to that for the WBC. It is suggested that the student master the WBC procedure before attempting to perform the RBC. To avoid duplication of material, the RBC is not presented in as detailed a manner as the WBC.

Reagents and Equipment

1. Pipets, one of the following:
   a. RBC Unopette (1:200 dilution).
   b. 20 µL pipet (40 × 75 mm test tubes with caps, and plain microhematocrit tube if this pipet is used).
   c. Thoma red count pipet (Fig. 3–10).
2. Red count diluting fluid.
   Trisodium citrate, 3.2% w/v   99 mL
   Formalin, 40%   1 mL
   This diluting fluid maintains the normal shape of the red cell. If there is auto-agglutination of the patient's red cells, omit the formalin in the above fluid and dilute the blood in 3.2% sodium citrate. Hayem's diluting fluid is not recommended because conditions such as hyperglobulinemia cause rouleaux and clumping of the red blood cells. If the RBC Unopette is employed, none of the above diluting fluids is needed.
3. Microscope.
4. Clean gauze or Kimwipes.
5. Hemocytometer and cover glass. Refer to Figure 3–7 and the explanation of the hemocytometer in the White Blood Cell Count section. The large middle square containing 25 smaller squares of equal size is used for the RBC.

a. The five small squares labeled 'R' are the areas to be counted for the RBC.

b. The large center square has a volume of 0.1 μL. Therefore, the volume of each of the 25 smaller squares is 0.004 μL, for a total volume of 0.02 μL for five small squares.

Specimen

Whole blood, using EDTA or heparin as the anticoagulant. Capillary blood may also be used.

Principle

To facilitate counting and prevent lysis of the red blood cells, whole blood is diluted with an isotonic diluting fluid.

Procedure

1. Dilution of blood. Prepare all dilutions in duplicate.
    a. RBC Unopette. Follow procedure outlined in the Unopette section.
    b. 20 μL pipet (1:201 dilution).
        1) Place exactly 4.0 mL of diluting fluid into a 10×75 mm test tube.
        2) Add 20 μL of well-mixed whole blood to the tube. Cap tube and mix.
        3) For a 1:200 dilution, remove 20 μL of diluting fluid from the 4.0 mL in step 1 above prior to adding the blood specimen.
    c. Thoma red count pipet. Draw the blood up to exactly the 0.5 mark in the red count pipet and dilute to the 101 mark with red count diluting fluid, thus making a 1:200 dilution of blood.
2. Clean the counting chamber.
3. Mix the diluted red blood cell counts for 3 minutes.
4. Fill the counting chamber (one red count dilution filling each side of the hemocytometer). Once the counting chamber is filled, allow approximately 3 minutes for the red blood cells to settle prior to counting.
5. Count the red blood cells.
    a. Carefully place the filled counting chamber on the microscope stage.

b. Using low power (10 $\times$ objective), place the large center square in the middle of the field of vision. Examine the entire large square for even distribution of red blood cells.

c. Carefully change to the high dry objective (40$\times$).

d. Move the counting chamber so that the small upper left corner square is completely in the field of vision. The square is further subdivided into 16 even smaller squares for ease of counting.

e. Count all red cells in this square, remembering to count the cells on two of the outer margins but excluding those lying on the other two outside edges.

f. Some of the red blood cells may be lying on their sides and, therefore, do not appear as round. These cells are to be included in the count.

g. If there are any white blood cells in the area being counted, do not include these cells in your count. (The white blood cell is usually much larger than the red blood cell and does not have as smooth an appearance.)

h. Count the red cells in each of the five small squares.

i. Count the red blood cells on the opposite side of the counting chamber in the corresponding five small squares.

6. Calculate the red blood cell count for each of the red counts performed and average the two results for the final report.

RBC/L =

$$\dfrac{\text{\# Cells in}}{\text{five squares}} \times \dfrac{\text{Correction}}{\text{for volume}} \times \dfrac{\text{Correction}}{\text{for dilution}} \times 10^6$$

For example:

# Cells in five small squares = 400
Dilution = 1:200
Volume counted = five small squares
Conversion to liter = $\times 10^6$

$$\text{RBC/L} = 400 \times \dfrac{1.0}{.02} \times 200 \times 10^6$$

$$= 4.0 \times 10^{12}$$

Discussion

1. In certain conditions, such as polycythemia, the red blood cell count may be extremely high, which makes it difficult

to obtain an accurate count. In this instance, make a larger dilution of blood. For a 1:301 dilution, add 20 μL of whole blood to 6.0 mL of diluting fluid.

2. For a patient who has severe anemia and in whom the RBC is low, make a 1:101 dilution by adding 20 μL of whole blood to 2.0 mL of diluting fluid.
3. Make certain the pipets, hemocytometer, and cover glass are free from dirt, lint, and dried blood. Ensure that the diluting fluid is free from blood and other contamination.
4. An RBC takes longer to perform than a WBC because of the larger number of cells. Therefore, proceed as quickly as possible once the cells have settled. Drying of the dilution in the counting chamber causes inaccuracies in the final cell count.
5. The range of error for a manual RBC is generally about 10 to 20%.

PREPARATION AND STAINING PROCEDURES FOR THE BLOOD SMEAR

There are three types of blood smear used in the laboratory: (1) the *cover glass smear*, (2) the *wedge smear*, and (3) the *spun smear*. The cover glass smear is generally thought to contain a more even distribution of white cells than the wedge smear. However, it is more time consuming, the technique is somewhat more difficult to master, cover glasses are too small for most automated stainers, they are harder to label and are easily broken. The spun smear uses the more easily handled and labeled glass slide and has the advantages of even distribution of the white cells and red blood cells free of distortion.

There are two additional types of blood smear used for specific purposes.

1. The *buffy coat smear* is for use on patient specimens when the patient's white blood cell count is less than 1.0×10^9/L and it is desirable to perform a 100-cell differential. This procedure concentrates the nucleated cells present in the blood.
2. *Thick blood smears* are commonly used when specifically looking for blood parasites such as malaria.

Once the blood smear is made, it is stained with Wright stain or Wright-Giemsa stain, so

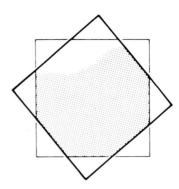

FIG. 3–11. Cover glass method of making a blood smear.

that a differential white blood cell count and morphology study may be performed. Smears using blood anticoagulated with EDTA should be made within 2 to 3 hours of blood collection.

Cover Glass Smears

1. Obtain two clean cover glasses, 22 mm square and 0.13 to 0.17 mm thick (number 1 or 1.5).
2. Hold one cover glass by its two adjacent corners with the thumb and index finger of one hand.
3. Place a small drop of blood on this cover glass.
4. With the other hand, hold a second cover glass in the same manner as the first.
5. Gently place the second cover glass over the cover glass containing the drop of blood (with the drop of blood in between the two cover glasses), so that the two cover glasses, one on top of the other, form a sixteen-sided figure (Fig. 3–11). As soon as the two cover glasses come together, the blood begins to spread.
6. Just before the spreading of blood is complete, separate the two cover glasses by a rapid, even, horizontal, lateral pull. Care should be taken to avoid squeezing the cover glasses together.
7. Allow the smears to air dry completely.
8. The cover glass smears are now ready for staining.

Discussion

1. The cover glasses must be scrupulously clean.
2. When obtaining blood from a finger tip puncture (or heel), the skin must not touch the cover glass.
3. As soon as the drop of blood is placed on the cover glass, the two cover glasses should be brought together without delay. If the drop of blood sits for longer than 3 to 5 seconds, clumping of the platelets and white blood cells, and rouleaux formation of the red blood cells occur.
4. Do not put too large a drop of blood on the cover glass. This results in smears too thick for accurate study.
5. A modified cover glass smear may be prepared on a glass slide by substituting a slide for one of the cover glasses. In this technique, place a drop of blood on the center of a glass slide. While holding a cover glass by opposite corners with the thumb and index finger, place it over the drop of blood on the glass slide. Just before the spreading of blood is complete, remove the cover glass from the slide by a rapid, even, lateral pull. The resultant blood smear on the slide is similar to a coverslip smear.

Wedge Blood Smears

1. Obtain a clean glass slide, one spreader slide, and, if using anticoagulated blood, a plain microhematocrit tube. (The spreader slide is merely a glass slide with specially ground ends to ensure even spreading of the blood.)
2. If anticoagulated blood is used, partially fill a microhematocrit tube with well-mixed blood. Carefully place a small drop of blood in the middle of the slide, approximately 1 cm from the labeled end.
3. When using blood from the finger or heel, place a drop of blood on the slide as described in step 2 above, being careful not to touch the skin of the finger (or heel) with the slide.
4. Place the slide on a flat table top with the drop of blood on the right (for right-handed people).
5. With the thumb and index finger of the

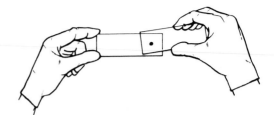

FIG. 3–12. Method of holding slides for preparation of blood smear.

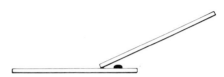

FIG. 3–13. Proper angle for spreader slide.

left hand, hold the two edges of the slide. With the right hand, hold the spreader slide with the thumb on the edge of one side and the other four fingers on the edge of the other side (Fig. 3–12). Place the end of the spreader slide slightly in front of the drop of blood. There should be an approximate 30° to 40° angle between the two slides (Fig. 3–13).
6. Draw the spreader slide back toward the drop of blood. As soon as the spreader slide comes in contact with the drop of blood, the blood will begin to spread to the edge of the spreader slide. If this does not occur, wiggle the spreader slide a little until it does so. (Be careful that blood does not get in front of the spreader slide.)
7. Keeping the spreader slide at a 30° to 40° angle and the edge of the slide firmly against the horizontal slide, push the spreader slide rapidly over the entire length of the slide. This step should be performed at the moment when the blood has spread to within a short distance of the edges of the slide.
8. When the blood smears have air dried, they are ready to be stained.

Discussion

1. The glass slides must be scrupulously clean.
2. As soon as the drop of blood is placed on

the glass slide, the smear should be made without delay. Any elapse of time results in an abnormal distribution of the white blood cells, with many of the larger cells accumulating at the thin edge of the smear. Rouleaux of the red blood cells and platelet clumping may also occur.

3. Common causes of a poor blood smear:
   a. Drop of blood too large or too small.
   b. Spreader slide pushed across the slide in a jerky manner.
   c. Failure to keep the entire edge of the spreader slide against the slide while making the smear.
   d. Failure to keep the spreader slide at the proper angle with the slide. (Increasing the angle results in a thicker smear [to be used when the specimen has a very low hematocrit], whereas a smaller angle gives a thin smear [may be used with specimens having an extremely high hematocrit].)
   e. Failure to push the spreader slide completely across the slide.
4. The Miniprep automatic blood smearing instrument affords the technologist a semiautomated method for preparing consistently high quality wedge smears. This instrument is described in Chapter 7.

Automated Spun Smear

The spun smear is prepared in a special instrument, such as the Hemaspinner (see Chapter 7). A clean glass slide is seated on a platen, and three to four drops of blood are placed in the middle of the slide. When the top of the instrument is closed, the platen spins at high speed for a period of time, during which excess blood is thrown from the slide into a catch basin, and the resultant slide is completely covered with a thin monolayer of cells. The more sophisticated spinners contain an optical system. During spinning, a beam of light passes up through the glass slide onto a sensor. When the cells have separated the proper amount, the sensor detects this and the platen automatically stops spinning. In this way, spreading of the blood is consistent from one smear to the next, regardless of the patient's hematocrit.

Buffy Coat Smear

1. Using a capillary pipet, fill a Wintrobe sedimentation tube with well-mixed whole blood.
2. Centrifuge the Wintrobe tube for 15 minutes at 1500 g.
3. Examine the centrifuged specimen, locating the buffy coat. Remove and discard all of the plasma except for a small amount near the buffy coat.
4. Using the capillary pipet, remove the small amount of remaining plasma, the entire buffy coat and a small amount of red blood cells.
5. Place the specimen on a glass slide and mix as well as possible. (Do not spread the specimen out too much on the slide.)
6. Transfer a small amount of the blood to each of two slides and immediately prepare wedge or cover glass smears.

Discussion

1. The amount of plasma mixed with the buffy coat and red cells should be approximately equal to the volume of the cellular portion of the mixture.
2. Alternatively, microhematocrit tubes may be used to centrifuge the specimen. After centrifugation, cut the hematocrit tube slightly above the buffy coat layer. Cut the sealed end of the hematocrit tube from the bottom of the tube. Allow the small plasma layer, buffy coat layer, and a few red blood cells to drain from the microhematocrit tube directly onto a glass slide. Mix this blood well and prepare wedge or cover glass smears.
3. The distribution of nucleated cells on a buffy coat smear does not always give an accurate differential count because of the fact that the nucleated cells will tend to sediment in layers according to cell type, during the centrifugation process. In cases of leukopenia, however, the differentials from well made buffy coat smears are thought to correlate relatively well with the standard blood smear.

Thick Blood Film

1. Place one large drop of well-mixed blood in the center of a glass slide.
2. Using the corner of a second slide, carefully spread the drop of blood over an area

the size of a dime. (To determine the correct thickness of the blood film, place the slide on a piece of newspaper. Spread the drop of blood until the newspaper print is just visible through the blood.)

3. Allow the blood film to completely air dry before staining. This will take at least 2 to 4 hours at room temperature, or preferably overnight. If the smear is not completely dry, the blood will be washed from the slide during the staining process since this type of smear is not fixed prior to staining.

Staining Procedure for Blood Smears

Romanowsky stains are routinely used to stain peripheral blood and bone marrow smears. Wright's, Giemsa, and the modified Wright's-Giemsa stains are the most commonly used in this country; Leishman, Jenner, and May-Grüwald are also included in this category of stains. Basically, the Romanowsky stains contain methylene blue (or its oxidation products, such as Azure B) and eosin B or eosin Y. They are considered polychromatic stains in that the dyes present produce multiple colors when applied to the cells and cellular elements. Azure B (trimethylthionin, a product of the oxidation of methylene blue) and eosin Y are the most important components of the stain. The quantity of dyes used to prepare the stain are controlled in order to yield a neutral compound. When the buffer solution is added to the stain, ionization occurs, during which time staining takes place. The eosin ions are negatively charged and stain the basic components of the cells an orange to pink color. The acid structures of the cells are stained varying shades of blue to purple by the positively charged azure B. Neutrophil granules are probably stained by the azure compounds.

Wright's stain is composed of oxidized methylene blue and eosin azures. Giemsa stain is thought to produce more delicate staining characteristics. It combines eosin Y with azure B and methylene blue in methanol with glycerin added as a stabilizer. Leishman's stain is similar to Wright's stain except for the method used to oxidize the methylene blue.

There is wide variability in the staining characteristics of these stains from one lot to the next, which is most likely due to contaminants present in the dyes. For this reason, the following procedure should be used as a guide only. Each laboratory should determine their optimum staining times based on the stain in use. For best results, blood smears should be stained within 2 to 3 hours of specimen collection.

Reagents and Equipment

1. Wright-Giemsa stain.

Wright stain powder	9.0 g
Giemsa stain powder	1.0 g
Glycerin	90 mL
Methanol (absolute, anhydrous, acetone free)	2,910 mL

(Mallinckrodt methanol is recommended for use in the Wright stain. The methanol used must contain less than 4% v/v of water.) Mix the above reagents in a large tightly stoppered brown bottle. The stain should be allowed to age for approximately 30 days prior to use. During this time, the stain should be shaken once a day. Incubation at 37°C speeds the aging process. The stain should be freshly filtered at the beginning of each day.

2. Sörenson's phosphate buffer.

Solution 1

Anhydrous monobasic potassium phosphate (KH_2PO_4), 0.067 M.	9.1 g

Dissolve and dilute to 1 L with distilled water.

Solution 2

Anhydrous dibasic sodium phosphate (Na_2HPO_4), 0.067 M.	9.5 g

Dissolve and dilute to 1 L with distilled water.

Mix solutions 1 and 2 together in the appropriate proportions according to the pH desired. For blood and bone marrow staining a pH of 6.8 is recommended, whereas a pH of 7.2 is used when looking for malaria parasites (in order to stain Schüffner's granules).

pH	Solution 1 (mL)	Solution 2 (mL)
6.6	63.0	37.0
6.8	50.8	49.2
7.0	38.9	61.1
7.2	28.0	72.0
7.4	19.2	80.8

3. Methanol, Mallinckrodt (absolute, anhydrous, acetone free).
4. Staining rack.

Procedure

1. Place the air dried blood smears on a level staining rack, with the smear side up.
2. Fix the smears by flooding the slides with methanol. Drain the excess methanol off the slides. (An alternative method is to dip the smears into a coplin jar containing methanol and then place the slides on the staining rack. However, the utmost care must be taken to change the methanol in the coplin jar several times a day and to keep the jar covered when not in use because methanol readily takes up water.)
3. Flood the slides with Wright-Giemsa stain and time for 4 minutes.
4. Without removing the stain, add an equal volume of phosphate buffer to the slide. Mix the two solutions on the slide by gently blowing back and forth over the solutions. A metallic green sheen should now form on top of this mixture. Time for 7 minutes.
5. Rinse the slide off thoroughly with a stream of tap or distilled water.
6. Wipe the back of the slides with a piece of gauze to remove any stain.
7. Stand the slides up on end to air dry. Never blot the smears dry.
8. A well-stained smear shows pink to orange red blood cells, pinkish gray reticulocytes, dark purple nuclei in the lymphocytes and neutrophils, a lighter purple nucleus in the monocyte, bright orange granules in the eosinophil, dark blue black granules in the basophil, and violet to purple platelet granules. The cytoplasm of the monocyte is a gray blue with fine reddish granules. The neutrophil has a light pink cytoplasm with lilac granules, and the lymphocyte shows varying shades of blue cytoplasm.

Discussion

1. Generally, when bone marrow smears are stained, the fixing and staining times must be increased. Fix the smears in methanol for 20 minutes and increase the staining time to 10 to 15 minutes.

2. The staining times for both peripheral blood and bone marrow smears vary from one laboratory to another, and may also change when a new lot of Wright stain is used.
3. The phosphate buffer controls the pH of the stain. If the pH is too acid, those cells or cell parts taking up an acid dye stain will stain pinker and the acid components that stain with the basic dye show very pale staining. If the stain-buffer mixture is too alkaline, the red blood cells will appear grayish-blue and the white cell nuclei will stain very deeply purple. Therefore, to stain all cells and cell parts well, the pH of the phosphate buffer is critical.
4. The staining rack must be exactly level to guard against uneven staining of the smear.
5. Insufficient washing of the smears when removing the stain and buffer mixture may cause stain precipitate on the dried smear.
6. Excessive rinsing of the stained smear will cause the stain to fade.
7. If it is desirable to restain a slide, the original stain may be removed with methanol. Flood the smear with methanol and rinse with tap water as many times as necessary to remove the stain and then restain the slide according to the previously described procedure. For best results, however, make a new smear.
8. For cover glass smears, after the stained smears have dried, mount the cover glass, blood side down, on a slide using a mounting medium.
9. This stain procedure may be carried out in coplin jars in which case the stain-buffer ratio and staining times will need to be adjusted.
10. The National Committee for Clinical Laboratory Standards (NCCLS) has recommended a standardized Wright's stain that will yield consistent results from one batch to the next. Pure azure B (CI 52010) (260 mg/100mL methanol) solution is combined with pure eosin Y (CI 45380) (130 mg/100mL methanol). One volume of the combined stains (1:1 ratio) is mixed with 10 volumes of Sörenson's phosphate buffer, pH 6.8. (The stock solutions of the individual stains must be

freshly prepared each week. The stain-buffer solution may only be used for 1 hour.) The prepared smears are immersed in the stain-buffer solution in coplin jars for 10 minutes, after which time they are rinsed quickly in distilled water and allowed to air dry.

DIFFERENTIAL CELL COUNT

The manual differential white blood cell count is performed to determine the relative number of each type of white blood cell present in the blood. At the same time, a study of red blood cell, white blood cell, and platelet morphology is performed. An approximation of the number of platelets is also made. The differential and smear review should be performed after the blood counts have been completed. In this way, examination of the smear may also be used to double check the white blood cell count. Obtaining an accurate manual white blood cell differential is somewhat difficult because of the fact that the white blood cells are not always randomly distributed. For routine testing, the wedge smear is the most widely used. Smears that are poorly made and/or are too thin will show an increased concentration of polymorphonuclear white cells, monocytes, and large abnormal cells at the edges and tail of the blood film. This will then cause a relative increased concentration of lymphocytes in the middle of the smear. It is therefore of utmost importance that the blood film be well prepared.

The normal range for the white blood cell differential should be determined by each laboratory. During infancy and childhood a mild lymphocytosis may be present. Adult normal values are reached by the age of 21. See Table 3–2 for an example set of reference ranges for the differential.

In disease states, a particular white blood cell type may show an absolute increase in number in the blood. Common diseases showing an increased number of a specific cell type are listed below.

1. *Neutrophilia* (absolute increase in the number of neutrophils):
   a. Appendicitis
   b. Myelogenous leukemia

TABLE 3–2. EXAMPLE OF REFERENCE RANGES FOR WHITE BLOOD CELL DIFFERENTIAL COUNT

Cell Type	%	Absolute Number ($\times 10^9$/L)
Neutrophil	35–71	1.5–7.4
Band	0–6	0.0–0.7
Lymphocyte	24–44	1.0–4.4
Monocyte	1–10	0.1–1.0
Eosinophil	0–4	0.0–0.4
Basophil	0–2	0.0–0.2

   c. Bacterial infections
2. *Eosinophilia* (absolute increase in the number of eosinophils):
   a. Allergies and allergenic reactions
   b. Scarlet fever
   c. Parasitic infections
   d. Eosinophilic leukemia
3. *Lymphocytosis* (absolute increase in the number of lymphocytes):
   a. Viral infections
   b. Whooping cough
   c. Infectious mononucleosis
   d. Lymphocytic leukemia
4. *Monocytosis* (absolute increase in the number of monocytes):
   a. Brucellosis
   b. Tuberculosis
   c. Monocytic leukemia
   d. Subacute bacterial endocarditis
   e. Typhoid
   f. Rickettsial infections
   g. Collagen disease
   h. Hodgkin's disease
   i. Gaucher's disease

Procedure for Examination of the Stained Blood Smear

1. Check the blood smear to ensure that it is well made. The tail of the film (Fig. 3–14) should be smooth. Place the slide (smear side up) on the microscope stage. (For consistency, when the wedge smear is used place the thick end of the smear on the same side of the microscope stage each time a differential is performed.)

Color Plates

Plate I

Normoblasts and megaloblasts contrasted (photomicrographs, ×1000; Wright stain).

    A, B, C, D, E, Normoblasts: A, pronormoblast; B, basophilic normoblast; C, early; D, late, poly-chromatophilic normoblasts; E, orthochromic normoblast with stippling.
    F–O. Various stages of megaloblasts (pernicious anemia): F, promegaloblast (left) and basophilic me-galoblast (right); G, H, I, J, K, mainly polychromatophilic megaloblasts; L, M, N, O, mainly or-thochromic megaloblasts, O being from the blood. All other cells are from the bone marrow. (From Wintrobe, M.M., et al.: Clinical Hematology, 8th ed. Philadelphia, Lea & Febiger, 1981.)

PLATE I

(Legend on opposite page)

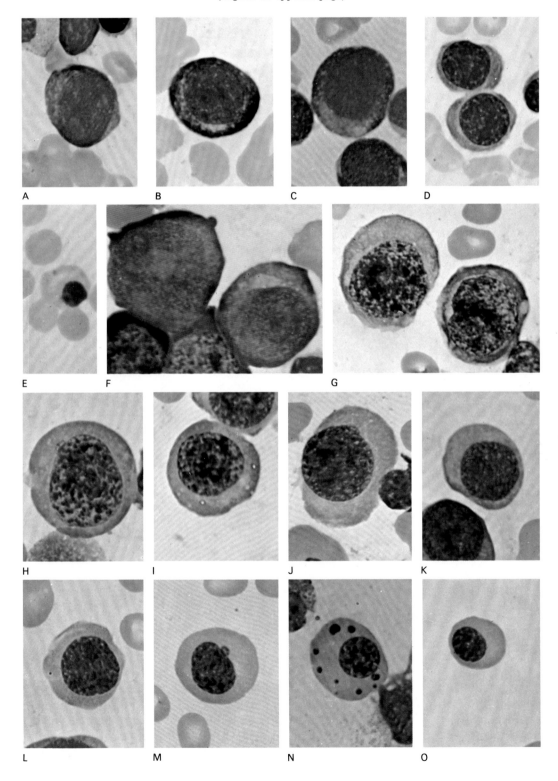

A   B   C   D

E   F   G

H   I   J   K

L   M   N   O

Plate II

Normal leukocytes from bone marrow and blood (photomicrographs, ×1000 [approx.]; Wright stain).

A, myeloblast; B, myeloblasts, with myelocyte and late metamyelocyte; C, two promyelocytes; D, promyelocyte; E, late promyelocyte or myelocyte; F, myelocyte; G, myelocyte; H, late myelocyte or early metamyelocyte; I, metamyelocyte; J, band neutrophil; K, band neutrophil; L, polymorphonuclear neutrophil; M, polymorphonuclear neutrophil; N, polymorphonuclear neutrophil; O, eosinophil; P, basophil; Q, monocyte; R, monocyte. (From Wintrobe, M.M., et al.: Clinical Hematology, 8th ed. Philadelphia, Lea & Febiger, 1981.)

PLATE II

(Legend on opposite page)

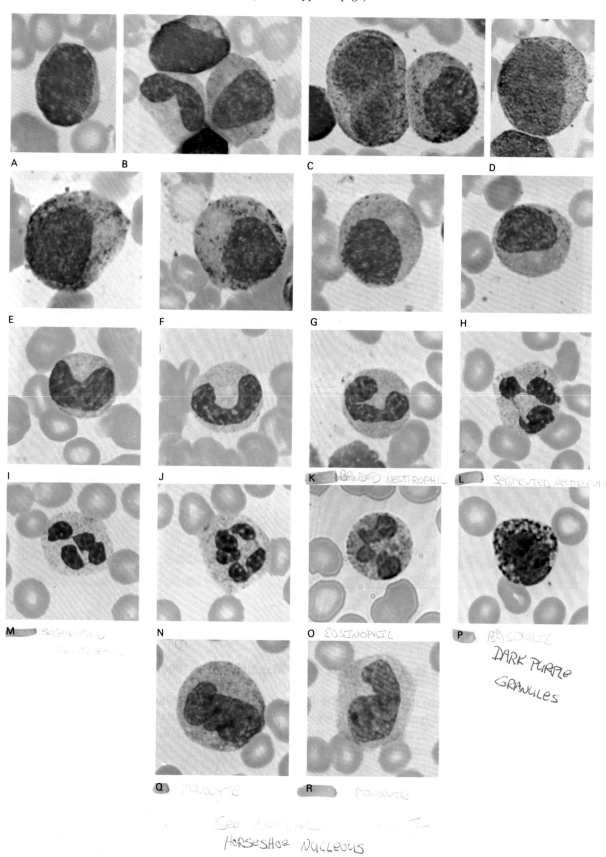

A

B

C

D

E

F

G

H

I

J

K   BANDED NEUTROPHIL

L   SEGMENTED NEUTROPHIL

M   SEGMENTED
    NEUTROPHIL

N

O   EOSINOPHIL

P   BASOPHIL
    DARK PURPLE
    GRANULES

Q   MONOCYTE

R   MONOCYTE

See _____
HORSESHOE NUCLEOUS

PLATE VIII

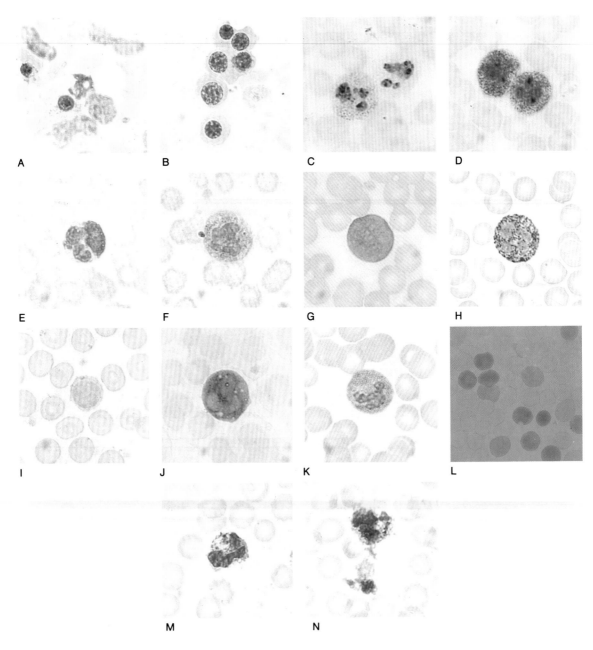

Plate VIII

Special Stains, NBT. (Stained as indicated. Magnification ×403.)

A–B, Iron (Prussian blue) stain (showing sideroblasts); C, leukocyte alkaline phosphatase stain (one neutrophil shows 0 activity, the second neutrophil shows 2+ activity); D, leukocyte alkaline phosphatase stain (both neutrophils show 4+ activity); E, peroxidase stain (neutrophil shows strongly positive staining); F, peroxidase stain (neutrophil shows very weak staining); G, periodic acid-Schiff stain (neutrophil); H, Sudan black B stain (neutrophil); I, acid phosphatase (note red staining granule in the cytoplasm of the lymphocyte); J, nonspecific esterase stain (monocyte); K, chloroacetate esterase stain (neutrophil); L, acid elution (normal RBC show little to no staining; the higher the hemoglobin F content of the red cell, the more intense the stain); M–N, NBT positive neutrophils (Wright's stain) (note black staining particles).

PLATE IX

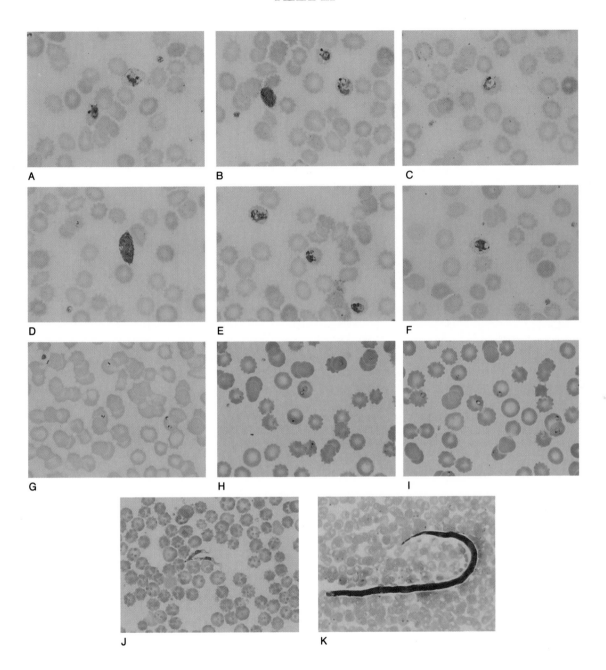

Plate IX

Blood parasites. (Photomicrographs, ×1000; Wright-Giemsa stain.)

A–F, Plasmodium vivax; G, Plasmodium falciparum; H–I, Babesia; J, Trypanosome (trypomastigote stage); K, Microfilaria.

PLATE X

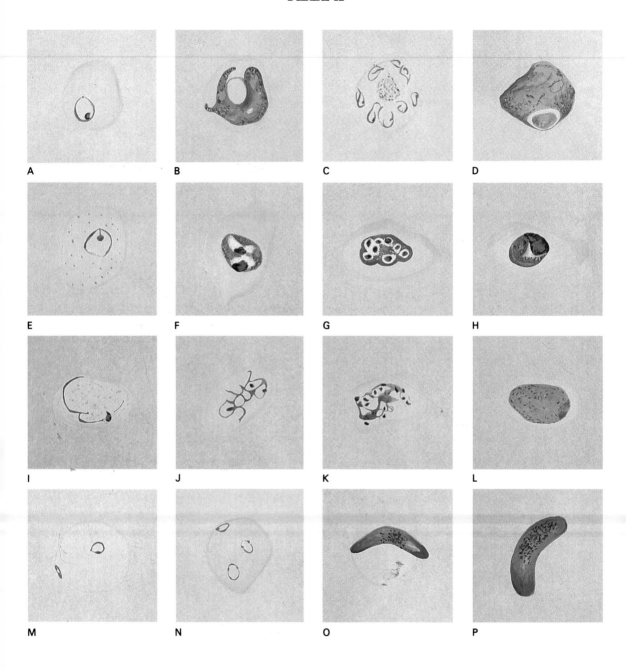

A–D, Plasmodium malariae: A, ring form (trophozoite); B, trophozoite; C, schizont; D, macro-gametocyte.

E–H, Plasmodium ovale: E, ring form (trophozoite); F, G, schizonts; H, gametocyte.

I–L, Plasmodium vivax: I, trophozoite; J, trophozoite (ameboid); K, schizont; L, macrogame-tocyte.

M–P, Plasmodium falciparum: M, double ring (trophozoite); N, multiple rings (trophozoite); O, macrogametocyte; P, microgametocyte.

FIG. 3–14. Wedge blood smear.

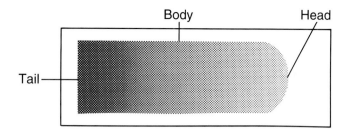

2. Examine the blood smear using the low power (10×) objective.
   a. The red and white blood cells and platelets must be correctly stained.
   b. Check that there is even distribution of the white blood cells on the smear.
   c. Estimate the white blood cell count (by noting the number of white cells/field and the number of white cells in relation to the red blood cell count). It should agree with the test result obtained. If it does not, the white count should be repeated.
   d. Examine the thin peripheral edge of the smear (the tail) (if the wedge smear is being used). If there is an increased number of white cells in this area, the differential cell count may be inaccurate. If there are clumps of platelets, the body of the smear may then show a decrease in platelets. In such situations, the blood smear should be discarded and another made.
   e. When scanning the blood smear, it is important to note anything unusual or irregular, such as large, abnormal looking cells or rouleaux formation of the red blood cells.
   f. Choose the area of the blood smear where the differential counting is to begin, place a drop of oil on the slide and carefully change to the oil immersion objective (100×).
3. Perform the differential cell count and, at the same time, examine the morphology of the white blood cells. There are several counting methods used, three of which are described below.
   a. Using the *cross-sectional* or *crenellation* technique the white cells are counted in consecutive fields as the blood film is moved from side to side as shown in Figure 3–15. Counting should begin in the thin area of the smear where the red blood cells are slightly overlapping and proceed into the thicker area. However, do not progress too far into the thick area if the white cells are not sufficiently spread for easy identification.
   b. In the *longitudinal* method the white cells are counted in consecutive fields from the tail toward the head of the smear as indicated in Figure 3–16. This is the ideal method if the smear is thin enough so that the white cells may be identified all the way to the beginning (head) of the smear. In this case, the strip of smear examined represents one complete section of blood. As many strips as necessary are counted until the desired number of white blood cells are counted.
   c. The *battlement* method uses a pattern of consecutive fields (Fig. 3–17) beginning near the tail on a horizontal edge: count three consecutive horizontal

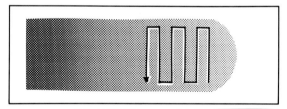

FIG. 3–15. Cross-sectional method of differential counting.

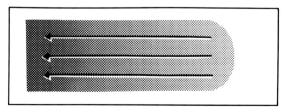

FIG. 3–16. Longitudinal method of differential counting.

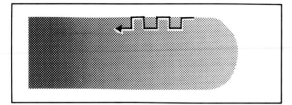

FIG. 3–17. Battlement method of differential counting.

Platelet Est. of	Report Platelet Est. as:
0–49,000/μL	Marked decrease
50,000–99,000/μL	Moderate decrease
100,000–149,000/μL	Slight decrease
150,000–199,000/μL	Low normal
200,000–400,000/μL	Normal
401,000–599,000/μL	Slight increase
600,000–800,000/μL	Moderate increase
Above 800,000/μL	Marked increase

A patient with a red blood cell count of 5.0×10^{12}/L and a platelet count of 300×10^9/L has 30 platelets for every 500 red blood cells. This must be kept in mind when performing a platelet estimate and adjustments made when the patient's red count is greater or less than 5.0×10^{12}/L. For example, if a patient's red count is 2.5×10^{12}/L and the platelet count is 300×10^9/L, there are 30 platelets for every 250 red blood cells, or 60 platelets for every 500 red blood cells. It is, therefore, helpful to know the patient's red blood cell count (hemoglobin or hematocrit) when performing a platelet estimate.

edge fields (moving away from the tail), count two fields toward the center of the smear, count two fields horizontally (moving away from the tail), count two fields vertically to the edge. Continue this pattern until the desired number of cells have been counted.

4. Identify each white blood cell seen and record on a differential cell counter until 100 white blood cells have been counted. If any nucleated red blood cells (NRBC) are seen during the differential count, enumerate them on a separate counter. These cells are not to be included in the 100-cell differential count, but are reported as the # of NRBC/100 WBC. (If any megakaryocytic cells or fragments, smudge cells, or epithelial cells are seen, these cells should also be enumerated in the same manner as the NRBC, and reported as the #/100 WBC.)

5. Examine the red blood cell morphology in a thin area of the slide where only a few of the red blood cells slightly overlap. Note any variations from normal and classify these irregularities as slight, moderate, or marked (or $1+$, $2+$, $3+$).

6. Examine the platelets on the smear for morphology and number present. Using the same fields on various parts of the smear, as in step 5 above for the red blood cell morphology, determine the approximate number of platelets per field. A normal (wedge) blood smear (normal red blood cell count and normal platelet count) should show approximately 8 to 20 platelets per field in this area. One method for reporting platelet estimates is to determine the average number of platelets per field (using 5 to 10 different fields) and multiply this result by 20,000 (for a wedge smear) to obtain an approximation of the platelet count. For example:

Discussion

1. When reporting a manual differential white cell count the results are reported as the percentage of each cell type present. Automated differential counters report the cells in percent and also as the actual number of each cell type/L of blood (absolute count). The most accurate and also the most preferred method of reporting is the absolute count because the result expressed in percent is a relative number and can be misleading to the clinician. For example, a differential showing 15% monocytes with a 9.0×10^9/L white count would be considered abnormal. However, if the white count is 1.5×10^9/L, the actual number of monocytes present is within the normal range. The absolute count is calculated as follows:

$$\frac{\text{Absolute \# of cells/L}}{} = \frac{\text{\% of cell type in}}{\text{differential} \times \text{WBC/L}}$$

2. When performing a differential, the following outline may be followed.
   a. White blood cells.

1) Check for even distribution and estimate the number present (also, look for any gross abnormalities present on the smear).
2) Perform the differential count.
3) Examine for morphologic abnormalities.
   b. Red blood cells.
   1) Examine for:
      a) Size and shape.
      b) Relative hemoglobin content.
      c) Polychromatophilia.
      d) Inclusions.
      e) Rouleaux formation or agglutination.
   c. Platelets.
   1) Estimate number present.
   2) Examine for morphologic abnormalities.

3. When studying a stained smear, do not progress too far into the thick area of the slide. The morphologic characteristics of the cells are difficult to distinguish in this area. Conversely, do not use the very thin portion of the smear where the red blood cells appear completely filled with hemoglobin and show no area of central pallor. The cells in this area are generally distorted and do not show a true morphologic picture.

4. When the white count is below $1.0 \times 10^9/$L, it may be difficult to find many white blood cells on the stained smear. In this situation, a differential may be performed by counting 50 white cells. A notation on the report must then be made that only 50 white blood cells were counted. (Alternatively, a buffy coat smear may be prepared.)

5. When the differential shows an abnormal distribution of cell types (as listed below):
   a. Over 10% eosinophils,
   b. Over 2% basophils,
   c. Over 11% monocytes, or
   d. More lymphocytes than neutrophils (except in children) a 200-cell differential may be performed. The results are then averaged (divided by 2) and a notation made on the report that 200 white blood cells were counted.

6. Before reporting platelets as decreased, scan the slide on low power, especially the feathered edge, for platelet clumps. Also recheck the tube of blood for a clot.

7. If the differential count shows the presence of immature granulocytic cells, this is termed a *shift to the left* and may be found in such disorders as leukemias and bacterial infections. A *shift to the right* refers to an increased number of hypersegmented neutrophils.

8. The differential is the most difficult laboratory test to learn, so do not hesitate to ask questions. Learning about cells and their morphologic features is a process that will continue for as long as you perform differentials.

9. There is a relatively large range of variability in the results of the 100-cell differential count. As the number of total cells counted increases, the amount of variability will decrease. The 95% confidence limit (± 2 S.D.) improves somewhat more remarkably when counting 200 white cells. Although the accuracy of the count improves with a 500 or 1000 cell count, the change is not as great as seen between 100 and 200 cell differential counts. (See below.)

Actual #	± 2 *S.D. when counting*			
of cell type	*100*	*200*	*500*	*1000*
2	0–8	0–6	0–4	1–4
25	16–35	19–32	21–30	22–28
45	35–56	38–53	40–50	41–49
60	54–68	56–66	57–63	58–63
80	71–90	73–87	76–85	77–83

(From: Nelson, D.A., and Morris, M.W.: Basic methodology, In: *Clinical Diagnosis and Management*, Henry, J.B., ed., Philadelphia, W.B. Saunders Co., 1984, p. 611.)

RED BLOOD CELL INDICES

The red blood cell indices are used to define the size and hemoglobin content of the red blood cell. They consist of the mean corpuscular volume (MCV), mean corpuscular hemoglobin (MCH), and mean corpuscular hemoglobin concentration (MCHC). With the widespread use of automated cell counters that routinely determine the red blood cell indices on each blood sample tested, the indices are commonly used as an aid in diagnosing and differentiating anemias.

Mean Corpuscular Volume (MCV)

The MCV is calculated from the red blood cell count and the hematocrit and indicates the average volume of the red blood cells in femtoliters (fL). If the MCV is less than 80 fL, the red blood cells are considered **microcytic.** If it is greater than 100 fL, the red blood cells are **macrocytic.** If the MCV is within the normal range, the red blood cells are termed **normocytic.**

$$MCV = \frac{\text{Volume of red blood cells in femtoliters (fL) of blood}}{RBC/L}$$

If: Hematocrit $= 45\%$ (or, .45 L)
RBC $= 5.0 \times 10^{12}/L$
1 μL $= 10^9$ fL
1 L $= 10^{15}$ fL

Then:

$$MCV = \frac{.45 \times 10^{15} \text{ fL/L}}{5.0 \times 10^{12}/L}$$
$$= .09 \times 10^3 \text{ fL}$$
$$= 90 \text{ fL}$$

Therefore, the formula:

$$MCV = \frac{Hct \times 10^3 \text{ fL}}{RBC/L}$$

Normal range for the MCV: 80 to 100 fL

Mean Corpuscular Hemoglobin (MCH)

The MCH is calculated from the hemoglobin and red blood cell count, indicates the average weight of hemoglobin in the red blood cell, and should always correlate with the MCV and MCHC. It is directly proportional to the size of the red blood cell and the concentration of hemoglobin in the cell. An MCH lower than 27 pg is found in microcytic anemia and also in the presence of normocytic, hypochromic red blood cells. An elevated MCH occurs in macrocytic anemias and in some cases of spherocytosis in which hyperchromia may be present. The MCH is much less valuable to the clinician than the MCV and MCHC.

$$MCH = \frac{\text{Weight of hgb in 1 L of blood}}{\text{\# of red cells in 1 L of blood}}$$

If: 1 g $= 10^{12}$ pg
1 L $= 10$ dL

Then:

$$MCH = \frac{Hgb \times 10 \times 10^{12} \text{ pg/L}}{RBC/L}$$

If: Hgb $= 15.0$ g/dL
RBC $= 5.0 \times 10^{12}/L$

Then:

$$MCH: = \frac{15 \times 10^{13} \text{ pg/L}}{5.0 \times 10^{12}/L}$$
$$= \frac{15 \times 10 \text{ pg/L}}{5.0/L}$$
$$= 30 \text{ pg}$$

Therefore, the formula:

$$MCH = \frac{Hgb \text{ (g/L)}}{RBC \text{ (/L)}} \text{ pg}$$

Normal range for the MCH: $= 27$ to 31 pg

Mean Corpuscular Hemoglobin Concentration (MCHC)

The MCHC is calculated from the hemoglobin and hematocrit and is an expression of the average concentration of hemoglobin in the red blood cells. It gives the ratio of the weight of hemoglobin to the volume of the red blood cell and is expressed as a percentage or in g/dL (or g/L). An MCHC below 31% indicates **hypochromia,** above 36%, **hyperchromia,** and red blood cells with a normal MCHC are termed **normochromic.** Please note that an MCHC above 38% should not occur. Such a result is usually due to incorrect calculation of the MCHC, or the patient's red blood cells may be agglutinated (cold agglutinin), thereby causing a falsely low red blood cell count (the hematocrit may also be falsely low if measured by electronic cell counters that calculate the hematocrit from the MCV and RBC). Alternatively, the MCHC will not fall below 22% when hypochromia is present. If the MCHC does fall below this value, it may be due to a lipemic plasma or an abnormal hemoglobin (such as C or S) causing an invalidly high hemoglobin.

$$MCHC = \frac{Hgb \text{ in g/dL}}{Hct \text{ (vol. of RBC in g/dL)}} \times \frac{100 \text{ (to}}{\text{convert to \%)}}$$

If: Hgb $= 15.0$ g/dL
Hct $= 45\%$ (or, 0.45)

Then:

$$MCHC = \frac{15.0 \text{ g/dL}}{45 \text{ g/dL}} \times 100\%$$
$$= 0.333 \times 100\%$$
$$= 33.3 \%$$

or,

$$MCHC = \frac{15.0 \text{ g/dL}}{0.45}$$

$$= 33.3 \text{ g/dL, or, } 333 \text{ g/L}$$

Therefore, the formula:

$$MCHC = \frac{Hgb \times 100\%}{Hct} \text{ or, } \frac{Hgb \text{ g/dL}}{Hct \text{ (expressed as a fraction)}}$$

Normal range for the MCHC = 31 to 36%
= 31 to 36 g/dL
(310 to 360 g/L)

Examples of Red Blood Cell Indices with Corresponding Red Blood Cell Morphology

1. Hgb = 14.0 g/dl   Hct = 41%
   RBC = 4.5 × 10¹²/L

   MCV = 91.1 fL   RBC are normocytic,
   MCH = 31.1 pg   normochromic.
   MCHC = 34.1%

2. Hgb = 9.8 g/dL   Hct = 30%
   RBC = 4.5 × 10¹²/L

   MCV = 66.7 fL   RBC are microcytic,
   MCH = 21.8 pg   normochromic.
   MCHC = 32.7%

3. Hgb = 9.0 g/dL   Hct = 30%
   RBC = 4.5 × 10¹²/L

   MCV = 66.7 fL   RBC are microcytic,
   MCH = 20.0 pg   hypochromic.
   MCHC = 30.0%

4. Hgb = 15.0 g/dL   Hct = 45%
   RBC = 4.0 × 10¹²/L

   MCV = 112.5 fL   RBC are macrocytic,
   MCH = 37.5 pg   normochromic.
   MCHC = 33.3%

5. Hgb = 11.8 g/dL   Hct = 41%
   RBC = 4.5 × 10¹²/L

   MCV = 91.1 fL   RBC are normocytic,
   MCH = 26.2 pg   hypochromic.
   MCHC = 28.8%

ERYTHROCYTE SEDIMENTATION RATE

The erythrocyte sedimentation rate (ESR) is a nonspecific measurement used to detect and monitor an inflammatory response to tissue injury (an acute phase response) in which there is a change in the plasma concentration of several proteins (termed acute phase proteins). This procedure, very simply, consists

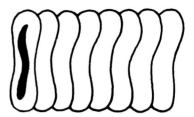

FIG. 3–18. Rouleaux formation of the red blood cells.

of allowing a specific amount of blood to sit in a vertical position for a period of time (usually 1 hour). The distance, in millimeters, that the red cells fall during this time period is the erythrocyte sedimentation rate and is reported in mm/hour.

The ESR is affected by three factors: erythrocytes, plasma composition, and mechanical/technical factors.

Erythrocytes

A factor of chief importance in determining the distance the red blood cells fall is the size or mass of the falling particle. The larger the particle, the faster its rate of fall. In normal blood, the red blood cells remain more or less separated. They are negatively charged and, therefore repel each other. In certain diseases, however, plasma protein concentrations may be altered, causing a reduction in the negative charge of the red blood cells and consequent formation of rouleaux (Fig. 3–18). This leads to a larger mass and an increased sedimentation velocity. Agglutination of the red blood cells due to changes in the erythrocyte surface also leads to an increased red blood cell mass and a more rapid sedimentation rate. Macrocytes tend to settle more rapidly than microcytes. Red blood cells which show an alteration in shape, such as sickle cells and spherocytes, are unable to aggregate or form rouleaux and the sedimentation rate is decreased. Anisocytosis and poikilocytosis reduce the ability of the red blood cell to form large aggregates and thereby tend to falsely lower an ESR. In severe anemia, the ESR is markedly elevated: The concentration of the erythrocytes in the blood is decreased, aggregation and rouleaux formation are increased, and they therefore, settle out more easily and rapidly. (A chart has been devised by Wintrobe and Landsberg [for use

slight, (2) sedimentation then occurs for a period of approximately 40 minutes at a more rapid and constant rate *(decantation phase),* and (3) during the last 10 minutes, the sedimentation rate is slow because of the accumulation of red blood cells in the bottom of the tube. The longer the tube the longer stage two will last, and therefore the higher the ESR result.

2. Although care may be taken in filling the sedimentation tube to the 0 mark, occasionally the upper level of the blood may only reach the 1- or 2-mm mark. In such a case, care should be taken when making the final reading. Subtract the 1 or 2 mm from the final result. For example, if the ESR tube is filled to the 2 mm mark and the red blood cells fall to the 18-mm mark, the ESR is reported as 16 mm/hour. If the level of blood falls below the 5-mm mark, the test should be repeated to ensure that valid results are obtained. If the upper level of the blood is below 0 due to leakage of the blood from the bottom of the tube (Westergren method) the test must be repeated from step 1. Leakage of blood from the bottom of the tube invalidates the test result.

3. All sedimentation racks should be equipped with leveling screws and a spirit level.

4. Sources of error:
   a. If the concentration of EDTA is greater than recommended, the ESR will be falsely low.
   b. If the ESR stands for more than 60 minutes, the results will be falsely elevated. If the test is timed for less than 60 minutes, invalidly low values are obtained.
   c. A marked increase (or decrease) in room temperature leads to increased (or decreased) ESR results.
   d. Tilting of the ESR tube increases the sedimentation rate.
   e. Bubbles in the blood cause invalid results.
   f. Fibrin clots present in the blood invalidate the test results.

5. The ESR should be set up within 2 hours of blood collection. If EDTA is used as the anticoagulant, the test may be set up within 6 hours if the blood has been refrigerated.

6. The Wintrobe ESR technique is thought to be more sensitive when the ESR is low, whereas the Westergren procedure more accurately reflects the patient's disorder when the results are high. The Westergren method has been chosen as the standard method by the International Committee for Standardization in Hematology.

7. When reading the ESR result on bloods with an extremely high white blood cell or platelet count, the buffy coat should be excluded from the reading.

8. If there is poor separation of the red blood cell and plasma layers this may be due to an increased number of reticulocytes and has been termed "stratified sedimentation."

9. The internal bore and the length of the graduated scale on the Westergren pipet are critical measurements. Any tube of a different size in these two dimensions will generally give results different from those obtained using the standard size pipet. If a smaller bore and/or length tube is used (for pediatric samples) a new set of normal values needs to be determined. It must also be kept in mind that even with the new set of normals, the results may still not be comparable with the reference technique.

10. Different types of ESR tubes are available for this procedure: plastic, tubes containing a cotton plug, and shorter and narrower tubes. Different plastics will have varying properties and must be checked against a standard method (see No. 11 below). Micro procedures have been described using tubes with a narrower bore. Results using these tubes are usually lower, and a new normal range would need to be established for this procedure. The overall length of the Westergren ESR pipet is not important but the graduated scale must be the same. If it is not, again, a new normal range would need to be established.

11. A reference procedure for the ESR has been described by the National Committee for Clinical Laboratory Standards, as outlined below.
    a. Undiluted, EDTA anticoagulated whole blood (5 mL) is required.

b. Prior to testing, the hematocrit of the blood sample is adjusted to 35% ± 1%. (If the specimen needs to be diluted, its own plasma must be used.)

c. The undiluted, well-mixed whole blood (hematocrit of 35% ± 1%) is drawn up in a standard glass Westergren pipet. The test is performed as described previously for the Westergren ESR method.

d. At the same time, the routine laboratory method for the ESR is set up on the remaining portion of blood.

e. At the end of 60 minutes, test results are read and recorded.

f. Refer to Table 3–3. Using the test result obtained for the reference method, the expected value for the routine ESR is determined, based on the method used. An acceptable result for the routine method will agree with the expected value within ± 2 S.D. The 2 S.D. value should be within 3 mm per hour for the Wintrobe and ZSR methods and within 6 mm/hour for the Westergren method.

g. Refer to the National Committee for Clinical Laboratory Standards: *Reference Procedure for the Erythrocyte Sedimentation Rate (ESR) Test* (H2-A2), Villanova, PA, 1988, for a more complete description and explanation of the above procedure.

12. Quality Control of the ESR: Approximately once per week or when any change has been made in the ESR procedure (new lot of tubes, testing location changed, etc.) the reference method, as described in item 11 above, should be performed against the laboratory procedure. Results should check within acceptable limits.

RETICULOCYTE COUNT

The red blood cell goes through six stages of development: pronormoblast, basophilic normoblast, polychromatophilic normoblast, orthochromic normoblast, reticulocyte, and mature red blood cell. The first four stages are normally confined to the bone marrow. The reticulocyte, however, is found in both the bone marrow and peripheral blood. In the bone marrow, it spends approximately 2 to 3 days maturing and is then released into the blood, where it ages for an additional day before becoming a mature red blood cell.

The reticulocyte count is an important diagnostic tool. It is a reflection of the amount of effective red blood cell production taking place in the bone marrow. Since the life span of a red cell is 120 days, ±20 days, the bone marrow replaces approximately 1% of the adult red blood cells every day. The normal value for a reticulocyte count is therefore 0.5 to 1.5/100 red blood cells (or, 0.5 to 1.5%), with a range of 25 to 75 × 10^9/L for the absolute count (multiply the red blood cell count by the percentage of reticulocytes). A decreased reticulocyte count is found in aplastic anemia and in conditions in which the bone marrow is not producing red blood cells. Increased reticulocyte counts are found in hemolytic anemias, individuals with iron deficiency anemia receiving iron therapy, thalassemia, sideroblastic anemia, and in acute and chronic blood loss.

Corrected Reticulocyte Count

A reticulocyte count should reflect the total production of red blood cells, regardless of the concentration of red cells in the blood (red blood cell count). As an example, compare the following two patients. Patient #1 has a hematocrit of 42% and a reticulocyte count of 1.0%. Patient #2 has a hematocrit of 21% and a reticulocyte count of 2.0%. Patient #2, theoretically, has ½ as many red blood cells as patient #1 but has the same number of reticulocytes as patient #1 because the reticulocytes are diluted by only ½ the number of red blood cells, as in patient #1. To compensate for this, a **corrected reticulocyte count** is calculated based on a normal hematocrit of 45%. The formula for this correction is:

$$\begin{array}{c} \text{Corrected} \\ \text{reticulocyte} \\ \text{count (percent)} \end{array} = \dfrac{\begin{array}{c}\text{Patient's}\\ \text{hematocrit}\end{array}}{\begin{array}{c}\text{Normal}\\ \text{hematocrit}\end{array}} \times \begin{array}{c}\text{Reticulocyte}\\ \text{count (percent)}\end{array}$$

In addition to correcting a reticulocyte count for an abnormally low hematocrit, consideration should also be given to the presence of marrow reticulocytes present in the peripheral blood. In this circumstance, the **reticulocyte production index** is calculated.

TABLE 3–3. COMPARATIVE REFERENCE VALUES FOR THE ROUTINE WESTERGREN, WINTROBE, AND ZSR METHODS (ALL BLOOD SAMPLES ADJUSTED TO A HEMATOCRIT OF 35%)

ESR-Ref	West.	Wint.	ZSR	ESR-Ref	West.	Wint.	ZSR
14	9	14	42	62	43	44	58
15	10	14	42	63	44	45	60
16	10	15	42	64	45	45	60
17	10	15	43	65	46	46	60
18	11	16	43	66	47	46	60
19	11	17	44	67	48	47	61
20	11	17	44	68	49	47	61
21	12	18	45	69	49	48	61
22	12	19	45	70	50	48	61
23	12	20	45	71	51	49	61
24	13	20	46	72	52	50	62
25	13	21	46	73	53	50	62
26	13	21	46	74	53	51	62
27	14	22	47	75	54	51	62
28	15	22	47	76	55	52	63
29	15	23	47	77	56	52	63
30	16	24	48	78	57	53	63
31	17	24	48	79	58	53	63
32	17	25	48	80	58	53	64
33	18	26	49	81	59	53	64
34	19	26	49	82	60	53	64
35	20	27	49	83	61	53	64
36	21	27	50	84	62	54	64
37	22	28	50	85	63	54	65
38	23	29	51	86	64	54	65
39	24	29	51	87	65	54	65
40	24	30	51	88	65	54	65
41	25	31	52	89	66	54	66
42	26	32	52	90	67	54	66
43	27	32	53	91	68	54	66
44	28	33	53	92	69	54	66
45	29	33	53	93	70	54	67
46	30	34	54	94	71	54	67
47	30	34	54	95	72	54	67
48	31	35	55	96	73	54	67
49	32	36	55	97	74	55	68
50	33	36	55	98	74	55	68
51	34	37	56	99	75	55	68
52	35	37	56	100	76	55	68
53	36	38	56	101	77	55	69
54	37	39	57	102	78	55	69
55	37	39	57	103	79	55	69
56	38	40	57	104	80	55	69
57	39	40	57	105	81	55	69
58	40	41	57	106	81	55	70
59	41	42	58	107	82	55	70
60	42	42	58	108	83	55	70
61	42	43	58				

National Committee for Clinical Laboratory Standards: Reference Procedure for the Erythrocyte Sedimentation Rate (ESR) Test, NCCLS Document H2-A2, Vol. 8, No. 3, 1988.

As previously stated, the reticulocytes spend approximately two to three days in the bone marrow before being released into the blood where they spend 1 day maturing in the peripheral circulation. Under some circumstances the marrow reticulocytes are released directly into the blood prior to maturation in the bone marrow. This is detected by nucleated red blood cells and/or polychromatophilic macrocytes (**shift cells**) present in the circulating blood. To correct for the increased time spent in maturation in the peripheral blood, the reticulocyte production index is calculated by dividing the corrected reticulocyte count by the number of days the reticulocyte most probably takes to mature in the blood. These times will vary, but are thought to be approximately one day in patients with a normal hematocrit, 1.5 days with a hematocrit of 35%, two days when the patient's hematocrit is in the range of 25%, and 3 days when the hematocrit level is at 15%. In patients with a normal hematocrit and showing no nucleated red cells or shift cells, the corrected reticulocyte count is divided by 1 (normal reticulocyte maturation time), and the reticulocyte production index is equal to the corrected reticulocyte count. If a patient has a hematocrit of 25% and has shift cells or nucleated red blood cells present in the peripheral blood, the corrected reticulocyte count may be divided by two in order to obtain the reticulocyte production index.

Reference

National Committee for Clinical Laboratory Standards, *Method for Reticulocyte Counting. Proposed standard.* Document #H16-P. NCCLS, Villanova, Pa., 1985.

Reagents and Equipment

1. New methylene blue stain solution.
   New methylene blue (CI 52030)   1.0 g
      (certified by the U.S. Biological
      Stain Commission)
   Sodium chloride   0.89 g
   Distilled water   100 mL
   Mix for at least 15 minutes, filter, and store at room temperature. Filter again on the day of use.
2. Glass slides.
3. Microhematocrit tubes.
4. Microscope.

Specimen

Whole blood (1 mL), using tripotassium EDTA as the anticoagulant. Capillary blood may also be used.

Principle

After the orthochromic normoblast loses its nucleus, a small amount of RNA remains in the red blood cell, and the cell is known as a reticulocyte. To detect the presence of RNA, the red blood cells must be stained while they are still living. This process is called **supravital staining.** Whole blood is incubated with new methylene blue. Smears of this mixture are then prepared and examined. The number of reticulocytes in 1000 red blood cells is determined. This number is divided by 10 to obtain the reticulocyte count in percent.

Procedure

1. Place three drops of filtered reticulocyte stain in a small test tube.
2. Add three drops of well-mixed whole blood to the tube containing the stain.
3. Mix the tube and allow to stand at room temperature, or incubate at 37°C, for 15 minutes. This allows the reticulocytes adequate time to take up the stain.
4. At the end of 15 minutes, mix the contents of the tube well.
5. Prepare several wedge or spun smears and allow to air dry.
6. Place the first slide on the microscope stage and, using the low power objective (10×), find an area in the thin portion of the smear in which the red blood cells are evenly distributed and are not touching each other. Carefully change to the oil immersion objective (100×) and further locate an area in which there are approximately 100 to 200 red blood cells per oil immersion field.
7. As soon as the proper area is selected, the reticulocytes may be counted. The red blood cells will be a light to medium green in color. The RNA present in the reticulocytes stains a deep blue. The reticulum may be abundant or sparse, depending on the cell's stage of development. The youngest reticulocyte shows

A

B

C

FIG. 3–21. Stages of maturation in the reticulocyte count.

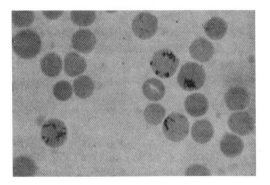

FIG. 3–22. Reticulocytes. (Supravital staining of the red blood cells with new methylene blue.) (Magnification ×1000.)

a larger amount of RNA (Fig. 3–21A), whereas the more mature reticulocyte shows only a small amount of RNA (Fig. 3–21C). Count all of the red blood cells in the first field on one cell counter. At the same time, enumerate the reticulocytes (Fig. 3–22) in the same field with a second cell counter. To be considered a reticulocyte the red cell must contain two or more blue-staining particles. Move the slide as described in the Differential Cell Count procedure, using the cross-sectional method, until all reticulocytes in 1000 red blood cells have been counted.

8. A second technologist may repeat the reticulocyte count in the same manner as described in step 7 on the second reticulocyte smear. The two results should agree within ±20% of each other. If they do not, repeat the reticulocyte count on the third smear.

9. Average the two results and calculate the reticulocyte count as shown below.

$$\% \text{ Reticulocytes} = \frac{\text{Number of reticulocytes in 1000 red blood cells}}{10}$$

10. Calculate the corrected reticulocyte count and the reticulocyte production index if applicable and/or desired.

Discussion

1. There are several methods for counting reticulocytes once the smears have been made: (1) A Miller disk may be placed inside the microscope eyepiece. This disk consists of two squares, as shown in Figures 3–23 and 3–24. The area of the smaller square (B) or (D) is one-ninth that of square A or C. When employing this method to count reticulocytes, the red blood cells in square B or D are counted in successive fields on the slide until a total of 20 fields have been counted. At

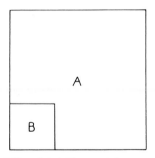

FIG. 3–23. Miller disk (older model).

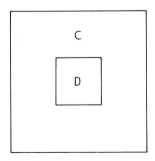

FIG. 3–24. Miller disk (newer model).

the same time, the reticulocytes in the large square A or C are enumerated. The reticulocyte count is then calculated by dividing the total number of reticulocytes counted by nine times the number of red blood cells counted in square B or D. The count may be performed in duplicate, using a second smear, and the results averaged to obtain the test value. (2) Place a small "window" in the eyepiece of the microscope. This makes the field smaller and the counting of cells easier. (Cut out a round piece of paper the same diameter as the eyepiece and cut a square hole in the center. Unscrew the top lens of the eyepiece, insert the paper, and replace the top lens.) (3) For reticulocyte counts less than 10%, count at least 100 reticulocytes (except in extremely low counts where this would not be practical). Instead of counting the number of red blood cells in every field, count the red blood cells in every 8 to 10 fields and also keep track of the number of fields examined. Calculate the reticulocyte count as follows:

$$\frac{\text{\# of RBC's}}{\text{examined}} = \frac{\dfrac{\text{\# of RBC's}}{\text{counted}}}{\dfrac{\text{\# of fields}}{\text{in which RBC's were counted}}} \times \frac{\text{\# of fields}}{\text{examined}}$$

$$\text{\% Reticulocytes} = \frac{\dfrac{\text{\# of retics.}}{\text{counted}}}{\dfrac{\text{\# of RBC's}}{\text{examined}}} \times 100$$

(4) Use of 15× eyepieces (instead of 10×) makes the field smaller and, at the same time, enables the technologist to see the reticulocytes much more clearly.

2. A tri-level reticulocyte control, Retic-Chex, is available from Streck Laboratories, Omaha, NE 68137.

3. When using EDTA as the anticoagulant, the blood may be stored for 24 hours prior to staining while still obtaining acceptable results. It is thought, however, that the reticulocyte count may tend to drop after 6 to 8 hours after obtaining the specimen.

4. Brilliant cresyl blue also stains reticulocytes but shows too much inconsistency in staining for routine use. Pure azure B, however, may be used in place of new methylene blue with good results (using the same stain concentration and procedure as described above).

5. The blood-to-stain ratio does not have to be exactly equal. For best results, a larger proportion of blood should be added to the stain when the patient's hematocrit is low. Add a smaller amount of blood to the stain when the patient has an unusually high hematocrit.

6. The time allowed for staining of the reticulocyte is not critical. It should not, however, be less than 10 minutes.

7. The presence of a high blood sugar (glucose) or the use of heparin as the anticoagulant may cause the reticulocytes to show pale staining.

8. It is advisable not to counterstain the reticulocyte smears with Wright stain because any precipitated stain may cause confusion in the identification of reticulocytes.

9. It is extremely important that the blood and stain be mixed well prior to making smears. The reticulocytes have a lower specific gravity than mature red blood cells and, therefore settle on top of the red blood cells in the mixture.

10. Red blood cells containing areas of high refractility may be noted on the smear. These cells should not be confused with reticulocytes. This condition is probably due to moisture in the air and poor drying of the smear.

11. There are several red blood cell inclusions that are stained by the new methylene blue stain, in addition to the RNA of the reticulocytes. Howell-Jolly bodies appear as one, sometimes two, round, deep purple staining structures. Heinz bodies stain a light blue green and are usually present at the peripheral edge of the red blood cell (Fig. 3–25). Pappenheimer bodies are most often confused with and most difficult to distinguish from reticulocytes. These purple staining deposits generally appear as several granules in a small cluster and will usually be a darker shade of blue than the reticulocyte. If Pappenheimer bodies are suspected, a Wright-stained smear may be examined to verify their presence. Hemoglobin H bodies will appear as round, greenish-blue inclusions.

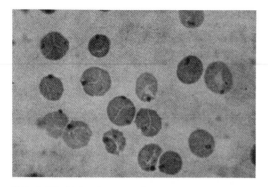

FIG. 3–25. Heinz bodies. (Supravital staining of red blood cells with new methylene blue. Compare with reticulocytes stained similarly.) (Magnification ×1000.)

12. The range of error in the reticulocyte count varies, depending on the number of reticulocytes counted. Using the previously outlined procedure, there is an error of approximately ±25% in the reticulocyte counts within the normal range. This decreases to ±10% in a reticulocyte count of 5% and decreases even further as the uncorrected reticulocyte count increases.

13. An automated procedure for counting reticulocytes using flow cytometry with fluorescent dyes is described in the Automation section. This method is more rapid, precise, and accurate than the manual procedure described here.

PLATELET COUNT

Platelet counts are important in helping to diagnose bleeding disorders. Platelets function primarily in hemostasis (the stoppage of bleeding) and in maintaining capillary integrity (injuries to capillary walls are plugged by platelets to inhibit bleeding and to maintain the sealing function of the capillary walls). The normal range for the platelet count is 150,000 to 400,000/µL (150 to 400 × 10⁹/L). An increased platelet count, **thrombocytosis,** is found in polycythemia vera, idiopathic thrombocythemia, chronic myelogenous leukemia, and following a splenectomy. A decreased platelet count, **thrombocytopenia,** occurs in thrombocytopenia purpura, aplastic anemia, acute leukemia, Gaucher's disease, pernicious anemia, and sometimes following chemotherapy and radiation therapy. A prolonged bleeding time and poor clot retraction are found when there is marked thrombocytopenia.

Platelets are difficult to count. They are small, disintegrate easily, and are hard to distinguish from dirt. They readily adhere to each other **(aggregation)** and also become easily attached to any foreign body **(adhesiveness).** The use of EDTA as an anticoagulant helps to decrease platelet clumping, but the mean platelet volume (MPV) will increase during the first hour in the tube. Although the MPV will be relatively stable for the next 8 hours, it is best to measure the MPV at 1 to 3 hours after obtaining the specimen. The platelets will eventually further increase in size. The larger platelet size may be due to its change from disc-shaped to a spherical form. Although fingertip (or heel) blood may be used, the results are generally less satisfactory and significantly lower than platelet counts performed on venous blood. (A significant number of the platelets are probably lost at the puncture site.)

There are two general methods for the direct counting of platelets. The phase microscope is employed in one method (outlined below) and an automated cell counter is the second procedure for enumerating platelets (the most accurate and reproducible). (See Automation section.)

Reference

Brecker, G., and Cronkite, E.P.: Morphology and enumeration of human blood platelets, J. Appl. Physiol., 3:365, 1950.

Reagents and Equipment

1. Platelet count Unopettes (containing ammonium oxalate). (Alternatively, the Thoma RBC pipet may be used.)

2. Ammonium oxalate, 1% (w/v), in distilled water (if Unopettes are not used). Store in refrigerator and filter before use.

3. Phase (thin, flat-bottomed) hemocytometer. (The hemocytometer used on a light microscope has a concave area on the underside, beneath the platform counting areas.) A thin disposable coverslip (#1 or #1½) should be used rather than the thick standard hemocytometer cover glass.

4. Glass slides.
5. Wright's stain and buffer.
6. Phase microscope.
7. Petri dish.
8. Filter paper.
9. Pipet rotator (if Thoma RBC pipet is used).

Specimen

Whole blood, using EDTA as the anticoagulant, is recommended. Blood from the fingertip (or heel) may be used if it is not feasible to draw venous blood. When obtaining a fingertip or heel specimen, the first small drop of blood following puncture should be wiped away. The platelet count should be obtained next, in duplicate, from a free-flowing drop of blood. The blood should not sit at the puncture site but should enter the diluting pipet as quickly as it flows from the wound in order to prevent platelet clumping or adhesion to the puncture site.

Principle

Whole blood is diluted with 1% ammonium oxalate, which hemolyzes the red blood cells. The platelets are then counted, using the phase hemocytometer and phase microscope. Results are double-checked by examination of the platelets on a Wright stained smear.

Procedure

1. Gently mix blood for approximately 2 minutes.
2. Check tube for clots. If present, a new specimen must be obtained.
3. Prepare a blood smear and Wright stain.
4. Make duplicate dilutions of the blood using platelet Unopettes. If the Thoma RBC pipet is used, draw blood up to the 1.0 mark and dilute to the 101 line with 1% ammonium oxalate. Prepare dilution in duplicate.
5. Mix the diluted blood samples for 10 to 15 minutes.
6. Clean the hemocytometer thoroughly and make certain it is completely free of all dirt and lint. The use of 95% (v/v) ethyl alcohol and a lint free cloth is recommended for this process.
7. Prepare a moist chamber as follows: obtain a Petri dish and a piece of filter paper

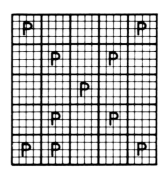

FIG. 3–26. Suggested squares to use for the platelet count.

of approximately the same diameter as the Petri dish. (Either the top or the bottom of the dish may be used.) Thoroughly moisten the filter paper and place in the top of the Petri dish so that it adheres to the dish.

8. When the diluted blood samples are adequately mixed, fill one side of the counting chamber with each dilution.
9. Place the moist chamber over the hemocytometer and allow the preparation to sit for 15 to 20 minutes. This allows time for the platelets to settle, and the moist cover prevents evaporation of the fluid in the counting chamber.
10. Place the hemocytometer on the phase microscope stage.
    a. Focus the large middle square of the hemocytometer under low power (10×).
    b. Carefully change to the 43× phase objective. The platelets appear as round or oval bodies with a light purplish sheen. When focusing up and down with the fine adjuster, the platelets may be seen to have one or more fine processes. Dirt and debris are distinguishable because of their high refractility.
    c. Count the platelets in 10 of the 25 small squares in the large central square. The suggested squares to use are those labeled with a P (Fig. 3–26).
    d. Enumerate the platelets in the same area on both sides of the counting chamber. The total number of platelets counted on each side should agree with each other by ± 10 when

the platelet count is in the normal range.

e. Add the two counts together and divide by 2 to determine the average number of platelets counted.

11. Calculate the number of platelets/L as shown below:

Plts/µL =   200

$$\frac{\text{Av \# plts counted} \times \text{Correction for dilution} \times \text{Correction for volume}}{}$$

Plts/L = plts/µL × 10⁶

12. A second technologist should scan a smear and estimate the platelet count. If the count does not reasonably agree with the estimate, the platelet count should be repeated. (If the platelets do not show even distribution on the smear, a second smear and platelet estimate may be made before repeating the count.)

Counted ÷ 10 × 10 × 200 ÷ 10 = _____ /µl

Discussion

1. If the concentration of EDTA exceeds 2 mg/mL of whole blood, the platelets may swell and then fragment, causing an invalidly higher count.

2. The blood should be diluted within 5 hours of obtaining the specimen, or within 24 hours if the blood has been stored at refrigerator temperature. Once the blood has been diluted with 1% ammonium oxalate, the dilution is stable for at least 8 hours.

3. As soon as the platelet count has been removed from the mixer, it should not stand for more than 8 to 10 seconds without being remixed.

4. It is imperative that the hemocytometer and pipets be scrupulously clean and the diluting fluid freshly filtered. There must be an even distribution of platelets in the counting chamber.

5. If clumps of platelets are noted in the platelet count, the procedure can be repeated because this may have been due to inadequate mixing. If poor technique was used in obtaining the blood specimen, a new sample should be obtained. Alternatively, a new specimen may be obtained using 0.109 M sodium citrate as the anticoagulant. If sodium citrate is used, final results must be multiplied by 1.1 to correct for the dilution of blood in the anticoagulant.

6. If fewer than 80 platelets are counted in the 10 small squares, all of the platelets in the large center square (25 small squares) on both sides of the hemocytometer should be counted. Then, if fewer than 50 platelets are counted per side, the platelet count may be repeated, diluting the original blood sample 1:20 using a white count pipet. For best results, a minimum of 100 platelets should be counted.

7. If the platelet count is extremely high, a dilution of 1:200 may be made, using the Thoma red count pipet.

8. With experience, it is possible to perform platelet counts by phase microscopy with a C.V. of 8% to 10%.

9. If a phase microscope is not available a routine bright light microscope may be used. The light in the microscopic field should not be too bright (move the condensor down). The platelets will appear as small, highly refractile bodies. When performing the platelet count on a bright light microscope, the blood should be diluted with Rees-Ecker diluting fluid (see below).

10. The Rees-Ecker platelet procedure utilizes brilliant cresyl blue staining solution: sodium citrate, 3.8 g; brilliant cresyl blue, 0.1 g; formaldehyde (37%), 0.2 mL; distilled water, 100 mL. This diluting fluid must be filtered before use. Follow the procedure as described above for diluting the blood and performing the count. This diluting fluid will not hemolyze the red blood cells. On the bright light microscope, platelets appear as small, round, oval, or elongated particles that are highly refractile and stain a light bluish color. The utmost care must be taken not to confuse the platelets with dirt or debris. Using this diluting fluid, the platelet count must be completed within 30 minutes of diluting in order to ensure against platelet disintegration.

11. The use of 15× eyepieces on the phase microscope greatly facilitates the counting of platelets.

EOSINOPHIL COUNT

Although the relative and absolute number of eosinophils in the blood may be determined from the WBC and differential white cell count, it is sometimes necessary to more accurately determine the total number of eosinophils/L of blood. The direct method for counting eosinophils is similar to the method used for the red and white blood cell counts.

The normal range for the eosinophil count is 50 to 350 $\times$ 10^6/L. A low eosinophil count (**eosinopenia**) is found in hyperadrenalism (Cushing's disease), shock, and following the administration of adrenocorticotropic hormone (ACTH). Increased numbers of eosinophils (**eosinophilia**) occur in allergic reactions, parasitic infestations, brucellosis, and certain leukemias. There may be considerable variation in the eosinophil count over a 24-hour period, with the lowest count generally present during late morning and the highest count present during the night (midnight and later).

There are two general methods for determining the absolute eosinophil count: the indirect method (white blood cell count multiplied by the percentage of eosinophils in the differential) and the direct method (described below). The most widely used procedure is to perform the eosinophil count by the direct method and double-check these results using the indirect method. This procedure is outlined below.

Reference

Randolph, T.G.: Differentiation and enumeration of eosinophils in the counting chamber with a glycol stain: A valuable technique in appraising ACTH dosage. J. Lab. Clin. Med., 34:1696, 1949.

Reagents and Equipment

1. Any one of the following diluting fluids may be employed.
   a. Phyloxine diluting fluid
Propylene glycol	50 mL
Distilled water	40 mL
Aqueous solution of phyloxine, 1%, w/v	10 mL
Aqueous solution of sodium carbonate, 10%, w/v	1 mL

Mix, filter, and store at room temperature. Stable for 1 month.
   b. Pilot's solution is prepared in the same manner as phyloxine diluting fluid (above) except that 100 units of heparin is added to the final mixture.
   c. Randolph's stain
      Solution 1
Methylene blue, 0.1% (w/v), in propylene glycol	50 mL
Distilled water	50 mL

      Solution 2
Phyloxine, 0.1% (w/v), in methylene blue	50 mL
Distilled water	50 mL

   Store solutions 1 and 2 at room temperature. Prior to use, mix equal volumes of both solutions together. This mixture is stable for 4 hours.
2. The eosinophil Unopette (contains phyloxine B as the diluting fluid) or the Thoma WBC pipet may be used.
3. Counting chamber. There are three counting chambers available for use in the eosinophil count.
   a. Hemocytometer with Neubauer ruling was previously described for the red and white blood cell counts. However, it is not recommended for the eosinophil count because of its relatively small volume.
   b. Fuchs-Rosenthal counting chamber (Fig. 3–27) consists of two platforms, or counting areas. The chamber is 0.2 mm deep. Each ruled counting area consists of 1 large square, 4 mm $\times$ 4 mm $\times$ 0.2 mm, or 3.2 μL in volume. The large square is divided into 16 smaller squares, each of which is 1 mm long and 1 mm wide. Each of these squares is further subdivided into 16 smaller squares.
   c. Speirs-Levy hemocytometer (Fig. 3–28) consists of four platforms, or counting areas. The chamber is 0.2 mm deep. Each counting area consists of 10 squares, 1 mm long and 1 mm wide, arranged in 2 horizontal rows of 5 squares. Each of these 10 squares is further subdivided into 16 smaller squares. The volume of 1 counting

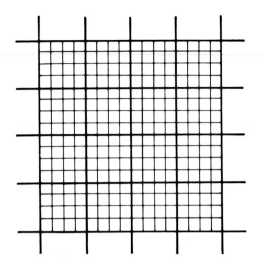

FIG. 3–27. Fuchs-Rosenthal counting chamber.

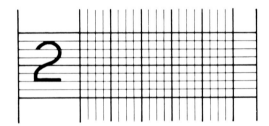

FIG. 3–28. Speirs-Levy counting chamber.

area is 2 mm × 5 mm × 0.2 mm, or 2.0 μL.
4. Microscope.
5. Moist chamber.
6. Glass slides.
7. Wright's stain and buffer.

Specimen

Collect 1 mL of whole blood using EDTA or heparin as the anticoagulant. Capillary blood may also be used.

Principle

Whole blood is diluted with stain solution. The phyloxine present in the diluting fluid serves to stain the eosinophils red; the sodium carbonate and water help to lyse the white blood cells (except the eosinophils); and the red blood cells are lysed by the propylene glycol. Heparin, if present in the diluting fluid, prevents clumping of the white blood cells. The sodium carbonate also enhances the staining of the eosinophil granules.

Procedure

1. If the eosinophil Unopette is used, draw the blood up in a 25-μL pipet and dilute in the Unopette (1:32 dilution). If using a Thoma white count pipet, draw the blood up to the 1.0 mark. Wipe off the outside of the pipet carefully. Draw the eosinophil diluting fluid up to the 11 mark to make a 1:10 dilution.
2. Repeat step 1, making a second dilution on the same specimen.
3. Mix both Unopettes (or Thoma pipets) for 2 minutes.
4. Fill one side of the counting chamber. Repeat, using the second dilution, and fill the opposite side of the chamber. (If the Speirs-Levy counting chamber is used, fill both counting areas on one side with the first dilution and the two opposite counting areas with the second dilution.)
5. Place a moist chamber (Petri dish with a piece of wet filter paper in the top) over the filled counting chamber.
6. Allow 15 minutes for the cells to settle. Lysis of the red and white blood cells and staining of the eosinophils also take place during this time.
7. Using the low-power objective (10×), count the eosinophils (stained red):
   a. Hemocytometer with Neubauer ruling: count the entire ruled area on both sides of the counting chamber. This gives a total volume counted of 1.8 μL.
   b. Fuchs-Rosenthal counting chamber: count the entire ruled area on both sides of the counting chamber. This gives a total volume counted of 6.4 μL.
   c. Speirs-Levy counting chamber: count the entire ruled area on two platforms, one on each side of the counting chamber. This gives a total volume counted of 4 μL.
8. Calculate the number of eosinophils/L as shown below:

$$\text{Eosinophils/L} = \frac{\text{Eosinophils}}{\text{counted}} \times \frac{\text{Correction}}{\text{for dilution}}$$

$$\times \frac{\text{Correction}}{\text{for volume of} \atop \text{chamber used}} \times 10^6$$

9. Double-check the direct eosinophil count:
   a. Perform a white blood cell count on the specimen of blood. Make two blood smears and Wright stain.
   b. Perform a 200-cell differential white count on the blood smear.
   c. Calculate the indirect eosinophil count as follows:

Eosinophils/L =
$$\frac{\text{Percent Eosinophils in differential}} {} \times \text{WBC/L}$$

   d. The results obtained should correlate with the eosinophil count by the direct method. If there is too large a variation, repeat the direct and indirect eosinophil counts.

Discussion

1. A single eosinophil count may be ordered on a patient, or, the eosinophil counts may be ordered in conjunction with the Thorn test for adrenal cortical function. This test, however, is rarely performed.
2. The indirect method for counting eosinophils is not as accurate as the direct method. Therefore, a close correlation between the results of the two methods is not always possible.
3. Once the eosinophil count is diluted, it should be counted within 30 minutes. The eosinophils will easily disintegrate in the diluting fluid if left diluted for too long a period of time. If the Unopette is used, the count should be completed within 1 hour of being diluted.
4. To improve the accuracy of the direct eosinophil count at least 100 eosinophils should be enumerated. In order to do this, the counting chamber may be filled and counted as many times as necessary. The C.V. of the eosinophil count when at least 100 cells are counted is about 10%.

SICKLE CELL TESTS

Sickle cell anemia and sickle cell trait are caused by hemoglobin S, an abnormal form of hemoglobin. In the presence of hemoglobin S, the red blood cells take on a sickle-like shape when the oxygen supply to the red cell is decreased. The degree of sickling depends on the concentration of hemoglobin S in the red blood cell. When the concentration of hemoglobin S is 80 to 100% (as in sickle cell anemia), sickling of the red cell occurs readily at only slightly reduced oxygen concentrations. When the concentration of hemoglobin S is only 20 to 40% (as in the sickle cell trait), oxygen concentrations must be much lower before sickling occurs. Other sickling hemoglobins include hemoglobins C_{HARLEM}, S_{TRAVIS}, and $C_{ZIGUINCHOR}$.

The sickling phenomenon may be demonstrated in the laboratory by depriving the red blood cells of oxygen. Further information on hemoglobin S is given in the Disease section of this book.

Sodium Metabisulfite Method

Reference

Daland, G.A., and Castle, W.B.: A simple and rapid method for demonstrating sickling of the red blood cells: The use of reducing agents. J. Lab. Clin. Med., 33:1082, 1948.

Reagents and Equipment

1. Sodium metabisulfite, 2% (w/v).
   Sodium metabisulfite   0.2 g
   Distilled water   10 mL
   Stable for 8 hours at room temperature.
2. Syringe (5 mL) filled with petroleum jelly.
3. 19-gauge needle.
4. Glass slide.
5. Cover glass.
6. Microscope.

Specimen

Whole blood, using EDTA or heparin as the anticoagulant. Capillary blood may also be used.

Principle

Whole blood is mixed with sodium metabisulfite, a strong reducing agent which deoxygenates the hemoglobin. Under these conditions, hemoglobin S present in the red blood cell causes the formation of sickle shaped red cells.

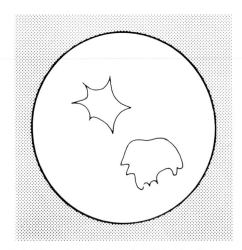

FIG. 3–29. Holly-leaf shaped red blood cells.

Procedure

1. Place one drop of the blood to be tested on a glass slide.
2. Add one to two drops of 2% sodium metabisulfite to the drop of blood (two drops if the hemoglobin is normal, a single drop if the hemoglobin is decreased) and mix well with an applicator stick.
3. Place a cover glass on top of the sample and press down lightly on it to remove any air bubbles and to form a thin layer of the mixture. Wipe off the excess sample.
4. Using a syringe and 19-gauge needle, carefully rim the cover glass with the petroleum jelly, completely sealing the mixture under the coverslip.
5. Examine the preparation for the presence of sickle cells after 1 hour, using the high dry objective (40×). (Take care that when the objective is changed to high dry, it does not come in contact with the petroleum jelly.) In some instances, the red blood cells may take on a 'holly-leaf' form, as shown in Figure 3–29. This shape is often found in the sickle cell trait, and, when present, the test is reported as positive.
6. If there is no sickling present at the end of 1 hour, allow the preparation to stand at room temperature for 24 hours and reexamine at that time.
7. When sickle cells or the 'holly-leaf' form of the red blood cells are present, the results are reported as positive. Normal looking red blood cells or slightly crenated red blood cells are reported as negative.

Discussion

1. The sickle cells or the 'holly-leaf' form of the cell must come to a point or points to be considered positive. Elongated cells with a rounded end must not be confused with sickle cells.
2. Sickling of the red blood cells is maximal at 37°C and decreases as the temperature lowers.
3. With this method, it is not possible to distinguish sickle cell trait from sickle cell anemia. (In sickle cell anemia, however, the sickling reaction occurs more rapidly than in sickle cell trait. This, however, must not be relied upon to differentiate between the two conditions.) If the sickle cell preparation is positive, it is advisable to perform a hemoglobin electrophoresis to determine the presence of the trait or the anemia and to positively identify the type of sickling hemoglobin present.
4. Either sodium metabisulfite or sodium bisulfite may be used interchangeably in this procedure.
5. It is advantageous to run a positive control each time this test is performed in case the reagent has deteriorated.
6. This test should not be performed on infants less than 6 months old.

Solubility Test

References

Nalbandian, R.M., Nichols, B.M., Camp, F.R., Jr., Lusher, J.M., Conte, N.F., Henry, R.L., and Wolf, P.L.: Dithionite tube test—a rapid, inexpensive technique for the detection of hemoglobin. Clin. Chem., *17*:1028, 1971.

National Committee for Clinical Laboratory Standards, *Solubility test for confirming the presence of sickling hemoglobins,* Document #H10-A, NCCLS, Villanova, Pa., 1986.

Reagents and Equipment

1. Stock solution

Dibasic potassium phosphate, anhydrous (K_2HPO_4)	216 g
Monobasic potassium phosphate, crystals (KH_2PO_4)	169 g

Saponin 10 g

Place approximately 500 mL of distilled water into a one liter volumetric flask. Add the dibasic potassium phosphate and mix until dissolved. Add the remaining reagents, one at a time, dissolving each one in the mixture before adding the next reagent. This solution is stable for approximately one month stored at 4°C.

2. Work ing solution
   Stock solution 10 mL
   Sodium hydrosulfite (dithionite) 50 mg
   ($Na_2S_2O_4$)

Prepare fresh, on the day of testing. Pre-prepared reagent is available commercially from most laboratory supply companies.
3. Test tubes, 12 × 75 mm.
4. Lined reader scale. This may be prepared by obtaining a piece of white cardboard and drawing 14- or 18-point black type parallel lines approximately 0.5 cm apart.
5. Pipets, 2.0 mL and 10 μL.
6. Positive and negative controls.

Specimen

Whole blood, using EDTA, heparin, or sodium citrate as the anticoagulant. Specimen may be up to 3 weeks old.

Principle

When red blood cells are added to the working solution, the red cells immediately lyse due to the saponin present. Hemoglobin S (and sickling hemoglobins), in the reduced state, in a concentrated buffer solution, forms liquid crystals and yields a turbid appearance.

Procedure

1. Centrifuge a small portion (1 mL) of whole blood at 1500 to 2000 g for 5 minutes. Remove the plasma and buffy coat layers.
2. Make certain the stock solution is at room temperature. Prepare the working solution and add 2 mL of the working solution to a 12 × 75 mm test tube for each patient and control to be tested.
3. Add 10 μL of the centrifuged red blood cells to each appropriately labeled tube. Mix.

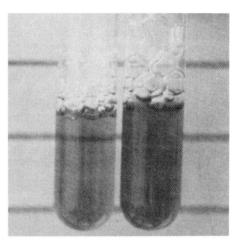

FIG. 3–30. Sodium dithionite tube test. (Negative results are indicated by the clear solution, where the black lines on the reader scale are visible through the test solution. Positive results are shown as a turbid solution, where the reader scale is not visible through the test solution.)

4. Allow tubes to stand at room temperature for 5 to 6 minutes.
5. Place the tube approximately 1 inch in front of the lined reader scale. If there is no sickling hemoglobin present, the solution will be clear and the lines on the reader scale will be visible through the solution. If a sickling hemoglobin is present, the solution will be turbid and the scale will not be visible through the solution (Fig. 3–30).
6. If the lines on the reader scale are visible through the test solution, report the results as negative. Failure to see the lines because of turbidity indicates a positive test.

Discussion

1. Whole blood may be used for this procedure, in which case, 20 μL of whole blood is added to 2.0 mL of working solution. However, when whole blood is used, the results are more liable to false negatives or false positives: hemoglobins of less than 7 g/dL will cause false negative results, whereas increased globulins, lipemia, and extremely high hemoglobins or white cell counts may cause false positive test results.

2. If the solubility test is positive, a hemoglobin electrophoresis should be performed on the specimen. Conversely, hemoglobin electrophoresis results showing the presence of hemoglobin S should be verified by a positive solubility test.

3. The purity of the saponin reagent is important. Fisher saponin has been found to be effective in this procedure. Also, care should be taken in handling the anhydrous dibasic potassium phosphate. This reagent absorbs moisture upon excessive exposure to the air.

4. The size of the test tube is important. Use of 10 × 75 mm test tubes may result in false negative results.

5. Infants less than 6 months old should not be tested by this method.

6. A positive solubility test may be found in hemoglobin Bart's.

7. Deterioration of reagents is an important factor in causing false negative and false positive results. It is, therefore, important to use positive and negative controls each time this procedure is performed. An incorrect result may also occur if the reagent is not at room temperature.

Hemocard Hb A and S Procedure

Isolab Inc. (Akron, Ohio) manufactures a monoclonal antibody based immunoassay for determining the presence of hemoglobin S (sickle cell anemia or trait). This procedure detects hemoglobin S in concentrations as small as 3.5% (in a blood sample with a hemoglobin of 7.5 g/dL). Where the minimum age for hemoglobin S detection is 3 to 6 months for other methods, the blood of newborns may be accurately tested using this procedure.

References

Isolab Inc.: Hemocard Hb A and S monoclonal antibody based assay, Isolines, 20, 1991.
Isolab Inc.: Hemocard Hemoglobin A and S, pkg. insert, Isolab Inc., Akron, OH, 1991.

Reagents and Equipment

1. The following materials are obtainable from Isolab Inc. All reagents should be stored at 2 to 8°C.

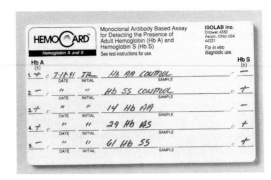

FIG. 3–31. HemoCard. (Courtesy of Isolab, Inc., Akron, OH.)

   a. Sample conditioner (contains methanol, surfactant, phosphate buffer, and sodium azide).

   b. Wash solution (contains the same reagents as the sample conditioner in addition to bromthymol blue and methyl red, sodium salt).

   c. Hb A reagent (contains bovine albumin and antibodies to hemoglobin A, which are adsorbed to metal sol particles).

   d. Hb S reagent (contains bovine albumin and antibodies to hemoglobin S, which are adsorbed to metal sol particles).

   e. HemoCard (Fig. 3–31).

   f. Hemoglobin A and hemoglobin S controls.

   g. Sample cups.

2. Pipets, 2.0 mL, 15 μL, 5 μL, and 2 μL.

3. Transfer pipets (pipet droppers capable of transferring volumes of 55 to 75 μL volumes).

4. Test tubes, 10 × 75 mm with caps.

Specimen

Whole blood using EDTA as the anticoagulant. Capillary blood may also be used, collecting blood in two heparinized microhematocrit tubes or the capillary specimen may be collected on filter paper (Schlelcher and Schuell, grade 903 or equivalent) by placing a drop of whole blood (minimum diameter of ⅛ inch) on the filter paper. Testing may also be performed on cord blood. Whole blood may be stored for 7 days at 2 to 8°C, or, may be frozen at −20°C for up to 30 days. Filter paper specimens may be stored in a plastic bag at 2 to 8°C for up to 60 days.

Principle

The red blood cells are hemolyzed using the sample conditioner reagent. The hemoglobin A and S reagents contain monoclonal antibodies (IgG), which specifically bind to the amino acids at or near the sixth position of the globin chain of hemoglobin A and hemoglobin S. The antibodies are adsorbed to suspended metal sol particles, which give the reagent its raspberry-like color. Hemoglobin S has a substitution of valine for glutamic acid at the sixth position on the β chain. Because of this, the hemoglobin S monoclonal antibody will react with this chain but the hemoglobin A reagent will not. In reverse, the hemoglobin S reagent will not react with hemoglobin A because it contains glutamic acid in the sixth position on the β chain, while the hemoglobin A reagent will react. Hemoglobin C has a substitution of lysine for glutamic acid at the sixth position and will therefore not react with either the hemoglobin A or hemoglobin S monoclonal antibody. However, other hemoglobin variants (other than hemoglobins S and C) will most likely give a false positive result for hemoglobin A because they have amino acid substitutions that do not occur at the sixth position. A positive result in this procedure is indicated by a raspberry red color on the HemoCard after being rinsed with the wash solution, because of the fact that the reagent (antibody) adheres to the globin chain.

Procedure

1. Label one 10 × 75 mm test tube for each sample to be tested. Place 2 mL of sample conditioner into each tube. Add 2 μL whole blood to the appropriately labelled tube.
2. Cap tube and mix well. Allow to stand at room temperature for a minimum of 10 minutes (maximum of 60 minutes).
3. Label two sample cups for each sample being tested (A and S). Add 5 μL of diluted sample to each appropriately labelled sample cup. (If the specimen is from a newborn, add 15 μL of the diluted sample to

the cup [due to low concentration of non-F hemoglobin]).
4. Add one drop of well mixed hemoglobin A reagent to the A sample cup for each sample being tested. Add one drop of well mixed hemoglobin S reagent to each S sample. Mix each cup carefully and allow to stand at room temperature for 2 minutes.
5. Using a dropper pipet, transfer the contents of the hemoglobin A sample cups to the corresponding hemoglobin A sample wells on the left side of the HemoCard. Add one drop of wash solution to each of the wells used. (Wipe away any sample that may have dropped on the surface of the card.)
6. Repeat step 5 above, adding the contents of the S cups to the hemoglobin S wells on the right side of the HemoCard. Add one drop of wash solution to each of the wells used.
7. Within 5 minutes or less, compare the hemoglobin A results to the hemoglobin A control well and the hemoglobin S results to the S control well. A positive result is indicated by a red or pink color in the well. If the well is white, gray, or greenish in color, the test is negative for that hemoglobin type.
8. Interpretation of results. Patients positive for hemoglobin S and positive for hemoglobin A are considered to have sickle cell trait. Results showing a positive hemoglobin S and a negative hemoglobin A are most probably indicative of sickle cell anemia. As noted above, exceptions to these interpretations will occur with other hemoglobin variants (non-A, S, C hemoglobins) giving false positive results for hemoglobin A because glutamic acid is in the sixth position of the amino acid chain.

Discussion

1. If the specimen was collected on filter paper, cut out a circle of the blood ⅛ inch in diameter and add to 2 mL of sample conditioner. Mix and allow specimen to sit at room temperature for 20 to 25 minutes. Remix and remove the filter paper. Testing should continue within the next 35 minutes. Mix just prior to use.

2. The hemoglobin concentration of the patient sample must be within the range of 7.5 to 22.5 g/dL in order to obtain valid test results. If the hemoglobin is less than 7.5 g/dL double the amount of specimen added to the sample conditioner, and if higher than 22.5 g/dL, half the amount of sample is used for testing.

3. Recently transfused blood will show up in this test. (A patient with sickle cell anemia, for example, who has recently received a blood transfusion will be positive for hemoglobin A.)

4. The results of this test should be confirmed using other methods, such as hemoglobin electrophoresis and agar gel.

5. Studies carried out by Isolab Inc. show that the limit of detectability for hemoglobin S (lowest concentration at which most of the hemoglobin S samples were positive) is 1.08%, although the test is only quality controlled to a detection limit of 3.5%.

SPECIAL HEMATOLOGY PROCEDURES

4

EXAMINATION OF THE BONE MARROW

Examination of the bone marrow is a widely used method of diagnosing many hematologic disorders. Because the bone marrow is the central area for the production of blood cells, it is therefore the best source for studying the production and maturation of these cells. It is a valuable tool for use in disorders wherein diagnostic cells are present in the bone marrow but absent in the peripheral blood. Such conditions are found in Gaucher's disease, multiple myeloma, Niemann-Pick disease, some megaloblastic anemias, and when tumor cells are metastasizing (spreading) from other organs of the body. When pancytopenia exists, a bone marrow examination is helpful to rule out the diagnosis of leukemia and, where possible, to determine the cause of the reduction in the formed elements of the blood. In addition to determining the presence of specific cells, the bone marrow procedure offers the opportunity for assessing the iron stores and cellularity of the marrow. When anemia is present, examination of the marrow is an aid in evaluating abnormalities in erythropoiesis. Alterations in the normal distribution of cells may be noted, and the marrow cells may also be studied with special staining techniques.

Bone marrow aspiration is performed by a physician and may be obtained by needle biopsy (most frequently performed method), a surgical biopsy, or a percutaneous (entering through the skin) trepine (a trepine is a small object/instrument used to remove a circular section of tissue) biopsy (i.e., a core of bone with accompanying marrow is obtained). Samples of bone marrow may be obtained from the sternum, the iliac crest, the spinous process of the lumbar vertebrae, and from the tibia in children under 2 years of age. The usual site of puncture in adults is the sternum, in the midline of the bone between the second and third ribs. The anterior or posterior iliac crest is also a common site for bone marrow biopsy. This area is advantageous in that there are no vital organs near the site of puncture and the patient is unable to see what is happening, which is helpful if the person is apprehensive.

Usually a 0.3 mL to 0.5 mL specimen is obtained. A small aspiration of marrow is generally representative of the entire bone marrow. As a rule, the marrow sample obtained will be unavoidably diluted with some peripheral blood. Smears of the aspirated marrow are prepared immediately after the specimen is obtained. In addition, histologic sections may be prepared, the specimen may be cultured for chromosomal analysis, and the marrow may be processed for electron microscopy studies. Once the slides are stained the smears are examined microscopically by the pathologist, with or without the aid of a technologist.

Preparation of the Bone Marrow for Study

The exact procedures to be followed in preparing the bone marrow for study will vary between laboratories and will depend on the clinical history and possible diagnosis of the patient. The most frequently used techniques are outlined below.

1. As soon as the bone marrow specimen is aspirated, it should be expelled onto a

127

glass slide or watch glass. A variety of smears may be prepared (all slides should be made as quickly as possible before the marrow specimen clots). (Alternatively, the marrow may be placed in a tube containing EDTA to prevent clotting. The specimen may then be returned to the laboratory for smear preparation. However, if the blood is anticoagulated smears should be prepared as soon as possible before cell morphology is altered by the anticoagulant.)

a. Prepare direct wedge or coverslip smear(s) by transferring a small drop of specimen to appropriate slides or coverslips. When the smears are made in this manner a characteristic marrow smear will show fat (small, irregular holes in the film) throughout the slide, and there should be numerous small marrow particles, most often found at the peripheral (feathered) end of the smear. Lack of these two characteristics usually indicates that there is little to no marrow in the specimen and it is primarily peripheral blood.

b. Prepare a particle smear. Place several marrow particles at one end of a clean glass slide (or add a small drop of marrow to the slide and aspirate the fluid portion of the specimen from the slide). Using a spreader slide, draw the slide back into the particles. As soon as the slide has come in contact with the particles push the spreader across the slide. This should deposit a trail of marrow cells on the slide behind the spreader.

c. Crushed particle smears may also be prepared. Transfer several of the marrow particles from the pool of marrow in the watch glass onto three or four slides or coverslips using the broken end of an applicator stick. Place a coverslip or slide over these particles and then gently pull apart with a smooth motion. If desired, the particles may be further crushed by squeezing the slides/coverslips together before pulling apart. However, distortion of the cells frequently occurs using the above procedures; also, the smear may be too thick for adequate staining.

d. When the pool of marrow remaining on the original slide has clotted, transfer this to a small bottle of suitable fixative for the cytology department, where stained sections of the clot can be made. The imprint of the specimen left on the slide may also be stained. This has been termed a "touch prep."

2. Several routine peripheral blood smears from the patient should be prepared on the same day as the bone marrow aspiration. (The fingerstick procedure may be preferrable in order to avoid any possible cellular distortion caused by an anticoagulant.) It is also helpful to obtain a complete blood count, platelet count, and reticulocyte count at the same time.

3. If an anticoagulated bone marrow specimen was prepared, it may be placed in a Wintrobe tube and centrifuged at $1500 \times$ g for 10 minutes. Once centrifuged, four layers may be seen (from top to bottom: fat, plasma, platelets and nucleated cells, red blood cells). The relative volume of fat and nucleated cells may be determined, although it should be noted that bone marrow may be diluted with peripheral blood by as much as 40 to 100%. Marrow concentrate (buffy coat) smears may then be prepared from this specimen:

a. Remove the plasma and fat layers from the Wintrobe tube. Using a clean, disposable dropper, withdraw the nucleated cell layer, dilute with an equal volume of the plasma, mix, and make several smears of this material.

4. The above smears may then be Wright-stained:

a. Thin direct smears.
b. Particle smears.
c. Crushed smears.
d. Concentrate (buffy coat) smears.
e. Peripheral blood smears.
(When Wright staining bone marrow smears, it is advisable to fix the smears in methanol for 20 to 25 minutes, especially when there is increased marrow cellularity. Increasing the staining times may also prove helpful.

5. It is often advisable to routinely stain a concentrate smear for iron (Prussian blue stain). Other stains in widespread use for bone marrow aspirates are the peroxidase, Sudan black B, and the periodic acid-Schiff, among others. The stains requested

depend on the possible diagnosis of the patient.

6. The sections of clot prepared by the cytology department are generally stained with the hematoxylin and eosin stain in addition to special stains as indicated.
7. Preparation of bone marrow smears from autopsy specimens. In order to better preserve the blood cells, the marrow obtained at postmortem examination may be suspended in bovine albumin prior to smear preparation.
   a. Obtain 5% bovine albumin (dilute one part bovine albumin with five parts of 0.85% w/v sodium chloride).
   b. Add 1 to 2 mL of 5% bovine albumin to a small piece of marrow. Mix gently.
   c. Centrifuge the mixture at moderate speed for 5 to 10 minutes. Remove the excess supernatant.
   d. Leave the volume of supernatant in the tube slightly less than the amount of centrifuged marrow.
   e. Mix the tube gently but well. Place a small drop of the mixture on each slide and prepare smears.

TABLE 4–1. NORMAL RANGES FOR THE BONE MARROW IN ADULTS

Cell	Percent
Myeloblast	0.3–4.0
Promyelocyte	1.0–5.0
Myelocytes	
Neutrophil	5.0–19.0
Eosinophil	0.5–3.0
Basophil	0.0–0.5
Metamyelocytes	13.0–32.0
Neutrophils	7.0–25.0
Eosinophils	0.5–4.0
Basophils	0.0–0.7
Lymphocytes	3.0–20.0
Monocytes	0.5–3.0
Megakaryocytes	0.1–3.0
Plasma cells	0.1–3.0
Reticulum cells	0.1–2.0
Pronormoblast	1.0–5.0
Basophilic normoblast Polychromatophilic normoblast Orthochromic normoblast	7.0–32.0
Mitotic cells	0.0–2.0
Myeloid:erythroid ratio	2:1–5:1

Examination of Marrow Slides

Bone marrow slides are studied and reported by the pathologist, with or without the aid of a technologist experienced in this area of hematology.

1. The histologic bone marrow section (prepared by the histology department) gives a better picture of the marrow architecture than the direct or particle smears. It also yields a more reliable estimate of the relative marrow cellularity and number of megakaryocytes present. Although not as well defined as in the marrow films, some abnormal cells may be detected, if present; differentiation between myeloid and erythroid cells is also possible.
2. The prepared bone marrow slides should first be examined macroscopically and those smears containing visible marrow particles chosen for study.
3. Microscopic examination of the Wright-stained smears.
   a. Using a particle smear (particles pulled across the slide) an estimate of the cellularity may be made using the low power (10×) objective. A hypocellular marrow will show less than 25% of the marrow occupied by cells, whereas in a hypercellular marrow the cells make up 75% or more of the marrow.
   b. The marrow slides should be scanned further using the low power (10×) objective to look for megakaryocytes, abnormal or malignant cells, mast cells, plasma cells, osteoblasts, and osteoclasts.
   c. Using the oil immersion (50× or 100×) objective, a differential count may be performed. At least 500 to 1000 cells should be counted. Because of the irregular distribution of marrow cells on the smear and the possibility of dilution with peripheral blood an accurate differential may be difficult to obtain. Results and normal value charts (Table 4–1) must therefore be interpreted accordingly. As the differential is being performed the cells should also be examined for morphologic abnormalities, abnormal cells, and abnormal maturation of the cells.

TABLE 4–2. APPLICATIONS OF CYTOCHEMICAL STAINS

Stain	Purpose
Leukocyte Alkaline Phosphatase (LAP)	Stains alkaline phosphatase present in the neutrophil, and to a small degree, in certain B Lymphocytes. Helpful in differentiating chronic myelogenous leukemia from a leukemoid reaction or polycythemia vera.
Peroxidase	Stains peroxidases present in the granulocytes and monocytes. Used to differentiate acute myelogenous and monocytic leukemias from acute lymphocytic leukemia.
Sudan Black B	Stains lipids present in the monocytes and granulocytes. Used to differentiate acute myelogenous and myelomonocytic leukemias from acute lymphocytic leukemia.
Chloroacetate Esterase	Stains esterases present in the granulocytes. Used to differentiate granulocytic cells from monocytic cells.
Nonspecific Esterase	Stains esterases in the monocytic cells, macrophages, megakaryocytes, and platelets. Used to differentiate monocytic leukemias from granulocytic leukemias.
Periodic Acid-Schiff	Stains mucoproteins, glycoproteins, and high molecular weight carbohydrates normally present in almost all blood cell types except pronormoblasts. Used to help in the diagnosis of DiGuglielmo's syndrome and may be an aid, when used in conjunction with other stains, to classify some acute leukemias.
Acid Phosphatase	Stains acid phosphatase present in the myelogenous cells, lymphocytes, plasma cells, monocytes, and platelets. Using L(+) tartaric acid, the stain is helpful in diagnosing hairy cell leukemia.

When the differential is complete the myeloid/erythroid ratio may be determined.

4. The patient's history, peripheral blood count, and smear should be studied. Reticulocyte and platelet counts may also prove helpful.
5. The Prussian blue stained concentrate smear may be examined, and an estimate made of the sideroblasts and particulate iron present.
6. Further special stains may be performed and examined based on the history of the patient and the appearance of the marrow smears. (See Tables 4–2 and 4–3.)

IRON STAIN (PRUSSIAN BLUE REACTION)

Siderotic granules are normally found in the cytoplasm of developing red blood cells in the bone marrow and represent iron (in the ferric state [Fe^{+3}]) not yet incorporated into hemoglobin. These granules may be stained with Perl's reagent (potassium ferrocyanide-hydrochloric acid) which is known as the Prussian blue reaction. Red blood cells that have one or more of these granules are termed **siderocytes**, whereas **sideroblasts** are nucleated red blood cells containing the siderotic granules. **Pappenheimer bodies** are thought to be structurally identical to siderotic granules and may be observed in Wright-stained blood smears as dark-staining dots in the red blood cell. Siderotic granules are found in 20 to 60% of the nucleated red blood cells in the bone marrow. They are also found in some marrow reticulocytes but are not normally present in the mature red blood cell of the peripheral blood.

Normally, all of the iron found in the cytoplasm of nucleated red blood cells is used in the production of hemoglobin. If, however, the synthesis of hemoglobin is disturbed

TABLE 4–3. CYTOCHEMICAL STAINING CHARACTERISTICS OF BLOOD/BONE MARROW CELLS AND PLATELETS (− = negative, + = positive, −/+ = negative to weakly positive)

Cell	LAP	Peroxidase	Sudan Black B	PAS	Chloroacetate	NonSpec. no Fl.	NonSpec. with Fl.	Acid Phosphatase	Acid Phosphatase with L(+)T
					Esterase Stains				
Myeloblast	−	−/+	−/+	−/+	−/+	−/+	−	−/+	−
Promyelocyte	−	+	+	−/+	+	−/+	−	−/+	−
Myelocyte	−	+	+	−/+	+	−/+	−	+	−
Neutrophil	+	+	+	+	+	−/+	−	+	−
Eosinophil	−	+	+	+	−	−	−	+	−
Basophil	−	−/+	−/+	+	−/+	−	−	−/+	−
Lymphocyte	−/+	−	−	−/+	−	−/+	−/+	−/+	−/+
Monocyte	−	−/+	−/+	−/+	−/+	+	−	+	−
Megakaryocyte	−	−	−	+	−	+	−/+	+	−
Platelet	−	−	−	+	−	+	−	+	−
Pronormoblast	−	−	−	−	−	−/+	−/+	+	−
Hairy Cells	−	−	−	−/+	−	−/+	−/+	+	+

this may result in iron stores remaining in the mature red blood cell, along with an increase in the size and number of these granules. In sideroblastic anemias, the granules may be arranged in a ring around the nucleus of the nucleated red blood cell (**ringed sideroblast**). The iron stores of the body and the serum iron level are related to the percentage of sideroblasts in the bone marrow. In iron deficiency anemia, in which the iron stores are markedly decreased, the number of marrow sideroblasts is also reduced. Siderocytes are usually present in the peripheral blood following splenectomy because the spleen, as one of its functions, removes the red blood cell from the circulation until heme synthesis is complete. The spleen may also remove these granules from the red blood cell. Siderocytes will also be increased in leukemia, alcoholism, hemolytic anemia, and megaloblastic anemia.

Reference

Lillie, R.D., and Fullmer, H.M.: *Histopathologic Technic and Practical Histochemistry,* New York, McGraw-Hill Book Co., 1976.

Reagents and Equipment

1. Methyl alcohol, Mallinckrodt (absolute anhydrous, acetone free).
2. Prussian-blue reagent.

Potassium ferrocyanide	2.0 g
Distilled water	36 mL
Hydrochloric acid, concentrated	4 mL

Use immediately after preparation.
3. Buffered neutral red, 1% w/v in acetate buffer, 0.1 N, pH 5.0.
4. Coplin jars, 2.
5. Coverslips.
6. Pro-texx mounting medium (Baxter, Scientific Products Division), or equivalent.

Specimen

Air dried blood or bone marrow slides.

Principle

Prussian-blue reagent stains nonheme iron (ferric [Fe^{+3}] ion) a vivid blue or green color. Nuclei and red cells are stained red or pink by the neutral red.

Procedure

1. Fix blood or bone marrow smears by flooding the slide with methanol for 30 seconds. Allow to air dry.
2. Place the smears in a coplin jar containing Prussian-blue reagent for 30 minutes.
3. Rinse the smears in distilled water.

4. Place the smears in a coplin jar containing neutral red and counterstain for 10 minutes.
5. Wash smears under running tap water.
6. Allow to air dry and coverslip.

Discussion

1. A positive control smear should be run each time this test is performed.
2. Wright-stained smears several years old may be effectively stained with Prussian-blue reagent.
3. This stain may be used for the detection of hemosiderin in urine, which will appear as blue staining intracellular (within the epithelial cells) or extracellular granules.

LEUKOCYTE ALKALINE PHOSPHATASE STAIN

Alkaline phosphatase activity is present in varying degrees in the neutrophil and band form of the granulocytes and, sometimes, to a very small degree in certain B lymphocytes. (See Plate VIII, C,D.) The amount of leukocyte alkaline phosphatase present will vary in different diseases and is useful in differentiating a leukemoid reaction (increased alkaline phosphatase activity) from chronic myelogenous leukemia (decreased activity).

Increased values for this test are found during pregnancy (the last trimester), in infections accompanied by neutrophilia, polycythemia vera, people receiving corticosteroids, aplastic anemia, multiple myeloma, myelosclerosis, and obstructive jaundice. In Hodgkin's disease the results of this stain closely parallel the progression of the disease, being elevated in untreated cases. In one type of lymphocytic lymphoma some lymphocytes will show alkaline phosphatase activity. Decreased scores for this test will be found in chronic myelogenous leukemia, paroxysmal nocturnal hemoglobinuria, sickle cell anemia, hereditary hypophosphatasemia, marked eosinophilia, sideroblastic anemia, and, rarely, in normal people. Normal alkaline phosphatase activity will be found in untreated hemolytic anemia, lymphosarcoma, viral hepatitis, and secondary polycythemia.

References

Ackerman, G.A.: Substituted naphthol AS phosphate derivatives for the localization of leukocyte alkaline phosphatase activity, Lab. Invest., *11*, 563, 1962.
Sigma Diagnostics: Alkaline Phosphatase, pkg. insert, Sigma Chemical Co., St. Louis, MO., 1988.

Reagents and Equipment

1. Acetone.
2. The following reagents are available from Sigma Chemical Co., St. Louis, MO.:
   a. Citrate concentrated solution. Store at room temperature. Do not use if contamination is evident.
      1) Citrate working solution. Dilute 2 mL of citrate concentrated solution to 100 mL with distilled water. Store in refrigerator.
      2) Citrate buffered acetone, 60% w/v, (fixative). Prepare just prior to use. Add 20 mL of the citrate working solution (must be at room temperature) to 30 mL of acetone while constantly stirring the mixture. Discard after using.
   b. Naphthol AS-MX phosphate alkaline solution (substrate). Store in refrigerator.
   c. Fast blue RR salt (capsules). Store below 0°C.
   d. Mayer's hematoxylin solution, 1 g/L. Store at room temperature.
3. Coplin jars, three.

Specimen

Fresh capillary blood is recommended. Prepare well-made fingerstick blood smears from the patient, from a positive control (pregnant woman in the last trimester or during the first several days post partum), and from a normal control (may be prepared by placing a blood smear in boiling water for 1 minute after it has been fixed [inactivates enzyme]). Alternatively, blood may be collected using heparin as the anticoagulant. (EDTA has an inhibitory effect on the stain reaction and will yield a falsely low result.) If anticoagulated blood is used, smears should be prepared as soon as possible after obtaining the specimen, and once made they should be stained within 8 hours. If this is not possible smears may be fixed and stored overnight in the freezer, in which case the smears must be air dried for 1 hour before fixing and then air-dried again for 3 hours after fixing prior to freezing.

Principle

The blood smears are fixed in citrate buffered acetone. When placed in the incubation solution containing naphthol AS-MX phosphate and fast blue RR, the alkaline phosphatase present in the white blood cells liberates naphthol AS-MX, which then couples with fast blue RR to form an insoluble blue compound (at the site of alkaline phosphatase activity) in proportion to the amount of enzyme present. The smears are then counterstained. The degree of reactivity is determined by scoring each of 100 neutrophils according to the amount of precipitated dye present.

Procedure

1. Prepare the staining solution immediately before use:
    a. Dissolve the contents of one capsule of fast blue RR in 48 mL of distilled water.
    b. Add 2 mL of naphthol AS-MX phosphate alkaline solution and mix.
    c. Place stain in a coplin jar. Discard stain after use.
2. After collection, place the air dried blood smears in a coplin jar containing citrate buffered acetone (fixative) for 30 seconds.
3. Carefully rinse the smears in running distilled water for 45 seconds. Do not allow smears to dry.
4. Place smears in the staining solution for 30 minutes at room temperature.
5. Wash smears in distilled water for 2 minutes. Do not allow smears to dry.
6. Counterstain with Mayer's hematoxylin for 10 minutes. Rinse smears in distilled water for 3 minutes.
7. Examine the smears microscopically in a relatively thin area of the smear using the oil immersion objective (100×). Count 100 consecutive neutrophils (and band forms) and grade each one from 0 to 4+ on the basis of the appearance (quantity and intensity) of the precipitated dye in the cell. The cytoplasm of the cells will be colorless to pale blue.

0 = No staining.
1+ = Faint and diffuse staining.
2+ = Pale, with a moderate amount of blue staining.
3+ = Strong blue precipitated staining.
4+ = Deep blue or brilliant staining with no visible cytoplasm.

8. The total rating for 100 neutrophils is determined by multiplying the number of cells in each group by its rating and adding these numbers together for the total LAP score. The normal range for this test will generally fall in the vicinity of 30 to 185, but should be determined by each laboratory.

Discussion

1. Delay in staining blood smears will cause gradual loss of alkaline phosphatase activity.
2. The entire staining procedure should be carried out with the slides protected from direct light as much as possible.
3. Glycerin gel may be used as a mounting medium if coverslipping is desired.
4. Control smears may be prepared in advance and stored in the freezer at −70°C for up to 1 year. Prepare smears as outlined previously (see Specimen). Wrap fixed, dry smears in Parafilm.
5. The reaction mixture should be between 18 and 26°C for optimal staining.
6. Naphthol AS-BI phosphate is also commonly used as a substrate for this stain.
7. Fast violet B salt (also obtainable from Sigma Chemical Co.) may be used in place of fast blue RR salt, in which case the smears must be rinsed in an alkaline tap water (or Scott's Tap Water [Sigma Chemical Co.]) following hematoxylin staining. The precipitated dye will be a violet color.

PEROXIDASE STAIN

Peroxidase is present in the primary azurophilic granules of the neutrophil and in the eosinophil and monocyte. (See Plate VIII, E.) No activity is found in the red blood cells or lymphocytes. The stain reaction in the myelogenous cells generally increases as the cell matures, with the greatest activity being present in the neutrophil. The eosinophil will also show intense peroxidase staining. The positive reaction in the monocyte is limited to finely granular staining throughout the cell.

The peroxidase stain is used for differentiating acute myelogenous or monocytic leukemia from acute lymphocytic leukemia and will generally show results similar to those of the Sudan black B stain. Auer rods will stain peroxidase positive. Blast cells that do not yet have granules may show positive staining of the peroxidase that has not yet been incorporated into granules. Normally, mature basophils show no peroxidase activity but will stain positively in patients with granulocytic leukemia. Neutrophils will show decreased peroxidase activity in cases of infection, acute myelogenous leukemia, and myelodysplastic conditions, whereas there will be increased activity in the mature neutrophils in chronic myelogenous leukemia.

References

Graham, R.C., Lundholm, U., and Karnovsky, M.J.: Cytochemical demonstration of peroxidase activity with 3-amino-9-ethylcarbazole, J. Histochem. Cytochem., *13*, 150, 1965.

Kaplow, L.S.: Substitute for benzidine in myeloperoxidase stains, Am. J. Clin. Pathol., *63*, 451, 1975.

Reagents and Equipment

1. Phosphate buffered formalin acetone fixative, pH 6.6 to 6.8.
2. Acetic acid, 0.02 M.
   Glacial acetic acid   1.16 mL
   Dilute to 1 liter with distilled water.
3. Sodium acetate, 0.02 M.
   Sodium acetate   2.72 g
   (CH$_3$COONa·3H$_2$O)
   Dilute to 1 liter with distilled water.
4. Acetate buffer, 0.02 M, pH 5.0 to 5.2.
   Acetic acid, 0.02 M   176 mL
   Sodium acetate, 0.02 M   800 mL
   Store in the refrigerator.
5. Hydrogen peroxide, 0.3%.
   Hydrogen peroxide, 30%   0.1 mL
   Distilled water   9.9 mL
   Prepare immediately before use.
6. Stain, pH 5.5. Prepare immediately before use.
   3-Amino-9-ethylcarbazole   10 mg
   (obtainable from Sigma Chemical Co., St. Louis, Missouri)

Dimethyl sulfoxide   6.0 mL
Acetate buffer, 0.02 M, pH 5.0
to 5.2   50 mL
Hydrogen peroxide, 0.3% v/v   0.4 mL
Filter before use. For more consistent results, allow stain to age at room temperature for 30 minutes prior to use.
7. Mayer's hematoxylin.
8. Glycerol gelatin mounting medium. (See Reagent section.)
9. Coplin jars, 3.
10. Coverslips.

Specimen

Fresh blood smears made from capillary blood are recommended, or, use fresh whole blood anticoagulated with EDTA or heparin.

Principle

When peroxidase is present in the white blood cells it will catalyze the oxidation of 3-amino-9-ethylcarbazole by the hydrogen peroxide present in the stain, to form an insoluble reddish-brown precipitate at the site of the peroxidase activity.

Procedure

1. Prepare thin blood or bone marrow smears and allow to air dry.
2. Place the smears in a coplin jar containing phosphate buffered formalin acetone for 30 seconds at room temperature.
3. Wash the smears under gently running tap water.
4. Place the smears in a coplin jar containing the stain mixture for 12 minutes.
5. Wash the smears under gently running tap water.
6. Counterstain the smears in a coplin jar containing Mayer's hematoxylin for 5 minutes.
7. Wash the smears under gently running tap water.
8. Allow the smears to air dry and immediately coverslip with glycerol gelatin mounting medium to prevent the stain from fading.
9. Examine the smears microscopically, using the oil immersion objective (100×). The presence of peroxidases is indicated by reddish-brown deposits present in the

cytoplasm of the granulocytes and monocytes. The cytoplasm of the neutrophils is packed with these red-brown granules. The monocytes show a small to moderate number of the granules. The eosinophil exhibits darkly stained granules, whereas the basophil and lymphocyte remain unstained. The early myeloblast may give a negative reaction.

Discussion

1. Light or faint staining of the reaction product may occur if the pH of the stain mixture is above pH 6.0.
2. Sigma Chemical Co. (St. Louis, MO) manufactures the Leukocyte Peroxidase stain kit (No. 390), which uses a combination of p-phenylene diamine and catechol reagents to produce a brown-black colored reaction. Other reagents used are 2,7-fluorenediamine, 2,6-dichlorophenol-indophenol, and o-toluidine. Previously, the most commonly used reagent was benzidine, which is no longer in use because of the chemical's carcinogenic properties.

PERIODIC ACID-SCHIFF (PAS) REACTION

The periodic acid-Schiff stain aids in the diagnosis of some acute lymphocytic leukemias and certain subtypes of acute myelogenous leukemias, and may also be helpful in distinguishing DiGuglielmo's disease. This stain indicates the presence of mucoproteins, glycoproteins, and high molecular weight carbohydrates. In blood cells it is primarily glycogen which stains positively. Normally, almost all blood cells, except erythroblasts, show positive staining. The intensity of the stain and the pattern of staining will vary with the cell type. (See Plate VII G.) It may be diffuse, granular, or a mixture of the two. Granulocytes normally show a diffuse staining pattern, while lymphocyte staining has a granular pattern. Granulocytes show a positive reaction in all stages of development, the mature neutrophils reacting the most strongly. Myelocytes and myeloblasts contain fewer positively stained granules. Eosinophil granules do not take up the stain, but the background cytoplasm stains positively. Lymphocytes contain a few fine or coarse, positively stained granules. Monocyte granules exhibit a small amount of positive staining, and nucleated red blood cells generally show no positively stained granules. Platelets will stain deeply. In disease states, the PAS staining reaction will differ from the normal and this is of some diagnostic value. In chronic lymphocytic leukemia, lymphosarcoma, and Hodgkin's disease, the lymphocytes contain an increased number of positively stained granules. In erythroleukemia (DiGuglielmo's disease) and thalassemia, the nucleated red blood cells often show a positive reaction. Some positive staining of the nucleated red blood cells has also been found in iron deficiency anemia, some hemolytic anemias, pernicious anemia, aplastic anemia, and polycythemia.

References

McManus, J.F.A.: Histological demonstration of mucin after periodic acid, Nature, *158*, 202, 1946.

Dacie, J.V., and Lewis, S.M.: *Practical Hematology*, 6th ed., New York, Churchill Livingstone Inc., 1984.

Reagents and Equipment

1. Alcoholic formalin fixative.
   Formaldehyde   10.0 mL
   Ethanol   90.0 mL
   Store in the refrigerator.
2. Periodic acid solution, 1% w/v. Store in refrigerator in a brown bottle. Stable for 3 to 4 months.
3. Schiff's reagent.
   Basic fuchsin   1.0 g
   Boiling distilled water   400 mL
   Allow the preceding solution to cool to 50°C and filter. Add 1.0 g of thionyl chloride ($SOCl_2$). Allow the mixture to stand in the dark for 12 hours. Add 2.0 g of activated charcoal to the mixture, shake for 1 minute, filter, and store in the dark at 0 to 4°C. (This reagent may be obtained commercially from Rowley Biochemical Institute, Rowley, MA, 01969.)
4. Mayer's hematoxylin.
5. Coplin jars.
6. Pro-texx mounting medium (Baxter, American Scientific Products), or equivalent.

Specimen

Air dried blood or bone marrow smears.

Principle

Carbohydrates present in the blood cells are oxidized to aldehydes by periodic acid. Schiff's reagent then reacts with the aldehydes to form an insoluble red colored precipitate (an aldehyde-fuschin-sulphurous acid compound).

Procedure

1. Fix smears in a coplin jar containing alcoholic formalin for 10 minutes.
2. Wash smears in running tap water for 15 minutes.
3. Place smears in a coplin jar containing 1% periodic acid for 20 minutes.
4. Wash smears in running tap water for 5 minutes.
5. Drain smears and place in a coplin jar containing Schiff's reagent for 30 minutes.
6. Rinse smears in tap water and then wash in distilled water for 5 minutes.
7. Counterstain smears in a coplin jar containing Mayer's hematoxylin for 5 minutes.
8. Rinse smears in running tap water for 15 minutes. Allow to air dry and coverslip.
9. Examine the smears microscopically, using the oil immersion objective (100×). The glycogen present in the cells will stain a bright reddish purple color.

Discussion

1. Blood or bone marrow smears that have been Wright-stained may be successfully stained according to the preceding procedure.
2. Smears several years old, whether Wright-stained or not, may also be stained by the PAS stain.
3. To make certain the Schiff's reagent is still effective it may be tested by adding a few drops of the reagent to 10 mL of formaldehyde (37%). The mixture should change to a light purple color. If it does not, this indicates that the Schiff's reagent is no longer good and it should be discarded.
4. Schiff's reagent is normally colorless. If it becomes pink it should be discarded.

SUDAN BLACK B STAIN

Sudan black B stains various lipids, among which are sterols, phospholipids, and neutral fats. As a stain, it is most often employed to distinguish acute myelogenous and myelomonocytic leukemias from acute lymphocytic leukemia. Lymphocyte granules do not stain. The myelogenous cells show coarse staining granules with faint staining in the myeloblast. The intensity of staining increases as the cells mature. (See Plate VIII, H.) Auer rods will stain intensely. The monocytic cells show positive staining of the finely scattered granules. This stain is similar to the peroxidase stain in the types of cells which stain positively. It is also similar in sensitivity to the peroxidase stain, but is more sensitive than the chloroacetate esterase in the staining of myeloblasts. It may be noted that vacuolated immature cells found in Burkitt's lymphoma may show positive staining of the lipid present in the vacuoles.

Reference

Sheehan, H.L., and Storey, G.W.: An improved method of staining leukocyte granules with Sudan black B, J. Path. Bact., *59*, 336, 1947.

Reagents and Equipment

1. Stock buffer solution.
   Crystalline phenol   16 g
   Ethanol   30 mL
   Add the preceding two reagents to 100 mL of distilled water containing 0.3 g of hydrated disodium phosphate ($Na_2HPO_4 \cdot 12H_2O$).
2. Stock Sudan black B solution.
   Sudan black B   0.3 g
   Ethanol   100 mL
   Prepare this solution several days prior to use. Allow it to sit at room temperature and shake frequently to ensure that all of the dye is dissolved. Filter before use.
3. Sudan black B staining solution.
   Stock buffer solution   20 mL
   Stock Sudan solution   30 mL
   Stable for 2 to 3 months.
4. Formaldehyde, 37%.
5. Buffered neutral red, 1% w/v in acetate buffer, 0.1 N, pH 5.0.
6. Ethyl alcohol, 70% v/v.

7. Coplin jars, 2.
8. PVP mounting medium.

Specimen

Air dried blood or bone marrow smears.

Principle

Sudan Black B stains various lipids such as sterols, phospholipids, and neutral fats. It may also stain some nonlipid components of the cells.

Procedure

1. Place torn up filter paper in the bottom of a coplin jar and moisten with 37% formaldehyde.
2. Place the air dried smears in the coplin jar and cover. Allow the smears to fix in the vapor for 10 minutes. Wash gently in tap water, allowing excess water to drain from the smear (avoid washing smear off slide).
3. Place the smears in a coplin jar containing Sudan black B staining solution for 30 minutes. (The time is variable, between 10 and 60 minutes depending on the age of the staining solution.)
4. Rinse each slide with 70% ethyl alcohol just long enough to remove the excess stain.
5. Wash the smears gently in running tap water for 2 minutes.
6. Place the smears in a coplin jar containing 1% neutral red and counterstain for 10 minutes.
7. Wash the slides very gently in tap water, air dry, and coverslip with PVP mounting medium.
8. Examine the smears microscopically, using the oil immersion objective (100×). The neutrophils and eosinophils will stain positively. The eosinophil granules will generally stain strongly around the edge of the granule but may retain an unstained central area. The monocytes will show scattered positive staining. The lymphocyte granules, platelets, and red blood cells remain unstained.

Discussion

1. Bone marrow or blood smears need not be fresh to obtain good results with the Sudan black B stain.

2. As the Sudan black B stain ages, it may be necessary to increase the staining time.
3. The granules are not readily decolorized by the 70% ethyl alcohol.

ACID PHOSPHATASE STAIN (WITH TARTRATE RESISTANCE)

The acid phosphatase stain is helpful in diagnosing hairy cell leukemia (leukemic reticuloendotheliosis). Normally, acid phosphatase activity is present in the myelogenous cells, lymphocytes, plasma cells, monocytes, and platelets. In this stain acid phosphatase is indicated by a red colored precipitate at the site of the enzyme's activity. In the presence of L(+) tartaric acid, the activity of acid phosphatase is inhibited and the above cells exhibit no activity (stain negatively). However, of the seven acid phosphatase isoenzymes (0, 1, 2, 3, 3b, 4, and 5) isoenzyme 5 (a pyrophosphatase present in large amounts in the hairy cells of leukemic reticuloendotheliosis), is resistant to L(+) tartaric acid, and will show a positive response for acid phosphatase in the presence of this chemical. The atypical lymphocytes of infectious mononucleosis, and, rarely, the lymphocytes in chronic lymphocytic leukemia and lymphosarcoma may show less than complete resistance to L(+) tartaric acid and may, therefore, stain very faintly positive.

Reference

Katayama, I., and Yang, J.P.S.: Reassessment of a cytochemical test for differential diagnosis of leukemic reticuloendotheliosis, Am. J. Clin. Path., 68, 268, 1977.

Reagents and Equipment

1. Phosphate buffered formalin acetone fixative, pH 6.6 to 6.8.
2. Sodium nitrite, 4% w/v. Prepare immediately before use.
3. Pararosanilin solution, 4% w/v in 20% (v/v) hydrochloric acid.
4. Saturated sodium hydroxide.
5. Solution A.
   Sodium nitrite, 4%   2.4 mL
   Pararosanilin solution,   2.4 mL
     4%, in 20% HCl
   Mix immediately before use in a 250 mL beaker.

6. Solution B.

Naphthol AS-BI phosphoric acid (obtainable from Sigma Chemical Co., St. Louis, Mo.)	40 mg
N,N-dimethyl formamide	4.0 mL
Acetate buffer, 0.1 N, pH 5.0	71.2 mL

   Prepare immediately before use.

7. Incubation mixture I.

   Add solution B to solution A. Mix and place 40 mL in a separate beaker. Adjust the pH of mixture I to pH 5.1 with saturated sodium hydroxide. Filter into a coplin jar in the 37°C water bath and use immediately.

8. Incubation mixture II.

L(+)tartaric acid	0.3 g
Incubation mixture I	40 mL

   Mix and adjust pH to 5.1 with saturated sodium hydroxide. Filter into a coplin jar in the 37°C water bath and use immediately.

9. Methyl green, 1% w/v, in acetate buffer, 0.1 N, pH 5.0.

10. PVP mounting medium.

11. 37°C water bath.

12. Coplin jars, 7.

13. Coverslips.

Specimen

Air dried blood or bone marrow smears, or use blood anticoagulated with heparin.

Principle

Acid phosphatase present in the cells hydrolyzes the naphthol AS-BI phosphoric acid in the incubation mixture releasing insoluble naphthol, which then couples with the pararosanilin, giving a red-colored precipitate at the site of the enzyme activity. In the presence of L(+) tartaric acid the activity of most acid phosphatase is inhibited. The exception is acid phosphatase isoenzyme 5 (present in hairy cell leukemia), which is resistant to L(+) tartaric acid.

Procedure

1. Prepare thin blood or bone marrow smears and allow to air dry. At least two smears should be prepared on each patient and normal control. Label one smear from each patient and normal control, I, and the second smear, II.

2. Place the slides in a coplin jar containing cold phosphate buffered formalin acetone for 30 seconds.

3. Wash smears in three changes of distilled water.

4. Place the labeled slide for each patient and normal control into the appropriate coplin jar containing incubation mixture I (prewarmed to 37°C) and into a coplin jar containing incubation mixture II (prewarmed to 37°C). Incubate the smears at 37°C for 60 minutes. (Make certain the level of water in the water bath is at or above the liquid level in the coplin jars.)

5. Wash smears in two changes of distilled water.

6. Place smears into a coplin jar containing 1% methyl green for 2 minutes.

7. Wash smears quickly in running tap water.

8. Allow the smears to air dry, mount, and coverslip in PVP mounting medium.

9. Examine the smears microscopically using oil immersion objective (100×). Those smears from incubation mixture I should show acid phosphate activity in the cytoplasm of the white blood cells and the platelets (varying degrees of reddish staining). The smears from incubation mixture II should show no acid phosphatase activity or only a minute amount of red staining. The "hairy" cells of leukemic reticuloendotheliosis exhibit positive red staining from both incubation mixtures I and II.

Discussion

1. If the stain cannot be performed immediately, the smears may be fixed and stored at −20°C for up to 2 weeks. Wrap the slides in Parafilm prior to storage.

2. An alternative method to the above uses Fast Garnet GBC (in place of pararosanilin) and yields a highly colored red precipitate This reaction may be more sensitive for cytologic specimens but will give less precise results on tissue sections.

3. Mayer's hematoxylin may also be used as a counterstain in place of methyl green.

NONSPECIFIC ESTERASE STAIN (WITH FLUORIDE INHIBITION)

White blood cells contain esterases, a group of lysosomal enzymes. The nonspecific and specific (chloroacetate) esterase stains are primarily utilized to differentiate granulocytic and monocytic leukemias. The nonspecific esterase stain, using α-naphthyl acetate as substrate, is more specific for monocytic cells and shows positive staining in the monocytes, macrophages, megakaryocytes, and platelets. (See Plate VIII, J.) In the presence of fluoride, however, the reaction is inhibited and these cells will then show no staining for nonspecific esterase activity. The lymphoblasts of acute lymphocytic leukemia may show a few weakly positive coarse granules which are not inhibited by fluoride. The nonspecific esterase stain is negative in acute myelogenous leukemia. In acute monocytic leukemia, generally 80 to 100% of the cells will stain positively, whereas in myelomonocytic leukemia, the monocytes will not stain as strongly and the granulocytes may show some positive staining that is not inhibited by fluoride (the monocyte staining will be inhibited). The erythroblasts present in erythroleukemia and DiGuglielmo's syndrome may stain positively for nonspecific esterase.

Reference

Yam, L.T., Li, C.Y., and Crosby, W.H.: Cytochemical identification of monocytes and granulocytes, Am. J. Clin. Path., *55*, 283, 1971.

Reagents and Equipment

1. Cold phosphate buffered formalin acetone, fixative, pH 6.6 to 6.8.
2. Pararosanilin, 4% w/v in 20% (v/v) hydrochloric acid.
3. Sodium nitrite, 4% w/v. Make fresh, just prior to use.
4. Phosphate buffer, M/15, pH 6.3.
Dibasic sodium phosphate (Na_2HPO_4)	1.183 g
Monobasic potassium phosphate (KH_2PO_4)	3.399 g

   Dilute to 500 mL with distilled water. Store in the refrigerator. Reagent must be at room temperature when used.
5. Sodium hydroxide, 1 N.
6. Sodium fluoride, 0.1 M.
Sodium fluoride	0.42 g

   Dilute to 100 mL with distilled water. Store at room temperature.
7. α-Naphthyl acetate in ethylene glycol monomethyl ether. Prepare just prior to use.
α-Naphthyl acetate	0.2 g
Ethylene glycol monomethyl ether	10.0 mL
8. Incubation mixture (A) without fluoride. Prepare just prior to use.
Pararosanilin (4% w/v in 20% HCl)	3.0 mL
Sodium nitrite, 4% w/v	3.0 mL

   Mix in a 200-mL beaker. Allow to sit for 1 minute and add:
Phosphate buffer M/15, pH 6.3	89.0 mL
α-Naphthyl acetate in ethylene glycol monomethyl ether	5.0 mL

   Mix. Remove 50 mL of this solution and place in a 100-mL beaker. This will be used to prepare the incubation mixture (B) with fluoride. Adjust the pH of incubation mixture A to approximately 6.1 (5.8 to 6.5), using 1 N sodium hydroxide. Filter directly into a coplin jar and use immediately.
9. Incubation mixture (B) with fluoride. Add 0.5 mL of 0.1 M sodium fluoride to 50 mL of incubation mixture (A) (which was set aside). Adjust the pH to 6.1 (5.8 to 6.5) using 1 N sodium hydroxide. Filter directly into a coplin jar and use immediately.
10. Buffered methyl green, 1% w/v in acetate buffer, 0.1 N, pH 5.0.
11. Pro-texx mounting medium (Baxter, Scientific Products Division), or equivalent.
12. Coplin jars.
13. Coverslips.

Specimen

Air-dried blood or bone marrow smears. Blood anticoagulated with EDTA or heparin may also be used.

Principle

The group of enzymes in the white blood cells called nonspecific esterases will hydrolyze α-naphthyl acetate to liberate a naphthyl compound, which then combines with pararosanilin to produce a red-staining precipitate at or near the site of enzyme activity.

Procedure

1. Prepare thin blood or bone marrow smears and allow to air dry. At least two smears should be prepared for each patient and normal control. Label one smear from each patient and normal control, A, and the second smear from each, B.
2. Fix the above smears in a coplin jar containing cold phosphate buffered formalin acetone for 30 to 60 seconds.
3. Wash smears in three changes of distilled water.
4. Allow smears to air dry for 10 to 30 minutes while making up the incubation mixtures.
5. Place the appropriately labeled slide for each patient and normal control into a coplin jar containing incubation mixture A and into a second coplin jar containing incubation mixture B. Incubate the smears at room temperature for 60 minutes.
6. Wash smears in three changes of distilled water.
7. Counterstain, by placing the smears in a coplin jar containing 1% methyl green for 1 to 2 minutes.
8. Wash smears in running tap water.
9. Allow the smears to air dry and coverslip.
10. Examine the smears microscopically using the oil immersion objective (100×). Nonspecific esterase activity is indicated by the presence of dark red-staining granules in the cytoplasm of the cell. Those smears from incubation mixture A (without fluoride) will show strong esterase activity in the cytoplasm of the monocyte, macrophages, megakaryocytes, and platelets. There may also be positive staining in some T-lymphocytes and plasma cells. Immature granulocytes and normal erythroblasts will show very weak to no nonspecific esterase activity. With fluoride, nonspecific esterase staining is inhibited in the monocytes, macrophages, megakaryocytes, and platelets.

Discussion

1. If the stain cannot be performed immediately, the unfixed smears may be stored in the dark at room temperature for up to 2 weeks without significant loss in activity.
2. An increase in the incubation time or an increase in the pH of the incubation medium may cause false positive staining of the granulocytic cells.
3. α-Naphthyl butyrate may also be used as a substrate in this procedure. The staining reaction, however, is more specific but at the same time less sensitive than when α-naphthyl acetate is used.

CHLOROACETATE ESTERASE STAIN

The chloroacetate esterase stain is specific for esterases found in the granulocytic cells. The myeloid cells normally stain strongly with even the myeloblast and promyelocytes frequently positive. Monocytes and basophils show negative to very weakly positive staining, whereas the remaining cells (lymphocytes, plasma cells, megakaryocytes, eosinophils, and nucleated red blood cells) are negative. Auer rods will generally stain positive, and a normal myeloblast will be more positively stained than a leukemic myeloblast. This stain may be performed in combination with the nonspecific esterase (on the same blood smear) to differentiate monocytic from granulocytic cells. (See Plate VIII, K.) The reactions of the chloroacetate esterase stain are similar to those of the Sudan black B and the peroxidase stains.

Reference

Yam, L.T., Li, C.Y., and Crosby, W.H.: Cytochemical identification of monocytes and granulocytes, Am. J. Clin. Path., 55, 283, 1971.

Reagents and Equipment

1. Cold phosphate buffered formalin acetone fixative pH 6.6 to 6.8.
2. Buffered methyl green, 1% w/v in acetate buffer, 0.1 N, pH 5.0.

3. Phosphate buffer, M/15, pH 7.4.

Dibasic sodium phosphate (Na_2HPO_4)	3.786 g
Monobasic potassium phosphate (KH_2PO_4)	0.907 g

Dilute to 500 mL with distilled water. Adjust the pH to 7.4.

4. Naphthol AS-D chloroacetate (0.2% w/v in N,N-dimethylformamide).

Naphthol AS-D chloroacetate	10 mg
N,N-dimethylformamide	5.0 mL

Prepare immediately before use.

5. Incubation mixture.

Phosphate buffer (M/15, pH 7.4)	47.5 mL
Naphthol AS-D chloro-acetate (0.2% w/v in N,N-dimethylformamide)	2.5 mL
Fast blue BB	30 mg

Mix and filter directly into a coplin jar. Prepare immediately before use.

6. Pro-texx mounting medium (Baxter, Scientific Products Division), or equivalent.
7. Coplin jars.
8. Coverslips.

Specimen

Air dried blood or bone marrow smears. Blood anticoagulated with EDTA or heparin may also be used.

Principle

Chloroacetate esterases present in the white blood cells will hydrolyze a substrate (naphthol AS-D chloroacetate) to liberate naphthol, which then combines with fast blue BB to form a blue colored precipitate at or near the site of enzyme activity.

Procedure

1. Prepare thin blood or bone marrow smears on the patient and the normal control and allow to air-dry.
2. Fix the smears in a coplin jar containing cold, phosphate buffered formalin acetone for 30 to 60 seconds.
3. Wash smears in three changes of distilled water.
4. Allow smears to air dry for 10 to 30 minutes while preparing the incubation mixture.
5. Place smears in a coplin jar containing the incubation mixture for 20 minutes.
6. Wash smears in three changes of distilled water.
7. Counterstain by placing the smears in a coplin jar containing 1% methyl green for 1 to 2 minutes.
8. Wash smears in running tap water.
9. Allow smears to air-dry and coverslip.
10. Examine the smears microscopically using the high immersion objective (100×). Chloroacetate esterase activity will show up as blue-staining granules in the granulocytic cells. Basophils show little to no chloroacetate esterase activity. Granulocytes, including promyelocytes, will show very strong activity, as do many, but not all, myeloblasts. Monocytes show little to no activity. Lymphocytes, eosinophils, plasma cells, megakaryocytes, and erythroblasts show no chloroacetate esterase activity.

Discussion

1. If the stain cannot be performed immediately, the unfixed smears may be stored in the dark at room temperature for up to 2 weeks without a significant loss in activity.
2. The nonspecific esterase stain and the chloroacetate esterase stain may be combined and performed on the same patient and control slides. For the combined nonspecific and chloroacetate esterase stains, perform steps 1 through 6 as outlined for the nonspecific esterase stain. Continue the procedure by performing steps 5 through 9 as described above for the chloroacetate esterase stain. The staining results for the combined stain are similar to the individual stain results. Nonspecific esterase activity is indicated by dark red granules in the monocytes, histiocytes, and megakaryocytes. Blue staining granules in the cytoplasm of the granulocytes indicates chloroacetate esterase activity.

NITROBLUE TETRAZOLIUM (NBT) NEUTROPHIL REDUCTION TEST

The nitroblue tetrazolium reduction test is helpful as a screening procedure for detecting metabolic defects of the neutrophil (e.g., chronic granulomatous disease). In these disorders markedly decreased values for the NBT reduction test are obtained. The procedure may also be used as an aid in differentiating bacterial from nonbacterial infections.

References

Okamura, K., Kato, H., Matsuda, N., and Takahashi, H.: An improved Nitroblue Tetrazolium test and its correlation with toxic neutrophils, Am. J. Clin. Pathol., 62, 27, 1974.

Park, B.H., Fikrig, S.M., and Smithwick, E.M.: Infection and nitroblue tetrazolium reduction by neutrophils, Lancet, 2, 532, 1968.

Sigma Chemical Co.: Nitroblue tetrazolium (NBT) reduction, histochemical demonstration in neutrophils, pkg. insert, Sigma Chemical Co., St. Louis, Mo., 1985.

Reagents and Equipment

1. The following reagents and equipment are available from Sigma Chemical Co.:
   a. Siliconized collection vial containing 20 units of heparin (#840–20).
   b. Nitroblue tetrazolium, 1 mg, with sodium chloride and phosphate buffer (#840–10). Store in the dark at 2 to 6°C. Reconstitute with 1.0 mL of distilled water. Mix vigorously. Once reconstituted the reagent is stable for 1 day stored in the refrigerator.
2. Plastic syringe, 5 mL.
3. Test tubes, plastic, 12 × 75 mm, with caps.
4. Pipets, 1.0 and 0.1 mL.
5. Water bath, 37°C.
6. Glass microscope slides.
7. Wright stain and buffer.

Specimen

Heparinized whole blood, 1.0 mL. Using a plastic syringe, carefully obtain 1.5 to 2 mL of whole blood making certain the specimen is not contaminated with tissue juice. Remove the needle from the syringe and slowly add 1.0 mL of the blood to the heparinized tube (containing 20 units of heparin). Cap the tube and gently mix by tilting for 30 seconds. Do not allow the blood to come in contact with the tube cap. Collect blood for a normal control at the same time the patient's blood is obtained. Specimen must be tested within 2 hours of collection, and should be refrigerated if not used immediately.

Principle

Increased enzyme activity normally present in neutrophils during a bacterial infection is capable of reducing colorless nitroblue tetrazolium to blue-black deposits of formazan. In chronic granulomatous disease, the neutrophils do not have the normal ability to kill certain organisms and are also unable to reduce nitroblue tetrazolium. In this procedure, blood is incubated with nitroblue tetrazolium, and smears are prepared and Wright-stained. The slides are examined microscopically for formazan-containing neutrophils. In healthy adults 10% or less of the neutrophils contain formazan. (Up to 17% of the neutrophils may contain the precipitated dye, however.) In the presence of a bacterial infection, as many as 70% of the neutrophils will normally reduce the nitroblue tetrazolium. Each laboratory, however, should determine its own normal range.

Procedure

1. Pipet 0.1 mL of NBT reagent into an appropriately labeled plastic test tube, 12 × 75 mm, for each specimen and control to be tested.
2. Add 0.1 mL of well-mixed whole blood to the above tube. Cap tube and mix thoroughly by very gently tilting, using a rolling motion.
3. Incubate each tube for 10 minutes at 37°C. At the end of this period, remove the tubes from the incubator and allow to stand at room temperature for an additional 10 minutes.
4. Mix the tubes very gently. Transfer a small drop of each mixture onto labelled microscopic slides and prepare a moderately thick blood smear. (A thick smear is prepared in order to avoid mechanical damage to the neutrophils.) Allow smears to air dry.
5. Wright stain the smears and allow the smears to air dry.
6. Using the oil immersion objective (100×), count 100 neutrophils, enumerating those neutrophils that contain the reduced nitroblue tetrazolium. The formazan appears as large black deposits in the neutrophil. The neutrophils counted must occur singly and have their cell membrane

intact. No other cell(s) or cellular material (except red blood cells) should be touching the neutrophil. Report results as the percent of neutrophils containing reduced nitroblue tetrazolium (% of NBT positive neutrophils). (See Plate VIII, M, N.)

Discussion

1. The absolute number of NBT positive neutrophils may be determined by performing a white count and 100 cell differential on the test blood. Calculate the absolute number of neutrophils by multiplying the neutrophil percentage by the white count. Multiply the absolute neutrophil count by the percentage of formazan-containing neutrophils to obtain the absolute NBT positive neutrophil count.
2. In chronic granulomatous disease, there is a 0 to negligible reduction of the nitroblue tetrazolium.
3. An increased concentration of heparin may give false positive results.
4. As an aid in detecting metabolic defects of neutrophil function, this procedure may be performed using a stimulating agent (a nonviable bacterial extract is available from Sigma Chemical Co. for this purpose [Stimulant—#840–15]). In this test, the procedure as described above is performed in exactly the same manner except that 0.1 mL of NBT solution is mixed with 0.05 mL of whole blood and 0.05 mL of stimulant. Normal results for this modification are quite variable but will usually be increased by an additional 10 to 50% NBT positive neutrophils. This modification may be performed simultaneously with the unstimulated procedure.
5. The whole blood specimens for this test should be treated *very* gently throughout the procedure to avoid break-up of the neutrophils.
6. A modification of the NBT test is described by Okamura (1974): Mix one volume of 0.1% NBT (w/v) in 0.9% sodium chloride) with one volume of glucose phosphate buffer (0.2% glucose and 0.6% sodium chloride in 0.067 M Sörenson's buffer, pH 7.2 [28.0 mL of solution 1: 0.91 g KH_2PO_4 dissolved and diluted to 100 mL, plus 72.0 mL of solution 2: 0.95 g Na_2HPO_4 dissolved and diluted to 100 mL]) and add to two volumes of heparinized whole blood. This mixture is incubated at 37°C for 15 minutes, gently mixing every 5 minutes. After incubation the blood is centrifuged in microhematocrit tubes at 1,500 rpm for 5 minutes. Buffy coat smears are then carefully prepared and Wright-stained. This procedure yields a stained smear that should contain a higher concentration of neutrophils that show less distortion and more preservation of the morphologic characteristics of the neutrophil.

HEINZ BODY PREPARATION

Heinz bodies represent precipitated hemoglobin and occur when the red cell glycolytic enzymes are not able to prevent oxidation of the hemoglobin molecule. They appear as single or multiple, round, oval, or serrated bodies, 1 to 3 μm in diameter, in the red blood cell. (See Plate VII, C.) They appear close to the cell membrane, to which they are generally attached. Heinz bodies will be found in the presence of an unstable hemoglobin, in certain red cell enzyme deficiencies (e.g., G-6-PD deficiency), and following ingestion of oxidative drugs where the quantity consumed is sufficient to neutralize the red blood cell reducing mechanisms. Drugs most commonly associated with the presence of Heinz bodies include sulfonamides, nitrofurans, antimalarials, dilantin, streptomycin, and fava beans, to name a few.

In the presence of an unstable hemoglobin, the spleen will generally remove the Heinz bodies from the red blood cell and they will, therefore, not commonly be seen in fresh blood, unless the patient has been splenectomized. Also, the following preparation will not show Heinz body formation after 15 minutes of staining, but Heinz bodies will most likely be present after 24 to 48 hours of incubation. Because normal aging of a red blood cell is accompanied by a decrease in the cell's enzyme systems, a few Heinz bodies will normally be seen with the stain.

Heinz bodies will not be seen on Wright-stained smears but are detected using supravital staining with new methylene blue, brilliant cresyl blue, methyl violet, or crystal violet. If this simple staining procedure is negative the test may be carried further, first exposing the blood to a reducing substance such as acetylphenylhydrazine. This method will detect those patients susceptible to Heinz body formation due to defective red cell reducing systems.

Reference

Beutler, E., Dern, R.J., and Alving, A.S.: The hemolytic effect of primaquine. VI. An in vitro test for sensitivity of erythrocytes to primaquine, J. Lab. & Clin. Med., 45, 40, 1955.

Specimen

Freshly drawn whole blood specimen, using heparin or EDTA as the anticoagulant. A normal control blood should be obtained at the same time the patient sample is drawn.

Stain for Heinz Bodies

Regents and Equipment

1. Test tubes, 10 × 75 mm.
2. Sodium chloride, 0.73%, w/v.
3. Crystal violet, 1%, w/v, in 0.73% sodium chloride.
   Crystal violet (color index 681)   2.0 g
   Dilute to 100 mL with 0.73% sodium chloride. Shake mixture for 5 minutes and filter. Dilute the filtered stain with an equal volume of 0.73% sodium chloride. This stain is stable at room temperature for approximately 5 months.
4. Coverslips.
5. Glass slides.

Principle

Whole blood is mixed with crystal violet stain. Slides are prepared and examined for the presence of Heinz bodies.

Procedure

1. Place five drops (one volume) of well-mixed whole blood into a labeled 10 × 75 mm test tube for each sample to be tested.
2. Add 10 drops (two volumes) of 1% crystal violet stain to each tube.
3. Mix well and incubate at room temperature for 15 minutes.
4. At the end of 15 minutes, and again after 24 hours of incubation remix the blood and stain solution. Place a small drop on each of two slides and cover with a cover glass. Allow approximately 10 minutes for the cells to settle. If desired, more permanent wedge smears may be prepared for examination, in place of the wet preparation.
5. Examine the red blood cells microscopically, using the oil immersion objective (100×). The Heinz bodies appear as purple, irregularly shaped bodies of varying sizes, from 1 to 3 μm in diameter. There may be more than one Heinz body present in a red blood cell, and they generally lie close to the cell membrane.

Discussion

1. The presence of Heinz bodies in a freshly drawn sample of blood may indicate:
   a. An oxidizing drug or chemical has been ingested in a quantity to overwhelm the normal red cell reducing system causing denaturation of the hemoglobin.
   b. A drug, such as primaquine, has been ingested by an individual with a red blood cell glycolytic enzyme deficiency, so that hemoglobin is not protected from oxidative denaturation.
   c. The patient has thalassemia or an unstable hemoglobin.

Heinz Body Preparation with Acetylphenylhydrazine

Reagents and Equipment

1. Phosphate buffer, pH 7.6.
   Potassium phosphate   9.1 g
     monobasic (KH_2PO_4)
   Dilute to 1 liter with distilled water.
   Sodium phosphate dibasic,   9.5 g
     anhydrous (Na_2HPO_4), or,
   Sodium phosphate dibasic   11.9 g
     ($Na_2HPO_4 \cdot H_2O$)
   Dilute to 1 liter with distilled water. For the working buffer, pH 7.6, mix 13 mL of monobasic potassium phosphate solution with 87 mL of dibasic sodium phosphate solution. Add 0.2 g of glucose. Store in the refrigerator. Stable for several months.

2. Acetylphenylhydrazine solution.
   Acetylphenylhydrazine   0.1 g
   Dilute to 100 mL with the working phosphate buffer, pH 7.6. This reagent should be used within 1 hour of preparation.
3. Pipets, 0.1 and 2.0 mL.
4. Water bath, 37°C.
5. All reagents and equipment as described for the Heinz body stain procedure.

Principle

Whole blood is mixed and incubated with acetylphenylhydrazine. A normal control blood is prepared in the same manner as the patient specimen. Heinz bodies will be formed when the red cells are exposed to the reducing substance (acetylphenylhydrazine). The blood specimens are then stained with crystal violet. Patients whose red cells have defective reducing systems will show greater than 32% of the red cells containing five or more Heinz bodies. Normally, fewer than 32% of the red cells will contain five or more Heinz bodies. (Each laboratory should determine its own normal range for this procedure.)

Procedure

1. Perform test on a normal control blood at the same time the patient sample is tested.
2. Place 2 mL of acetylphenylhydrazine solution into a labeled 10 × 75 mm test tube for each sample to be tested.
3. Add 0.1 mL of well-mixed whole blood to the above tube. Gently shake mixture two to three times to mix. Using a 0.1 mL pipet whiffle the mixture (force air through the mixture), three times, using the 0.1 mL pipet.
4. Place tubes in the 37°C water bath for 2 hours.
5. After 2 hours incubation, whiffle mixture (bubble air through it) four to five times, using the 0.1 mL pipet.
6. At the end of 4 hours incubation, gently shake the mixture and place five drops into a 10 × 75 mm test tube. Add 10 drops of 1% crystal violet stain. Allow to incubate (stain) at room temperature for 10 to 15 minutes.
7. Gently shake the mixture and place a small drop on each of two slides. Coverslip

and allow cells to settle for about 10 minutes. As an alternative procedure, wedge smears may be prepared for examination.
8. Using the oil immersion objective, count 200 red blood cells, enumerating those red cells which contain five or more Heinz bodies. Divide the total number of these cells (with more than five Heinz bodies) by two in order to determine the test result (percentage of red blood cells with five or more Heinz bodies).

Discussion

1. The following conditions are critical to the accurate performance of this procedure.
   a. The phosphate buffer should be at pH 7.6. At an increased pH there will be faster development of Heinz bodies, while a decreased pH slows down Heinz body formation.
   b. The amount and speed of Heinz body development will increase with increased concentrations of acetylphenylhydrazine. A decrease in the ratio of reagent to red blood cells will decrease formation. Therefore, in the presence of anemia, the concentration of red blood cells should be adjusted to near normal values (remove plasma from specimen) in order to obtain valid results.
   c. The amount of oxygenation (determined by the amount of whiffling) greatly influences the final test result. The more oxygenation, the greater the development of Heinz bodies. Because of this, capillary blood should not be used in this procedure.
   d. The acetylphenylhydrazine solution is relatively unstable and should be used as soon as possible after preparation.
2. In this method, Heinz body formation is increased in G-6-PD deficiency, 6-phosphogluconate dehydrogenase deficiency, glutathione reductase deficiency, glutathione synthetase deficiency, glutathione peroxidase deficiency, and triosephosphate isomerase deficiency.

BLOOD SMEAR PREPARATION AND EXAMINATION FOR PARASITES

Several parasites are associated with the blood. In most laboratories, *malaria* is studied in hematology. The organisms actually invade the red blood cell, and detection and diagnosis are made using a Wright or Giemsa stained smear. A large portion of the organism's life cycle takes place in the blood. Malarial parasites belong to the genus Plasmodium. There are four species that affect humans: Plasmodium falciparum (the most pathologic), Plasmodium vivax (the most prevalent), Plasmodium ovale, and Plasmodium malariae. Malaria is transmitted by the infected Anopheles mosquito. It normally occurs between latitudes of 45° North and 40° South and causes fever, anemia, and splenomegaly in the infected patient. *Babesia* is a blood parasite of animals, most notably cattle, dogs, horses, and rodents. It is transmitted to humans through the bite of an infected tick and is found most frequently in New England, but has been seen in other parts of the United States. The remaining parasites sometimes seen in the blood are generally studied in Parasitology. The hematology technologist, however, should be familiar with them because they may be found on routine examination of a blood smear. Several species of flagellates will be seen in the blood of an infected person. These organisms belong to the genera of *Trypanosoma* and *Leishmania*. Trypanosomas gambiense and rhodesiense are found in Africa, are the cause of sleeping sickness, and are transmitted through the bite of the tsetse fly. Trypanosoma cruzi is found in the southern United States, Mexico, and Central and South America. It is the cause of Chaga's disease and is transmitted via the reduvid bug ("kissing bug"). Trypanosoma rangeli is also transmitted by species of the reduvid bug and is found mostly in Central and South America. Leishmania is found primarily in portions of Europe, Africa, Asia, and Central and South America. Several species infect humans: Leishmanias braziliensis, mexicana, donovani, and tropica. The parasite is transmitted by the sand fly. There are at least seven known species of *filaria* that infect humans: Wucheria bancrofti, Loa loa, Dipetalonema perstans, Brugia malayi, and three species of Mansonella. Filariae will be found in parts of Africa, Asia, Central and South America, and the tropics and subtropics. The parasite infection is transmitted to humans by mosquitos and flies.

Although only a few of the parasites described above occur naturally in the United States, infections are being found more frequently in this country than previously. This is due to increasing world travel by more people. Obtaining a travel history from the patient is therefore important. Malaria and Babesia are diagnosed through study of thick and thin Wright and Giemsa stained blood smears. A rapid concentration procedure for malaria is described below. This procedure may also be used for the diagnosis of trypanosome infections. Various other concentration techniques (not covered in this text) are available for the isolation of the leishmanias, trypanosomes, and filariae. These organisms may also be detected on Wright and Giemsa stained smears.

Blood Smear Preparation and Stain

Specimen Collection

Capillary blood (finger or heel) is recommended. If this is not possible collect 1 mL of fresh whole blood anticoagulated in EDTA. Specimens should be obtained at different times depending on the infection suspected.

Malaria. Blood should first be collected as soon as malaria is suspected. It is most helpful to obtain blood specimens midway between the attacks (paroxysms), because the smears will usually contain the parasites in more advanced stages in which there are increased identifying characteristics. A malaria infection can be life threatening, and testing should be available at any time in the hematology laboratory. Blood specimens must be obtained prior to beginning treatment.

Trypanosomes. These parasites are most often found in the blood during the early, acute phase of the infection. This will be during the first month for Trypanosoma cruzi, which may also be found in the blood during periods of fever (febrile stages). The African trypanosomes may be present in the blood at the beginning of the infection for several months to as long as a year.

Filaria. The appropriate time to obtain specimens for microfilariae will depend on the species. Wucheria bancrofti and Brugia malayi are nocturnal and specimens should be collected at night, whereas blood is obtained around noon time for Loa loa.

Concentration Technique for Malaria

1. Using fresh EDTA anticoagulated whole blood, fill four microhematocrit tubes and spin for 2 to 3 minutes in the microhematocrit centrifuge.
2. With a small file, score each microhematocrit tube 1 to 2 mm below the buffy coat layer (in the red cell portion). Break the hematocrit tubes at this junction.
3. Using the portion of the hematocrit tube containing the red cells, buffy coat, and plasma, gently tap the hematocrit tube on a slide to express the red cells and buffy coat. Also add a small amount of plasma.
4. Using the corner of a second slide, mix the red cells, buffy coat, and plasma together. As soon as mixed, prepare a wedge smear.

Blood Smear Preparation

1. Thin smears. Make two or three thin wedge blood smears from fingertip blood or blood anticoagulated with EDTA. Air dry smears.
2. Thick smears. Make two or three thick smears by placing a large drop of blood on a glass slide. Using the corner of a second slide, carefully spread the drop of blood over an area the size of a dime. (To determine the correct thickness of the blood smear, place the slide on a piece of newspaper. Spread the blood until the small newsprint is just visible through the smear). Allow the smears to air dry, protected from dust, for 8 to 12 hours, or overnight.
3. Buffy coat smears. Prepare as described above.

Reagents and Equipment

1. Dibasic Sodium phosphate, 0.067 M.
   Anhydrous dibasic sodium
   phosphate (Na_2HPO_4)   9.5 g
   Dissolve in a small amount of distilled water and dilute to 1 L with distilled water.
2. Monobasic potassium phosphate, .067 M.
   Anhydrous monobasic potassium
   phosphate (KH_2PO_4)   9.1 g
   Dissolve in a small amount of distilled water and dilute to 1 L with distilled water.
3. Triton X-100, 10% (v/v) aqueous solution.
   Triton X-100   10.0 mL
   Dilute to 100 mL with distilled water. Kept tightly stoppered, this reagent will keep indefinitely. (Triton X-100 will improve the staining properties of Giemsa stain, and is also effective in the staining of Schüffner's dots.)
4. Buffered distilled water, pH 7.2.
   Dibasic sodium phosphate,
   0.067 M   72.0 mL
   Monobasic potassium phosphate,
   0.067 M   28.0 mL
   Triton X-100, 10% (v/v)   1.0 mL
   Dilute above mixture to 1 L with distilled water. (If the pH of the mixture is checked, it must be done prior to adding the Triton X-100.) This reagent may be stored for 1 week at room temperature. Storage for longer periods requires verification of the correct pH prior to use.
5. Giemsa staining solution.
   Liquid Giemsa stain   2 mL
   Buffered distilled water, pH 7.2   38 mL
   Prepare fresh daily. (Different lot numbers of Giemsa stain will vary in their staining characteristics. The staining times and dilution with buffered water should be checked for each new lot of stain prior to use.)
6. Methanol.
7. Coplin jar.

Procedure

1. Fix the thin smears and buffy coat smears with methanol for several seconds. Do not fix the thick smears.
2. Place the smears in a coplin jar containing Giemsa staining solution for 30 minutes.
3. At the end of 30 minutes, rinse the smears in running tap water and allow to air dry.
4. Examine the smears microscopically. The cells on the thick, unfixed smears will be lysed, making examination easier. The thick blood film is used for the detection of the blood parasite and consists of white cell nuclei and platelet debris.

Discussion

1. Slides should be precleaned with 70 to 90% ethyl alcohol just prior to use.
2. To ensure staining of the red cell stippling

found in malaria, blood smears should be prepared within 1 hour of obtaining the specimen.

3. Thick smears must be dried at room temperature (25°C). Heating the smear to speed up drying will cause parts of the smear to become fixed and interfere with lysis of the cells. The smears may be stained before 8 hours, but extra care must be taken that the blood does not wash off the slide. Use of a fan will cut drying time in half.

4. The Giemsa stain should contain azure B. Azure A is not as effective a stain for blood parasites.

5. The pH of the buffered water should be between 7.0 and 7.2.

6. Field's stain, using methylene blue and Azure B, is also used as a malarial stain.

Examination of the Smear for Parasites

Malaria. Examine the stained smears microscopically, using the oil immersion objective (100×). The concentration of malarial parasites in the blood may be as low as one parasite/100,000 red blood cells, or one parasite/400 high oil immersion fields on a thin blood smear, which could take about 1 hour to examine. However, this same volume of blood may be examined on a thick blood smear in 5 minutes. The thick smear is useful for detecting the parasite, whereas the thin smears show the morphologic characteristics and should be used for identification of the organism. Mixed infections of malaria are sometimes found and are much more difficult to diagnose. The mixed infection currently found most often is Plasmodia falciparum and vivax. The identification of a species of malaria requires the consideration of three factors: the appearance of infected erythrocytes, the appearance of the parasites, and the stages found. See Table 4–4 for differentiating characteristics of the four species. (Color Plate IX, A–G, X.)

Babesia. Examine the stained smears microscopically using the high oil immersion objective. Diagnosis of this infection is made by finding pleomorphic, ring-like forms in the red blood cells. They frequently appear as a single reddish chromatin dot with delicate tufts of blue cytoplasm and will vary in size from 1 to 4 μm in diameter. These forms are very similar to, and can be mistaken for, the ring forms of Plasmodium falciparum. The Babesia parasite, however, is smaller than the ring forms of malaria; they are very fragile and do not contain pigment. A single red cell may contain four or five organisms; the formation of a *tetrad* of four organisms (merozoites) is a characteristic finding. (See Color Plate IX, H, I.)

Flagellates. There are two or more stages in the development of these parasites: amastigote, promastigote, epimastigote, and trypomastigote. Some of the organisms may show only two of these stages in their development, whereas others will show more. Morphologically they are differentiated on the basis of the size, shape, and origin of the flagellum. In human infections of Leishmania only the amastigote stage may be seen in the peripheral blood. This organism is oval in shape and is 2 to 5 μm in size, has pale blue cytoplasm with a reddish staining nucleus, a red kinetoplast, and a short flagellum that does not extend to the outside. The amastigote will be found in the white blood cells, most notably monocytes and macrophages. The different species are morphologically indistinguishable. Diagnosis of this infection is usually made by identification of the amastigote stage in blood cells, tissue sections, or tissue impressions. In trypanosome infections in the trypomastigote stage may be seen in the blood. Depending on the species it will vary from 14 to 33 μm in length. Trypanosoma rangeli may be even longer. This stage has a central nucleus and a small kinetoplast at the posterior (blunt) end. The flagellum courses through the body and extends to the outside. Diagnosis of this infection is usually made by identification of the parasite in the blood. (See color Plate IX, J.)

Filaria. Adult filaria, located in different areas of the body, will release microfilariae into the blood. These organisms will vary in length from 150 to 350 μm and in width from 3 to 10 μm. Diagnosis is made by identification of the parasite in the blood or skin. Differentiation of species depends on their location in the body (skin or blood), the time of day or night during which they are found in the

TABLE 4–4. DISTINGUISHING CHARACTERISTICS OF PLASMODIUM SPECIES

Characteristic	P. vivax	P. falciparum	P. malariae	P. ovale
Stages present in the blood	All stages: A wide variety may be seen	Ring and gametocyte only except in severe infections	All, not at the same time, only a few rings and gametocytes	All
Ring form				
Size # in Red cells	Large 2 or more frequently seen	Small, delicate Multiple forms in one red cell	Small, compact 1	Small, compact 1
# Chromatin dots	1 to 2	1 to 2	1	1
Trophozoite characteristics	Ameboid, appears spread out, large	Usually not seen, medium sized	Compact with dense cytoplasm	Small, compact
Mature schizont (# merozoites)	12–24 (average of 16)	Usually not seen, 8–24	6–12	6–12, average of 8
Size of infected red blood cell	Enlarged, may be irregularly shaped	Normal	Normal	Enlarged, oval with irregular border (fimbriated)
Stippling	Shüffner's granules	Occasional Maurer's dots	Rare Ziemann's dots	Shüffner's granules
Pigment	Golden brown	Large, brown granules	Abundant and conspicuous, dark brown	Dark brown
Other differentiating characteristics	Trophozoite often fills most of red cell	Crescent- or sausage-shaped gametocytes	Gametocytes not very numerous	Shüffner's granules prominent

blood, and their morphology. They will vary in length, width, presence or absence of a sheath, shape of the tail, and the location of tail nuclei. Microscopic examination should be made on low power (10×). More magnification will be needed, however, to identify their characteristics. (See Color Plate IX, K.)

RED CELL ZINC PROTOPORPHYRIN

Measurement of zinc protoporphyrin in red blood cells may be used as a diagnostic test for iron deficiency anemia and as a screening procedure for lead poisoning.

During the development of heme, iron is inserted into protoporphyrin IX. In iron deficiency anemia where there is insufficient iron, or, in chronic lead poisoning where the utilization of iron is defective, zinc is incorporated into the protoporphyrin IX ring, which then attaches to a heme site on globin, forming a nonfunctional molecule that remains for the life of the red blood cell. Measurement of the zinc protoporphyrin level in the red blood cells may therefore be used as an indicator of lead poisoning or iron deficiency.

The test described below uses the Protofluor-Z Hematofluorometer (Helena Laboratories, Beaumont, Texas) (Fig. 4–1) and is a

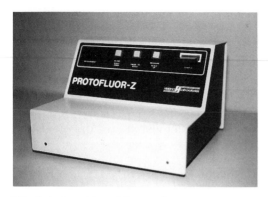

FIG. 4–1. ProtoFluor-Z Hematofluorometer.

quick and easy procedure to perform. Using this method as described, the normal range for iron deficiency anemia is approximately 30 to 80 μmol ZPP/mol Heme (or, 15 to 36 μg ZPP/dL of whole blood). However, each laboratory should determine its own normal ranges. When screening for lead poisoning, a blood lead assay should be performed when the ZPP level is at or above 70 μmol/mol Heme.

References

Helena Laboratories: ProtoFluor® Reagent System, pkg. insert, Beaumont, Texas, 1987.

Helena Laboratories: *ProtoFluor-Z Hematofluorometer Operator's Manual*, Beaumont, Texas, 1990.

Labbe, R.F., and Rettmer, R.L.: Zinc protoporphyrin: A product of iron-deficient erythropoiesis, Semin. Hematol., *26*, 40, 1989.

Reagents and Equipment

1. The following reagents and equipment are available from Helena Laboratories:
   a. ProtoFluor reagent contains stabilizers and a cyanide salt in a water solution. It may be stored at room temperature or at 2 to 6°C. Cloudiness is indicative of reagent deterioration.
   b. Low and High ProtoFluor Calibrators contain zinc protoporphyrin, preservatives, and stabilizers and are ready for use as packaged.
   c. ProtoFluor coverslips, 24 mm × 24 mm.
   d. ProtoFluor Z Hematofluorometer.
2. Test tubes, 10 × 75 mm.
3. Pipets, 0.05 and 0.1 mL.

4. Microhematocrit tubes.
5. Sodium chloride, 0.85% (w/v).
6. Bovine albumin, 22%.
7. 12 mL centrifuge tubes.
8. Zinc protoporphyrin controls. Store at 2 to 6°C. (Available from Kaulson Laboratories, Inc., W. Caldwell, New Jersey.)

Specimen

Whole blood, 1 mL, collected in heparin, sodium citrate, or EDTA. Blood up to 1 week old may be used unless it is hemolyzed. Capillary blood may also be collected by filling two to three heparinized microhematocrit tubes.

Principle

ProtoFluor reagent is added to anticoagulated whole blood in order to completely oxygenate the hemoglobin (incomplete oxygenation of the hemoglobin will yield falsely low test values). A drop of this mixture is placed on a coverslip and inserted into the Hematofluorometer. Light with a wavelength of 415 nm is focused onto the blood mixture. At the same time, a portion of this light beam is deflected onto a photocell for measurement to allow for correction of any variation in the light intensity. The light that comes in contact with the blood specimen causes the zinc protoporphyrin present in the red blood cells to emit light of a wavelength of 595 nm. This light is collected onto a photomultiplier tube, which produces a current in proportion to the amount of light reaching it. The current produced is directly proportional to the μmol of zinc protoporphyrin/mol heme. The result is unaffected by the hematocrit.

Procedure

1. Allow reagent, calibrators, and controls to warm to room temperature. Turn on the Hematofluorometer 30 minutes prior to testing. If the instrument is already on from previous testing, turn the instrument off and then on again in order to reset the electronics.
2. Check the back of the instrument to verify that it is set in the correct mode for the desired units of reporting. (Top setting is for results in μg/dL [patient hematocrit of

42% or above], bottom setting is μg/dL [patient hematocrit lower than 42%], and the middle setting is for μmol ZPP/mol heme.)

3. Blank the instrument when ready for testing:
   a. Insert the Sample Holder into the instrument (end with hole facing forward, with the recessed area facing up) until it "clicks" into position.
   b. Press the Measure button. The display will read '---' ("H35" or "H42") for about 5 seconds, followed by the blank reading, which should be 000 ±3. If the value displayed is any higher this may indicate a problem for which Service would need to be called.
   c. Remove the Sample Holder from the instrument.
   d. Remove a single coverslip from the box, handling it only by the edges. Examine it to make certain it is free of any dirt, fingerprints, or scratches. Place the coverslip in the Sample Holder.
   e. Insert Sample Holder (with coverslip) into the instrument. Press the Blank button. The reading on the Display should be between 4 and 14. If the results are outside of these limits, repeat using a second coverslip.
   f. Press Measure. The reading on the Display should now read 000 ±1, which indicates that the instrument is blanked (zeroed) on that coverslip. It is only necessary to blank the first one or two coverslips.

4. Calibrate the instrument:
   a. Place a clean coverslip in the Sample Holder (or use the one from the above step) and insert into the instrument. Press the Measure button. The optimal reading for use with the calibrators is 000. Remove the Sample Holder from the instrument.
   b. Place one drop of High Calibrator in the center of the coverslip (in the Sample Holder). Using the tip of the vial spread the drop so that it covers the sample area (minimum diameter of 8 to 10 mm). Make certain there are no bubbles.
   c. Carefully insert the Sample Holder into the instrument. Press the Measure

button. The reading on the display should be within 10 units of the assay. Set the instrument to the exact assay value by pressing the Press To Scale button and simultaneously pressing the Scale Up or Scale Down button until the correct assay value is displayed.
   d. Remove the Sample Holder from the instrument and discard the coverslip.
   e. Place a new coverslip in the Holder and take a reading (press Measure button).
   f. Remove the Sample Holder and place a new drop of High Calibrator on the coverslip. Take a reading (press Measure). The reading should be within ±3 of the assay value. If it is not repeat the above described procedure.
   g. Remove the Sample Holder from the instrument and discard the coverslip containing the High Calibrator.
   h. Repeat steps 4a and b above using the Low Calibrator. Insert the Sample Holder into the instrument. Press the Measure button. The reading on the display should be within ±3 of the assay value for the Low Calibrator. If it is not, press the Measure button two more times, taking a reading each time. If two of the three readings are within ±3 of the assay value the instrument is considered set correctly. If the readings are not within range, the instrument must be recalibrated as described above using the High Calibrator. Do not make any adjustments using the Low Calibrator.

5. Patient and control testing:
   a. Mix the patient (or control) sample well.
   b. Place 0.05 mL of whole blood (patient or control) into a labeled 10 × 75 mm test tube. Add 0.1 mL of ProtoFluor reagent to the tube and mix well. (Once reagent has been added to the patient sample, testing must be completed within 5 minutes.)
   c. Place one drop of the test mixture in the center of the coverslip in the Sample Holder. Spread the drop evenly over the sample area.
   d. Immediately, place the Sample Holder in the instrument and take a reading by pressing the Measure button. (If the

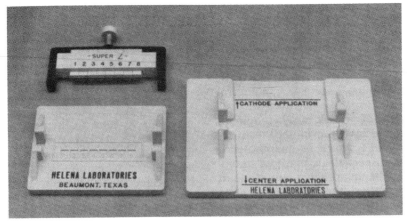

FIG. 4–2. Equipment used in hemoglobin electrophoresis by cellulose acetate. Sample applicator (top left), sample plate (left), and aligning base (right).

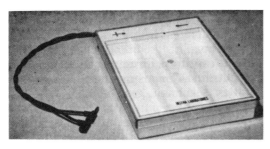

FIG. 4–3. Electrophoresis chamber. (Courtesy of Helena Laboratories, Beaumont, Texas.)

7. Sample well plate (holds hemolysate samples to be tested) (Fig. 4–2).
8. Aligning base (holds cellulose acetate strip for inoculation). (Fig. 4–2).
9. Electrophoresis chamber (Fig. 4–3).
10. Large filter paper (for blotting cellulose acetate strips).
11. Test tubes, 10 × 75 mm.
12. Pipet, 5 μL.
13. Disposable pipet droppers.
14. Squeeze bottle of distilled water for rinsing applicator and sample well plate.
15. Small shallow pans, five, for buffer, stain, and acetic acid rinse.
16. Hemostats, two pair.
17. Acetic acid, 5% (v/v).
18. DC-regulated power supply (Fig. 4–4).
19. Microhematocrit tubes, plain.
20. Glass slides, 1 × 3 inch.
21. Sodium chloride, 0.85% (w/v).
22. Known control samples. These may be liquid or frozen red cell hemolysates and

may be prepared from blood with known abnormal hemoglobins, or purchased from any one of several commercial laboratory distributors.

Specimen

Whole blood (0.5 mL) using EDTA or heparin as the anticoagulant. Capillary blood may also be used (three to four microhematocrit tubes, three-quarters filled). Whole blood samples may be stored in the refrigerator for up to 1 week, or, once the hemolysate has been prepared, it may be frozen for several months.

Principle

Electrophoresis is the movement of charged particles in an electric field. In an alkaline buffer (pH 8.2 to 8.6) hemoglobin is a negatively charged molecule and will migrate

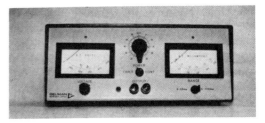

FIG. 4–4. Power supply. (Courtesy of Gelman Instrument Co., Ann Arbor, Michigan.)

toward the anode (+). The various hemoglobins move at different rates depending on their net negative charge, which in turn is controlled by the composition (amino acids) of the hemoglobin molecule (globin chain).

The red cell hemolysate (red blood cell membranes are destroyed to free the hemoglobin molecules for testing) is placed on a cellulose acetate membrane, which is positioned in an electrophoresis tray with the inoculated hemolysate near the cathode (−). One end of the cellulose acetate strip is immersed in the buffer (pH 8.2 to 8.6) on the cathode side and the other end is placed in the buffer on the anode (+) side. An electric current of specific voltage is allowed to run for a timed period. During electrophoresis, the hemoglobin molecules migrate toward the anode because of their net negative charge. The difference in the net charge of the hemoglobin molecule determines its mobility and manifests itself by the speed with which it migrates to the positive pole. The cellulose acetate membrane is then stained in order to color the proteins (hemoglobins). By noting the distance each hemoglobin has migrated and comparing this distance with the migration distance of known controls, the types of hemoglobins may be identified.

Procedure

1. Preparation of hemolysate
   a. *Using washed red blood cells.* Place ½ to 1 mL of well-mixed whole blood into an appropriately labeled 10 × 75 mm test tube. Wash red cells one to three times with sodium chloride (0.85%, w/v): fill tube with sodium chloride and centrifuge at 1200 to 1500 g for 5 minutes; remove supernatant; repeat cell washing two more times. Place one drop of washed, packed red blood cells into an appropriately labeled 10 × 75 mm test tube. Add six drops of hemolysate reagent. Mix and allow to sit for 5 minutes for complete hemolysis of the red cells. If the hemolysate is cloudy, place in the freezer for about 10 minutes. Upon thawing the hemolysate should be crystal clear.
   b. *Using whole blood.* Place one drop of whole blood into a 10 × 75 mm test tube. Add three drops of hemolysate reagent. Mix and allow to stand for 5 minutes. If the hemolysate is not crystal clear, freeze and thaw specimen as described in step a above.
   c. *Using microhematocrit tubes.* Centrifuge two microhematocrit tubes. Using a file, cut the packed red cell layer into three or four sections, discarding the plasma and buffy coat portions and the sealed end. Place the open sections containing the red cells, into a 10 × 75 mm test tube. Repeat this procedure for the second microhematocrit tube, placing the red cells in the same tube with the sections from the first hematocrit. Add eight drops of hemolysate reagent to the tube. Mix vigorously by drawing across the top of a test tube rack numerous times. Allow to sit for 10 minutes for hemolysis to occur.
   d. *Using capillary blood collected on filter paper* (available from Rochester Paper Co., Rochester, MI, as ROPACO #1023, 0.038 inch). The specimen is collected by placing a large drop of blood (minimum of 12 mm diameter) onto the filter paper. The specimen may then be stored in the refrigerator. To prepare hemolysate, cut out a circular sample of the blood 1 cm in diameter. Place in a test tube and add two drops of hemolysate reagent. Mix and allow to elute for 30 minutes. Remove filter paper. The hemolysate may now be tested or may be frozen for future testing.

2. Fill a pan with approximately 40 mL of buffer solution.

3. Holding a cellulose acetate strip at the edge with a clean, dry hemostat, slowly and uniformly immerse it into the buffer solution. This should take 10 to 15 seconds. If the membrane is immersed too quickly, white areas appear on the cellulose acetate and it must be discarded. Allow the entire strip to soak in the buffer for a minimum of 5 minutes prior to use. (Make certain your hands are clean and free of any oil or grease if you touch the cellulose acetate strip prior to the last step of this procedure [staining].)

4. Pour 100 mL of buffer into each of the

outer compartments of the electrophoresis chamber. Moisten two disposable paper wicks in the buffer and drape one over each of the two middle support bridges, ensuring that one side is immersed in the buffer and that there are no air bubbles under the wicks.

5. Place 5 μL of each hemolysate into its own well in the sample well plate. Place the known control hemolysate in well number 1 and/or 2. Cover the sample well plate with glass slide if the hemolysates will not be inoculated within 5 minutes.

6. Prime the sample applicator: Remove the slide from the sample well plate, place the sample applicator on the sample plate, and depress the tips into the wells three or four times. Apply the hemolysate to a blotter. Replace the applicator over the sample well plate.

7. Remove the cellulose acetate strip from the buffer, and carefully blot the strip between two pieces of filter paper in order to remove the excess surface buffer only. Proceed quickly to the next step.

8. With the mylar (plastic) backing facing up, label the strip C (for cathode) in the appropriate corner and write each sample number for the specimen being tested at the edge of the strip corresponding to its inoculation site.

9. Place a drop of buffer on the middle of the aligning base (prevents slippage of the strip). Quickly turn the strip over (cellulose acetate side up) and place it in the aligning base with the bottom edge lined up with the line marked 'cathode application.'

10. Depress the applicator tips into the sample wells three or four times. Quickly transfer the applicator to the aligning base. Press the button down and hold it on the strip for 5 seconds.

11. Quickly place the strip, cellulose acetate side down and with the long side of the strip on the horizontal, in the chamber with the application site nearest the cathode (−) side. Place one or two glass slides on top of the strip to act as a weight. Carefully place the cover on top of the chamber.

12. Attach the electrode terminal pins to the power supply. Turn the power supply on

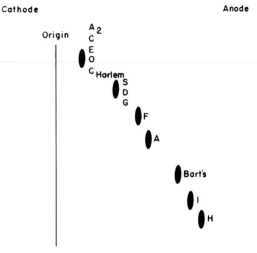

FIG. 4–5. Electrophoretic mobility of various hemoglobins at pH 8.2 to 8.4.

and electrophorese for 25 minutes at a setting of 350 volts.

13. At the end of 25 minutes, turn the power supply off, carefully remove the strips from the chamber, and blot the side edges to remove the excess buffer.

14. Place the strips in a pan containing Ponceau S stain for 5 minutes.

15. Remove the strip from the stain and place it in a 5% acetic acid solution for about 2 minutes to rinse the excess stain off. Agitate the membrane gently.

16. Repeat step 15, two or three more times, in clean 5% acetic acid until all of the excess stain is removed. The strip should return to its white color, with only the hemoglobin taking up the stain.

17. After the last acetic acid wash, remove the excess moisture by blotting on filter paper. Allow 5 to 10 minutes for air-drying.

18. Identify the hemoglobin types present in the patient samples by comparing their migration distances with the known controls. See Figure 4–5 for the mobilities of various hemoglobins. Some abnormal hemoglobins have identical electrophoretic migration distances on cellulose acetate in an alkaline buffer (pH 8.4). For this reason it is recommended that citrate agar gel electrophoresis be performed when an abnormal hemoglobin is detected by this method.

Discussion

1. If the Ponceau S stain is kept tightly covered, it may be used for approximately 1 month. The staining time in this procedure is not critical.
2. The buffer solution used for soaking the cellulose acetate strips may be used for soaking up to 12 strips or for 5 working days (whichever occurs first) if it is kept covered when not in use.
3. Fresh chamber buffer should be used daily.
4. If a specimen migrates as hemoglobin S, perform a sickle cell test. The results should be positive. If the sickle cell test is negative (and the blood migrates as hemoglobin S), the abnormal hemoglobin is most probably D. Agar gel electrophoresis should then be performed for further identification.
5. Three cellulose acetate strips may be run in the electrophoresis chamber at one time.
6. Generally, when eight samples are inoculated on a strip, distortion may occur in the first and eighth samples. For consistently good results, use only the second through seventh slots in the sample well plate.
7. If semiquantitative results are desired, the cellulose acetate strip is cleared in order to develop a transparent background. It is then placed in a scanning densitometer (specifically designed for this purpose) and read at a wavelength of 525 nm. For accurate quantitation of hemoglobin F and hemoglobin A_2, the alkali denaturation or radial immunodiffusion test for hemoglobin F, and a quantitative test specifically for hemoglobin A_2, should be performed.
8. There may be a small amount of hemoglobin that distributes itself along the pathway of the migrating hemoglobin. This is called *trailing*. A small amount of this trailing is not unusual. Excessive amounts may be due to (1) denaturation of the hemoglobin because of excessive heat, (2) samples that are too old, (3) too large a sample of hemolysate used, or (4) a dirty membrane.
9. Neutral pH electrophoresis uses a 0.05 M phosphate buffer (pH 6.9 to 7.1) and is used for differentiating hemoglobin H and hemoglobin Bart's from other fast-moving hemoglobins. At an alkaline pH these hemoglobins will show diffuse bands, and their exact positions may be difficult to determine. However, at a neutral pH, the hemoglobin bands are much sharper. The hemolysate is applied to the center of the cellulose acetate strip, and after electrophoresing for 30 minutes at 150 volts hemoglobin H will migrate a greater distance toward the anode than any other hemoglobin. Bart's hemoglobin will also migrate toward the anode but not as far as H will. Fresh blood must be used for this procedure because hemoglobin H is unstable and will easily denature. A known H, Bart's, and normal hemoglobin control should be used when performing this procedure.
10. Acid and alkaline globin chain electrophoresis may also be used to assist in the identification of unknown hemoglobins. In these two procedures 2-mercaptoethanol and urea are used to dissociate the heme and globin chains of the hemoglobin molecule. At the alkaline pH (8.8 to 9.5) or acid pH (6.0 to 6.2) the different globin chains will migrate to specific positions on cellulose acetate. At least two different known hemoglobins should be used as a control in the procedure; results are compared with the migration distances of the known globin chains. (Because the fumes from the 2-mercaptoethanol are irritating this procedure should be performed under a fume hood.)

CITRATE AGAR ELECTROPHORESIS

Citrate agar electrophoresis is used to confirm variant hemoglobins and further differentiates hemoglobin S from D and G, and hemoglobin C from hemoglobins E, O_{Arab}, and C_{Harlem}. The procedure should not be used as a screening procedure because many abnormal hemoglobins migrate with hemoglobin A. However, this procedure is the method of choice when examining newborns (cord blood specimens) and infants under 3 months of age for some abnormal hemoglobins such as S and C because the test is able to detect quantities of hemoglobin not easily seen by other techniques.

References

Helena Laboratories: Titan IV citrate hemoglobin electrophoresis procedure, pkg. insert, Beaumont Tex., Helena Laboratories, 1983.

National Committee for clinical Laboratory Standards: *Citrate Agar Electrophoresis for Confirming Identification of Variant Hemoglobins*, (H23-T), NCCLS, Villanova, PA, 1988.

Reagents and Equipment

1. The following reagents and supplies are obtainable from Helena Laboratories. (Items e, f, g, i, j, and k are the same as those listed for the cellulose acetate hemoglobin electrophoresis procedure.)
   a. Citrate buffer, 0.05 M, pH 6.0 to 6.3, (contains sodium citrate and citric acid). Dilute one package of citrate buffer to 1 L with distilled water. Stable for 1 month stored at 2 to 6°C. Discard if the dry powder is discolored or if the solution is cloudy.
   b. Citrate agar plates (Titan® IV) (1.5% [w/v] agarose in citrate buffer with an added preservative).
   c. Zip Zone® sponge wicks.
   d. o-Tolidine, 0.2% (w/v) (or O-Diansidine 0.2% [w/v]) in methanol.
   e. Electrophoresis chamber.
   f. Zip Zone® sample applicator (with the spring removed).
   g. Zip Zone® sample well plate.
   h. Titan® IV aligning base.
   i. Microdispenser (for measuring 5 μl amounts).
   j. Hemolysate reagent.
   k. AFSC hemoglobin control.
2. DC-regulated power supply.
3. Pipets, 1, 5, and 10 mL.
4. Test tubes, 10 × 75 mm.
5. Polypropylene centrifuge tubes, 15 mL.
6. Acetic acid, 5% (v/v).
7. Sodium nitroferricyanide, 1% (w/v).
8. Hydrogen peroxide, 30%.
9. Parafilm.
10. Glass slides, 1 × 3 inch.

Specimen

Whole blood using EDTA as the anticoagulant. If capillary blood is being used, collect four to six hematocrit tubes three-fourths filled with blood. Whole blood may be refrigerated for up to 1 week before testing.

Principle

A red blood cell hemolysate is prepared in order to destroy the red blood cell membrane and free the hemoglobin. The patient's hemolysate, along with known controls, is placed on a slide containing a thin layer of agar. This slide is placed, agar side down, across the support bridges of an electrophoresis tray. An electric current of specific voltage is applied for a timed period. At the conclusion of electrophoresing the agar slide is placed in a heme-specific stain. By noting the distance each hemoglobin has migrated and comparing this distance with the migration distance of known controls, the different types of hemoglobins present may be identified. The migration distances of the different hemoglobins are based on the electrophoretic charge of the molecules and their adsorption (characteristics) to the agar compound. There are four major zones of hemoglobin migration on the agar at this acid pH: the negatively charged molecules of hemoglobins C and S move toward the anode (+), while hemoglobins A and F (positively charged) migrate to the cathode (hemoglobin A remains close to the site of inoculation). The results of this procedure are correlated with migration characteristics on the cellulose acetate hemoglobin electrophoresis.

Procedure

1. Remove the necessary number of Titan® citrate agar plates from the refrigerator and allow to warm to room temperature.
2. Prepare the patient sample hemolysates by adding one drop of patient whole blood to 19 drops of hemolysate reagent. Mix vigorously and make certain the resultant dilution is crystal clear. Prepare the control hemolysate by adding one drop of hemolysate reagent to one drop of the Helena AFSC control. Mix well. (If the patient sample has a hemoglobin value of less than 8 g/dL, add 10 drops of hemolysate reagent to one drop of whole blood.)
3. Fill the electrophoresis tray with cold citrate buffer, pH 6.0 to 6.3 (use of cold

buffer will yield sharper hemoglobin bands): Place approximately 100 mL of buffer into each of the outer compartments of the electrophoresis chamber. Thoroughly wet two of the sponges in the citrate buffer and place one in each of the outer chambers, against the inner chamber wall, such that the top surface protrudes approximately 2 mm above the wall.

4. Using the microdispenser (5 μL pipet), add 5 μL of each hemolysate to the appropriate well of the sample plate. (Samples run in the first and last positions on the agar gel plate may not electrophorese as well as the centrally located samples. For this reason, it may be preferable to use only sections 2 through 7.) Cover the sample well plate with a glass slide if the hemolysates are not to be inoculated within 2 minutes. Position the sample applicator directly over the sample well plate.

5. Prime the sample applicator by lowering the tips into the sample wells several times. Apply this first loading to a piece of filter paper or blotter. This action primes the applicator to ensure more uniform inoculation onto the agar.

6. Remove the citrate agar plate from the plastic bag, peel off the tape around the cover, and remove cover. Label the plate by writing the sample numbers on one side edge of the plate. Also, label the right end of the plate with a "+" for anode and the other end of the plate "−" for cathode. Immediately, place the agar gel plate in the Titan IV aligning base so that the set of grooves for the applicator will be centrally located to the plate.

7. Load the applicator by depressing the tips into the wells of the sample plate several times. Place the applicator in the set of grooves closest to the center of the plate and slowly and carefully lower the applicator tips down onto the top surface of the agar. Allow the applicator tips to remain on the agar surface for 1 minute so that the hemolysates soak into the agar. Be extremely careful that the applicator tips do not at any time break the surface of the agar.

8. Very quickly, place the agar plate, gel side down, labeled "+" side at the anode, in the electrophoresis chamber so that the gel layer makes good contact with the top surface of the sponges.

9. Carefully place the cover on the electrophoresis chamber. Attach the electrode terminal pins to the power supply. Turn the power supply on and electrophorese for 45 minutes at 50 volts.

10. Approximately 10 minutes before electrophoresing is complete, prepare the stain. Mix together:

5% Acetic acid	10.0 mL
O-Tolidine (or O-Diansidine), 0.2%	5.0 mL
1% Sodium nitroferri-cyanide	1.0 mL
Distilled water	0.9 mL
Hydrogen peroxide	0.1 mL

11. At the conclusion of the electrophoresing period, remove the plates from the electrophoresis chamber. Place each plate, agar side up, on a level surface (near a sink is advisable). Using a disposable dropper pipet, carefully flood each plate with a thin layer of stain and allow to sit until all hemoglobin components are stained (generally takes 2 to 5 minutes using fresh stain).

12. When staining is complete, carefully rinse the plates under running tap water. Place each plate, agar side down, on a blotter or filter paper until the moisture is absorbed (10 to 15 minutes).

13. When most of the moisture has been removed, allow the slides to air dry and read. The top may be replaced on the agar gel plate once all moisture has been removed, and the plate may then be stored for future reference, if desired.

14. Identify the hemoglobin types present in the patient samples by comparing the migration distances with the known controls. See Figure 4–6 for the mobilities of various hemoglobins. The interpretation of agar gel results must be correlated with the hemoglobin types found on cellulose acetate hemoglobin electrophoresis.

Discussion

1. For best results, the hemoglobin concentration of the patient hemolysates should be slightly less than 1 g/dL. Cord blood

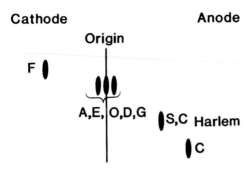

FIG. 4–6. Electrophoretic mobility of various hemoglobins on agar gel at pH 6.0 to 6.3.

hemolysates should have a concentration of approximately 4 g/dL.

2. The same hemolysate used for the cellulose acetate procedure may also be used for agar gel electrophoresis by adding one drop of the original hemolysate (cellulose acetate) to four drops of hemolysate reagent.

3. On agar gel the mobility of the hemoglobins will tend to vary more than on cellulose acetate and is more dependent on the concentration of hemoglobin, size of inoculation, and composition of the buffer.

4. Amido black, 1% (w/v), may be used as an alternative stain. Dissolve 10 g of amido black 10B in 100 mL of glacial acetic acid. Dilute to 1 L with distilled water. After staining, rinse and decolorize using 5% acetic acid until the agar background is free of stain.

HEMOGLOBIN A$_2$

Very small amounts of hemoglobin A$_2$ (up to about 3.5%) are normally found in the adult. Elevated levels (up to 8%) generally indicate β-thalassemia trait, although some patients with homozygous β thalassemia may show an increased hemoglobin A$_2$. Decreased levels may be found in iron deficiency anemia, hemoglobin H disease, hereditary persistence of fetal hemoglobin, sideroblastic anemia, and in carriers of α thalassemia.

The anion exchange microchromatography procedure outlined below is an accurate and easily performed method for hemoglobin A$_2$ quantitation.

Reference

Helena Laboratories: *Beta-Thal Hemoglobin A$_2$ Quik Column™ Procedure*, Beaumont, Tex., Helena Laboratories, 1984.

Reagents and Equipment

1. Beta-Thal HbA$_2$ Quik Column™ test kit (available from Helena Laboratories) contains the following:
   a. Beta Thal HbA$_2$ Quik Columns™ (Fig. 4–7) containing DEAE cellulose (diethylaminoethylcellulose) resin in a 0.2 M glycine buffer. Small amounts of potassium cyanide and sodium azide are also present. Store at 2 to 6°C. If discoloration (bright yellow or yellow-green color) develops the column should be discarded.
   b. HbA$_2$ Developer (contains 0.2 M glycine and potassium cyanide). Refrigerate when not in use. Must be clear and colorless.
   c. Hemolysate Reagent-C containing Triton X-100 and preservatives. Store at 2 to 6°C. Must be clear and colorless.
2. Additional materials needed (also obtainable from Helena Laboratories):
   a. Rack for holding the columns during testing.
   b. Total Fraction tubes (15 mL).
   c. HbA$_2$ Collection tubes (3 mL).
   d. Normal and abnormal hgb A$_2$ controls.
3. Pipets, 0.05, 0.2, and 1.0 mL.
4. Disposable pasteur pipets.
5. Parafilm.
6. Distilled water.
7. Test tubes, 10 × 75 mm and 13 × 100 mm.
8. Stopwatch.

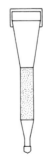

FIG. 4–7. HbA$_2$ Quik Column™.

9. Spectrophotometer, 415 nm.

Specimen

Whole blood (minimum of 0.1 mL) anticoagulated with EDTA. Fresh blood is desirable, but hemolysates stored up to 10 days at 2° to 6°C may be used.

Principle

A hemolysate is prepared from the patient's red blood cells (freeing the hemoglobin from the red cells). A specific amount of hemolysate is then added to the top of the resin column. The DEAE resin is a preparation of cellulose attached to positively charged molecules, thus giving the cellulose a positive charge. When the hemolysate is added to the column, the pH of the buffer present determines the net negative charge of the hemoglobins, which then bind to the positively charged cellulose resin. The hemoglobins are selectively removed from the cellulose according to the pH (or ionic strength) of the developer. In this procedure, the hemoglobin A_2 (originally bound to the resin) is released from the resin and eluted by the developer as it passes through the column. Most other abnormal and normal hemoglobins remain bound to the resin in the column. The eluted hemoglobin A_2 is then measured spectrophotometrically and compared with the amount of total hemoglobin in the specimen to calculate the percent of hemoglobin A_2 present.

Procedure

1. Allow all reagents to warm to room temperature. (The cellulose resin column will yield best results if allowed to sit at room temperature for a minimum of 2 hours, preferably 4 hours, prior to testing.)
2. Prepare the patient hemolysate.
   a. Pipet 0.05 mL of well-mixed whole blood into a 10 × 75 mm test tube for each patient to be tested.
   b. Add 0.25 mL of Hemolysate Reagent-C to each tube. Vigorously mix each tube by drawing across the top of a test tube rack several times.
   c. Allow each mixture to sit for 5 to 10 minutes to allow for complete hemolysis of the red cells. If the hemolysate is not crystal clear, quickly freeze and thaw the mixture as many times as necessary to accomplish complete lysis of the red blood cells.
3. Label one Quik Column™ tube, one Total Fraction (TF) tube, and one A_2 Collection tube for each patient and control to be tested. Place the resin columns and the A_2 collection tubes in the top and bottom portions of the rack respectively. Place the labeled TF tubes in a separate rack.
4. When the hemolysates are ready for testing, prepare the resin columns for use:
   a. Carefully invert the column tube two times in order to remove any resin that may be adhering to the cap or side of the tube.
   b. Remove the top screw cap and, using a pasteur pipet, carefully resuspend the resin by aspirating and expelling the resin several times. Perform this procedure carefully so as not to disturb the filter at the bottom of the resin column. Start a stopwatch. Proceed to the next step immediately before the resin begins to settle.
   c. Carefully loosen and remove the small plastic cap at the bottom of the tube and place the tube in the rack, allowing it to drain into a 13 × 100 mm empty test tube. Proceed to the next step quickly.
   d. Carefully watch the resin repack as the buffer drains out. The top portion of the mixture will quickly become clear, the middle portion will be cloudy, and, as the resin begins packing a definite line of demarcation will form between the packed resin and the second (cloudy) portion. As soon as the cloudy portion disappears and there are only two layers seen (packed resin on bottom and clear liquid portion on top) (approximately 2 minutes 15 seconds will have elapsed on the stopwatch), carefully aspirate and remove all of the clear buffer portion on top, using a pasteur pipet. Discard. (The stopwatch may be discontinued at this point. Its primary purpose is to standardize the repacking time of the resin column.)

e. The above steps must be accomplished without delay so that the resin does not become too tightly packed. If more than 2 minutes 15 seconds elapse the column may need to be resuspended: Replace the small cap on the bottom of the tube, pour the drained buffer back into the tube, and repeat above procedure.

5. Immediately after the excess buffer is removed from the top of the resin column in the above step, the sample must be applied to the column:

a. Carefully, apply 0.1 mL of the sample hemolysate to the top of the resin column, ensuring that the resin is not disturbed. The sample must not run down the inside of the tube, the pipet tip must not touch the top of the resin, and no bubbles should form in the sample. Start the stopwatch as soon as the sample has been added to the column.

b. Add 0.1 mL of the patient's hemolysate to the appropriately labeled TF tube. Fill the tube to the 15 mL line with distilled water and mix.

6. Allow the sample to completely absorb into the resin. When 1 to 2 minutes have elapsed on the stopwatch, the top of the resin should have a dull mat-like finish indicating complete absorption of the hemolysate.

7. Wipe the bottom of the Quik Column tube and place the tube directly above the appropriately labeled A_2 Collection tube. Slowly add 2.5 mL of HbA_2 developer to the top of the column without disturbing the resin or hemolysate. Halt the stopwatch. Less than 5 minutes should have elapsed since step 5 was completed. This timing is critical because the top of the resin column must not be allowed to dry out.

8. Allow 30 minutes for the developer to drain through the column. If this step takes much longer than 45 minutes, there may be a problem with the resin column and the test should be repeated using a new Quik Column™ tube.

9. Repeat steps 4 through 8 above for each patient and control.

10. When all of the Developer has passed through the resin columns, fill the A_2 Collection tubes to the 3-mL mark with distilled water. Mix.

11. Set the spectrophotometer at a wavelength of 415 nm and set 0.00 absorbance using distilled water. Record the absorbance reading for each total hemoglobin (TF tube) and hemoglobin A_2 sample.

12. Calculate the concentration of hemoglobin A_2 for each specimen and control:

$$\text{Hgb } A_2 = \frac{\text{O.D. of } A_2}{\text{O.D. of Total hgb} \times 5} \times 100$$

Discussion

1. Several abnormal hemoglobins (S, C, E, O, D, and S-G hybrid), if present, will be eluted along with the hemoglobin A_2 in the above procedure. This will be evident when the results of the procedure show greater than 10% hemoglobin A_2. In these cases the Sickle-Thal Quik Column™ kit (available from Helena Laboratories) may be used. This procedure is similar to the one described above. The resin column is slightly different in this test kit and allows elution of hemoglobin A_2 in the presence of hemoglobins A, F, S, and numerous other abnormal hemoglobins. In addition, an HbS developer reagent is included in the kit that allows for quantitation of hemoglobin S, if present. This test kit may also be used routinely for quantitating hemoglobin A_2.

2. The final test dilutions are stable for 4 hours.

3. Each laboratory should determine its own normal range for this test procedure.

4. The preparation of the Quik Columns™ in step 4 above are critical. Also, any bubbles or disturbance present in the resin will cause erroneous results. The top of the resin should not be allowed to dry out at any time during the procedure.

5. If developer is added to the column too quickly, results will be invalidly low, or if the developer does not flow through the column correctly, the test should be repeated using a new column.

6. If a patient heterozygous for β-thalassemia also has iron deficiency, the hemoglobin A_2 may be within the normal range.

7. If the patient has received a transfusion recently this test should not be performed.

8. Slightly elevated hemoglobin A_2 results may be found in patients with an unstable hemoglobin.

QUANTITATION OF HEMOGLOBIN F

Three procedures for quantitating hemoglobin F are outlined on the following pages. Although results of less than 2% are considered normal for these methods, each laboratory should determine its own normal range for the procedure tested.

Approximately 65 to 90% of the total hemoglobin at birth is hemoglobin F. By the age of 4 months there is approximately 10% hemoglobin F present, and by 6 to 12 months of age the level of hemoglobin F is less than 2%. Increased amounts of fetal hemoglobin are present in hereditary persistence of fetal hemoglobin (usually above 15%), sickle cell anemia (may range from normal to 20%), acquired aplastic anemia, and other hemoglobinopathies. Hemoglobin F may also be elevated in megaloblastic anemia, paroxysmal nocturnal hemoglobinuria, leukemia, myelofibrosis, and refractory anemias, and during pregnancy. Patients with β-thalassemia trait will usually show levels of 2 to 5% hemoglobin F, whereas patients homozygous for β-thalassemia will have hemoglobin F levels of 15 to 100%. The alkali denaturation method of Betke is considered accurate for concentrations of hemoglobin F up to 10 or 15%. The Singer alkali denaturation procedure is the most accurate for hemoglobin F concentrations of 10 to 40%. Results will tend to be invalidly low above 10 to 15% in the Betke method or above 40% using the Singer procedure. A radial immunodiffusion (RID) procedure (Helena Laboratories) is also described.

Betke Method of Alkali Denaturation

Reference

Betke, K., Marti, H.R., and Schlict, I.: Estimation of small percentages of fetal hemoglobin, Nature, *184*, 1877, 1959.

Reagents and Equipment

1. Cyanmethemoglobin (HiCN) regent.
2. Saturated ammonium sulfate.
   Ammonium sulfate   160 g
   Add 200 mL of distilled water.
   Mix the above solution until all possible ammonium sulfate goes into solution. Mix frequently over the next several hours and allow to stand overnight. Remix solution and add more ammonium sulfate, if necessary, until no more reagent will go into solution. A small amount of reagent must always be present, undissolved, in the bottom of the bottle. When using this reagent, handle bottle carefully so that the undissolved reagent in the bottom of the bottle is not unnecessarily disturbed.
3. Sodium hydroxide, 1.2 N.
4. Sodium chloride, 0.85%, w/v.
5. Carbon tetrachloride (CCl_4).
6. Whatman #42 filter paper.
7. Graduated centrifuge tube, polypropylene, 15 mL.
8. Normal and abnormal hemolysate controls.
9. Test tubes, 13 × 100 mm.
10. Water bath, 20°C.
11. Spectrophotometer, 540 nm.

Specimen

Whole blood (2 to 3 mL) anticoagulated with EDTA. Prepare the red blood cell hemolysate on the same day the specimen is obtained. The hemolysate may then be frozen at −20°C for up to 7 days, possibly longer.

Principle

A red blood cell hemolysate is prepared to lyse the red blood cells and free the hemoglobin. This test utilizes the characteristic of fetal hemoglobin to resist denaturation in an alkaline solution. The hemolysate is added to cyanmethemoglobin reagent and then exposed to an alkaline reagent, sodium hydroxide, for a specified period. During this time, normal hemoglobin is denatured or destroyed, but the fetal hemoglobin remains intact. Ammonium sulfate is added to halt the denaturation process and to precipitate the denatured hemoglobin. The solution is filtered, measured spectrophotometrically, and compared with the spectrophotometric readings of the original cyanmethemoglobin solution to determine the percent of hemoglobin F present.

Procedure

1. Preparation of hemolysate.
   a. Place 2 to 3 mL of the patient's whole blood into a graduated, polypropylene centrifuge tube. Prepare a normal and abnormal control hemolysate in the same manner.
   b. Fill tubes with 0.85% sodium chloride to wash the red blood cells. Centrifuge at 1200 to 1500 g for 5 minutes. Remove the supernatant.
   c. Wash the red blood cells two more times by repeating step b above.
   d. Remove 1 mL of washed red blood cells from each tube and place in a clean, labeled, polypropylene centrifuge tube. Add 1 mL of distilled water to each tube. Mix. Add 0.5 mL of CCl_4 to each tube. Stopper tubes.
   e. Vortex, or vigorously shake, each tube for 5 minutes.
   f. Centrifuge the tubes at 1500 g for 25 to 30 minutes. Carefully remove tubes from the centrifuge.
   g. Remove the upper hemolysate layer from each tube, being careful not to disturb the lower stroma and CCl_4 layers.
   h. Determine the hemoglobin content of the hemolysate. It should be between 9 and 11 g/dL. Adjust, if necessary, using distilled water.
2. Pipet 0.5 mL of the patient's hemolysate and the normal and abnormal control hemolysates into respective tubes containing 9.5 mL of cyanmethemoglobin reagent. Label tubes "Total Hgb." This gives a hemoglobin concentration of approximately 0.5 g/dL.
3. Mix and transfer 2.8 mL of each of the preceding cyanmethemoglobin solutions into each of two labeled test tubes. (Each test is performed in duplicate.) Label tubes "Hgb F." Place the test tubes in a 20°C water bath for 5 to 10 minutes to reach the proper temperature.
4. Add 0.2 mL of 1.2 N sodium hydroxide to the first test tube and rapidly mix. Allow to incubate for exactly 2 minutes.
5. At exactly 2 minutes, add 2 mL of saturated ammonium sulfate to the tube, directly into the solution, and quickly mix the tube to stop the reaction. Allow the tube to stand at room temperature for 5 to 10 minutes.
6. Repeat steps 4 and 5 above for each patient and control sample in step 3.
7. Filter each of the preceding solutions through Whatman #42 filter paper. If the filtrate is not absolutely clear, refilter the solution using the same filter paper.
8. Prepare the total hemoglobin specimen for the patients and controls: add 0.4 mL of each of the "Total Hgb" solutions (step 2) to 6.75 mL of distilled water. Prepare this dilution in duplicate.
9. Transfer the filtrates and total hemoglobin solutions to cuvettes and read in a spectrophotometer at a wavelength of 540 nm, using cyanmethemoglobin reagent to set the instrument at 0 optical density. Record the absorbance of all specimens. The optical density readings should fall within a range of 0.05 to 0.50 for maximum sensitivity. If the filtrate is too concentrated, dilute it, using distilled water.
10. Calculate the results as follows:

$$\% \text{ Hemoglobin F} = \frac{\text{O.D. Hemoglobin F}}{\text{O.D. Total Hgb} \times 10} \times 100$$

The optical density of the total hemoglobin is multiplied by 10 because this solution is 10 times more dilute than the Hgb F solution.

Singer Method of Alkali Denaturation

Reference

Singer, K., Chernoff, A.I., and Singer, L.: Studies on abnormal hemoglobin. 1. Their demonstration in sickle cell anemia and other hematologic disorders by means of alkali denaturation, Blood, 6, 413, 1951.

Reagents and Equipment

1. Potassium hydroxide, 0.083 N, pH 12.7.
   Potassium hydroxide   2.34 g
   Dissolve and dilute to 500 mL with distilled water. Store in refrigerator in a plastic bottle.

2. Precipitating solution: ammonium sulfate, 50% saturated (with hydrochloric acid).

Saturated ammonium sulfate (Prepare as described for the Betke method)	400 mL
Distilled water	400 mL
Hydrochloric acid, 10 N	2 mL

Combine above reagents.
3. Sodium chloride, 0.85% (w/v).
4. Carbon tetrachloride.
5. Test tubes, 10 × 100 mm.
6. Whatman #42 filter paper.
7. Graduated polypropylene centrifuge tubes, 15 mL.
8. Normal and abnormal controls.
9. Waterbath, 20°C.
10. Spectrophotometer, 540 nm.

Specimen

See Betke method of alkali denaturation.

Principle

The red blood cell hemolysate is incubated with potassium hydroxide, which destroys (denatures) normal and nonfetal hemoglobin. Addition of the precipitating solution stops this reaction and precipitates the denatured hemoglobin. The non-altered hemoglobin (F) is then measured spectrophotometrically.

Procedure

1. Prepare a red blood cell hemolysate as described in step 1 for the Betke method.
2. Pipet 1.6 mL of 0.083 N potassium hydroxide into appropriately labeled tubes, two for each patient and control to be tested. These are the "Hgb F" tubes.
3. Place tubes in a waterbath at 20°C (19 to 21°C) for 10 minutes to allow solutions to reach the proper temperature.
4. Label two additional test tubes for each patient and control with the name and "Total" (represents the total hemoglobin).
5. Pipet 5.0 mL of distilled water into each of the "Total" tubes.
6. Add 0.02 mL of the appropriate hemolysate to each "Total" test tube.
7. Label another set of tubes (two for each patient and control) into which the "Hgb F" tubes will be filtered.
8. When the potassium hydroxide has reached 20°C (step 3) add 0.1 mL of the first hemolysate to the appropriately labeled tube, at the same time starting a stopwatch. Rinse the pipet in the solution six to eight times and then mix the tube well. After exactly 1 minute add 3.4 mL of precipitating solution and thoroughly mix by capping the tube and inverting at least six times. Immediately filter the mixture into the appropriately labeled "Hgb F" tube.
9. Repeat step 8 for each specimen and duplicate.
10. Transfer the filtrates and total hemoglobin solutions to cuvets and read in a spectrophotometer at a wavelength of 540 nm, using distilled water to set the instrument at 0 optical density. Record all readings.
11. Calculate the results as follows:

$$\% \text{ Hemoglobin F} = \frac{\text{O.D. Hgb F}}{\text{O.D. Total}} \times 0.203 \times 100$$

Note: 0.203 is the conversion factor for the hemolysate dilutions:

$$\text{Hgb F dilution} = 0.1{:}5.1 \text{ or } 1{:}51$$

$$\text{Total dilution} = 0.2{:}5.02 \text{ or } 1{:}251$$

$$\frac{51}{251} = 0.203$$

Discussion (Alkali Denaturation Methods)

1. The following aspects of the test are critical and must be carried out as indicated in the procedure.
   a. Concentration of sodium/potassium hydroxide.
   b. Incubation time and temperature.
   c. The hemoglobin concentration of the hemolysate should be within 9 and 11 g/dL.
   d. The filtrate must be crystal clear.
   e. Concentration of the ammonium sulfate.
2. When performing the Betke method, if the hemolysate has a hemoglobin concentration of less than 9 g/dL, the "Total Hgb" dilution (as prepared in step 2) may

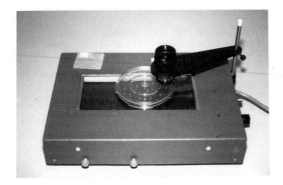

FIG. 4–8. HbF QUIPlate, Titan IEP VuBox, and QUIP Comparator.

be altered to compensate for this. The following calculations may be used:

$$\frac{A}{10.0} = \frac{0.5}{C} \quad \text{then:} \quad B = 10 - C$$

where: A = hgb in g/dL of the hemolysate
B = amount of cyanmethemoglobin reagent to be used in step 2 above
C = amount of hemolysate to add to the cyanmethemoglobin reagent (step 2)

3. If control results do not fall within range the test should be repeated using newly prepared alkaline and precipitating reagents, and the pH of the reagents should also be checked.

Radial Immunodiffusion Procedure for Hemoglobin F

Reference

Helena Laboratories, HbF QUIPlate, pkg. insert, Beaumont, Texas, 1988.

Reagents and Equipment

1. The following are obtainable from Helena Laboratories, Beaumont, Texas:
   a. HbF QUIPlate is composed of 1.5% agarose in tris buffer (0.1 M) with a monospecific antihuman hemoglobin F antiserum (0.1% sodium azide is present as a preservative). Store in the refrigerator according to package insert. Plates must be tightly covered. (See Fig. 4–8)
   b. Hemoglobin F standards: 0.5%, 5.0%, and 10.0%. Store in the refrigerator.
   c. Hemoglobin F QUIPlate controls.
   d. Hemoglobin F diluent.
   e. QUIPlate (or linear) graph paper.
   f. Titan IEP VuBox, or equivalent. (A light source, on top of which the agar plates are examined for determination of results at the conclusion of testing.) (See Fig. 4–8.)
   g. QUIP Comparator. (An ocular containing a micrometer. The opaque-appearing rings are enlarged for better viewing and measured using the micrometer). (See Fig. 4–8.)
2. Pipets: 0.005, 0.2, 1.0, 2.0, and 10 mL.
3. Humidity chamber (plastic box with a snug fitting lid).
4. Test tubes, 13 × 100 mm.
5. Distilled water.

Specimen

Whole blood, 1 mL, anticoagulated with EDTA. Samples stored at 2 to 6°C for up to 5 days may be used.

Principle

In the radial immunodiffusion (RID) procedure, prepared agar plates containing antiserum specific for hemoglobin F are used. These plates contain standard-sized wells (holes) cut in the gel. A specific amount of diluted patient hemolysate (standard or control) is added to a well and allowed to incubate. During this time period the hemoglobin F present in the sample (standard or control) diffuses through the agar and reacts with the antiserum, producing a precipitin ring around the well. The diameter of each precipitin ring squared is proportional to the amount of hemoglobin F present in the sample. The standards are used to prepare a reference curve. The values for the unknown samples and quality control specimens are then calculated from this curve.

Procedure

1. Remove the HbF QUIPlate from the refrigerator and allow to come to room temperature while preparing the patient samples.

2. Determine the hemoglobin concentration in g/dL for each patient specimen to be tested.

3. Dilute each specimen to a hemoglobin concentration of 1.0 g/dL using distilled water. Determine the dilution as follows:

T = total volume of blood and distilled water
D = volume of distilled water to add to 0.2 mL whole blood (to obtain a concentration of 1.0 g/dL of hemoglobin)

$$T = \frac{0.2 \text{ mL (whole blood)} \times \text{(hgb. in g/dL)}}{1.0 \text{ g/dL hgb}}$$

D = T − 0.2 mL

4. Mix dilutions to ensure complete hemolysis. (The diluted samples must be crystal clear.)

5. Remove the cover from the QUIPlate by placing thumb and fingers on the plate flanges and then twist the two sections apart. Remove any excess moisture from the plate or wells if present.

6. Log in each standard, control, and patient sample in order to assign it a well number.

7. Add exactly 0.005 mL (5 μL) of sample to the appropriate well (one standard, control, or patient/well).

8. Replace cover on plate (top and bottom flanges should not align with each other).

9. Place plate in the humidity chamber, close, and leave at room temperature (15 to 30°C) for a minimum of 24 hours.

10. At the end of 24 hours determine the diameter of the precipitin ring for each standard, control, and patient specimen:
   a. Remove the plate from the humidity chamber.
   b. Remove the top from the plate.
   c. Place the ocular directly over the first well (without touching the agar) and position your eye as close as possible to the ocular in order to obtain the most accurate and reproducible reading.
   d. Determine the diameter of each precipitin ring to the closest 0.1 mm. Record results.

11. Square each ring diameter reading.

12. Using graph paper plot the standard curve: % hemoglobin F on the X-axis and the diameter squared on the Y-axis. The three points (of the standards)

should form a straight line. Draw the best fit straight line through these points.

13. For each control and patient sample, read the % hemoglobin F from the graph, using the squared precipitin diameter value.

Discussion

1. The above procedure accurately quantitates hemoglobin F concentrations up to 10%. For results above 10% specimen testing must be repeated, making a further dilution of the specimen using hemoglobin F diluent:
   a. Prepare (dilute) patient specimen with distilled water as described in steps 2 and 3 above.
   b. Vortex both the diluted patient sample and the hemoglobin F diluent.
   c. Prepare a 1:5 and/or a 1:10 dilution of the patient specimen using hemoglobin F diluent:
      1) 1:5 (5 μL of specimen + 20 μL diluent)
      2) 1:10 (5 μL of specimen + 45 μL diluent)
   d. Mix dilutions well.
   e. Repeat testing as described above (steps 4 through 13).
   f. Correct results for the dilution used: for the 1:5 dilution, multiply results by 5, and for the 1:10 dilution, multiply results by 10.

2. If the well in the agar plate is damaged results will be erroneous.

3. The plates must be allowed to incubate for a minimum of 24 hours, or, they may be tightly covered and stored at room temperature for a maximum of 14 days following incubation. If refrigerated they may be stored for up to 28 days before being read.

4. If the curve is not linear or if control results are not within range, an application error may have been made, the plates may not have been incubated long enough, the QUIPlate may have deteriorated, or the well(s) may be damaged.

5. If not all of the wells on the agar plate were used, the cover may be replaced (tightly) and the plate refrigerated. These wells may be used within 14 days without

running a new reference curve (any controls must be tested, however). After 14 days the plate may still be used but a new reference curve must be prepared.

ACID ELUTION TEST

The acid elution test is employed to assess the distribution of hemoglobin F in the red blood cell: to determine whether hemoglobin F is present in the same amount in all red blood cells, or whether it is present in varying amounts in only some of the red blood cells. This information is useful in helping to diagnose hereditary persistence of fetal hemoglobin and in determining the presence of fetal red cells in the maternal circulation during pregnancy.

References

Division of Host Factors, Center for Infectious Diseases, CDC: *Laboratory Methods for Detecting Hemoglobinopathies,* Atlanta, Centers for Disease Control, 1984.

Shepard, M.K., Weatherall, D.J., and Conley, C.L.: Semiquantitative estimation of the distribution of fetal hemoglobin in red cell populations, Bull. Johns Hopkins Hosp., *110*, 293, 1962.

Sigma Diagnostics, Fetal hemoglobin, pkg. insert, St. Louis, MO, 1988.

Reagents and Equipment

1. Ethyl alcohol, 80% (v/v). Stable in the refrigerator for 1 month (or 100 slides), unless the solution becomes cloudy.
2. Citric acid-phosphate buffer, pH 3.2 to 3.3.
   Dibasic sodium phosphate, 0.2 M

Dibasic sodium phosphate (Na_2HPO_4)	14.2 g

   Dilute to 500 mL with distilled water. Stable for 6 months when stored in the refrigerator.
   Citric acid, 0.1 M

Citric acid ($C_6H_8O_7 \cdot H_2O$)	10.5 g

   Dilute to 500 mL with distilled water. Stable for 6 months when stored in the refrigerator.
   Prior to use, prepare the citric acid-phosphate buffer:

Dibasic sodium phosphate, 0.2 M	13.3 mL
Citric acid, 0.1 M	36.7 mL

Check the pH of this mixture on a pH meter. The pH must be within 3.2 and 3.3.
3. Erythrosin B (eosin B) stain, 0.1% (w/v), aqueous solution. Eosin yellowish, 1.25% (w/v), may be used as an alternative (0.5 g of eosin yellowish in 120 mL of absolute alcohol and 280 mL of distilled water). Add two to three drops of glacial acetic acid.
4. Ehrlich's acid hematoxylin.

Hematoxylin, crystalline	4.0 g
Ethyl alcohol, 80% (v/v)	200 mL
10% aqueous solution of sodium iodate	8 mL
Distilled water	200 mL

   Heat the above solution until it boils, cool until lukewarm, and add the following:

Glycerine	200 mL
Aluminum sulfate	6.0 g
Glacial acetic acid	200 mL

   Mix, and store at room temperature. (Mayer's hematoxylin may also be used.)
5. Coplin jars.
6. Waterbath, 37°C.

Specimen

Obtain four blood smears from the fingertip (toe or heel), or make blood smears from venous blood collected in EDTA anticoagulant. Obtain a similar blood specimen for a normal and abnormal control at the same time the patient's blood is collected. For best results blood should be less than 6 hours old, although successful staining has been achieved on specimens refrigerated for up to 2 weeks. The smears should be fixed within 2 hours of preparation.

Principle

Blood smears are fixed with ethyl alcohol and then incubated in a citric acid-buffer solution. In an acid medium (pH 3.2 to 3.3), hemoglobin F is resistant to elution from the red blood cell, while other types are removed from the red cells. The slides are stained with hematoxylin (stains the white cell nuclei) and erythrosin B (stains the red cells). The smears are then reviewed microscopically to determine the presence of hemoglobin F, and the percentage of red blood cells containing fetal hemoglobin may be assessed.

Procedure

1. Prewarm citric acid-phosphate buffer. Place 50 mL of the buffer solution into a coplin jar and cover. Incubate at 37°C for 30 minutes. (Make certain the level of water in the incubator is level with, or above, the level of buffer in the coplin jar.)

2. Preparation of blood smears.
   a. Patient—Make several thin (a monolayer of cells) blood smears.
   b. Normal control—Make two thin blood smears from a normal adult.
   c. Positive control—Mix two drops of cord blood with two drops of normal, ABO compatible, whole blood. Make two thin blood smears. (As an alternative, use cord blood, alone, as the positive control.)

3. Allow the blood smears to air-dry for at least 10 minutes.

4. Fix blood smears (patient and controls) in 80% ethyl alcohol for 5 minutes.

5. Rinse the smears carefully in distilled water and allow to air-dry.

6. Place the dry smears in the prewarmed citric acid-phosphate buffer solution for 5 minutes. At 1 and 3 minutes (of incubation), carefully lift each slide out of the buffer solution and immediately replace. This action will provide a gentle stirring of the solution.

7. After 5 minutes, remove the slides from the citric acid-phosphate buffer solution and carefully rinse with distilled water. Air-dry.

8. Stain the dry smears in acid hematoxylin for 3 minutes. Rinse with distilled water and remove as much of the water as possible from the smears by gently tapping one end of the slide on an absorbent material.

9. Counterstain the smears with erythrosin B for 4 minutes. Rinse with distilled water, allow to air-dry, and coverslip (if desired).

10. Examine the slides microscopically, (oil immersion objective [100×]), for the presence of hemoglobin F. Red cells containing large amounts of hemoglobin F will stain a deep pink. The intensity of the pink staining is directly proportional to the concentration of hemoglobin F.

Cells containing normal amounts (less than 2%) of hemoglobin F will stain as very pale ghost cells.

11. To determine the percentage of red blood cells containing fetal hemoglobin:
    a. Count the number of red blood cells in three to five microscopic fields and determine the average # of red cells/field.
    b. Examine 20 to 25 microscopic fields, counting the number of red cells containing hemoglobin F.
    c. Calculate the percentage of RBC containing hemoglobin F as shown below:

$$\text{\# hgb F RBC/field} = \frac{\text{\# hgb F RBC counted}}{\text{\# of fields counted}}$$

$$\text{\% RBC with hgb F} = \frac{\text{\# hgb F RBC/field}}{\text{Av. \# RBC/field}} \times 100$$

Discussion

1. Reticulocytes may resist elution and would, therefore, give the appearance of cells containing hemoglobin F.

2. In hereditary persistence of fetal hemoglobin, the amount of hemoglobin F in each cell is constant and, therefore, all of the red blood cells are consistently stained. Conversely, in diseases such as sickle cell anemia, thalassemia, acquired aplastic anemia, and several other hemoglobinopathies, the amount of hemoglobin F present in the red blood cells varies. This shows up as an inconsistent staining of the red cells.

3. The pH of the citric acid-phosphate buffer is critical. A pH below 3.1 may cause elution of hemoglobin F from the red cells, while a pH above 3.3 may retard the elution of non-F hemoglobin from the cells.

4. A temperature above 25°C during fixation in the ethyl alcohol will inhibit elution of normal hemoglobin.

5. Ethyl alcohol concentrations above 80% may cause the elution of hemoglobin F, while concentrations below 80% may cause morphologic alterations.

6. Positive control smears may be prepared in advance. Add cord blood to EDTA (1 drop of 2% EDTA/1 mL of whole blood).

Prepare blood smears and fix in 80% ethyl alcohol. Place fixed smears in tightly sealed cardboard slide boxes and store at −20°C. These smears should be good for 1 year, prepared and stored in this manner.
7. A reagent kit is available for this test from Sigma Diagnostics, St. Louis, MO.

HEMOGLOBIN H PREPARATION

Patients suspected of having thalassemia trait, who have an MCV below 80 fL and are not iron deficient, who have a normal hemoglobin electrophoresis, and who show normal levels of hemoglobins F and A_2, may have α thalassemia. In this disorder, there is an excess of β chains (due to a deficiency in the production of α chains) that form β_4 tetramers (hemoglobin H). Due to the small amount of hemoglobin H formed, it will generally not be seen on cellulose acetate hemoglobin electrophoresis. However, in the presence of an oxidant, such as brilliant cresyl blue, this abnormal hemoglobin will precipitate within the red cell and form many small inclusions. (See Plate VII, E.) Unstable hemoglobins may also be detected and stained with this method. In addition, inclusion bodies may be found in the red cells of some patients with enzyme deficiencies (e.g., G-6-PD deficiency) and after exposure to oxidant drugs. Normal hemoglobin will not denature or precipitate in this procedure and will therefore be negative for inclusion bodies.

References

Jones, J.A., Broszeit, H.K., LeCrone, C.N., and Detter, J.C.: An improved method for detection of red cell hemoglobin H inclusions, Am. J. Med. Tech., 47, 94, 1981.

Raven, J.L., and Tooze, J.A.: α-thalassaemia in Britain, Br. Med. J., 4, 486, 1973.

Reagents and Equipment

1. Microhematocrit tubes, non-heparinized.
2. Microhematocrit centrifuge.
3. Clay, to seal the end of the microhematocrit tube.
4. Water bath, 37°C.

5. Small file to cut microhematocrit tubes.
6. Glass slides, 25 × 75 mm.
7. Test tubes, 12 × 55 mm.
8. Microscope.
9. Citrate saline solution.
   Sodium citrate   0.4 g
   ($Na_3C_6H_5O_7 \cdot 2H_2O$)
   Dissolve and dilute to 100 mL with 0.9% (w/v) sodium chloride.
10. Brilliant cresyl blue, 1%, w/v, in citrate saline solution. Filter before use. Store at room temperature. Stain is good for 1 month.

Specimen

Whole blood, using EDTA (or ACD) as the anticoagulant. Excess amounts of anticoagulant may interfere with the staining process. Fresh blood samples, less than 8 hours old are preferable.

Principle

Red blood cells containing hemoglobin H are removed more quickly from the circulation by the reticuloendothelial system. Therefore, the red cells containing hemoglobin H, which are present in the blood, are relatively young cells, and, when centrifuged, will lie near the top of the red cell layer. In this procedure, the blood is centrifuged in several microhematocrit tubes. The top layers of red blood cells are removed and incubated with brilliant cresyl blue stain. During incubation, hemoglobin H (an unstable hemoglobin) present in the red cell will denature and precipitate within the cell. The hemoglobin H bodies and any other denatured hemoglobin will be stained by the brilliant cresyl blue. Smears are made, air-dried, and examined for the presence of hemoglobin H bodies (Plate VII, E).

Procedure

1. Fill four microhematocrit tubes with well-mixed whole blood. Seal tubes. Centrifuge in the microhematocrit centrifuge for 5 minutes.
2. Using a file, score each hematocrit tube approximately 3 mm above, and 5 mm below, the plasma-red cell interface.
3. Place each of the 4 hematocrit sections into a 12 × 55 mm test tube. Add 1 drop

of 1% brilliant cresyl blue stain. Mix tube vigorously by drawing back and forth over the top of a test tube rack.

4. Incubate blood and stain mixture at 37°C for 2 to 3 hours.
5. Fill a microhematocrit tube with the blood-stain mixture. Centrifuge for 5 minutes.
6. With the file, score and break the hematocrit tube midway between the clay seal and the interface of the plasma-stain and red cell layers. Discard the lower red cell portion. While holding the index finger over the top of the hematocrit tube, allow all of the red cells and a small amount of stain to be expelled from the hematocrit tube onto a glass slide. Mix well and make two wedge smears.
7. The smears may be coverslipped with Protexx mounting medium (or equivalent) if desired.
8. Examine approximately 50,000 red cells (200 oil immersion fields containing 200 to 300 red blood cells per field). Hemoglobin H bodies are multiple, evenly distributed, bodies in the red cell that may be described as resembling the even pattern of a golf ball. The H bodies stain a bluish-green in color (in contrast to the blue-purple of a reticulocyte).
9. Results are reported as positive or negative for hemoglobin H bodies.

Discussion

1. In hemoglobin H disease, 10 to 100% of the red cells may contain these inclusion bodies. However, in α thalassemia trait only a few red blood cells (0.01 to 1% of the red cells) will be seen with H bodies.
2. In order to detect other unstable hemoglobins by this technique, the blood-stain mixture should be incubated for longer periods of time (from 4 to 24 hours) since these unstable hemoglobins require longer incubation for denaturation and precipitation.
3. Heinz bodies may stain with this procedure and may be differentiated from the H bodies by the fact that they are larger, fewer in number, and most often appear along the membrane of the red cell.
4. Diagnosis of an unstable hemoglobin should also be confirmed by other tests,

such as the heat precipitation, isopropanol precipitation, and hemoglobin electrophoresis.

5. The above procedure may be carried out by omitting the centrifugation sections (steps 1 and 5), because this portion of the test is only meant to increase the sensitivity of the procedure.
6. Individual lots of brilliant cresyl blue dye will vary in their staining abilities. It is therefore advisable to use a slightly longer staining time. A normal control should be used with each set of tests. It is also helpful to run a positive control if one is available.

HEAT PRECIPITATION TEST

The reader is referred to the Isopropanol Precipitation Procedure described previously for the detection of an unstable hemoglobin. The heat precipitation method described here may be used to verify the results of the isopropanol procedure. Normally, less than 5% of the hemoglobin precipitates out when this test is performed by the following procedure.

References

Dacie, J.V., and Lewis, S.M.: *Practical Hematology*, New York, Churchill Livingstone, Inc., 1991.
Schneiderman, L.J., Junga, I.G., and Fawley, D.E.: Effect of phosphate and non-phosphate buffers on thermolability of unstable haemoglobins, Nature, *225*, 1041, 1970.

Reagents and Equipment

1. Tris buffer, 0.1 M, pH 7.4.
2. Cyanmethemoglobin (HiCN) reagent.
3. Sodium chloride, 0.85% (w/v).
4. Carbon tetrachloride.
5. Centrifuge tubes, polypropylene, 15 mL.
6. Waterbath, 50°C.
7. Spectrophotometer, 540 nm.
8. Disposable pipet droppers.
9. Test tubes, 10 × 55 mm, with caps.
10. Test tubes, 13 × 100 mm.

Specimen

Whole blood, using EDTA or heparin as the anticoagulant. A normal control blood must be collected at the same time the patient's blood is obtained. Blood specimens should be less than 72 hours old and should be refrigerated until tested.

Principle

A red blood cell hemolysate is mixed with tris buffer, pH 7.4, and incubated at 50°C for 2 hours. A duplicate mixture is refrigerated. Most unstable hemoglobins will precipitate out more rapidly than normal hemoglobins at this elevated temperature (50°C). The hemoglobin content of the heated and refrigerated supernatants are then determined, and the percentage of unstable hemoglobin (which precipitated during incubation) is calculated.

Procedure

1. Prepare patient and control hemolysates immediately before use, according to the directions outlined for the Isopropanol Precipitation Test (step 1 a through i).
2. Label one 13 × 100 mm test tube for each patient and control to be tested and place 5.0 mL of tris buffer in each tube.
3. Add 0.5 mL of each hemolysate into the appropriately labeled tube containing tris buffer. Mix.
4. Label two 10 × 55 mm test tubes for each patient and control. Label one tube with an "H" (heat) and one tube with an "R" (refrigerate).
5. Transfer 2 mL of the patient's tris buffer-hemolysate mixture into the appropriately labeled "H" and "R" tubes. Stopper tubes. Repeat, for each patient and control. Place all of the tubes marked "H" in the 50°C waterbath. Incubate tubes for 2 hours. Place the "R" tubes in the refrigerator for 2 hours.
6. At the end of the 2-hour incubation, remove tubes from the waterbath and refrigerator. Centrifuge all tubes at 1200 to 1500 g for 10 minutes.
7. While the above tubes are centrifuging, label one 13 × 100 mm-test tube for each of the tubes (one "H" an one "R" tube for each patient and control). Pipet 10 mL of cyanmethemoglobin reagent into each tube.
8. Add 0.5 mL of each supernatant to the appropriately labeled tubes (step 7

above). Mix and allow tubes to stand for 10 minutes.
9. Centrifuge tubes at 1200 to 1500 g for 10 minutes.
10. Carefully remove the supernatant and read the absorbance in a spectrophotometer at a wavelength of 540 nm, using a blank prepared by adding 0.5 mL of tris buffer to 10.0 mL of cyanmethemoglobin reagent.
11. Calculate the results for the patient and the normal control as shown below:

Percent unstable hgb
$$= \frac{\text{Absorbance of 'R'} - \text{Absorbance of 'H'}}{\text{Absorbance of 'R'}} \times 100$$

12. Report results as the percent of unstable (precipitated) hemoglobin.

Discussion

1. Tris buffer is more sensitive to unstable hemoglobins than the phosphate buffer as described in some procedures. As a result, false negative results may occur with the use of phosphate buffer in this method.
2. The diagnosis of an unstable hemoglobin should be confirmed by other tests such as the Isopropanol Precipitation test, tests for inclusion bodies.
3. Increased waterbath temperatures over 50°C will cause false positive results.

ISOPROPANOL PRECIPITATION TEST

Because of the type(s) of amino acid substitution(s) or deletion(s), many of the unstable hemoglobins show normal electrophoretic migration. These hemoglobins may be detected by the isopropanol precipitation or heat denaturation test. Using the following procedure hemoglobins will begin to show precipitation in a 17% isopropanol solution after about 40 minutes, whereas unstable hemoglobins will begin to precipitate after 5 minutes and show heavier flocculation at 20 minutes.

References

Carrell, R.W., and Kay, R.: A simple method for the detection of unstable haemoglobins, Br. J. Haematol., 23, 615, 1972.

Division of Host Factors, Center for Infectious Diseases: *Laboratory Methods for Detecting Hemoglobinopathies*, Atlanta, Centers for Disease Control, 1984.

Reagents and Equipment

1. Isopropanol-tris buffer, pH 7.4.
   Tris (hydroxymethyl)   12.11 g
   aminomethane
   Isopropyl alcohol, 100%   170 mL
   Dilute to 1 liter with distilled water. Adjust to pH 7.4 using concentrated HCl. Store at room temperature. This solution may be used for approximately 1 month.
2. Water bath, 37°C.
3. Test tubes, 10 × 75 mm, with caps.
4. Centrifuge tubes, polypropylene, 15 mL.
5. Sodium chloride, 0.85%, w/v.
6. Distilled water.
7. Carbon tetrachloride (CCl_4).
8. Pasteur pipets.
9. Pipets, 0.2 mL and 2.0 mL.
10. Vortex mixer.
11. Parafilm.
12. Timer.

Specimen

Whole, anticoagulated blood. The type of anticoagulant used is not critical. A normal control blood should be collected at the same time the patient's specimen is obtained. A cord blood specimen may be used as a positive control (test in the same manner as the patient). Blood may be stored at 2 to 6°C for up to 1 week prior to testing. However, if specimen has been at room temperature for 48 hours, it will yield false positive results.

Principle

A red blood cell hemolysate is prepared, added to a 17% solution of isopropanol, and incubated at 37°C. The specimens are examined at 5 minutes and 20 minutes for precipitation of unstable hemoglobin. The isopropanol solution weakens the internal bonding of hemoglobin, causing a faster rate of precipitation of unstable hemoglobins than normal hemoglobin. All hemoglobins will eventually denature in this solution; however, the more unstable the hemoglobin the faster it will precipitate.

Procedure

1. Prepare hemolysate immediately before use:
   a. Place 2 to 3 mL of patient's whole blood into a graduated, polypropylene centrifuge tube.
   b. Fill tubes with 0.85% sodium chloride to wash the red blood cells. Centrifuge at 1200 to 1500 g for 5 minutes. Remove the supernatant.
   c. Wash the red blood cells two more times by repeating step b above.
   d. Remove 1 mL of washed red blood cells from each tube and place in a clean, labeled, polypropylene centrifuge tube. Add 1 mL of distilled water to each tube. Mix. Add 0.5 mL of CCl_4 to each tube and stopper.
   e. Vortex, or vigorously shake, each tube for 5 minutes.
   f. Centrifuge the tubes at 1500 g for 25 to 30 minutes. Carefully remove tubes from the centrifuge.
   g. Remove the upper hemolysate layer from each tube, being careful not to disturb the lower stroma and CCl_4 layers.
   h. The final hemoglobin concentration of each hemolysate should be between 9 and 12 g/dL.
   i. Perform testing immediately.
2. For each patient and control to be tested, place 2.0 mL of the isopropanol-tris buffer solution into a 10 × 75 mm test tube. Stopper each tube and place in the 37°C water bath for 10 minutes in order to prewarm. Be certain the liquid in the tubes is completely immersed in the water of the incubator. (To save time, place the test tubes in the water bath just prior to the last centrifugation in the preparation of the hemolysate.)
3. Add 0.2 mL of each hemolysate to the appropriately labeled test tubes of buffer in the water bath. Stopper each tube and gently invert two times to mix.
4. Check each test tube at 5, 20, and 45 minutes for evidence of precipitation or flocculation. When examining the test tubes, extreme care must be taken not to mix the solution too much. (The precipitate will quickly break up if the solution is physically mixed.) Carefully remove the

test tube from the water bath, very gently tilt the tube horizontally, and examine the solution for precipitation against a light source.

5. Interpretation of results.
   a. Negative for unstable hemoglobin: No precipitation or flocculation at 5 minutes or 20 minutes. Precipitation should begin to appear at 45 minutes.
   b. Positive for unstable hemoglobin: precipitation present at the 5 minute reading, with definite flocculation at 20 minutes.
   c. The normal control should be negative for hemoglobin precipitation at 5 and 20 minutes. To ensure that the buffer solution is effective, precipitation should begin appearing at 45 minutes in a normal specimen. If these results are not obtained for the normal control, fresh buffer reagent should be prepared and the entire test repeated. (The 5 and 20 minute readings must be taken because false negative results may occur by continuing the patient incubation until the normal control precipitates.)

Discussion

1. Toluene and chloroform should not be used in the preparation of hemolysates for unstable hemoglobin testing.
2. The concentration of isopropanol (17%) in the buffer solution is critical as is the temperature of the 37°C water bath.
3. The pH of the buffer solution must be at least 7.2.
4. The presence of any red cell stroma in the hemolysate will give false positive results.
5. Small amounts of an unstable hemoglobin may be lost in the hemolysate preparation. This may lead to some false negative results in patients having only a small amount of an unstable hemoglobin.
6. Specimens containing increased amounts of hemoglobin F, and old samples containing an increase in methemoglobin, may give false-positive results by the above procedure.
7. The diagnosis of an unstable hemoglobin should be confirmed by other tests such as the heat precipitation procedure, tests for inclusion bodies, etc.

OSMOTIC FRAGILITY TEST

The osmotic fragility test is a measure of the ability of the red cells to take up fluid without lysing. This procedure is employed to help diagnose different types of anemias, in which the physical properties of the red blood cell are altered. The primary factor affecting the osmotic fragility test is the shape of the red cell, which, in turn, depends on the volume, surface area, and functional state of the red blood cell membrane. The larger the amount of red cell membrane (surface area) in relation to the size of the cell, the more fluid the cell is capable of absorbing before rupturing (it is more resistant to hemolysis and has decreased fragility). The target cell has the largest surface area (amount of membrane) for its size and therefore shows decreased fragility. As the red cell takes in fluid it becomes more round (spherocytic). It therefore follows that the spherocyte has the smallest surface area for its volume, ruptures the most quickly, and has increased fragility.

Increased osmotic fragility (decreased resistance) is found in hemolytic anemias and hereditary spherocytosis, and whenever spherocytes are found. Decreased osmotic fragility (increased resistance) occurs following splenectomy and in liver disease, sickle cell anemia, iron-deficiency anemia, thalassemia, and polycythemia vera, and conditions in which target cells are present. Reticulocytes show decreased osmotic fragility; the older red cells are also more fragile.

References

Dacie, J.V., and Lewis, S.M.: *Practical Hematology*, 6th ed., New York, Churchill Livingstone, Inc., 1991.

Parpart, A.K., Lorenz, P.B., Parpart, E.R., Gregg, J.R., and Chase, A.M.: The osmotic resistance (fragility) of human red cells, J. Clin. Invest., 26, 636, 1947.

Reagents and Equipment

1. Buffered sodium chloride stock solution (osmotically equivalent to 10% sodium chloride).

Sodium chloride	90 g

   (Dry for 24 hours in a desiccator with calcium chloride prior to weighing out.)

Dibasic sodium phosphate (Na_2HPO_4)	13.65 g

Monobasic sodium   2.43 g
  phosphate ($NaH_2PO_4 \cdot 2\ H_2O$)
Dilute to 1 liter with distilled water. This solution is stable for several months at room temperature if kept well stoppered.

2. Buffered sodium chloride working solution.
    Buffered sodium chloride   20 mL
      stock solution
    Distilled water   180 mL
3. Distilled water.
4. Erlenmeyer flask (250 mL) and glass beads (3 to 4 mm in diameter), if defibrinated whole blood is used.
5. Pipets, 10, 5, and 0.05 mL.
6. Test tubes 13 × 100 mm.
7. Parafilm.
8. Centrifuge.
9. Spectrophotometer.

Specimen

Heparinized venous blood, or, 15 to 20 mL of defibrinated whole blood. A normal control blood should be collected in the same manner and at the same time the patient's blood is drawn. The test should be set up within 2 hours of collection, or within 6 hours if the blood is refrigerated.

Principle

If red blood cells are placed in an isotonic solution (0.85% sodium chloride), fluid will neither enter nor leave the red blood cell. If red cells are placed in a hypotonic solution (e.g., 0.25% sodium chloride), however, fluid enters the red blood cell until the cell either ruptures or an equilibrium is reached. A spherocyte, which is almost round, swells up in a hypotonic solution and ruptures much more quickly than a normal red blood cell or more quickly than cells having a large surface area per volume, such as target cells or sickle cells. The fragility of the red blood cell is said to be increased when the rate of hemolysis is increased. When the rate of hemolysis is decreased, the fragility of the red blood cells is considered decreased. In the osmotic fragility test, whole blood is added to varying concentrations of buffered sodium chloride solution and allowed to incubate at room temperature. The amount of hemolysis in each saline concentration is then determined by reading the supernatants on a spectrophotometer. A normal control blood is run at the same time the patient's blood is being tested.

Procedure

1. Prepare dilutions of buffered sodium chloride and place in the appropriately labeled test tube (Table 4–5).
2. Mix the preceding dilutions well, using Parafilm to cover each test tube while mixing.
3. Transfer 5 mL of each dilution to a second set of test tubes labeled #1 through #14. This set of dilutions will be used for the normal control blood.
4. If defibrinated blood is to be used, proceed as follows:
  a. Place 15 to 20 mL of whole blood into an Erlenmeyer flask containing 15 glass beads.
  b. Gently rotate the flask until the hum or noise of the beads on the glass can no longer be heard (about 10 minutes).
  c. Repeat steps 4a and 4b for the normal control blood.
5. Add 0.05 mL of the patient's heparinized or defibrinated blood to each of the 14 test tubes. Repeat, adding the normal control blood to the set of 14 control test tubes.
6. Mix each test tube immediately by gentle inversion.
7. Allow the test tubes to stand at room temperature for 30 minutes.
8. Remix the test tubes gently and centrifuge at 1200 to 1500 g for 5 minutes.
9. Carefully transfer the supernatants to cuvettes and read on a spectrophotometer at a wavelength of 540 nm. Set the optical density at 0, using the supernatant in test tube #1, which represents the blank, or 0% hemolysis. Test tube #14 represents 100% hemolysis.
10. Calculate the percent hemolysis for each supernatant as follows:

Percent hemolysis
$$= \frac{\text{O.D. of supernatant}}{\text{O.D. supernatant tube \#14}} \times 100$$

11. The results of the test may then be

TABLE 4–5. DILUTIONS AND NORMAL RANGES FOR THE OSMOTIC FRAGILITY TEST

Test Tube #	1% Buffered Sodium Chloride (mL)	Distilled Water (mL)	Final Concen. Buff. Sodium Chloride (%)	% Hemolysis
1	10.0	0.0	1.00	0
2	8.5	1.5	0.85	0
3	7.5	2.5	0.75	0
4	6.5	3.5	0.65	0
5	6.0	4.0	0.60	0
6	5.5	4.5	0.55	0
7	5.0	5.0	0.50	0–5
8	4.5	5.5	0.45	0–45
9	4.0	6.0	0.40	50–90
10	3.5	6.5	0.35	90–99
11	3.0	7.0	0.30	97–100
12	2.0	8.0	0.20	100
13	1.0	9.0	0.10	100
14	0.0	10.0	0.00	100

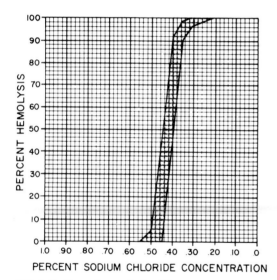

FIG. 4–9. Normal osmotic fragility curve.

graphed, with the percent hemolysis plotted on the ordinate (vertical axis) and the sodium chloride concentration on the abscissa (horizontal axis) as shown in Figure 4–9 (shows normal range).

12. Normal results are shown in Table 4–5.

Discussion

1. Instead of determining the amount of hemolysis on the spectrophotometer, the test may be read visually. In this method, the first test tube (the highest concentration of sodium chloride) showing a trace of hemolysis in the supernatant determines the beginning of hemolysis. The first test tube, having the highest concentration of sodium chloride in which hemolysis is complete, determines complete hemolysis. Normally, hemolysis should be complete in 0.3% sodium chloride, and beginning hemolysis should not occur in a concentration over 0.45% sodium chloride.

2. The pH of the blood-saline mixture is important and should be 7.4.

3. There are many sources of technical error in this procedure. It is, therefore, important to report the control results and interpret the patient's test in light of the normal control values.

4. If anticoagulated blood is used for this test, use only heparin as the anticoagulant, in order to avoid adding more salts to the blood.

5. Becton-Dickinson manufactures a Unopette test kit for determination of the red cell osmotic fragility test. This reagent set is made up of 10 buffered saline concentrations (0.85%, 0.65%, 0.60%, 0.55%, 0.50%, 0.45%, 0.40%, 0.35%, 0.30%, and 0.0%) contained in Unopette reservoirs. Each Unopette contains 1.98 mL of a buffered saline reagent with preservative (to inhibit bacterial growth). For testing, 20

μL of well-mixed whole blood (heparinized or defibrinated) is added to each Unopette dilution, mixed, incubated at room temperature for exactly 20 minutes, re-mixed, transferred to 12 × 75 mm test tubes, centrifuged at 2000 RPM for 5 minutes, and the supernatants read on a spectrophotometer at a wavelength of 540 nm. The normal ranges for this method are similar to those for the procedure outlined above.

6. The exact amount of whole blood added to each buffered saline dilution is not critical. The important point is that the same amount of whole blood be added to each saline dilution.

7. If hemolysis is present in the 0.85% sodium chloride tube, the test should be repeated using a new specimen. If the normal control also shows hemolysis at this concentration, or does not reflect a normal set of results, the buffered sodium chloride stock and working solutions should be discarded and re-prepared.

OSMOTIC FRAGILITY TEST WITH INCUBATION

The osmotic fragility of red cells after 24 hours of incubation at 37°C is more sensitive to slight differences in the red blood cell fragility and is also a measure of the red cells' ability to take up fluid without lysing. There are, however, other factors to be considered. Normally, after incubation, the red blood cells have increased osmotic fragility due to an accumulation of sodium in the red cells which is greater than the loss of potassium. This is determined by the membrane properties of the red cell and the metabolic activity of the cell. The metabolism of the red cell during incubation is stressed due to a lack of glucose. Those red cells with an abnormal membrane (hereditary spherocytosis, elliptocytosis) show an abnormal increase in osmotic fragility. Red cells having a glycolytic deficiency (pyruvate kinase deficiency) will show variable results: if the deficiency is severe, the osmotic fragility may increase greatly, or the fragility may decrease due to a greater loss of potassium in proportion to the increases in sodium in the red cell. Thalassemias major and minor generally show markedly reduced fragility due to a large loss of potassium. Iron deficiency anemia usually shows a less marked decrease in osmotic fragility. Abnormal results in the incubated osmotic fragility indicate an abnormality but are not always diagnostic of a specific disorder.

Reference

Dacie, J.V., and Lewis, S.M.: *Practical Hematology*, 6th ed., New York, Churchill Livingstone, Inc., 1991.

Reagents and Equipment

1. Water bath 37°C.
2. Sterile screw cap vials, 10 mL (two/specimen), if defibrinated whole blood is used.
3. See Osmotic Fragility Test. All reagents and equipment listed will be needed for this procedure.

Specimen

Heparinized venous blood or 15 to 20 mL of defibrinated whole blood. A normal control blood should be collected in the same manner and at the same time the patient's blood is drawn.

Procedure

1. Place unopened heparinized tube of patient and normal control blood in the 37°C water bath and incubate for 24 hours.
2. If defibrinated blood is to be used, proceed as follows:
   a. Place 15 to 20 mL of whole blood into a sterile Erlenmeyer flask containing 15 sterile glass beads.
   b. Gently rotate the flask until the hum or noise of the beads on the glass can no longer be heard (about 10 minutes).
   c. Place 5 mL of the patient's defibrinated blood into each of two sterile screw-cap vials. Repeat, using the control blood.
   d. Incubate the above specimens of blood at 37°C for 24 hours.
3. At the end of the 24 hours of incubation, number two sets of test tubes #1 through 17.

TABLE 4-6. DILUTIONS AND NORMAL RANGES FOR THE INCUBATED OSMOTIC FRAGILITY TEST

Test Tube #	1% Buffered Sodium Chloride (mL)	Distilled Water (mL)	Final Concen. Buff. Sodium Chloride (%)	% Hemolysis
1	10.0	0.0	1.00	0
2	9.0	1.0	0.90	0
3	8.5	1.5	0.85	0
4	8.0	2.0	0.80	0
5	7.5	2.5	0.75	0
6	7.0	3.0	0.70	0–5
7	6.5	3.5	0.65	0–10
8	6.0	4.0	0.60	0–40
9	5.5	4.5	0.55	15–70
10	5.0	5.0	0.50	40–85
11	4.5	5.5	0.45	55–95
12	4.0	6.0	0.40	65–100
13	3.5	6.5	0.35	75–100
14	3.0	7.0	0.30	85–100
15	2.5	7.5	0.25	90–100
16	2.0	8.0	0.20	95–100
17	1.0	9.0	0.10	100

4. Prepare the dilutions (see Table 4–6) of buffered sodium chloride and place in the appropriately labeled test tubes.
5. Mix the preceding dilutions well, using Parafilm to cover each test tube while mixing.
6. Transfer 5 mL of each dilution to the second set of labeled test tubes. This is to be used for the normal control blood.
7. Gently mix the incubated blood samples. (Pool the contents of the two patient test tubes together and combine the contents of the two control test tubes, if defibrinated blood was used. Do not pool the samples if one appears to be contaminated.) The blood should not be grossly hemolyzed.
8. Add 0.05 mL of the patient's incubated blood to each of the 17 test tubes. Repeat, adding the normal incubated control blood to the set of 17 control test tubes.
9. Mix each test tube immediately by gentle inversion.
10. Allow the test tubes to stand at room temperature for 30 minutes.
11. Remix the test tubes gently and centrifuge at 1200 to 1500 g for 5 minutes.
12. Carefully transfer the supernatants to cuvettes and read on a spectrophotometer at a wavelength of 540. Set 0 optical density using the supernatant in test tube #1, which represents the blank, or 0% hemolysis. Test tube #17 represent 100% hemolysis.
13. Calculate the percent hemolysis for each supernatant:

Percent hemolysis

$$= \frac{\text{O.D. of supernatant}}{\text{O.D. supernatant tube \#17}} \times 100$$

14. The results of the test should be graphed with the percent hemolysis plotted on the ordinate (vertical axis) and the sodium chloride concentration on the abscissa (horizontal axis) as shown in Figure 4–10 (shows normal range).
15. Normal results are shown in Table 4–6.

Discussion

1. It is important to maintain the sterility of the blood during incubation at 37°C. Bacterial contamination may produce hemolysis and inaccurate test results. For this reason the defibrinated blood is divided into two tubes prior to incubation. If one tube is contaminated it should be discarded and the second, noncontaminated tube used for testing.

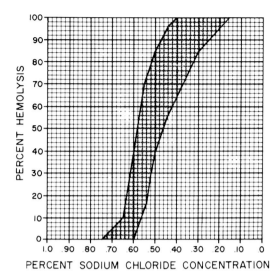

FIG. 4–10. Normal curve for the incubated osmotic fragility test.

2. The Becton-Dickinson Unopette test kit for the red cell osmotic fragility test may also be used in this procedure, in the same manner as outlined for the non-incubated osmotic fragility test.

AUTOHEMOLYSIS TEST

The autohemolysis test is increased in hereditary spherocytosis. In the past, this procedure was used in differentiating several types of congenital nonspherocytic hemolytic anemias using glucose and ATP. The development of less complicated and more specific enzyme assays have made the test unnecessary for this purpose.

Reference

Dacie, J.V., and Lewis, S.M.: *Practical Hematology*, New York, Churchill Livingstone, Inc., 1991.

Reagents and Equipment

1. Water bath, 37°C.
2. Sterile glass beads, 3 to 4 mm in diameter.
3. Cyanmethemoglobin (HiCN) reagent.
4. Glucose solution, 10%.

Glucose	10.0 g
Sodium chloride, 0.85% (w/v)	100 mL

This solution must be sterile. Autoclave or sterilize by Seitz filtration.
5. Sterile 0.85% sodium chloride (w/v).
6. Sterile screw-cap test tubes.
7. Sterile Erlenmeyer flask, 125 mL.
8. Sterile pipets, 2.0 and 0.1 mL.

Specimen

Whole defibrinated blood (15 to 20 mL) from the patient and a normal control.

Principle

One portion of sterile, defibrinated blood is incubated for 48 hours at 37°C. A second sample of the defibrinated blood is incubated with a specific amount of glucose. The percentage of hemolysis in each specimen is then determined spectrophotometrically. Normally, and in certain disorders such as hereditary spherocytosis, the amount of autohemolysis is reduced in the presence of glucose. In other pathologic states, the addition of glucose does not effectively decrease the autohemolysis. The degree of hemolysis that takes place in this procedure (with and without glucose) is a function of the metabolism and membrane properties of the red blood cell.

Procedure

1. The entire test procedure must be run under sterile conditions.
2. Defibrinate the patient and control bloods according to the following procedure:
   a. Add 15 to 20 mL of whole blood to a 125 mL sterile Erlenmeyer flask containing 15 sterile glass beads.
   b. Gently rotate the flask until the hum or noise of the beads on the glass can no longer be heard (about 10 minutes).
3. Label eight sterile screw cap tubes, #1 through #8.
4. Place 2 mL of the patient's defibrinated blood into test tubes #1, 2, 3, and 4. Place the remainder of the patient's defibrinated blood in an empty sterile screw cap tube and centrifuge at 1500 × g for 10 minutes. Remove the serum and place in

a sterile screw cap tube in the refrigerator.

5. Repeat step 4 above, adding 2 mL of control blood to tubes #5, 6, 7, and 8.

6. Add 0.1 mL of 0.85% sodium chloride to tubes #1, 2, 5, and 6. Gently mix the tubes.

7. Add 0.1 mL of 10% glucose solution to test tubes #3, 4, 7, and 8. Mix the tubes gently.

8. Incubate the eight test tubes at 37°C for 24 hours.

9. At the end of 24 hours, gently mix the test tubes by carefully inverting them 5 to 10 times. Incubate the tubes for an additional 24 hours.

10. At the end of 48 hours, inspect each test tube for contamination (a greenish discoloration or bad odor).

11. If there is no contamination, pool test tubes #1 and 2 together, #3 and 4 together, #5 and 6 together, #7 and 8 together.

12. Perform a duplicate hematocrit on each of the four specimens. Average the duplicate readings and record the results.

13. Pipet 0.02 mL of well-mixed blood from each test tube to four appropriately labeled tubes containing 5.0 mL of cyanmethemoglobin reagent (1:251 dilution).

14. Centrifuge the four tubes of pooled blood at 1500 × g for 10 minutes.

15. Remove the supernatant serums from each tube and pipet 0.5 mL of each serum into appropriately labeled test tubes containing 5.0 mL of cyanmethemoglobin reagent (1:11 dilution).

16. Pipet 0.5 mL of the nonincubated (refrigerated) patient's serum into an appropriately labeled test tube containing 5.0 mL of cyanmethemoglobin reagent. Repeat, pipetting 0.5 mL of the nonincubated (refrigerated) control serum into a second test tube containing 5.0 mL of cyanmethemoglobin reagent.

17. Record the optical density readings of the following solutions diluted with cyanmethemoglobin reagent, using a spectrophotometer set at a wavelength of 550 nm and using the cyanmethemoglobin reagent as the solution blank (0 O.D.):

a. Patient's incubated whole blood.
b. Patient's incubated serum without glucose.
c. Patient's incubated serum with glucose.
d. Patient's nonincubated serum.
e. Control's incubated whole blood.
f. Control's incubated serum without glucose.
g. Control's incubated serum with glucose.
h. Control's nonincubated serum.

18. Calculate the percent hemolysis for the control and patient bloods incubated with, and without, glucose according to the following formula:

$$\% \text{ Hemolysis} = (D_2 - D_3) \times \text{Dilution factor of serum} \times \frac{100 - \text{hematocrit}}{D_1 \times \text{Dilution factor or blood}}$$

D_1 = The optical density of diluted whole blood.
D_2 = The optical density of the diluted serum after incubation.
D_3 = The optical density of the diluted nonincubated serum.
Dilution factor of serum = 11.
Dilution factor of whole blood = 251.

19. Interpretation of test results. Normally, there is less than 4.0% hemolysis in the blood specimen with no added glucose, and less than 0.5% hemolysis in the specimen with added glucose. In hereditary spherocytosis and triosephosphate isomerase deficiency, autohemolysis in the absence of added glucose is generally greatly increased. With the addition of glucose, however, autohemolysis is usually reduced in a similar proportion as normal blood. Increased hemolysis present in both specimens (with and without glucose) may indicate pyruvate kinase deficiency or a deficiency in the glycolytic pathway.

Discussion

1. There may be considerable methemoglobin formation in the preceding procedure. Therefore, the cyanmethemoglobin method must be employed for measuring the amount of hemoglobin in the serum.

2. Hemolysis may be increased by bacterial contamination.

ASCORBATE-CYANIDE SCREENING TEST

The ascorbate-cyanide test is a nonspecific screening procedure for detecting deficiencies in the pentose phosphate pathway. Positive results will be found, most commonly, in glucose-6-phosphate dehydrogenase deficiency, but the procedure also detects deficiencies in glutathione, glutathione peroxidase, and glutathione reductase.

Jacob and Jandl Method

References

Jacob, H.S., and Jandl, J.H.: A simple visual screening test for glucose-6-phosphate dehydrogenase deficiency employing ascorbate and cyanide, N. Engl. J. Med., *274*, 1162, 1966.

Deacon-Smith, R.: The ascorbate cyanide test and the detection of females heterozygous for glucose-6-phosphate dehydrogenase deficiency, Med. Lab. Sciences, *39*, 139, 1982.

Reagents and Equipment

1. Ascorbate and glucose tubes for testing. Place:

Sodium ascorbate	10.0 mg
Glucose	5.0 mg

   into each of several 13 × 100 mm test tubes. (One tube is used for each test and control.) These tubes may be stoppered and stored at −20°C indefinitely.
2. Iso-osmotic phosphate buffer, pH 7.4.
   Solution 1

Monobasic sodium phosphate (NaH$_2$PO$_4$·2H$_2$O)	23.4 g

   Dilute to 1 liter with distilled water.
   Solution 2

Dibasic sodium phosphate (Na$_2$HPO$_4$)	21.3 g

   Dilute to 1 liter with distilled water.
   For iso-osmotic phosphate buffer, pH 7.4, mix together:

Solution 1	18 mL
Solution 2	82 mL

3. Sodium cyanide.

Sodium cyanide	500 mg
Distilled water	50 mL

   Iso-osmotic phosphate buffer 20 mL.
   Adjust the above mixture to a pH of 7.0 using 3 N hydrochloric acid. Dilute to 100 mL with distilled water. This solution is stable at room temperature indefinitely.
4. Pipets, 2.0 and 0.1 mL.
5. Water bath, 37°C.

Specimen

Collect 3 mL of whole blood, using heparin or EDTA as the anticoagulant. A normal control blood should be collected at the same time the patient's blood is obtained. (EDTA is the anticoagulant of choice.)

Principle

Sodium cyanide and sodium ascorbate are added to aerated whole blood (oxyhemoglobin). Hydrogen peroxide is generated by a reaction between sodium ascorbate and oxyhemoglobin. The inhibiting effect of catalase (present in the red cell) on hydrogen peroxide is blocked by the added sodium cyanide. Unless the hydrogen peroxide is reduced by glutathione peroxidase (in the pentose phosphate pathway) it will convert the oxyhemoglobin to a brown pigment (including methemoglobin formation). In a normal blood, the added glucose will be utilized by the pentose phosphate pathway to reduce the hydrogen peroxide. If there is an enzyme deficiency present in this pathway, hydrogen peroxide will not be reduced and the blood will become brown in color.

Procedure

1. Aerate both patient and control bloods to a bright red color by gently swirling the blood under air.
2. Add 2 mL of well-mixed whole blood to a test tube containing sodium ascorbate and glucose. Repeat, for each specimen and control to be tested.
3. Mix each tube well.
4. Add 0.1 mL of sodium cyanide solution to each of the preceding test tubes.
5. Gently mix the tubes and place, unstoppered, in a 37°C water bath for 2 to 4 hours.
6. During the incubation, gently shake each mixture at the end of 2, 3, and 4 hours and inspect the color of the solutions each time.
7. The normal control mixture should be a red color. If the patient's mixture is red, the test result is normal. If, however, the patient's solution has turned a brown color, the test is positive, and there is probably an enzyme deficiency in the pentose phosphate pathway, most often a glucose-6-phosphate dehydrogenase deficiency. (Generally, the color change is not very great when positive results are obtained.

A certain amount of experience is required to correctly detect the end point. As soon as the tube of blood is shaken, note the color of the film of blood as it moves down the side of the test tube.) If EDTA is used as the anticoagulant and the result is positive, the color change to brown is most evident within 2 hours of incubation. With the use of heparin, however, this color change will take 3 to 4 hours.

Discussion

1. If the blood specimen has a hematocrit below 20%, the volume of blood added to the ascorbate tube should be adjusted so that the amount of red blood cells added is equivalent to a hematocrit of 30 to 40%. For example, if the hematocrit is 20%, add 3 to 4 mL of whole blood to the ascorbate tube. As an alternative method, an appropriate amount of plasma may be removed from the whole blood until a hematocrit reading of 30 to 40% is attained.
2. Patients with half the normal level of G-6-PD activity (heterozygotes) may or may not show positive results within 2 hours.
3. To increase the sensitivity of this test, the red blood cells may be stained and examined for inclusions at the conclusion of the test. Add two drops of the test mixture to eight drops of 0.5% methyl violet (in 0.85% sodium chloride) (filter before use) and incubate at room temperature for 10 minutes. Prepare several blood smears, allow to air dry, and examine the red cells for inclusions. Normal blood will show inclusion bodies in less than 5% of the red cells. A specimen from a patient heterozygous for glucose-6-phosphate dehydrogenase deficiency will show an increased number of red cells containing inclusion bodies. Homozygotes will show inclusions in virtually all of the red blood cells.
4. Due to normally decreased concentrations of gluthathione peroxidase in newborns, this age group may also show positive results when tested by this procedure.

GLUCOSE-6-PHOSPHATE DEHYDROGENASE FLUORESCENT SCREENING TEST

When red blood cells are exposed to an oxidant drug, the activity of the pentose phosphate pathway increases. If one of the enzymes in this pathway (for example, glucose-6-phosphate dehydrogenase) is decreased or absent, reduced glutathione cannot be produced and oxidation of the hemoglobin takes place.

References

Beutler, E.: A series of new screening procedures for pyruvate kinase deficiency, glucose-6-phosphate dehydrogenase deficiency, and gluthathione reductase deficiency. Blood, *28*, 553, 1966.

Dow, P.A., Petteway, M.B., and Alperin, J.B.: Simplified method for G-6-PD screening using blood collected on filter paper, Am. J. Clin. Pathol., *61*, 333, 1974.

Sigma Diagnostics: Glucose-6-Phosphate Dehydrogenase (G-6-PDH) Deficiency, pkg. insert, St. Louis, Sigma Chemical Co., 1989.

Reagents and Equipment

1. The following reagents are obtainable from Sigma Chemical Co., St. Louis:
   a. Phosphate buffer, 0.075 M, pH 7.4 (contains 0.05% sodium azide as a preservative). Store in refrigerator. Discard if solution becomes cloudy.
   b. G-6-PDH screening test substrate, containing glucose-6-phosphate, nicotinamide-adenine dinucleotide phosphate (NADP), and a hemolytic reagent. Reconstitute with 2.0 mL of phosphate buffer, 0.075 M, pH 7.4. Allow to stand for 1 to 2 minutes. Mix carefully by inversion. Use as quickly as possible. (When reconstituted, this reagent is stable for approximately 2 weeks when frozen.)
   c. G-6-PDH normal and deficient controls (normal, #G6888; deficient, #G5888).
2. Test tubes, 12 × 75 mm.
3. Microhematocrit tubes (without anticoagulant).
4. Pipets, 2 mL, 0.2 mL, and 10 μL.
5. Filter paper, 32 cm, No. 1.
6. Long wave ultraviolet lamp (should emit light in the range of 320 to 400 nm). (Available from various laboratory suppliers.)
7. Water bath, 37°C.
8. Timer.

Specimen

Whole blood, 1 mL, using EDTA, heparin, or ACD (acid citrate dextrose) as the anticoagulant. (Specimens may be stored at 4°C for several days without loss of G-6-PDH activity.)

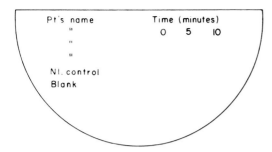

FIG. 4–11. Folded filter paper for G-6-PD procedure.

Principle

When red blood cells containing glucose-6-phosphate dehydrogenase (G-6-PDH) are mixed with the test reagent (containing glucose-6-phosphate and NADP), the following reaction occurs:

$$\text{Glucose-6-phosphate} + \text{NADP} \xrightarrow{\text{G-6-PDH}} \text{NADPH} + \text{6-phosphogluconate}$$

The resultant NADPH fluoresces under long wave ultraviolet light. NADP does not fluoresce.

Procedure

1. Reconstitute one vial of the G-6-PDH substrate as described previously.
2. Label one 12 × 75 mm test tube for each patient and control to be tested. (If a negative control is not available, 0.85% w/v sodium chloride may be used, or a normal blood may be diluted 1:5.)
3. Pipet 0.2 mL of G-6-PDH substrate into each of the preceding test tubes.
4. Fold a piece of 32 cm filter paper in half as shown in Figure 4–11.
5. Pipet 10 µL of whole well-mixed blood from the first specimen and add to the appropriately labeled test tube containing the G-6-PDH substrate. Rinse the pipet several times. Mix the contents of the test tube and, using a microhematocrit tube, quickly place a drop of the mixture on the filter paper (diameter of the drop should be 10 to 15 mm) under the 0 column (0 time) across from the appropriate name. Place the test tube in a 37°C water bath and set a clock for 5 minutes.
6. Repeat step 5 for each specimen and control. (Add 10 µL of 0.85% sodium chloride to the blank.)

7. At the end of the first 5-minute incubation period, place 1 small drop of each mixture in the appropriate line in the 5 minute column on the filter paper. Reset the clock for a second 5-minute incubation period. At the completion of the incubation period, place a small drop of each mixture in the appropriate column on the filter paper.
8. Allow 10 to 15 minutes for the sample applications to dry. In a dark room, place the filter paper under a long-wave ultraviolet light and observe for fluorescence. Record the results, using + for the presence of fluorescence, and − for lack of fluorescence, and ± for weak fluorescence (outer rim fluoresces, whereas the center of the spot does not).
9. Interpretation of results. There should be little to no fluorescence at 0 time. (The reaction occurs very quickly causing possible fluorescence at 0 time.) Normal G-6-PDH activity is indicated by maximum fluorescence at 10 minutes. Little or no fluorescence is seen in the 10-minute column on patients with a gross G-6-PDH deficiency. The normal control should show strong fluorescence at 10 minutes, whereas the negative control should show no fluorescence. Patients with a mild deficiency (about 50%) generally show a dull fluorescence or about half that seen with the normal control. In the presence of a more marked deficiency (less than 20%), no fluorescence will be present.

Discussion

1. Blood specimens may be collected on filter paper for use in this procedure. Place a drop of blood (from finger or heel stick) on a piece of filter paper (diameter of drop on filter paper should be 10 to 15 mm) and allow to dry. This specimen may be stored at room temperature for at least 5 days. When ready for testing, the spot of blood is cut from the filter paper, added to 0.2 mL of G-6-PDH substrate, and mixed. Test at 5 and 10 minutes as previously described.
2. False normal results may occur in the presence of elevated platelet or white blood cell counts. Removal of the buffy

coat from a centrifuged specimen is recommended in these cases (when the WBC is above 20,000/μL).

3. Reticulocytes normally contain a high concentration of G-6-PDH. Therefore, if the patient has had a recent hemolytic episode the test results may be falsely normal. In this case, the blood may be centrifuged and the red cells at the bottom of the specimen removed for testing.

4. Hemoglobin has a quenching effect on fluorescence. If the patient's hematocrit is greater than 50%, half as much specimen should be used. Conversely, if the hematocrit is less than 20%, use double the amount of specimen in the test procedure.

5. This test may be performed at room temperature. However, the amount of fluorescence will be less than if the specimens have been incubated at 37°C.

6. The 32 cm filter paper should be folded in half (not torn in half). The drops placed on the filter paper generally seep through one layer of the filter paper and, unless they are protected, may pick up contamination from the counter top (from a previous drop).

7. If the G-6-PDH substrate has deteriorated (a) a dried spot may show fluorescence, and/or (b) the amount of fluorescence may be decreased when incubated with a normal specimen.

8. Once the drop of mixture has been placed on the filter paper, the reaction will continue until the drop completely dries.

9. No fluorescence or decreased fluorescence will be present as long as the drop is moist. Once dried, the fluorescent spots on the filter paper are stable for several hours but will begin to fade within 24 hours. Fluorescence of the dried spots may be retained for several weeks by wrapping the filter paper in foil with a dessicant and storing in the refrigerator.

10. This test may be used to differentiate normal and grossly deficient levels of the enzyme. Quantitative assays should be performed when abnormal or questionable results are obtained by this procedure.

11. Sigma Chemical Co. also offers a kit for the quantitative determination of G-6-PDH.

PYRUVATE KINASE TEST

Pyruvate kinase is an enzyme in the Embden-Meyerhof pathway. A deficiency in this enzyme causes congenital nonspherocytic hemolytic anemia and is probably the most common cause of this type of anemia. Crenated and irregularly contracted red blood cells may also be found in this deficiency.

References

Beutler, E.: A series of new screening procedures for pyruvate kinase deficiency, glucose-6-phosphate dehydrogenase deficiency, and glutathione reductase deficiency, Blood, *28*, 553, 1966.

Sigma Diagnostics: Pyruvate Kinase Deficiency, Qualitative, Visual Fluorescence Determination in Red Cells, pkg. insert, St. Louis, Sigma Chemical Co., 1987.

Reagents and Equipment

1. Pyruvate kinase deficiency screening test reagent. Reconstitute with 2.0 mL of distilled water. Allow to stand for 2 minutes. Mix gently. Reconstituted reagent may be stored at 0°C for approximately 5 days. (Available from Sigma Chemical Co., St. Louis.)
2. Test tubes, 12 × 75 mm.
3. Microhematocrit tubes.
4. Pipets, 2.0 mL, 0.2 mL, 0.1 mL, and 20 μL.
5. Sodium chloride, 0.85% w/v.
6. Filter paper, 32 cm, No. 1.
7. Long-wave, ultraviolet lamp.
8. Water bath, 37°C.
9. Timer.

Principle

The pyruvate kinase reagent contains phosphoenolpyruvate, adenosine diphosphate (ADP), and reduced nicotinamide-adenine dinucleotide (NADH). When red blood cells containing pyruvate kinase and lactate dehydrogenase (LDH) are added to the test reagent, the following reactions occur:

Phosphoenolpyruvate

$$+ \text{ADP} \xrightarrow{\text{Pyruvate kinase}} \text{ATP} + \text{Pyruvate}$$

$$\text{Pyruvate} + \text{NADH} \xrightarrow{\text{LDH}} \text{Lactate} + \text{NAD}$$

Under long-wave, ultraviolet light, NADH fluoresces, whereas NAD does not fluoresce. Normally, all fluorescence should disappear within 30 minutes after the patient's red blood cells have been mixed with the pyruvate kinase test reagent.

Specimen

Whole blood, 1 mL, using EDTA, heparin, or ACD as the anticoagulant. For a fingerstick specimen, obtain about 1 mL of whole blood, using heparinized microcollection tubes. Obtain a specimen for a normal control at the same time. (Pyruvate kinase activity in the red blood cells is stable for 2 to 3 weeks when the blood is stored at 4°C.)

Procedure

1. Place approximately 1 mL of patient's whole blood into an appropriately labeled tube. Repeat, using a normal control blood. Centrifuge at 1200 to 1500 g for 5 minutes. Remove the supernatant plasma and buffy coat.
2. Place 0.4 mL of 0.85% sodium chloride into 12 × 75 mm test tubes appropriately labeled for each of the preceding specimens in addition to a tube labeled as the blank (represents a deficient specimen).
3. Carefully remove 0.1 mL of packed red blood cells from the bottom of the tube. (Do not contaminate the red cells with any cells from the buffy coat.) Wipe off the outside of the pipet and transfer the red blood cells to the appropriately labeled tube containing 0.4 mL of sodium chloride. Rinse the pipet several times with the mixture. Repeat this step for each specimen.
4. Reconstitute the pyruvate kinase reaction mixture.
5. Pipet 0.2 mL of pyruvate kinase reaction mixture into appropriately labeled 12 × 75 mm test tubes (one tube for the normal control, one tube for the blank, and one tube for each patient).
6. Fold a piece of 32 cm filter paper in half and label with the patients' name, control and blank as shown in Figure 4–11 for the glucose-6-phosphate dehydrogenase test procedure. Insert reading times of 0, 10, 20, and 30 minutes.

7. Pipet 20 μL of well-mixed diluted red blood cell suspension into the appropriately labeled test tube containing 0.2 mL of reaction mixture. Mix the test tube and, using a microhematocrit tube, quickly place a drop of the mixture on the filter paper under the 0 column (0 time). Place the test tube in a 37°C water bath. Set the clock for 30 minutes.
8. Repeat step 7 for each specimen and control, working as quickly as possible. (Use only one clock.) Add 20 μL of 0.85% sodium chloride to the blank in place of the red blood cell suspension.
9. When 10 minutes have elapsed on the clock, place one drop of each mixture in the 10-minute column. (Each drop should be about 10 to 15 mm in diameter.) Repeat at 20 and 30 minutes.
10. Allow 10 to 15 minutes for the sample applications to dry. In a dark room, place the filter paper under a long-wave ultraviolet light and observe for fluorescence. Record the results, using + for the presence of fluorescence, − for lack of fluorescence, and ± for weak fluorescence (outer rim fluoresces, whereas the center of the spot does not).
11. Interpretation of results. There should be strong fluorescence at 0 time. With normal pyruvate kinase activity, all NADH should be oxidized to NAD and there will be no fluorescence at 30 minutes. Any fluorescence present at 30 minutes or after indicates decreased pyruvate kinase activity. The normal control blood should show no fluorescence at 30 minutes, whereas the blank mixture shows fluorescence throughout the 30 minutes. Normally, fluorescence disappears within 10 to 20 minutes.

Discussion

1. Pyruvate kinase is present in the plasma, white blood cells, and platelets. Because this procedure is used to test the pyruvate kinase activity of the red blood cells, it is important that no plasma or white blood cells contaminate the red blood cell suspension. The red cells may be washed 1 time using 0.85% sodium chloride if desired.

2. Hemoglobin has a quenching effect on fluorescence.
3. See G-6-PDH Fluorescent Screening Test, under Discussion—#6, #8, #9, and #10 are applicable to this procedure.
4. Reticulocytes contain increased pyruvate kinase activity.
5. People who are heterozygous for pyruvate kinase deficiency will have approximately 50% of normal activity.

GLUTATHIONE REDUCTASE TEST

Glutathione reductase is a red blood cell enzyme. It functions in the pentose phosphate pathway to catalyze the reaction of the transfer of electrons from NADPH to glutathione in forming reduced glutathione. A severe hemolytic anemia, frequently drug-induced, is caused by a deficiency in glutathione reductase.

References

Beutler, E.: A series of new screening procedures for pyruvate kinase deficiency, glucose-6-phosphate dehydrogenase deficiency, and gluthathione reductase deficiency, Blood, 28, 553, 1966.

Sigma Chemical Co.: Glutathione Reductase Deficiency, pkg. insert, St. Louis, Sigma Chemical Co., 1986.

Reagents and Equipment

1. Glutathione reductase deficiency screening test reagent. Reconstitute with 2.0 mL of distilled water. Allow to stand for 2 minutes. Mix gently. Reconstituted reaction mixture can be frozen for 5 days without losing activity. (Available from Sigma Chemical Co., St. Louis, Mo.)
2. Test tubes, 12 × 75 mm.
3. Microhematocrit tubes.
4. Pipets, 2.0 mL, 0.2 mL, and 20 μL.
5. Filter paper, 32 cm., No. 1.
6. Long-wave, ultraviolet lamp.
7. Sodium chloride, 0.85% w/v.
8. Water bath, 37°C.
9. Timer.

Specimen

Whole blood using EDTA, heparin, or ACD as the anticoagulant. For fingerstick specimens, obtain 6 or 7 heparinized microhematocrit tubes (about three-fourths full). As soon as each tube is collected, allow the blood to flow back and forth several times to ensure complete anticoagulation. Obtain a normal control specimen at the same time. (Whole blood may be stored at refrigerator temperatures for 3 weeks without loss of glutathione reductase activity.)

Principle

The glutathione reductase reagent contains oxidized glutathione (GSSG) and reduced nicotinamide-adenine dinucleotide phosphate (NADPH). When red blood cells containing glutathione reductase (GSSG-R) are added to the reaction mixture, the following reactions occur:

$$GSSG + NADPH \xrightarrow{GSSG-R} \text{Reduced glutathione} + NADP$$

Under long-wave ultraviolet light, NADPH shows fluorescence, whereas NADP does not. Generally, in normal patients, fluorescence begins to disappear within 20 minutes after the patient's red blood cells have been mixed with the glutathione reductase test reagent. In blood samples from patients with decreased activity of glutathione reductase, fluorescence may continue for 1 hour or longer.

Procedure

1. Reconstitute the glutathione reductase test reagent.
2. Pipet 0.2 mL of glutathione reductase reagent into the appropriately labeled 12 × 75 mm test tubes (one tube for the normal control, one tube for the blank, and one tube for each patient).
3. Fold a piece of 32 cm filter paper in half and label with the patient's name, control and blank, as shown in Figure 4–11 for the glucose-6-phosphate dehydrogenase test procedure. Insert reading times of 0, 20, 40, and 60 minutes.
4. Pipet 20 μL of whole, well-mixed blood from the first specimen into the appropriately labeled test tube containing 0.2 mL of reaction mixture. Rinse the pipet several times. Mix the test tube and, using a microhematocrit tube, quickly place a drop of the mixture on the filter paper under the 0 column (0 time). Place the

tube in the 37°C water bath. Set the timer for 60 minutes.

5. Repeat step 4 for each specimen, working as quickly as possible. (Use only 1 clock.) (Add 20 µL of 0.85% sodium chloride to the blank in place of the whole blood.)
6. When 20 minutes have elapsed on the clock, place 1 small drop of the mixtures in the 20 minute column. Repeat at 40 and 60 minutes.
7. Allow 10 to 15 minutes for the sample applications to dry. In a dark room, place the filter paper under a long-wave, ultraviolet light and observe for fluorescence. Record the results, using + for the presence of fluorescence, − for lack of fluorescence, and ± for weak fluorescence (outer rim fluoresces, whereas the center of the spot does not).
8. Interpretation of results. There should be strong fluorescence at 0 time. With normal glutathione reductase activity, all NADPH is generally oxidized to NADP and there is little to no fluorescence at 20 minutes. Fluorescence at 60 minutes indicates a severe deficiency. The normal control blood should show almost no fluorescence at 20 minutes, whereas the blank mixture does show fluorescence in all samples.

Discussion

1. Hemoglobin has a quenching effect on fluorescence.
2. See G-6-PDH Fluorescent Screening Test, under Discussion—#6, #8, #9, and #10 are applicable to this procedure.

QUANTITATION OF METHEMOGLOBIN

Methemoglobin (Hi) is a form of hemoglobin in which the ferrous ion has been oxidized to the ferric state and is, therefore, incapable of reversibly combining with oxygen (and, therefore, cannot transport the oxygen molecule). Normally, a small amount of methemoglobin is continuously being formed in the red cell, but is, in turn, reduced by the red blood cell enzyme systems. Increased amounts may be found in both hereditary and acquired disorders. The hereditary form of methemoglobinemia is found (1) in disorders in which the red blood cell reducing systems are abnormal and unable to reduce methemoglobin back to oxyhemoglobin, or (2) in the presence of hemoglobin M, where the structure of the polypeptide chains making up the hemoglobin molecule is abnormal (there is a tendency toward oxidation of hemoglobin, with a decreased ability to reduce it back to oxyhemoglobin). The acquired causes of methemoglobinemia are mainly due to certain drugs and chemicals, such as nitrates, nitrites, quinones, chlorates, sulfonamides and aniline dyes.

Methemoglobin is normally present in the blood in a concentration of 0.03 to 0.13 g/dL, but a normal range should be determined by each laboratory. Slightly higher levels are present in infants and heavy smokers.

References

Williams, W., Beutler, E., Erslev, A.J., and Lichtman, M.A.: *Hematology*, McGraw-Hill, New York, 1990.
Evelyn, K.A., and Malloy, H.T.: Microdetermination of oxyhemoglobin, methemoglobin, and sulfhemoglobin in a single sample of blood, J. Biol. Chem., *126*, 655, 1938.

Reagents and Equipment

1. Phosphate buffer, 0.067 M, pH 6.6.
   Solution 1 (potassium dihydrogen phosphate, 0.067 M)
Monobasic potassium phosphate (KH_2PO_4)	9.1 g
Distilled water	1 L
   Solution 2 (dibasic sodium hydrogen phosphate, 0.067 M)
Dibasic sodium phosphate (Na_2HPO_4)	9.5 g
Distilled water	1 L
   For phosphate buffer, 0.067 M, pH 6.6, mix:
Solution 1	63.0 mL
Solution 2	37.0 mL
2. Phosphate buffer, 0.017 M (pH 6.6).
Phosphate buffer (0.067 M, pH 6.6)	1 volume
Distilled water	3 volumes
   Add approximately 0.2 g of saponin.
3. Sodium cyanide, 10% w/v.
Sodium cyanide	10 g
Distilled water	100 mL
4. Potassium ferricyanide, 20% w/v.
Potassium ferricyanide	20 g
Distilled water	100 mL

5. Acetic acid, 12% v/v.
6. Neutralized sodium cyanide. Prepare this reagent under a fume hood, just prior to use. Place four drops of 10% sodium cyanide in a small (12 × 75 mm) test tube. While carefully shaking the tube, add four drops of 12% acetic acid. Stopper tube as soon as possible. This reagent must be used within 1 hour of preparation.
7. Test tubes, 13 × 125 mm.
8. Pipets, 5 mL, 50 μL, and 20 μL.
9. Spectrophotometer.

Specimen

Fresh anticoagulated whole blood, using EDTA or heparin as the anticoagulant. This test should be performed within 1 hour of blood collection. However, once the blood has been diluted in the buffer reagent, it may be stored at 2 to 6°C for a maximum of 24 hours.

Principle

Whole blood is diluted with a phosphate buffer solution. Methemoglobin has a maximum absorbance at a wavelength of 630 nm. The diluted specimen is read in a spectrophotometer at 630 nm and the absorbance reading noted (D_1). Neutralized sodium cyanide is added to the mixture, converting the methemoglobin to cyanmethemoglobin, and read on the spectrophotometer (D_2). The change in optical density is directly proportional to the amount of methemoglobin present. The methemoglobin in g/dL is then calculated using a factor, previously determined, for the spectrophotometer used.

Procedure

1. Determination of calculation factor, F. Before the methemoglobin results can be calculated, a calibration factor for the spectrophotometer being used must be determined. This is done one time only, or whenever a different spectrophotometer is used for the procedure.
   a. Obtain a whole blood sample and determine the hemoglobin concentration in g/dL.
   b. Place 5.0 mL of 0.017 M phosphate buffer into each of two test tubes. Add 50 μL of the whole blood specimen to one tube and mix. The second tube is to be used as the blank.
   c. Add 20 μL of freshly prepared 20% potassium ferricyanide to both tubes. Mix and allow to stand for 2 minutes.
   d. Read on the spectrophotometer at 630 nm, using the blank to set the optical density at 0, and record the absorbance (D_x).
   e. Add 20 μL of neutralized sodium cyanide to both tubes. Mix and allow to stand for 2 minutes. Read on the spectrophotometer as above and record the optical density (D_y).
   f.
   $$F = \frac{Hgb\ (g/dL)}{D_x - D_y}$$

2. Procedure for testing patient specimen.
   a. Label and place 5 mL of 0.017 M phosphate buffer into one tube for each specimen and control to be tested and one additional tube to serve as a blank.
   b. Add 50 μL of whole blood to the appropriately labeled tube and mix well. Allow to sit at room temperature for 5 minutes.
   c. Read on the spectrophotometer at a wavelength of 630 nm, using the blank to set the optical density at 0. Record the absorbance of the solution (D_1).
   d. Add 20 μL of neutralized sodium cyanide reagent to each tube including the blank, and mix. Allow to sit for 2 minutes. Read as in step c above and record the optical density (D_2).
   e. Calculation of results:

   $$Methemoglobin\ (g/dL) = (D_1 - D_2) \times F$$

Discussion

1. Sulfhemoglobin is not measured at any time during the above procedures.

SERUM HAPTOGLOBIN TEST

The major breakdown (hemolysis) of red blood cells occurs in the reticuloendothelial system. Approximately 10% of red blood cell destruction, however, occurs intravascularly. In this circumstance, free hemoglobin is released directly into the blood and undergoes dissociation into α, β dimers, which are then bound to a serum globulin called *haptoglobin*. The binding of the α and β dimers to the haptoglobin prevents renal excretion of the pigment. This complex is removed from the plasma by the reticuloendothelial system. Normally, haptoglobin is present in amounts sufficient to bind 30 to 200 mg of hemoglobin per dL of plasma. The haptoglobin decreases and begins to disappear when hemolysis is increased to twice the normal rate. Increased amounts of haptoglobin are found in pregnancy, chronic infections, malignancy, Hodgkin's disease, rheumatoid arthritis, tissue damage, and systemic lupus erythematosus. Reduced levels of haptoglobin will be found in hemolytic anemia, liver disease, and infectious mononucleosis. There will be little to no haptoglobin present in the newborn but it will begin to appear at about 6 weeks of age and subsequently increase to normal levels.

References

Colfs, B., and Vekeyden, J.: A rapid method for the determination of serum haptoglobin, Clin. Chem. Acta., *12*, 470, 1965.

Dacie, J.V., and Lewis, S.M.: *Practical Haematology*. New York, Churchill Livingstone, 1991.

Lathem, W., and Worley, W.E.: The distribution of extracorpuscular hemoglobin in circulating plasma. J. Clin. Invest., *38*, 474, 1959.

Reagents and Equipment

1. Phosphate buffer, 0.05 M, pH 7.0.
   Solution 1
   Dibasic sodium phosphate   7.1 g
   (Na_2HPO_4)
   Dilute to 1 L with distilled water.
   Solution 2
   Monobasic sodium
   phosphate   3.45 g
   ($NaH_2PO_4 \cdot H_2O$)
   Dilute to 500 mL with distilled water.
   For phosphate buffer, 0.05 M, pH 7.0, mix:
   Solution 1   1 L
   Solution 2   500 mL
   Store in the refrigerator.
2. O-dianisidine reagent. Prepare just before using.
   O-dianisidine   0.5 g
   Ethyl alcohol, 95% (v/v)   70 mL

3. Acetate buffer, pH 4.7.
   Sodium acetate ($Na_2C_2H_3O_2 \cdot 3H_2O$)
   (27.22 g/L of distilled water)   53.5 mL
   Acetic acid (11.3 mL of glacial acetic acid diluted to 1 L with distilled water)
   46.5 mL
4. Hydrogen peroxide, 3% (v/v).
5. Staining reagent. Prepare just before using.
   O-dianisidine reagent   70 mL
   Acetate buffer   10 mL
   Hydrogen peroxide, 3% (v/v)   2.5 mL
   Dilute to 100 mL with distilled water.
6. Tweezers, one pair.
7. Microzone electrophoresis cell. (Obtainable from Beckman Instruments, Palo Alto, Calif.)
8. Cellulose acetate membranes (Beckman Instruments).
9. Sample applicator (Beckman Instruments).
10. DC-regulated power supply.
11. Drying oven, capable of reaching 100 to 110°C.
12. Glass drying plates (same size as the cellulose acetate membranes).
13. Acetic acid, 5% (v/v).
14. Ethyl alcohol, 95% (v/v).
15. Clearing solution. Prepare immediately before using.
    Ethyl alcohol, 95% (v/v)   75 mL
    Glacial acetic acid   25 mL
    It may be necessary to vary the amounts of glacial acetic acid and ethyl alcohol depending on the membranes used.
16. Triton-X wetting agent.
17. Sodium chloride, 0.85% (w/v).
18. Chloroform.
19. Glycerin.
20. Graduated centrifuge tubes, 15 mL.
21. Parafilm.
22. Hemoglobin solutions of 0.25, 0.50, 1.0, and 2.0 g/dL.
    a. Preparation of the hemolysate
       1) Place 3 to 4 mL of normal, whole anticoagulated (EDTA) blood in a 15-mL graduated centrifuge tube.
       2) Centrifuge at 1000 $\times$ g for 5 minutes. Remove plasma and discard.
       3) Fill tube to the 15-mL mark with 0.85% sodium chloride, mix, and centrifuge at 1000 $\times$ g for 5 minutes. Remove the supernatant sodium chloride.

4) Wash the red blood cells two more times.
5) Add one drop of Triton-X wetting agent, mix tube well, and allow to stand for 15 minutes to ensure complete hemolysis of the red blood cells.
6) Add a volume of chloroform equal to one-half the volume of the red blood cells. Use stopper and shake the tube vigorously for 1 minute.
7) Centrifuge for 5 minutes at 1000 × g.
8) Carefully remove the upper layer of the hemolysate.
9) Add an equal volume of glycerin to the hemolysate and mix. One may use a stopper and place the mixture in the freezer until ready for use.

b. Determine the exact hemoglobin concentration of the hemolysate (cyanmethemoglobin method). Using distilled water, adjust the hemoglobin concentration to 10 g/dL.

c. Prepare the following dilutions as indicated:
1) Hemoglobin concentration of 2.0 g/dL: 2.0 mL of hemolysate (10 g/dL) plus 8.0 mL of distilled water.
2) Hemoglobin concentration of 1.0 g/dL: 2.0 mL of hemoglobin solution (2.0 g/dL) plus 2.0 mL of distilled water.
3) Hemoglobin concentration of 0.5 g/dL: 2.0 mL of hemoglobin solution (1.0 g/dL) plus 2.0 mL of distilled water.
4) Hemoglobin concentration of 0.25 g/dL: 2.0 mL of hemoglobin solution (0.5 g/dL) plus 2.0 mL of distilled water.

Specimen

Clotted blood, 6 mL. Collect a blood specimen from a normal control at the same time the patient's blood is obtained. (Hemolyzed serum cannot be used in this procedure.)

Principle

The patient and control serums are incubated with varying concentrations of hemoglobin solutions. During this time, the haptoglobin present in the serum binds the hemoglobin, depending on the amount of haptoglobin available. The serum-hemolysate is then electrophoresed, during which time any free hemoglobin present will separate from the hemoglobin-haptoglobin complex. One may ascertain the approximate amount of haptoglobin present in the serum by noting at which hemoglobin concentration a second band of free hemoglobin appears.

Procedure

1. Incubate the patient and control specimens of whole blood at 37°C until the clot begins to retract. Centrifuge the specimens at 1500 × g for 10 minutes. Remove the supernatant serum and place in appropriately labeled test tubes. (If the test will not be performed at this time, freeze the serum.)
2. Number eight test tubes, #1 through #8, and set up the serum-hemolysate dilutions as shown in Table 4–7.
3. Incubate the above eight tubes at 37°C for 30 minutes.
4. Fill both sides of the electrophoresis cell with phosphate buffer.
5. Fill a small tray (of a size to accommodate one cellulose acetate membrane) with approximately 40 mL of buffer solution.
6. Using tweezers, place a cellulose acetate membrane in the tray of buffer. The membrane should be allowed to float on the surface of the buffer to allow capillary action to draw the buffer up evenly through the membrane. As soon as the entire membrane has become wet, immerse it completely in the buffer by carefully agitating the tray. Remove the membrane from the buffer using the tweezers. Carefully blot the membrane between two pieces of filter paper or blotters by passing a hand lightly over the top blotter once.
7. Immediately suspend and mount the wet membrane on the bridge of the electrophoresis cell, ensuring that the membrane lies evenly and that each end hangs freely in opposite chambers containing the buffer.
8. Replace the upper lid of the microzone

TABLE 4–7.   SERUM-HEMOLYSATE DILUTIONS FOR HAPTOGLOBIN TEST

Tube #	Normal Control Serum (mL)	Patient Serum (mL)	0.02 mL Hemolysate (g/dL)	Final Hgb. Concen. (mg/dL)
1	0.18		0.25	25
2	0.18		0.50	50
3	0.18		1.00	100
4	0.18		2.00	200
5		0.18	0.25	25
6		0.18	0.50	50
7		0.18	1.00	100
8		0.18	2.00	200

cell to guard against drying of the membrane.

9. Attach the connecting cables of the power supply to the electrode terminal pins. Do not turn on the power supply yet.

10. Allow the membrane to equilibrate for about 2 minutes before applying the blood samples.

11. Apply a 75 μL sample of hemolysate to the cellulose acetate strip (on the cathode side). It may be necessary to deposit more than one sample of the serum-hemolysate in the same place on the strip, depending on the size of each inoculation.

12. Rinse the applicator tip with a thin stream of distilled water and blot dry.

13. Repeat step 11, applying each serum-hemolysate sample in one of the eight positions on the cellulose acetate membrane.

14. As soon as all samples have been applied to the membrane, turn on the power supply to 150 V for 40 minutes.

15. At the end of 40 minutes, turn off the power supply and remove the plugs from the electrode terminal pins.

16. Carefully remove the membrane from the bridge without allowing any buffer to splash or run over the membrane.

17. Immediately immerse the membrane in a pan containing freshly prepared stain for 5 minutes.

18. Remove the membrane from the stain and wash in distilled water.

19. Place the membrane in a pan containing

5% acetic acid for approximately 5 minutes.

20. Allow the excess acetic acid to drain from the membrane and place it in 95% ethyl alcohol for exactly 1 minute.

21. Drain the excess ethyl alcohol from the membrane and place it in the clearing solution for exactly 30 seconds. While the membrane is immersed in the clearing solution, place the glass drying plate directly over the membrane. As soon as 30 seconds have elapsed, hold the membrane and glass together at one end. Lift this end from the clearing solution first, allowing the membrane to become positioned on the glass plate. Make certain the membrane lies flat on the glass plate and contains no air bubbles.

22. Place the glass plate (with membrane) in the drying oven at 100 to 110°C for 10 to 15 minutes.

23. Carefully remove the glass plate and membrane from the oven and allow to cool. The membrane should be completely transparent when removed from the oven.

24. When the glass plate has cooled sufficiently, loosen one corner of the membrane and carefully peel it from the glass, taking care that it does not tear.

25. The membrane may then be placed in a storage envelope (in between two pieces of plastic) to preserve it and avoid curling at the edges.

26. Interpretation: the free hemoglobin and hemoglobin bound to haptoglobin migrate as shown in Figure 4–12. The lowest concentration of hemoglobin showing a free hemoglobin band determines

CATHODE   ANODE

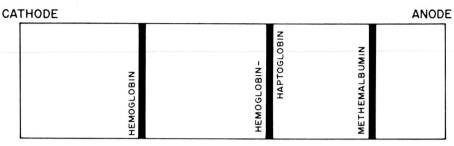

FIG. 4–12. Electrophoretic migration of free hemoglobin, hemoglobin-haptoglobin, and methemalbumin.

the amount of haptoglobin present in the serum. For example, if the serum-hemolysate mixture from tube #8 shows a hemoglobin-haptoglobin band and a free hemoglobin band, but hemolysate #7 shows only a hemoglobin-haptoglobin band, 100 to 200 mg/dL of haptoglobin is reported as present in the serum.

Discussion

1. If the freshly incubated serum sample is allowed to stand, methemalbumin is formed. In this situation, the methemalbumin will be present on the membrane as a band located on the right of the hemoglobin-haptoglobin band.
2. This same general procedure may be used to quantitate the amount of haptoglobin present in the serum more accurately, if a densitometer is available. For this method, incubate the patient's serum with a hemoglobin solution (1 volume hemolysate with 9 volumes of serum). Determine the exact concentration of the hemolysate (it should be 3.5 to 4.0 g/dL). Perform the procedure as described earlier beginning with step 3, and electrophorese one sample/patient or control. Using the densitometer, scan the dried membrane at 450 μm and a 0.3-mm slit width. The haptoglobin is calculated as follows:

Haptoglobin (mg/dL) =
$$\frac{\% \text{ Haptoglobin} \times \dfrac{\text{hemoglobin concentrate}}{10}}{10} \times 1000$$

Dilution of hemoglobin = 10
Conversion factor (g/dL to mg/dL) = 1000

3. Numerous methods are available for measuring the amount of serum haptoglobin: paper, agar gel, starch gel, and acrylamide gel electrophoresis, in addition to radioimmunodiffusion and nephelometry.

SUGAR WATER SCREENING TEST

The sugar water test is a simple screening procedure for paroxysmal nocturnal hemoglobinuria (PNH), an acquired disorder in which the patient's red blood cells are abnormally sensitive to destruction by normal constituents in plasma. Usually this disorder is characterized by red cell hemolysis during sleep (nocturnal hemoglobinuria).

If the sugar water test is positive, the sucrose hemolysis procedure should be performed before a diagnosis of PNH is made.

Reference

Hartmann, R.C., Jenkins, D.E., Jr., and Arnold, A.B.: Diagnostic specificity of sucrose hemolysis test for paroxysmal nocturnal hemoglobinuria, Blood, *35*, 462, 1970.

Reagents and Equipment

1. Sugar water solution, pH 7.4 $\pm$ 0.1.
   Sucrose (commercial granulated sugar)   9.5 g
   Distilled water   100 mL
   Prepare fresh.
2. Cyanmethemoglobin reagent.
3. Test tubes, 12 × 75 mm and 13 × 100 mm.
4. Pipets, 10, 2, 1, and 0.2 mL.
5. Spectrophotometer, 540 nm.

Specimen

Citrated whole blood: 1 part 0.109 M sodium citrate to 9 parts whole blood. Obtain a blood specimen for the normal control at the same time the patient's blood is collected.

Principle

Whole blood is mixed with a sugar water solution and incubated at room temperature. PNH red blood cells are abnormally susceptible to lysis by complement and under the conditions of this test will show hemolysis. The presence of hemolysis in this test, therefore, indicates a positive result for paroxysmal nocturnal hemoglobinuria.

Procedure

1. Pipet 1.8 mL of sugar water solution into each of two 12 × 75 mm test tubes, labeled patient and control.
2. Add 0.2 mL of well-mixed control and patient's whole blood to the respective test tubes.
3. Invert each test tube gently to mix.
4. Incubate both tubes at room temperature for 30 minutes.
5. While the tubes are incubating, label 13 × 100 mm test tubes, "Total" and "Test" for each patient and control. Label one tube as the blank. Pipet 9.5 mL of cyanmethemoglobin reagent into each tube.
6. At the end of the 30-minute incubation, remix each tube very gently. Remove 0.5 mL of the mixture from each tube and add to the appropriately labeled "Total" tube containing cyanmethemoglobin reagent. Mix well by inversion. Allow to sit at room temperature for 10 minutes.
7. Centrifuge the remaining blood-sugar water mixtures at 1200 to 1500 g for 5 minutes.
8. Add 0.5 mL of each supernatant to the appropriately labelled "Test" tube containing cyanmethemoglobin reagent. Add 0.5 mL of the sugar water reagent to the tube labeled "Blank." Mix all tubes well by inversion and allow to sit at room temperature for 10 minutes.
9. Transfer each mixture to a cuvet and read in a spectrophotometer at a wavelength of 540 nm, setting the blank at 0.0 optical density. Record the O.D. readings for each sample.
10. Calculate the percent of hemolysis for each specimen as shown below.

$$\text{Percent Hemolysis} = \frac{\text{O.D. Test}}{\text{O.D. Total}} \times 100$$

11. Interpretation of results. Hemolysis of 5%, or less is considered negative and within normal limits. Hemolysis of 6 to 10% is borderline. Positive results will show greater than 10% hemolysis, and must be confirmed by the sucrose hemolysis test and/or the acid-serum test.

Discussion

1. Prior to performing the test it is suggested that a small portion of the patient and control bloods be centrifuged (e.g., microhematocrit) to make certain there is no initial hemolysis present in the plasma.
2. In the presence of anemia, hemolysis may be slightly increased in PNH negative specimens.
3. The use of defibrinated blood may cause false positive results due to hemolysis of the traumatized red blood cells.
4. The test should be performed within 2 hours of obtaining the specimen.

SUCROSE HEMOLYSIS TEST

The sucrose hemolysis test is used as a confirmatory test for paroxysmal nocturnal hemoglobinuria (PNH) when the sugar water test is positive.

Reference

Hartmann, R.C., Jenkins, D.E., Jr., and Arnold, A.B.: Diagnostic specificity of sucrose hemolysis test for paroxysmal nocturnal hemoglobinuria, Blood, *35*, 462, 1970.

Reagents and Equipment

1. Sodium phosphate,   7.8 g
   50 mmol/L (NaH$_2$PO$_4$ · 2H$_2$O)
   Dissolve and dilute to 1 liter with distilled water.
2. Sodium phosphate,   7.1 g

50 mmol/L (Na_2HPO_4)
Dissolve and dilute to 1 liter with distilled water.

3. Sucrose solution (isotonic).

Sucrose (reagent grade)	92.4 g
NaH_2PO_4 (50 mmol/L)	91 mL
Na_2HPO_4 (50 mmol/L)	9 mL

Mix and adjust pH to 6.1, if necessary, using dilute NaOH or HCl. Dilute to 1 liter with distilled water. Reagent is stable at refrigerator temperature for 2 weeks.

4. Cyanmethemoglobin reagent.
5. Test tubes, 12 × 75 mm and 13 × 100 mm.
6. ABO compatible serum (or serum from type AB blood) from a normal donor. Specimen must be fresh.
7. Sodium chloride, 0.85% w/v.
8. Pipets, 10, 2, 1, 0.2, and 0.1 mL.
9. Spectrophotometer, 540 nm.

Specimen

Citrated whole blood: 1 part 0.109 M sodium citrate to 9 parts whole blood. Obtain a blood specimen (preferably the same blood type) for the normal control at the same time the patient's blood is collected.

Principle

Washed red blood cells are incubated in an isotonic sucrose solution containing normal ABO compatible serum. At low ionic concentrations, red blood cells absorb complement components from serum. Because PNH red blood cells are much more sensitive than normal red cells they will hemolyze under these conditions. The normal red blood cells will not. At the end of the incubation period the mixture is examined for hemolysis.

Procedure

1. Place 1 mL of patient and control bloods in respective 12 × 75 mm test tubes. Wash red cells by adding 0.85% sodium chloride to each tube. Centrifuge specimens at 1200 to 1500 g for 5 minutes. Carefully remove supernatant. Wash the red blood cells a second time in the same manner.

2. Prepare a 50% solution of red cells for both patient and control: add 3 drops of washed red blood cells to 3 drops of 0.85% sodium chloride. Mix.

3. Into appropriately labeled 12 × 75 mm test tubes (one tube for each patient and control, and one tube for the blank), pipet 1.7 mL of sucrose solution. Add 0.1 mL of ABO compatible serum (or serum from a type AB donor) to each tube.

4. Add 0.2 mL of the 50% suspension of red cells to each appropriately labeled tube. Gently mix each tube by inversion.

5. Incubate all tubes at room temperature for 30 minutes.

6. While the tubes are incubating, label 13 × 100 mm test tubes, "Total" and "Test" for each patient and control, and 1 tube for the blank. Pipet 9.5 mL of cyanmethemoglobin reagent into each tube.

7. At the end of the 30-minute incubation, remix each blood-sucrose tube very gently. Remove 0.5 mL of the mixture from each tube and add to the appropriately labeled "Total" tube containing cyanmethemoglobin reagent. Transfer 0.5 mL from the tube labeled blank to the cyanmethemoglobin tube labeled blank. Mix well by inversion. Allow to sit for 10 minutes.

8. Centrifuge the remaining blood-sucrose mixtures at 1200 to 1500 g for 5 minutes.

9. Add 0.5 mL of each supernatant to the appropriately labeled "Test" tube containing cyanmethemoglobin reagent. Mix all tubes well by inversion and allow to sit for 10 minutes.

10. Transfer above mixtures to a cuvet and read in a spectrophotometer at a wavelength of 540 nm, setting the blank at 0.0 optical density. Record the O.D. readings for each sample.

11. Calculate the percent hemolysis for each specimen as shown below.

$$\text{Percent Hemolysis} = \frac{\text{O.D. Test}}{\text{O.D. Total}} \times 100$$

12. Interpretation of results. Hemolysis of 5%, or less is considered negative and within normal limits. Hemolysis of 6 to 10% is thought to be borderline. Positive results will show greater than 10% hemolysis.

Discussion

1. Increased hemolysis (generally less than 10%) may be found in some patients with leukemia or myelosclerosis, whereas patients with PNH show 10% to 80% hemolysis (will only rarely be as low a 5%).
2. Results of the sucrose hemolysis test should correlate with the acid serum test.

ACID-SERUM TEST

Paroxysmal nocturnal hemoglobinuria (PNH) may be reliably diagnosed by means of the acid-serum test.

Ham Method

References

Ham, T.H.: Studies on destruction of red blood cells, Arch. Intern. Med., 64, 1271, 1939.

Dacie, J.V., and Lewis, S.M.: *Practical Haematology*, New York, Churchill Livingstone, Inc., 1991.

Sirchia, G., Soldano, F., and Mercuriali, F.: The action of two sulfhydryl compounds on normal human red cells. Relationship to red cells of paroxysmal nocturnal hemoglobinuria, Blood, *25*, 502, 1965.

Reagents and Equipment

1. Glass beads, 3 to 4 mm in diameter.
2. Sodium chloride, 0.85% (w/v).
3. Test tubes, 12 × 75 mm.
4. Hydrochloric acid, 0.2 N.
5. Water bath, 37°C.
6. Water bath, 56°C.
7. Erlenmeyer flasks, 125 mL.
8. Ammonium hydroxide, 0.04% (v/v), or cyanmethemoglobin (HiCN) reagent.
9. Graduated centrifuge tubes, 15 mL.

Specimen

Whole blood, 10 ml, to be defibrinated. Collect blood to use as a normal control and process in the same manner as the patient's specimen. (The normal control [serum and cells] may be obtained from blood allowed to clot at room temperature. Patient blood, however, must not be allowed to clot in the normal manner, since PNH red cells would most likely lyse while the blood was sitting at room temperature or 37°C.) (The control blood must be of the same ABO blood group, or, one compatible with the patient's blood group.)

Principle

The red blood cells of patient's with PNH are unusually susceptible to lysis by complement. In this procedure the patient's red blood cells are mixed with normal serum, with the patient's own serum, and with normal serum inactivated to destroy the complement. A weak acid is added to the inactivated serum tube, to one of the normal serum tubes, and to the patient's serum tube in order to adjust the pH of the mixture for maximum hemolytic activity. Normal red blood cells are incubated in acidified serum samples also, as a normal control. After incubation, all tubes are inspected for hemolysis. Normally, there will be no lysis of the red blood cells in any of the tubes of this test. In PNH, however, the patient's red blood cells will hemolyze in the presence of noninactivated, acidified, normal serum and in the patient's own noninactivated, acidified serum.

Procedure

1. Defibrinate the patient and control blood:
   a. Using a syringe obtain 10 mL of whole blood from the patient (or control) and place in Erlenmeyer flask containing 10 glass beads.
   b. Gently rotate the flask until the hum or noise of the beads on the glass can no longer be heard (about 10 minutes).
2. Decant the blood into a graduated centrifuge tube and spin at 1500 × g for 5 minutes.
3. Separate the serum from the red cells and save each.
4. Repeat steps 1, 2, and 3 for each specimen and control to be tested.
5. Number eight 12 × 75 mm test tubes for each patient to be tested. Pipet 0.5 mL of normal control serum into tubes #1 through #6. Add 0.5 mL of patient's serum to tubes #7 and #8. Place tubes #3 and #6 in a 56°C water bath for 30

TABLE 4–8. ACID SERUM TEST RESULTS INDICATING PAROXYSMAL NOCTURNAL HEMOGLOBINURIA

Tube	0.05 mL RBC	0.5 mL Serum	0.5 mL Inactivated Serum	mL of 0.2 N HCl	Hemolysis
1	P	N			Trace
2	P	N		0.05	+
3	P		N	0.05	0
4	N	N			0
5	N	N		0.05	0
6	N		N	0.05	0
7	P	P		0.05	+
8	P	P			Trace

minutes (to inactivate the serum and destroy the complement).

6. While the serum is incubating, wash the red cells: Fill each graduated centrifuge tube containing the red blood cells (step 3 above) with 0.85% sodium chloride. Mix and centrifuge at 1500 × g for 5 minutes. Remove the supernatant and wash the red cells two more times. After the last wash, note the volume of the packed red blood cells.

7. Add an equal volume of 0.85% sodium chloride to the packed red cells in each tube. Mix. This represents a 50% suspension of red cells.

8. Add 0.05 mL of the patient's red blood cells to tubes #1, 2, 3, 7 and 8. Add 0.05 mL of normal control red blood cells to tubes #4, 5, and 6. (See Table 4–8.) Mix all tubes gently.

9. Add 0.05 mL of 0.2 N hydrochloric acid to tubes #2, 3, 5, 6, and 7. Mix tubes gently.

10. Place all tubes in the 37°C water bath for 1 hour.

11. At the end of 1 hour, centrifuge the 8 tubes (per patient) at 800 × g for 2 minutes, and examine the supernatants for hemolysis.

12. The percent hemolysis present in each tube may be quantitated as follows.
   a. For each patient, add 0.05 mL of the original cell suspension (in step 7) to 0.55 mL of 0.85% sodium chloride. This mixture represents 100% hemolysis for those tubes to which 0.05 mL of hydrochloric acid was added.

Label tubes appropriately. To represent 100% hemolysis for the other tubes which contain no hydrochloric acid (and, therefore, a lesser volume), add 0.05 mL of the red blood cell suspension to 0.5 mL of 0.85% sodium chloride. Label tube.

   b. Add 5 mL of 0.04% ammonium hydroxide (or cyanmethemoglobin reagent) to 12 test tubes and label #1 through #12.

   c. Add 0.3 mL of the supernatants to the respectively numbered test tubes containing ammonium hydroxide (or cyanmethemoglobin reagent).

   d. To tube #9, add 0.3 mL of the cell suspension representing 100% hemolysis (for the acidified mixtures). Add 0.3 mL of the red cell suspension representing no addition of acid, to tube #10.

   e. To tube #11 add 0.3 mL of normal preincubated serum. This represents 0% hemolysis for those tubes using normal serum. Tube #12 represents 0% hemolysis for the tubes containing the patient's serum and must have 0.3 mL of the preincubated patient's serum added.

   f. Read the above solutions in a spectrophotometer at a wavelength of 540 nm, using tube #11 or #12 (whichever is appropriate) to set the instrument at 0 optical density.

   g. Calculate the percent hemolysis as shown below (use the appropriate tube to represent 100% hemolysis):

Percent Hemolysis =

$$\frac{\text{O.D. of test}}{\text{O.D. of tube representing}} \times 100$$
$$\text{100\% hemolysis}$$

   h. A positive test will usually show 10 to 50% hemolysis (with a range from 5 to 80%).

13. Interpretation of test results.

   a. Normal—no hemolysis in any tubes.

   b. Paroxysmal nocturnal hemoglobinuria—hemolysis present in tubes #2 and #7. There may also be a trace of hemolysis present in tubes #1 and #8. There should be no hemolysis in tubes #3 or #6 since the complement in the serum has been destroyed. Tubes #4 and #5 contain normal red cells so there should be no hemolysis in these tubes. Rarely, there may be decreased or no hemolysis in tube #7 (patient's serum) possibly due to complement depletion.

   c. In the rare disorder, dyserythropoietic anemia type II (also termed HEMPAS, or **h**ereditary **e**rythroblast **m**ultinuclearity with a **p**ositive **a**cid **s**erum test), tube #2 will show hemolysis. However, in these patients the red cells will not be lysed by their own serum and, therefore, tube #7 will show no lysis. Also, the sucrose hemolysis test will be negative.

Discussion

1. Hemolysis in test tubes #2, 3, and 7 may indicate the presence of markedly spherocytic red blood cells. This can be differentiated from paroxysmal nocturnal hemoglobinuria because lysis of the spherocytes is unaffected by heating the serum at 56°C.
2. Inactivating the serum in test tubes #3 and #6 at 56°C destroys the hemolytic system. Therefore, lysis present in these tubes rules out the possibility of a positive test for PNH.
3. When the patient has received blood transfusions, less lysis occurs because of the presence of normal transfused red blood cells.
4. A positive control should be run with this test and may be prepared by treating normal red blood cells with 2-aminoethylisothiouronium bromide (AET). Normal blood is collected in ACD anticoagulant and the red cells washed two times with 0.85% sodium chloride (w/v). An 8% (w/v) aqueous solution of AET is prepared and the pH of the solution adjusted to 8.0 with 5 N sodium hydroxide. Four volumes of 8% AET (pH 8.0) is added to one volume of packed washed red blood cells, placed in a flat bottomed beaker, mixed well, and incubated at 37°C for 19 minutes. At the end of this period, the red cells are washed repeatedly with relatively large amounts of 0.85% sodium chloride until the supernatant is clear. (Each time the cells are washed the red cells should be mixed well to ensure resuspension before centrifuging. After the first wash the red blood cells will be clumped together and the mixing and resuspension are very important.) At the end of the last wash, remove as much of the supernatant as possible. The red cells are then ready for use as a positive PNH control.

LUPUS ERYTHEMATOSUS PREPARATION (L.E. PREP)

Antinuclear antibodies (antinuclear factors [ANF]) occur in the serum of patients with a number of disorders including systemic lupus erythematosus (SLE). This antinuclear antibody is also termed the LE factor and is a component of the globulin fraction of serum protein. Several methods are available for detection of the LE factor: (1) immunofluorescence, (2) radioimmunoassay, (3) a serologic procedure using coated latex particles, and (4) demonstration of LE cells in which the LE factor in the serum causes lysis of neutrophil nuclei, with subsequent phagocytosis of the nuclear material by other neutrophils (described below).

References

Dacie, J.V., and Lewis, S.M.: *Practical Haematology*, New York, Churchill Livingstone, Inc., 1991.

Magath, T.B., and Winkle, V.: Technic for demonstrating "L.E." (lupus erythematosus) cells in blood, Am. J. Clin. Path., *22*, 586, 1952.

Zinkham, W.H., and Conley, C.L.: Some factors influencing the formation of L.E. cells. A method for enhancing L.E. cell production, Bullet. Johns Hopkins Hosp., *98*, 102, 1956.

L.E. Cell Technique Using Heparinized Blood

Reagents and Equipment

1. Glass beads, 4 mm in diameter.
2. Test tube rotator.
3. Wintrobe ESR tubes, 3 to 4.
4. Glass slides.
5. Wright stain.
6. Disposable dropper pipets with a long narrow tip for filling the Wintrobe tubes.
7. Incubator or water bath, 37°C.

Specimen

Five mL of whole blood using heparin as the anticoagulant. Make certain the blood to heparin ratio is correct. (Heparin concentration must be the minimum amount to prevent clotting.)

Principle

In order for the LE factor (present in a patient's plasma) to lyse the neutrophil nuclei, the cells must first be damaged to allow for liberation of the nuclei from the cells. Also, the LE factor is not able to act upon healthy, living white blood cells. For this reason, glass beads are added to whole blood which is then mixed for a period of time in order to damage some of the neutrophils. The blood is then incubated to allow for lysis of the neutrophil nuclei. The whole blood is centrifuged and buffy coat smears prepared, stained and examined for phagocytized nuclear material (L.E. cells).

Procedure

1. Add 5 to 10 glass beads to the tube of blood and mix on a mechanical rotator for 30 minutes.
2. Incubate tube of blood at 37°C for 30 minutes.
3. Fill three to four Wintrobe tubes with the well mixed blood and centrifuge at 200 × g for 10 minutes.
4. Discard the plasma from each of the tubes. Remove the buffy coat and prepare three to four smears. Wright stain.
5. Examine each smear for the presence of L.E. cells (Figs. 4–13 and 4–14). Report

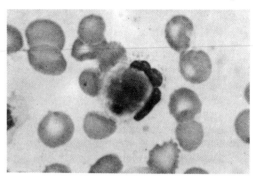

FIG. 4–13. L.E. cell. (Magnification ×1000.)

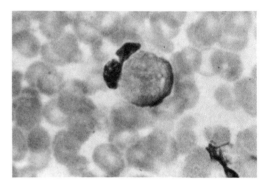

FIG. 4–14. L.E. cell. (Magnification ×1000.)

results as positive or negative. The slides should be examined for at least 10 minutes. The smear should be studied using the low oil objective (50×), or on low power (10×) when enough experience has been gained. All suspicious cells should be examined under the high oil immersion objective (100×). The characteristic L.E. cell is a neutrophil containing a large spherical body in its cytoplasm. Usually, the neutrophil nucleus is pushed to one side of the cell and appears to wrap itself around the ingested material. The inclusion shows no nuclear structure and stains as a pale purple homogeneous mass with a velvety appearance. In rare instances, the ingesting cell may be a monocyte or eosinophil. The L.E. phenomenon also includes **rosettes**, which consist of free lysed nuclear material surrounded by neutrophils. These are readily seen using the low power objective (10×). The **tart cell**, which may be confused with the L.E. cell, is usually a monocyte which has ingested another cell or the nucleus of another cell. In this case, the ingested material resembles a lymphocyte nucleus or phagocytized material with a definite nuclear pattern. Another form of ingested material found in the tart cell is an intensely stained body termed a **pyknotic nucleus**. The significance of these cells is not known. Their presence in an L.E. preparation does not signify a positive test for systemic lupus erythematosus.

L.E. Cell Technique Using Clotted Blood

Reagents and Equipment

1. Wire sieve and pestle.
2. Petri dish.
3. Wintrobe ESR tubes, three to four.
4. Glass slides.
5. Wright stain.
6. Disposable dropper pipets with a long narrow tip for filling the Wintrobe tubes.
7. Incubator or water bath, 37°C.

Specimen

Clotted whole blood, 10 ml.

Principle

Clotted blood is allowed to sit at room temperature for 2 hours. The clot is then macerated by forcing it through a sieve. The trauma produced when the blood is forced through the strainer causes extrusion of nuclei from the polymorphonuclear cells. The LE factor present in the blood lyses the nuclear material, which is then phagocytized by other neutrophils. This forms the L.E. cell.

Procedure

1. Place 10 mL of whole blood in a plain test tube and allow the blood to clot.
2. Incubate the tube of clotted blood at room temperature for 2 hours.
3. Place the sieve over a petri dish.
4. Transfer the clot and serum to the sieve and mash the clot through the sieve, using the pestle.
5. Transfer the blood from the petri dish to three or four Wintrobe tubes.
6. Incubate the filled Wintrobe tubes at 37°C for 2 hours.
7. Centrifuge the Wintrobe tubes at 200 × g for 10 minutes.
8. Remove the serum from each of the tubes, using a disposable dropper. Remove the buffy coat from each tube and prepare three to four blood smears. Wright stain.
9. Examine smears as described in step 7 above for the procedure using heparinized blood.

Discussion

1. The presence of one L.E. cell is not a substantial basis for reporting a positive result. Several typical L.E. cells should be seen before a positive report is made.
2. If a patient has severe leukopenia, a false-negative result may be obtained due to the decreased number of neutrophils present. Therefore, because the LE factor is present in the serum, 5 mL of patient's serum may be added to 5 mL of washed red and white blood cells (type O blood) obtained from a normal individual. The test should then be carried out as previously described.
3. Occasionally, false-positive results are obtained in patients with drug reactions, hepatitis, and rheumatoid arthritis.
4. This test is positive only in about 75% of the patients with systemic lupus erythematosus. False-negative results may also be obtained on patients with the disease who are receiving adrenocorticosteroid therapy.

SERUM VISCOSITY TEST

Viscosity is that property of a fluid that resists the force causing it to flow. The viscosity of serum is primarily a function of the concentration of protein and is determined by comparing it with the viscosity of distilled water. This result is normally in the range of 1.4 to 1.8. An increased serum viscosity is most often found in an IgM monoclonal gammopathy (Waldenström's macroglobulinemia) and in some lymphomas and IgA and IgG myelomas. The severity of the clinical abnormalities are often better correlated with the viscosity of the serum than with the level of the protein involved. Therefore, therapy

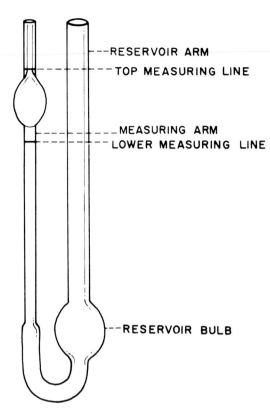

--RESERVOIR ARM

--TOP MEASURING LINE

--MEASURING ARM

--LOWER MEASURING LINE

--RESERVOIR BULB

FIG. 4–15. Ostwald viscometer.

may be followed by serum viscosity measurements.

Reference

Fahey, J.L., Barth, W.F., and Solomon, A.: Serum hyperviscosity syndrome, JAMA, *192*, 464, 1965.

Reagents and Equipment

1. Water bath, 37°C (optional).
2. Rubber tubing.
3. Stopwatch.
4. Sodium chloride, 0.85% (w/v).
5. Distilled water.
6. Ostwald viscometer (Fig. 4–15). (Alternatively, a red blood cell pipet or a 1 mL volumetric pipet may be used in place of the viscometer.)
7. Support stand with clamp (to hold viscometer or pipet).

Specimen

Collect approximately 12 mL of whole blood and allow to clot. This test requires 5 mL of serum if the Ostwald viscometer is used. (The 1 mL pipet or red blood cell pipet requires less than 2 mL of serum.) The specimen (serum) may be refrigerated for up to 2 days prior to testing.

Principle

Serum viscosity is determined by comparing the rate of flow of serum to the rate of flow of distilled water through a viscometer (pipet). The patient's serum is placed in a viscometer and the time required for the serum to flow from one mark to a second mark is measured. This time is then compared with the time required for distilled water to flow the same distance in the viscometer (pipet).

Procedure

1. Centrifuge the clotted blood at 3000 × g for 10 minutes. Remove the serum and centrifuge a second time. Place the serum in a test tube.
2. Suspend the viscometer in a 37°C water bath by means of a laboratory stand.
3. Place 5 mL of patient's serum in the reservoir bulb through the reservoir arm.
4. Allow several minutes for the serum to reach 37°C. During this time, remove any air bubbles in the serum by gently blowing through the aspirator attached to the top of the measuring arm.
5. Using suction, draw the serum up into the measuring arm above the highest line. Release the suction.
6. As the serum flows down through the measuring arm, start the stopwatch as soon as the top of the serum is even with the top measuring line.
7. Time the passage of serum between the two measuring lines: as soon as the upper border of the serum is even with the lower measuring line, stop the watch. Record the flow time of the serum.
8. Repeat steps 5 through 7 two more times and average the three readings.
9. Remove the serum and rinse the viscometer several times with 0.85% sodium chloride followed by two rinses with distilled water.

10. Repeat steps 2 through 8, using 5 mL of distilled water in place of the patient's serum.
11. Calculate the results as shown below:

Relative serum viscosity

$$= \frac{\text{Flow time of serum}}{\text{Flow time of distilled water}}$$

Discussion

1. The flow time of distilled water through the Ostwald viscometer is generally about 59 seconds.
2. The viscometer, when it is not in use, should be sealed with Parafilm.
3. This procedure may be performed at room temperature if a 37°C water bath is not available.
4. If a pipet is used in place of the viscometer it must be supported in a vertical position; the test may be performed at room temperature.
5. Symptoms of the hyperviscosity syndrome are generally present in the patient when the relative serum viscosity is between 6 and 7, but may also be present with a test result as low as 4.

REAGENTS
(Special Hematology-Reagents)

Acetate Buffer, 0.1 N, pH 5.0

Sodium acetate   4.797 g
  (CH₃COONa·3H₂O)
Acetic Acid, 1 N   14.75 mL
Dissolve the sodium acetate in 1 N acetic acid and dilute to 1 liter with distilled water. Refrigerate.

Acetic Acid, 1 N

Glacial acetic acid   6 mL
Dilute to 1 liter with distilled water.

Barbital Buffered Saline Solution, pH 7.35

Sodium diethylbarbiturate   5.875 g
Sodium chloride   7.335 g
Distilled water   785 mL

Hydrochloric acid, 0.1 N   215 mL
Store in the refrigerator.

Buffered Methyl Green, 1% w/v, in Acetate Buffer (0.1 N, pH 5.0)

Methyl green   1.0 g
Acetate buffer, 0.1 N, pH 5.0 100 mL
Adjust the pH from 4.2 to 4.5 with 1 N sodium hydroxide or 1 N hydrochloric acid. Filter. Store at room temperature.

Buffered Neutral Red, 1% w/v in Acetate Buffer (0.1 N, pH 5.0)

Neutral red   1.0 g
Acetate buffer, 0.1 N, pH 5.0 100 mL
Warm the above solution and mix until the stain is dissolved. Filter when cooled to room temperature.

Glycerol Gelatin

Gelatin   20 g
Distilled water   105 mL
Glycerin   125 mL
Heat the above, while mixing, to dissolve the gelatin. Store in a jar. Refrigerate. Prior to use, remove a small portion and heat until liquified.

Hydrochloric Acid, 1 N

Hydrochloric acid,   97.85 mL
  concentrated (37.25% purity)
Dilute to 1 liter with distilled water.

Mayer's Hematoxylin

Hematoxylin   1 g
Aluminum ammonium sulfate   50 g
  (ammonium alum)
Chloral hydrate   50 g
Dilute to 1 liter with distilled water. Add 0.2 g of sodium iodate (ripening agent) and mix well. Store reagent at room temperature for 7 days in order to ripen before use.

Pararosanilin, 4% w/v in 20% (v/v) Hydrochloric Acid

Pararosanilin hydrochloride	1.0 g
Distilled water	20 mL
Hydrochloric acid, concentrated	5 mL

Gently warm the above while mixing in order to dissolve as much pararosanilin as possible. Allow the mixture to cool, filter, and store in a brown bottle at room temperature.

Phosphate Buffered Formalin Acetone Fixative, pH 6.6 to 6.8

Dibasic sodium phosphate (Na_2HPO_4)	0.1 g
Monobasic potassium phosphate (KH_2PO_4)	0.5 g

Dissolve the above in 150 mL of distilled water and add:

Acetone	225 mL
Formaldehyde, 37%	125 mL

Store in the refrigerator.

Sodium Hydroxide, 1 N

Sodium hydroxide	40 g

Dilute to 1 liter with distilled water.

Sodium Nitrite, 4% w/v

Sodium nitrite	4.0 g

Dilute to 100 mL with distilled water. Prepare immediately before use.

Tris buffer, 0.1 M, pH 7.4

Tris-(2-amino-2[hydroxy-methyl]1,3-propandiol)	12.1 g

Dissolve reagent in 800 mL of distilled water. Adjust pH to 7.4 using 0.1 N hydrochloric acid. Dilute to 1 liter with distilled water. Store in the refrigerator. Warm to room temperature before using.

COAGULATION

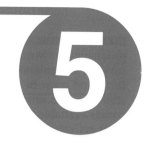

The above outline serves as a guide for the reader. The topics are presented in the order as written. However, the sequence of events in the complex process of clot formation and dissolution do not occur in the order as outlined above. An attempt has been made here to present the material in a manner that may be more easily understood. The numbers to the right of each subject (in parentheses) indicates the chronological order in which the events might be thought of as occurring.

Introduction

Hemostasis is the process that (1) retains the blood within the vascular system during periods of injury, (2) localizes the reactions involved to the site of injury, and (3) repairs and re-establishes blood flow through the injured vessel. It is a system in dynamic balance that, when tipped by deficiencies (congenital or acquired) of the procoagulant portion or excesses of the fibrinolytic portion, results in uncontrolled bleeding (hemorrhage); when tipped by deficiencies (congenital or acquired) of the fibrinolytic portion or uncontrolled activation of the procoagulant portion, the result is excessive clot formation or persistance of clot (thrombosis). The hemostatic process requires the interaction of numerous components: blood vessels, endothelium, platelets, coagulation factors, inhibitors, and fibrinolytic substances. Hemostasis is a highly complex mechanism consisting of many reactions occurring simultaneously, which, even today, is not completely understood. A basic knowledge of hemostasis and fibrinolysis is necessary in order to understand the principles of coagulation testing.

During *primary hemostasis* there is constriction of the damaged blood vessels, which decreases the blood flow through the injured blood vessel. Platelets clump together and adhere to the injured vessel to form a platelet plug and further inhibit bleeding.

During *secondary hemostasis* the coagulation factors present in the blood (and tissue factor) interact, forming a fibrin meshwork (clot) to more efficiently stop the bleeding. During this process, naturally occurring inhibitors present in the blood will block activated coagulation factors so that widespread coagulation does not occur. The normal circulation of blood will also serve to transport coagulation factors to and from the injured area. When a clot has formed, slow breakdown (lysis) of the clot begins, and final repair to the injured site takes place.

Coagulation Mechanism

The coagulation mechanism may be thought of as a complex series of cascading reactions involving development of enzymes from

cofactor to enhance the activation of factor X by IXa with phospholipid and calcium ions. Based on its characteristics, factor VIII may be symbolized as follows: (1) factor VIII, factor VIIIC, and factor VIII:C stands for the coagulant property of the factor, that portion of the molecule that is measured by standard factor VIII assays, and it is markedly decreased in classic hemophilia (hemophilia A); (2) factor VIII antigen (factor VIII:Ag) represents the antigenic properties of factor VIII measured by immunoassays.

von Willebrand factor functions in primary hemostasis, acts as a carrier for the coagulant portion of the factor VIII complex, and constitutes greater than 90% of this complex. It is synthesized in the megakaryocytes and endothelial cells and is also present in the α granules of the platelets. Based on its characteristics von Willebrand factor may be symbolized as follows: (1) vWf or von Willebrand factor, which represents that portion of the factor responsible for a normal bleeding time, or normal platelet adhesiveness in-vitro; (2) von Willebrand factor antigen (vWf:Ag) was previously termed the factor VIII related antigen (VIIIR:Ag) and is measured by immunoassays; (3) ristocetin co-factor activity, which is that property of the factor which causes platelet aggregation in the presence of ristocetin.

Factor IX (antihemophilic B factor) is a single chain glycoprotein synthesized in the liver, and requires vitamin K for its production. It is decreased in the plasma of patients with Christmas disease (hemophilia B). It is stable at 4°C for several weeks. It has a half-life of approximately 24 hours and is present in serum.

Factor X (Stuart factor) is a glycoprotein. It is synthesized in the liver and requires vitamin K for its production. It is relatively heat stable and may be stored for up to 2 months at 4°C. It has a half-life of approximately 40 hours. It may be activated by both the intrinsic and extrinsic coagulation systems.

Factor XI (plasma thromboplastin antecedent) is a β-2 globulin that is thought to circulate in plasma in a complex with high molecular weight kininogen. It is probably synthesized in the liver, is relatively stable at room temperature, and has a half-life of approximately 45 hours.

Factor XII (Hageman factor) is a single chain

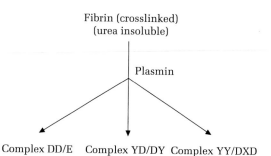

Fibrin (crosslinked) (urea insoluble)

Plasmin

Complex DD/E   Complex YD/DY   Complex YY/DXD

FIG. 5–2. Degradation of cross-linked fibrin by plasmin.

polypeptide. The actual site of production is not known. It is stable in that it can be stored (in oxalated plasma) at 4°C for almost 3 months. It is relatively heat stable and remains in serum after 30 minutes at 60°C.

Factor XIII (fibrin stabilizing factor) is heat stable and has a half-life of 3 to 12 days. Although its site of production is not known, it is thought that the liver may play a role.

Prekallikrein (Fletcher factor) is a single chain γ globulin. It is produced in the liver but is not dependent on vitamin K for its production. This factor is present in serum and is not adsorbed out of the plasma by barium sulfate and aluminum hydroxide.

High molecular weight kininogen (HMWK) (Fitzgerald Factor) is a single chain glycoprotein, has a half-life of 6.5 days, and is present in serum. It is produced in the liver, is not vitamin K dependent, and is present in barium sulfate and aluminum hydroxide adsorbed plasma.

Fibrinolysis

The primary purpose of fibrinolysis is to digest fibrin clots as they are formed in order to keep the vascular system free of deposited fibrin and fibrin clots. Fibrinolysis occurs when plasminogen is converted into plasmin, which dissolves the fibrin (or fibrinogen) into smaller fragments termed *fibrin(ogen) degradation products* (see Figs. 5–2 and 5–3).

Plasminogen. Plasminogen is a single chain glycoprotein found in the plasma in a concentration of 20 to 40 mg/dL and in all other body fluids in lesser amounts. It is produced by the liver. During the clotting process, it

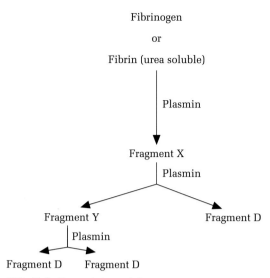

Fibrinogen

or

Fibrin (urea soluble)

$\downarrow$ Plasmin

Fragment X

Plasmin

Fragment Y   Fragment D

Plasmin

Fragment D   Fragment D

FIG. 5–3. Degradation of fibrinogen and noncross-linked fibrin by plasmin.

forms complexes with fibrin and is absorbed into the clot.

Plasminogen activators. Activation of plasminogen is carried out by plasminogen activators. Intrinsic activators are present in the blood and include factor XIIa, kallikrein, and HMWK. Tissue-type plasminogen activator (t-PA), secreted by the endothelial cells, and urokinase-like plasminogen activator (u-KA), produced by the kidney, are extrinsic activators. There are three therapeutic activators that are used for treatment of thromboemboli: streptokinase, urokinase, and tissue-like plasminogen activator (t-PA). These drugs will induce a high degree of fibrin(ogen)-olysis.

Fibrinolysis mechanism. During formation of a clot, small amounts of plasminogen become bound to the fibrin and are incorporated into the fibrin clot. Plasminogen activator (t-PA) is released from surrounding endothelial cells as a result of various stimuli (such as thrombin). The t-PA has a high affinity for fibrin and thereby absorbs onto the fibrin clot and activates the plasminogen present to form plasmin. As the clot begins to dissolve the partially degraded fibrin binds additional plasminogen, which is activated to plasmin so that fibrinolysis continues.

Degradation of fibrin. Degradation of non-cross-linked fibrin produces almost the same degradation products as those formed from fibrinogen (Fig. 5–3). Degradation of cross-linked fibrin, however, is slower than that of fibrinogen (and non-crosslinked fibrin), and the products formed are different because of the bonding present in the cross-linked fibrin (Fig. 5–2). The smallest complex formed (DD/E) is composed of fragment DD (termed a *D-dimer*) and fragment E. Other complexes formed are YD/DY and YY/DXD. Further breakdown of these complexes may be prevented in-vivo by fibrinolytic inhibitors.

Inhibitors of fibrinolysis. The primary inhibitor of plasmin is α_2 *antiplasmin*. It is present in the plasma and also in platelets. Its inhibitory effect on free plasmin in the blood is very fast. However, plasmin is inactivated by this inhibitor relatively slowly when the plasmin is bound to fibrin. α_2 *Macroglobulin* is also an inactivator of plasmin. *Thrombospondin*, released by the platelets, inhibits activation of fibrin-bound plasminogen. There are also naturally occurring inhibitors to plasminogen activators: *plasminogen activator inhibitor-1 (PAI-1)* and *plasminogen activator inhibitor-2 (PAI-2)*. PAI-1 is secreted into the blood by the endothelial cells and is also present in platelets. It inactivates t-PA and urokinase. Antistreptokinase antibodies, when present, will inactivate therapeutic streptokinase.

Control of fibrinolysis. The fibrinolytic system must be regulated so that unwanted clots are dissolved but not broken down prematurely before bleeding has ceased and the healing process begun. Because of its location in the clot, plasmin is inaccessible to the α_2 antiplasmin. However, any plasmin that escapes from the clot into the plasma will be immediately neutralized by this inhibitor. PAI-1, stored in platelets in the area of the clot, may be released and thereby inhibit the action of t-PA, preventing premature lysis of the clot. Also, thrombospondin, released from platelets following stimulation by thrombin, inhibits activation of the fibrin-bound plasminogen.

Limiting Mechanisms of Hemostasis

Normally, blood does not clot as it circulates through the blood vessels. When injury occurs a platelet-fibrin plug is formed at the site of injury. As time passes, this clot is dissolved and replaced by regenerating tissue. The clot that is formed is normally present only for that period of time necessary because of the activity of several mechanisms: (1) The normal circulation of blood through the injured area not only acts as a transportation system to bring the necessary substances to the area for platelet and fibrin plug formation, but also serves as a means of diluting out and carrying away the active coagulants formed in the area. (2) Naturally occurring inhibitors to coagulation are present in the blood and serve to contain this process. (3) During clot formation, plasminogen is activated to degrade the formed clot (fibrinolysis).

Inhibitors of Coagulation

The surfaces of the endothelium and platelet are a major site of coagulation inhibition.

Protein C is a glycoprotein produced in the liver and is the major inhibitor of blood coagulation. Activated protein C is a strong anticoagulant and degrades factors Va and VIIIa and stimulates fibrinolysis by inactivating plasminogen activator inhibitors.

Protein S is also produced in the liver and serves as a cofactor for protein C. It is present in the plasma in a free form that represents approximately 40% of the total protein S. The remaining 60% is bound to the complement protein C4 binding protein (C4BP) and is not functionally active. The ratio of free to bound amounts may shift in disease states such as inflammation when the amount of free protein S decreases and the concentration of the bound form increases. Only the free protein S serves as a cofactor for protein C.

As thrombin is formed during coagulation, some binds to *thrombomodulin* on the endothelial surface. This modifies the action of thrombin to act more as an inhibitor than as an activator of the clotting mechanism by activating protein C. Once activated, protein C binds with protein S. This complex then degrades factors Va and VIIIa and binds with plasminogen activator inhibitors, rendering them ineffective. In this reaction, thrombomodulin greatly enhances the ability of thrombin to activate protein C.

Antithrombin III is also produced in the liver and is a major inhibitor of thrombin. By itself, it acts very slowly. Heparin binds to antithrombin III and greatly enhances the rate of activity. Heparan sulfate from blood vessel walls may be the in-vivo source of heparin for normal enhancement of antithrombin III. This complex also inhibits factors IXa, Xa, XIa, XIIa, kallikrein, and plasmin (fibrinolytic system).

Heparin cofactor II whose activity is greatly enhanced by heparin, also inhibits thrombin.

α_2-*Macroglobulin* forms a complex with thrombin, kallikrein, and plasmin, thus inhibiting their activities.

Extrinsic pathway inhibitor (EPI), also called *lipoprotein associated coagulation inhibitor (LACI)*, inhibits the VIIa-tissue factor complex.

C1-inhibitor is the principle inactivator of factor XIIa and plasma kallikrein. It also inhibits factor XIa and plasmin.

α_1 *Antitrypsin* is a weak inhibitor of thrombin and factors Xa and XIa.

Activated protein C inhibitor will inhibit the activity of protein C. Its action is greatly enhanced by the presence of heparin.

Primary Hemostasis

Platelets

Platelets play a central role in hemostasis.

Structure of the platelet. The outer surface of the platelet is called the *glycocalyx*. The plasma *membrane* contains 30 or more glycoproteins, of which some of the major ones are glycoproteins Ib, IIb/IIIa complex, I, IIa, and IV. *Microtubules* are located beneath the membrane and give the platelet its structural support. Between the membrane and the microtubules are contractile *microfilaments*, which are primarily composed of actin and myosin. There is an *canalicular system* that is open to the outside of the platelet. The *dense tubular system* is the site of arachidonic acid metabolism and provides small amounts of calcium to the resting platelet. Mitochondria, glycogen, α granules, dense bodies, lysosomes, and peroxisomes are all present within the platelet cytoplasm. The α *granules* contain platelet fibrinogen, factor V, von Willebrand factor, platelet factor 4, β thromboglobulin, platelet-derived growth factor, thrombospondin, fibronectin, and albumin, among other substances. *Dense bodies* are composed of ATP,

ADP, calcium, serotonin, and several other components. *Peroxisomes* have peroxidase activity.

When vascular injury occurs, platelets function in both primary hemostasis (platelet adhesion, secretion, aggregation) and in secondary hemostasis (coagulation). *(1) Platelet adhesion:* When vascular injury occurs platelets come in contact with the subendothelium (collagen, fibronectin) and adhere to portions of it. This is termed *platelet adhesiveness* and most likely occurs because of the presence of von Willebrand factor (vWf) (present in the plasma and subendothelium) being deposited on the injured tissues. The vWf binds to glycoprotein sites (Ib and IIb/IIIa complex) on the platelet membrane. *(2) Platelet secretion:* Following activation, the platelet undergoes a shape change most probably caused by contraction of the microtubules. The platelet changes from a disk-shape to a spherical shape with the extrusion of numerous pseudopods. At the same time, the platelet granules move to the center of the platelet and fuse with the open canalicular system connected to the outside of the platelet. In this way, the contents of the granules (ADP, serotonin, β thromboglobulin, platelet factor 4, vWf, platelet-derived growth factor, etc.) are extruded to the outside. *(3) Platelet aggregation:* Simultaneously with platelet release, platelet stimulating agents (collagen, ADP, epinephrine, thrombin) bind to the platelets, causing them to adhere to one another (*platelet aggregation*). Prostaglandins are produced by the activated platelet and will cause platelet aggregation and the platelet release reaction. Phospholipases in the platelet membrane will be activated by collagen and epinephrine, which, in turn, will hydrolyze the phospholipids in the membrane to release arachidonic acid. Cyclo-oxygenase (from the platelets) metabolizes arachidonic acid to form prostaglandin endoperoxides, which are converted to thromboxane A_2 (a vasoconstrictor and a platelet stimulator, causing platelet secretion and aggregation). Fibrinogen is necessary as a cofactor for platelet aggregation. The fibrinogen binding sites on the platelet surface are exposed when the platelet is stimulated in the presence of small amounts of calcium or magnesium. Several prostaglandins (PGD_2, PGI_2, and PGE_1) act as inhibitors to platelet function. They bind to receptors on the platelet surface and may function to limit the size of the hemostatic plug. *(4) Coagulation:* Platelets also play an important role in the production of the fibrin clot. Platelet factor 3 (PF3) (phospholipid) is available on the surface of the platelet, in addition to surface receptors for factors Va and Xa. This therefore makes possible the conversion of prothrombin to thrombin on the platelet surface. In addition, it is thought that platelets provide surface for the activation of factor X by factor IXa in the presence of factor VIII. Activated platelets may also assist in the activation of factors XII and XI. Clot retraction follows clot formation and requires activated platelets in the presence of calcium ions and factor XIII. It is thought that the activated platelets interact directly with the fibrin formed.

Endothelium

Blood vessels are lined by endothelial cells. When injury first occurs, contraction of the vessel walls takes place, reducing the blood flow through the injured area. What triggers vasoconstriction is poorly understood. Thromboxane A_2, produced and secreted by the platelets, is a strong vasoconstrictor. Activation of factor XII causes production of substances that result in smooth muscle contraction, and fibrinopeptide B (a component of fibrinogen that is released by the action of thrombin) also has these capabilities. Vasoconstrictors may also be produced and released by the injured tissue.

Normal, intact endothelium does not stimulate or support the activated platelet or contribute to the coagulation process. The intact endothelium will produce prostacyclin (prostaglandin I_2), which prevents platelet aggregation on normal uninjured vascular endothelium. It also has anticoagulant properties. Glycosaminoglycans on the surface of the endothelium speed up the inactivation of activated coagulation factors, whereas thrombomodulin, also located on the surface of the endothelium, binds excess thrombin. This complex, thrombin-thrombomodulin, activates protein C in the plasma. Healthy endothelial cells may also secrete von Willebrand factor and tissue plasminogen activator (t-PA) and inhibitor. However, when the endothelium is injured, it will secrete tissue factor, and will stimulate platelet adhesion and activation.

The endothelial cells assist in the activation of platelets, the limiting of the coagulation mechanism, and the dissolution of the clot.

COAGULATION SCREENING PROCEDURES

The detection and diagnosis of a hemostatic disorder should begin with a physical examination and a clinical history of the patient and his or her family. The drug/medication history is very important. If an abnormality is present, this will frequently yield a clue as to the type of disorder. Liver disease, renal failure, cancer, vitamin K deficiency, and alcoholism are some of the disorders in which hemostatic abnormalities may be present secondarily to the primary disease. Screening procedures should test the vasculature, platelets, coagulation mechanism, and fibrinolysis. The most valuable screening test is a comprehensive and careful clinical history.

An abnormality in primary hemostasis may present with easy bruisability and/or bleeding of the mucous membranes. A bleeding time should be performed, along with a platelet count and review of a peripheral blood smear for platelet morphology and estimate of numbers. Results of the bleeding time should be correlated with the platelet count. When these two test results do not agree (e.g., prolonged bleeding time, normal platelet count) von Willebrand's disease or other functional platelet disorders may be suspected and further appropriate testing (such as platelet aggregation studies) may then be performed.

Patients with factor deficiencies will usually exhibit bleeding from larger blood vessels. The prothrombin time (PT) is used to evaluate the extrinsic coagulation system, and when abnormal, indicates a defect in that pathway. The activated partial thromboplastin time (APTT) is sensitive to factor deficiencies in the intrinsic coagulation pathway. As a cautionary note, mild deficiencies may have a normal screening test. If there is a positive history, a normal PT or APTT does not rule out a deficiency. Also, a normal

bleeding time may be found in a mild case of von Willebrand's disease.

If a factor deficiency is suspected, it is important to perform a test for circulating anticoagulants in order to rule out the presence of an inhibitor. If this test is negative for an inhibitor, the APTT (or PT) substitution test may then be performed to identify the exact factor deficiency. A factor assay should be performed to determine the activity of the deficient factor. In the presence of a circulating anticoagulant (inhibitor) the prothrombin time and/or the activated partial thromboplastin time will be prolonged, depending on the specific factor inhibitor present. If there is a lupus inhibitor the activated partial thromboplastin time is more often abnormal. The thrombin time or quantitative fibrinogen (functional) tests for functional fibrinogen.

The presence of fibrinogen degradation products may be detected by use of the FDP test. The D-dimer procedure is performed for detection of the cross-linked fibrin degradation product (D-dimer). Circulating fibrin monomer-fibrinogen complexes may be detected using the ethanol gelation test. The euglobulin clot lysis procedure will test for fibrinolysis.

In summary, the routine screening procedures used to detect a coagulopathy are the platelet count, bleeding time, prothrombin time, activated partial thromboplastin time, and thrombin time (or quantitative fibrinogen). The tourniquet test may be used to test for vascular (capillary) integrity. Further studies are performed if any of these test results are abnormal. The exact tests to be performed will depend on which test result(s) (which portion of the hemostatic mechanism) was abnormal.

The prothrombin time is used to monitor oral anticoagulant therapy in patients with deep vein thrombosis or with a high risk of developing thrombosis. Heparin is frequently administered to hospitalized patients with thrombosis, and the dosage monitored by use of the activated partial thromboplastin time.

COAGULATION TESTING REQUIREMENTS

Coagulation specimens require special attention. Poor techniques used in collection, processing, or storage will cause misleading and inaccurate results.

Specimen Collection

1. A clean venipuncture is absolutely necessary. Any contamination of the blood with tissue fluid leads to incorrect results. (a) For routine coagulation procedures, the vacutainer blood collection system is adequate. When this system is used, the tube for coagulation studies should be the second or third tube filled. If only coagulation tests are ordered, a plain tube should be filled with 2 to 3 mL of blood first and then the coagulation tube filled. The first tube may then be discarded upon returning to the laboratory. (b) When obtaining a blood specimen for special coagulation procedures, a two-syringe technique may be applied using plastic syringes. Withdraw approximately 2 mL of blood into the first syringe. Quickly and carefully disconnect this syringe from the needle (leaving the needle in the patient's vein) and connect the second syringe to the needle. Proceed with the venipuncture, discarding the blood in the first syringe. (Prior to performing the two-syringe venipuncture, make certain the first syringe is easily removed from the needle but fits snugly enough so that blood will not leak out at the connection.) (c) Capillary specimens are generally not used for coagulation testing because of the difficulty in obtaining a blood specimen without trauma and free of tissue juice.
2. When phlebotomizing the patient it is important to release the tourniquet as soon as the blood enters the first tube (or the syringe, if used). When using vacutainer tubes care must be taken to allow the tube to fill until there is no vacuum remaining. The anticoagulant-to-blood ratio is important in coagulation studies. The tube must be filled to within $\pm 10\%$ of its expected volume. Greater or lesser amounts of blood will yield incorrect coagulation test results.
3. All test tubes used for coagulation studies should have a "noncontact" surface. That is, the inside surface of the tubes should not be of a material (such as glass or soda lime) that will react or activate the coagulation factors. Most vacutainer tubes for collecting coagulation studies have a siliconized surface.
4. The anticoagulant of choice for coagulation studies is 0.109 M sodium citrate (buffered or nonbuffered). Alternatively, 0.129 M sodium citrate may be used, but is not the recommended concentration. The ratio of blood to anticoagulant is 9 parts blood to 1 part sodium citrate. It is critical that the proper amount of blood ($\pm 10\%$) be added to the anticoagulant. The presence of a buffer in the anticoagulant maintains a more stable pH.
5. Blood specimens with a high hematocrit will contain less plasma in relation to the total volume of blood in the tube. As a result, when the blood has been centrifuged, the plasma fraction will contain an increased concentration of anticoagulant (sodium citrate). (The 0.5 mL of anticoagulant will be diluted with less plasma.) During testing, as calcium is added to the test mixture, it may combine with the excess anticoagulant present instead of being available for the coagulation reaction. Therefore, whenever a patient's hematocrit is 55% or higher the amount of sodium citrate in the collection tube should be decreased (or the amount of anticoagulant may be held constant, and the volume of blood collected increased). The following formula may be used to determine the proper amount of sodium citrate.

Amount of sodium citrate
$$= \frac{100 - \text{Hematocrit}}{595 - \text{Hematocrit}} \times \text{mL of whole blood used}$$

For example, when a patient has a hematocrit of 60%, 0.34 mL of 0.109 M sodium citrate should be placed in the tube and 4.5 mL of whole blood added. When altering the amount of anticoagulant (or specimen) the sample must be obtained using a syringe.

Specimen Processing

1. Each blood specimen should be checked for clots prior to testing. Because the tubes must be centrifuged with their tops on, the red cell layer may be checked for clots after the plasma has been removed. The presence of a clot irrespective of how small it is renders the specimen unacceptable for coagulation testing.
2. Unless otherwise noted, the coagulation

specimen should be centrifuged within 1 hour of obtaining the sample. It is desirable to complete testing within 2 to 4 hours, depending on the specific procedure.

3. All pipets, test tubes, and reaction cups which come in contact with the test plasma should have a "noncontact" surface (e.g., plastic, siliconized).

4. The plasma specimen should be in a stoppered container at all times, except when testing. This prevents loss of CO_2 and a resultant pH change of the plasma.

5. For most coagulation procedures, unless noted under specimen requirements, if the specimen will be tested within 2 hours of collection it may be kept at room temperature. If there is to be a delay beyond 2 hours it is advisable to keep the specimen on ice. Exceptions to this rule are specimens for prothrombin time, factor VII assay, and platelet function studies. These specimens should be maintained at room temperature. Factor VII may become activated by the cold. Also, plasma for the euglobulin clot lysis procedure must be tested or frozen within 30 minutes of collection.

6. With the exception of platelet function studies, plasma for coagulation testing should be platelet poor (plasma platelet count less than $15,000/\mu L$). Centrifugation for 15 minutes at $2500 \times g$ will routinely produce acceptable platelet-poor plasma. Use of commercially available serum-plasma separators (Sure-Sep, Organon Teknika, Durham, NC) produces excellent quality platelet-poor plasma acceptable for coagulation testing. In addition, several small table top high speed centrifuges are available for more rapid centrifugation of plasma samples. Platelet-poor plasma may be obtained using speeds of $13000 \times g$ for 2 minutes. These centrifuges cost less than $2000 and are excellent for rapid turnaround of test results when necessary.

7. An alternative method to crushed ice for keeping specimens cold is the commercially available Kryorack (Streck Laboratories, Inc., Omaha, Nebraska). This test tube holder contains an aqueous solution within a sealed unit (Fig. 5–4) and is available in various sizes. When placed at

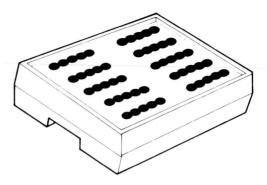

FIG. 5–4. Kryorack ice bath.

freezer temperatures ($-18°C$) for 8 hours, it maintains a temperature for the test tubes of less than $8°C$ for 8 hours at room temperature. The tubes do not come in contact with water or ice, affording a more convenient method of refrigerating plasma.

8. Hemolyzed plasma is indicative of a traumatic venipuncture and should not be used for coagulation studies. Results will not be dependable. Also, automated instruments may not be able to detect the end point on some lipemic or icteric plasma samples.

Plasma Storage

1. Platelet-poor plasma may be stored at $-40°C$ or lower for at least several weeks without loss of most factors. The plasma should initially be frozen (in covered plastic containers) very quickly using liquid nitrogen or temperatures at $-80°C$ to $-40°C$.

2. When thawing frozen plasma it should be done rapidly in a $37°C$ incubator or water bath. Remove the plasma from the incubator as soon as it is thawed. Plasma cannot be refrozen.

Coagulation Testing

1. Most coagulation studies are carried out at $37°C$. It should be noted that specimens incubated in dry heat take slightly longer to reach $37°C$ than those incubated in a water bath. It is essential, when required, that the specimens and reagents reach the

proper temperature of 37°C before proceeding with the test. Overheating or prolonged heating at 37°C, however, may lead to destruction of some of the coagulation factors and, therefore, a prolonged clotting time. The temperature of the incubator should not fluctuate more than ±0.5°C.

2. Accurate timing of clotting times is extremely important. Many of the procedures are timed to within one-tenth of a second, so that the initial starting and stopping of the stopwatch must be done precisely.

3. There are four general techniques in widespread use for reading the end point of clotting procedures. The *tilt tube* method requires gentle tilting of the tube back and forth at the rate of about once per second until a fibrin web is formed. The nichrome *wire loop* technique employs the use of a wire loop that is passed through the mixture at the rate of two sweeps per second until a formed clot adheres to the loop. (In these first two techniques, a light source without glare is important. A black background also facilitates the end point readings.) The third and fourth procedures employ the use of automation: a clot is detected either by use of a *moving probe* immersed in the mixture that is triggered by clot formation or by the change in *optical density* of the mixture when a clot forms.

4. The appearance of the clot formed frequently depends on its rate of formation. Normal, or only slightly prolonged clotting times show a pronounced clouding of the mixture that is easy to see with the human eye. Prolonged clotting times, however, form more slowly and may first appear as very fine fibrin threads. The mixture becomes cloudy (opaque) very slowly; it is often difficult to detect when final end point occurs. Automated coagulation analyzers based on optical density should be able to read this latter type of clot formation.

5. Historically, almost all coagulation procedures have been performed in duplicate and the two numbers averaged for a final result. This is time consuming and expensive. Because of more accurate and precise pipets and instrumentation now in use,

this double testing is becoming unnecessary. Each laboratory should check the accuracy and precision of their methods in an effort to change over to single sample testing. Alternatively, sample and reagent volumes may be reduced on some instrumentation so that duplicates may be performed using the same plasma/reagent volumes as for a single sample.

COAGULATION TIME OF WHOLE BLOOD

In the past, the Lee and White clotting time was used as a screening test to measure all stages in the intrinsic coagulation system and to monitor heparin therapy. It is, however, a time-consuming test, has poor reproducibility, is sensitive to only extreme factor deficiencies, and is insensitive to high doses of heparin. It is, therefore, of limited use in today's laboratory. Severe hemophilia, afibrinogenemia, and severe fibrinolytic states cause a prolonged clotting time, as do circulating anticoagulants (inhibitors), and heparin.

The normal range for the test described below is 5 to 15 minutes, but each laboratory should determine its own normal values.

Lee and White Method

Reference

Lee, R.I., and White, P.D.: A clinical study of the coagulation time of whole blood, Am. J. Med. Sci., *145*, 495, 1913.

Reagents and Equipment

1. Water bath, 37°C.
2. Glass test tubes, 13 × 100 mm.
3. Stopwatch.
4. Plastic syringe (10 mL) and 20-gauge needle.

Specimen

Fresh whole blood, 4 mL. A two-syringe technique is preferrable, drawing 1 to 2 mL of blood in the first syringe and discarding.

Principle

The coagulation time of whole blood is the length of time required for a measured amount of blood to clot under certain specified conditions.

Procedure

1. Label three 13 × 100 mm test tubes with the patient's name, and number them, #1, #2, and #3.
2. Perform a clean, untraumatic venipuncture using a 20-gauge needle and withdraw 4 mL of blood.
3. Remove the needle from the syringe, and carefully place 1 mL of blood in test tube #3, 1 mL in tube #2, and 1 mL in tube #1. The last 1 mL of blood may be discarded. Start the stopwatch as soon as the blood is placed in tube #3.
4. Place the three test tubes in a 37°C water bath.
5. At exactly 5 minutes, tilt test tube #1 gently to a 45° angle. Repeat this procedure every 30 seconds, until the test tube can be completely inverted without spilling the contents (that is, until the blood is completely clotted).
6. Record the time it took the blood in test tube #1 to clot.
7. Thirty seconds after the blood in test tube #1 is clotted, proceed with tube #2, and repeat the preceding procedure, tilting the test tube every 30 seconds, until a clot is formed. Record the results. Repeat this procedure for test tube #3.
8. Since agitation and handling speed up coagulation, the clotting time of test tube #3 is the reported result.

Discussion

1. The activated clotting time test uses 2 mL of whole blood placed in a gray stoppered B-D vacutainer tube containing diatomaceous earth. (Blood should be drawn using the two-syringe technique.) The procedure is carried out at 37°C and the tube tilted after the first minute, and, thereafter at 5 to 10 second intervals until the clot forms. Using this procedure coagulation is normally complete in less than 101 seconds.

2. Poor venipuncture technique, causing hemolysis or tissue thromboplastin to mix with the blood, shortens the clotting time.
3. Bubbles entering the syringe when the blood sample is being obtained increase the rate of coagulation. Unnecessary agitation of the blood shortens the coagulation time.
4. Always tilt the tube in the same direction and at the same angle so that the blood is moving in the same pathway up the side of the tube each time.
5. At the completion of the clotting time, one tube should remain in the 37°C water bath to be checked after 2 and 4 hours for clot retraction. Also, this same tube may be allowed to remain in the water bath overnight and checked the next day for clot lysis.

PROTHROMBIN TIME

The prothrombin time (PT) is a useful screening procedure for the extrinsic coagulation mechanism including the common pathway (detects deficiencies in factors II, V, VII, and X). The PT will also be prolonged when the fibrinogen concentration is less than 80 mg/dL and in cases of dysfibrinogenemia. As a general rule, only a 30% concentration of factors V, VII, and X are needed for a normal PT. This test is least sensitive to deficiencies in factor II. The PT is frequently used to follow the course of oral anticoagulant therapy. Factors II, VII, IX, and X are inhibited by oral anticoagulants, with factor VII showing decreased activity first. Common causes of a prolonged prothrombin time are vitamin K deficiency, certain liver diseases, specific coagulation deficiencies, disseminated intravascular coagulation, circulating anticoagulants, presence of fibrin(ogen) split products, some dysproteinemias, and oral anticoagulant therapy.

The normal prothrombin time is in the range of 10 to 12 seconds. These values, however, differ according to the method and reagents (and reagent lot numbers) used in the performance of the test and must be determined by each laboratory.

International Normalized Ratio (INR). When patients are receiving oral anticoagulants, the ratio of the patient's prothrombin time to that of the normal control is useful in monitoring this therapy. However, different thromboplastins will not have the same sensitivity. The prothrombin time ratio will therefore be affected by the reagent used and the method of clot detection. As a result, the World Health Organization (WHO) with the International Commission on Standardization in Hematology and the International Committee on Thrombosis and Hemostasis devised a method of monitoring patients on oral anticoagulants using the International Normalized Ratio (INR). An international reference thromboplastin reagent has been developed for use in standardizing the prothrombin time ratio. Manufacturers of thromboplastin calibrate each lot number of their reagent against the standard WHO thromboplastin reagent. The results of this calibration are used to develop the *International Sensitivity Index (ISI)* for each batch of reagent. This number then allows the calculation of the INR, which is defined as the prothrombin time ratio had the test been performed using the international standard thromboplastin reagent.

$$INR = \left(\frac{\text{Patient's prothrombin time}}{\text{Mean PT of the normal range}}\right)^{ISI}$$

With the INR it is possible to obtain more consistent and meaningful results on patients receiving anticoagulant therapy. Using the INR should decrease or eliminate the differences seen between laboratories (between thromboplastin reagents). For example, if the same plasma sample was tested in laboratory A and laboratory B, two different results may be obtained, which should calculate out to similar INRs:

	Lab. A	Lab. B
Prothrombin Time	17.0 sec.	27.0 sec.
Mean of normal range	10.0 sec.	12.0 sec.
Reagent ISI	1.9	1.2
Calculated INR	2.7	2.7

The ISI for each thromboplastin is published by the manufacturer. A table is usually included for looking up the INR (using the prothrombin time ratio and the ISI). Alternatively, most hand-held calculators can quickly formulate this result.

References

Quick, A.J.: *Bleeding Problems in Clinical Medicine*, Philadelphia, W.B. Saunders Co., 1970.

Organon Teknika Corp.: International Normalized Ratio (INR), pkg. insert, Organon Teknika, Durham, NC, 1989.

Reagents and Equipment

1. Water bath, 37°C.
2. Thromboplastin-calcium chloride reagent. Keep refrigerated when not in use.
3. Normal and abnormal plasma controls.
4. Test tubes, 13 × 100 mm.
5. Stopwatch.

Specimen

Citrated plasma: 1 part 0.109 M sodium citrate to 9 parts whole blood. Testing should be performed within 2 hours after specimen is drawn when the plasma is maintained at room temperature and within 2 to 5 days when the plasma is stored at −20°C.

Principle

The calcium in whole blood is bound by sodium citrate, thus preventing coagulation. Tissue thromboplastin, to which calcium has been added, is mixed with the plasma, and the clotting time is noted. (Factor VII reacts with the tissue factor [thromboplastin] in the presence of calcium ions to activate factor X. The coagulation mechanism continues from there.)

Procedure

1. Centrifuge specimen as soon as possible after blood collection to obtain platelet-poor plasma.
2. Testing should proceed immediately, or cap the centrifuged or plasma tube and complete the procedure within 2 hours.
3. Pipet 0.2 mL of thromboplastin-calcium reagent into the appropriate number of 13 × 100 mm test tubes. Warm the test tubes in the water bath for at least 1 minute, until they have reached 37°C. The incubation period for this mixture is not critical once it reaches 37°C.
4. Incubate the plasma for 2 to 3 minutes,

until it reaches 37°C. Plasma should be incubated for no longer than 5 minutes after reaching 37°C.

5. Forcibly pipet 0.1 mL of patient's plasma into the test tube containing 0.2 mL of thromboplastin-calcium mixture and simultaneously start the stopwatch.

6. Mix the contents of the tube, remove the tube from the water bath, and wipe dry. Gently tilt the tube back and forth until a clot forms, at which point the timing is stopped.

7. Each test and control plasma should be performed in duplicate when manual methods are used. The results should agree with each other within ± 0.5 seconds when the prothrombin time is below 30 seconds. Duplicate tests on a prothrombin time above 30 seconds should agree within 2 to 4 seconds, depending on the degree of prolongation.

8. Average the two clotting times and report the patient's results along with the normal range for the test as performed in your laboratory.

Discussion

1. The prothrombin time may also be performed by automated procedures using mechanical or optical density methods of clot detection.

2. A control plasma should be run with each batch of tests performed. A normal and an abnormal plasma control must be run each time a new lot number of thromboplastin-calcium mixture is opened and at least once per day. The abnormal control should be in the same range as the majority of patients on oral anticoagulant therapy.

3. When preparing reagents and controls careful attention must be paid to the methods of reconstitution and use. Manufacturer's directions should be strictly adhered to.

4. Patients receiving oral anticoagulants for thromboembolic disorders generally have prothrombin times that yield an INR of 2.0 to 2.5. In certain conditions this ratio may be increased to as high as 4.5.

5. Normal plasma control values must fall within the laboratory's normal range. If the control results fall outside of this

range, results must not be reported. Usually, fresh reagents will need to be prepared. The plasmas must be retested when the problem has been resolved. If retesting cannot be performed within the 2-hour time period, the plasma samples should be frozen.

ACTIVATED PARTIAL THROMBOPLASTIN TIME

The activated partial thromboplastin time (APTT) is a most useful procedure for routine screening of coagulation disorders in the intrinsic system, for detecting the presence of circulating anticoagulants (inhibitors), and for monitoring heparin therapy. It measures those factors present in the intrinsic coagulation mechanism except for platelets and factor XIII. (Factor VII is not measured because it is in the extrinsic system.) It is somewhat insensitive to decreases in fibrinogen in which only levels of 60 to 80 mg/dL or lower will cause a prolonged APTT.

The normal range for the APTT may vary widely from one laboratory to another and depends on the reagents used and the clot detection method employed. It is, therefore, important that each laboratory determine its own normal range for the specific instrumentation and type and lot number of reagents used. The normal mean value for the APTT will generally fall between 25 and 35 seconds.

Reference

Organon Teknika Corp.: Automated APTT, pkg. insert, Organon Teknika, Durham, NC, 1990.

Reagents and Equipment

1. Water bath, 37°C.
2. Calcium chloride, 0.025 M.
3. Partial thromboplastin containing an activator.
4. Normal and abnormal control plasmas.
5. Test tubes, 13 × 100 mm.
6. Stopwatch.
7. Ice bath.

Specimen

Citrated plasma: 1 part 0.109 M sodium citrate to 9 parts whole blood.

Principle

The calcium in whole blood is bound by the sodium citrate anticoagulant to prevent coagulation. The plasma, after centrifugation, contains all intrinsic coagulation factors except calcium and platelets. Calcium, a phospholipid substitute for platelets (partial thromboplastin), and an activator (to ensure maximal activation), are added to the plasma. The time required for the plasma to clot is the activated partial thromboplastin time.

Procedure

1. Centrifuge specimen as soon as possible after collection to obtain platelet poor plasma.
2. Incubate a sufficient amount of 0.025 M calcium chloride at 37°C.
3. Pipet 0.2 mL of control plasma (or patient's plasma) into a 13 × 100 mm test tube.
4. Pipet 0.2 mL of partial thromboplastin (containing activator) into the test tube containing the control (or patient's) plasma.
5. Mix the contents of the tube quickly and place in a 37°C water bath for 5 minutes.
6. After exactly 5 minutes, forcibly pipet 0.2 mL of prewarmed calcium chloride into the tube, and simultaneously start stopwatch.
7. Mix the test tube immediately after adding calcium chloride. Allow the test tube to remain in the water bath while gently tilting the tube every 5 seconds. At the end of 20 seconds, remove the test tube from the water bath. Quickly wipe off the outside of test tube with a clean gauze so that the contents of the tube can be clearly seen.
8. Gently tilt the test tube back and forth until a clot forms, at which point the timing is stopped.
9. When manual testing is performed, control and patient plasma specimens should be run in duplicate, and the results averaged to obtain the final report. The two results should check within ± 1.5 seconds of each other when the APTT is less than 45 seconds, within 5 seconds when the results are between 50 and 100 seconds, and within 8 to 10 seconds when

the APTT is above 100 seconds. If formation of the clot has not started by the end of 2 minutes, the test may be stopped and the results reported as greater than 2 minutes.
10. Report the patient results in seconds along with the normal range for the test as determined for your laboratory. (Normal control results must always fall within the normal range, otherwise, there is a problem with reagents, equipment, or the technique being used, and the entire test must be repeated.)

Discussion

1. When the APTT is abnormally prolonged, there may be a deficiency in one of the coagulation factors or an inhibitor (circulating anticoagulant) present. To differentiate between these two abnormal states, the test for circulating anticoagulants may be performed to determine if the abnormal APTT is due to an inhibitor or to a factor deficiency. The sensitivity of the APTT to factor deficiencies and inhibitors (including the lupus anticoagulant) depends on the APTT reagent used.
2. The partial thromboplastin time (PTT) is performed in exactly the same manner as the APTT except that an activator is not included in the thromboplastin reagent. Normal results for the PTT are in the range of 40 to 100 seconds, with a result of 120 seconds or longer being considered abnormal. The activator in the APTT allows for maximum activation of the contact factors and gives more consistent and reproducible results.
3. The PTT and APTT are much more sensitive to coagulation factor deficiencies than is the whole blood clotting time.
4. If there are sufficient stopwatches available, it is possible to do more than one test at a time by starting each of the 5 minute incubations at 3-minute intervals.
5. Incubation of the plasma at 37°C for more than 5 minutes may cause a decrease in factors V and VIII, and therefore, invalidly prolonged clotting times.
6. An abnormally shortened APTT may be caused by partial clotting of the blood as a result of a traumatic venipuncture, high

levels of factor VIII, disseminated intravascular coagulation, or the presence of platelets in the plasma.

7. A control plasma should be run with each group of tests performed. In addition, a normal and an abnormal plasma control should be run each time a new lot number of reagent is used and at least once per shift. The abnormal control should be in the same range in which heparinized patients are being monitored.

PLASMA RECALCIFICATION TIME
(Plasma Clotting Time)

The plasma recalcification time is a measure of the intrinsic coagulation mechanism. In the procedure outlined here, a deficiency in platelets or platelet activity is not detected. A decrease in any of the clotting factors present in the intrinsic system will cause a prolonged clotting time.

The normal plasma recalcification time on platelet poor plasma is in the range of 90 to 250 seconds and should be determined by each laboratory.

Reference

Sirridge, M.S., and Shannon, R.: *Laboratory Evaluation of Hemostasis and Thrombosis,* 3rd Ed. Philadelphia, Lea & Febiger, 1983.

Reagents and Equipment

1. Water bath, 37°C.
2. Calcium chloride, 0.025 M.
3. Test tubes, 13 × 100 mm.
4. Stopwatch.
5. Pipets, 0.2 mL.

Specimen

Citrated plasma: 1 part of 0.109 M sodium citrate to 9 parts whole blood. Obtain blood for use as a normal control at the same time the patient's specimen is obtained.

Principle

Calcium chloride (to replace the calcium bound by the anticoagulant) is added to platelet-poor plasma and the clotting time determined.

Procedure

1. Immediately after collection, centrifuge blood to obtain platelet poor plasma.
2. Prewarm calcium chloride and each test plasma to a temperature of 37°C.
3. Place four 13 × 100 mm test tubes into the 37°C water bath (two tubes for each patient and control).
4. Pipet 0.2 mL of patient's plasma into the first tube. Add 0.2 mL of calcium chloride and simultaneously start a stopwatch. Gently mix the tube.
5. Allow the tube to remain in the 37°C water bath for 90 seconds, gently tilting the test tube every 30 seconds.
6. After 90 seconds, remove the test tube from the water bath and gently tilt at a rate of once per second. Stop the watch as soon as a clot forms, and record the results.
7. Repeat steps 4, 5, and 6 for each patient and control. It is recommended that all testing be performed in duplicate and the results averaged.

Discussion

1. The plasma recalcification time varies according to the number of platelets present in the plasma. As the number of platelets increases, the plasma recalcification time shortens. It is therefore important to centrifuge the blood in the prescribed manner.
2. The plasma recalcification time may be performed on platelet rich plasma, in which case the normal range is about 90 to 160 seconds.
3. A modification of the plasma clotting time is called the *activated recalcification time* and employs the use of 0.1 mL of platelet rich plasma, 0.1 mL of 0.025 M calcium chloride, and 0.1 mL of 1% Celite as an activator. The normal clotting time by this procedure is less than 50 seconds.

STYPVEN TIME
(Russell's Viper Venom Time)

The Stypven time is used to detect deficiencies in prothrombin, fibrinogen, and factors V and X. It differs from the prothrombin time in that deficiencies in factor VII are not detected.

The normal Stypven time is usually in the range of 6 to 10 seconds when performed by the following procedure. Each laboratory, however, should determine its own normal range.

References

Wellcome Research Laboratories: Russell Viper Venom, pkg. insert, Beckenham, England, Wellcome Research Laboratories, 1977.

Triplett, D.A., Harms, C.S.: *Procedures for the Coagulation Laboratory,* Chicago, American Society of Clinical Pathologists, 1981.

Reagents and Equipment

1. Russell viper venom. (Obtainable from Burroughs Wellcome Co., Research Triangle Park, NC.) Reconstitute with 2.0 mL of sodium chloride, 0.85% (w/v). Reagent may be used for 1 week after reconstitution if stored in the refrigerator.
2. Platelin. (Obtainable from Organon Teknika Corp., Durham, NC.) Reconstitute according to directions on vial. Reagent may be used for 1 week after reconstitution when stored in the refrigerator.
3. Calcium chloride, 0.025 M.
4. Water bath, 37°C.
5. Normal control plasma.
6. Test tubes, 12 × 75 mm.
7. Pipets, 0.1 mL.
8. Stopwatch.

Specimen

Citrated plasma: 1 part 0.109 M sodium citrate to 9 parts whole blood. Testing should be performed within 2 hours of blood collection. If this is not possible, refrigerate plasma and test within 4 hours or freeze plasma at −20°C if testing is to be performed after 4 hours.

Principle

Russell viper venom (Stypven) is a thromboplastin-like substance that activates factor X. When this reagent is added to plasma, together with platelets (Platelin) and calcium chloride, the coagulation process is begun at the point of factor X activation, with subsequent conversion of prothrombin to thrombin and fibrinogen to fibrin. In this way, deficiencies in factors V, X, prothrombin, and fibrinogen may be detected.

Procedure

1. Centrifuge specimen as soon as possible after collection to obtain platelet poor plasma.
2. Warm the Stypven reagent to 37°C.
3. Combine equal volumes of Platelin and calcium chloride and prewarm to 37°C.
4. Into a 12 × 75 mm test tube in the 37°C water bath, pipet 0.1 mL of patient's plasma and 0.1 mL of Stypven reagent. Mix and allow the tube to incubate for 30 seconds.
5. At the end of 30 seconds, add 0.1 mL of prewarmed Platelin-calcium chloride mixture to the tube and simultaneously start a stopwatch.
6. Record the clotting time.
7. Each patient and control sample should be tested in the above manner in duplicate.

Discussion

1. If the prothrombin time is normal, the Stypven time need not be performed.
2. In a factor VII deficiency, the prothrombin time would be prolonged and the Stypven time normal.
3. The above procedure may also be used to assay for factors V and X: Prepare dilutions of the reference, control, and patient plasmas as outlined in the Factor VII Assay procedure. Perform the Stypven time on each dilution. Draw the reference curve and calculate the control and patient results as outlined for the Factor VII Assay. The Stypven time is sensitive to factors V and X and generally gives reproducible results using this procedure.

REPTILASE TIME

Reptilase is an enzyme found in the venom of the Bothrops atrox snake. It is capable of converting fibrinogen to fibrin and is unaffected by heparin. This procedure is, therefore, helpful in testing for functional fibrinogen when the thrombin time is prolonged because of heparin. Both the thrombin and Reptilase times will be prolonged when the fibrinogen level is decreased, in dysfibrinogenemia, during streptokinase therapy, and in the presence of fibrin(ogen) degradation products.

The normal range for the test outlined below is approximately 10 to 15 seconds, but should be determined for each laboratory.

References

Sigma Diagnostics: Atroxin® (Bothrops atrox venom) Determination of Plasma Clotting Time, pkg. insert, St. Louis, Sigma Diagnostics, 1989.

Funk, C., Gmür, J., Herold, R., and Straub, P.W.: Reptilase®-R—A new reagent in blood coagulation, Br. J. Haem., *21*, 43, 1971.

Reagents and Equipment

1. Atroxin® (buffered Bothrops atrox venom). (Available from Sigma Diagnostics, St. Louis, MO.) Reconstitute with 1.0 mL of distilled water. Mix by swirling. Do not shake. Stable in the refrigerator for 1 month after reconstitution.
2. Plastic test tubes, 12 × 75 mm.
3. Pipets, 0.2 mL and 0.1 mL.
4. Water bath, 37°C.
5. Ice bath.
6. Stopwatch.

Specimen

Citrated plasma: 1 part 0.109 M sodium citrate to 9 parts whole blood. Testing should be performed within 4 hours of collection. If this is not possible freeze specimen at −20°C.

Principle

When Atroxin® (Reptilase) is added to plasma, it acts by releasing fibrinopeptide A from the fibrinogen molecule. The resultant monomers polymerize end-to-end, forming a clot.

Procedure

1. Centrifuge specimen to obtain platelet-poor plasma.
2. Incubate a sufficient amount of Atroxin® (0.1 mL per test) at 37°C.
3. Pipet 0.2 mL of patient plasma (or control) into a 12 × 75 mm test tube and incubate for 2 to 3 minutes (until the specimen reaches 37°C).
4. Add 0.1 mL of Atroxin® to the tube containing the prewarmed plasma and simultaneously start a stopwatch.
5. Mix the contents of the tube and record the clotting time. Test the duplicate in the same manner.
6. Repeat steps 3, 4, and 5 above for each specimen and control.
7. Duplicate clotting times should agree within ±10%. If they do not, repeat test. Average results and report.

THROMBIN TIME

The thrombin time measures the availability of functional fibrinogen. Prolonged thrombin times are found when the fibrinogen level is below 75 to 100 mg/dL, when the function of fibrinogen is impaired, and in the presence of heparin, fibrin(ogen) degradation products, and thrombolytic agents (such as streptokinase). The thrombin time is a sensitive test in detecting heparin inhibition. It may be normally prolonged in the newborn and in multiple myeloma (the abnormal globulin interferes with the polymerization of fibrin).

The normal range for the thrombin time depends on the concentration of thrombin, and the ionic strength of the thrombin diluent. The normal thrombin time for the procedure described below is between 10 and 14 seconds, but must be determined by each laboratory.

References

Organon Teknika Corp.: Thromboquick™ thrombin reagent, pkg. insert, Organon Teknika Corp., Durham, NC, 1990.

Harrison, R.L., and Birotte, R.: The thrombin clotting time, Am. J. Clin. Pathol., *89*, 81, 1988.

Reagents and Equipment

1. Purified water.
2. Thromboquick™ thrombin reagent (Organon Teknika Corp.) contains 3 to 4 units of thrombin per mL, buffer, calcium chloride, and stabilizers. Reconstitute with 3.0

mL of purified water. Mix gently. Once reconstituted, it may be stored at 2 to 8°C for 2 weeks.

3. Normal and abnormal control plasmas.
4. Water bath, 37°C.
5. Nichrome wire loop.
6. Stopwatch.
7. Plastic test tubes, 13 × 100 mm.

Specimen

Citrated plasma: 1 part 0.109 M sodium citrate to 9 parts whole blood. Specimen should be stored at 2 to 8°C as soon as collected, and the test performed within 4 hours. The platelet poor plasma may be frozen (quickly at −20°C or lower). (Prior to testing, rapidly thaw plasma to prevent protein denaturation.)

Principle

A measured amount of thrombin is added to plasma. The length of time for a fibrin clot to form is recorded as the thrombin time.

Procedure

1. Centrifuge blood to obtain platelet-poor plasma.
2. Incubate a sufficient amount of thrombin reagent at 37°C (0.4 mL/patient or control). Testing should be performed in duplicate.
3. Place 0.2 mL of patient's plasma or normal control into a 13 × 100 mm test tube in the water bath and warm to 37°C.
4. Add 0.2 mL of thrombin reagent to the test plasma, simultaneously starting the stopwatch.
5. With a nichrome wire loop, sweep through the mixture, two times per second, until a clot is formed. Stop the watch and record the thrombin time.
6. Run a normal control with each series of thrombin times. Duplicate tests performed on the same plasma sample should check within ±1.5 seconds of each other. Report the average of the two results.

Discussion

1. Whenever thrombin is used, plastic or siliconized glassware and pipets should be employed for testing.

2. This test may be adapted to clot detection instruments.
3. Lipemic, hemolyzed, or icteric plasma may be tested by the previously described procedure without the results being affected. If photo-optical instruments are used for clot detection, results may be affected, however.

PREKALLIKREIN (FLETCHER FACTOR) SCREENING TEST

A deficiency of prekallikrein may be detected using a modification of the activated partial thromboplastin time (APTT).

Reference

Hattersley, P.G., and Hayse, D.: The effect of increased contact activation time on the activated partial thromboplastin time, Am. J. Clin. Path., *66*, 479, 1976.

Reagents and Equipment

1. Water bath, 37°C.
2. Calcium chloride, 0.025 M.
3. Activated partial thromboplastin (APTT) reagent, containing kaolin, silica, or celite as the activator. Ellagic acid should not be used as an activator because it does not correct the APTT in a prekallikrein deficiency.
4. Normal control plasma.
5. Test tubes, 12 × 75 mm.
6. Stopwatch.

Specimen

Citrated plasma: 1 part 0.109 M sodium citrate to 9 parts whole blood. Immediately after blood collection, place the tube of blood in a cup of crushed ice and deliver to the laboratory.

Principle

Patients with a Fletcher factor deficiency will have a prolonged APTT. If the plasma + APTT reagent mixture is incubated for 10 minutes (instead of the routine 3 or 5 minutes) the prolonged APTT will be shortened to normal, or almost normal, if the deficiency is due to Fletcher factor.

Procedure

1. Centrifuge the specimen as soon as possible after collection to obtain platelet-poor plasma. Remove the plasma from the cells and proceed with testing.
2. Perform an APTT on the patient and normal control plasma specimens. If the patient results are normal, a prekallikrein deficiency is not considered to be present. If the patient results are prolonged, proceed with step 3.
3. Perform an APTT on the patient and normal control plasma specimens, incubating the plasma + APTT reagent mixture for 10 minutes (instead of the usual 3 or 5 minutes). Add calcium chloride and determine the clotting time.
4. Interpretation of results. The APTT performed in step 3 (10 minute incubation) should correct to a normal, or almost normal, clotting time in the presence of a prekallikrein deficiency. If the APTT is not corrected by the increased incubation time, a problem other than a prekallikrein deficiency is assumed to be present. The normal plasma control should remain within or near the normal range with the 10 minute incubation period.

Discussion

1. Normal clotting occurs with concentrations of prekallikrein of 1.5 to 2.0% and above.
2. To confirm a prekallikrein deficiency, an APTT may be performed on a 1:1 dilution of patient's plasma with prekallikrein deficient substrate. The APTT should not correct using this substrate. If it does correct, a prekallikrein deficiency does not exist.

FACTOR XIII SCREENING TEST

Factor XIII, known as the fibrin stabilizing factor, is responsible for converting the fibrin clot to a more stable form. It is thought to exist in the plasma in an inactive state and is activated by thrombin during the fibrinogen-to-fibrin conversion. Activated factor XIII causes the formation of covalent bonds between the fibrin monomers, thus stabilizing the fibrin polymer. When factor XIII is present, the fibrin clot formed is insoluble in 5 M urea and 1% monochloroacetic acid when left standing for 24 hours. A deficiency in this factor is rare. Generally, a 1% level of factor XIII is sufficient to make a clot insoluble in 5 M urea.

Reference

Losowsky, M.S., Hall, R., and Goldie, W.: Congenital deficiency of fibrin-stabilising factor, Lancet, 2, 156, 1965.

Reagents and Equipment

1. Urea, 5.0 M.
   Urea, 30 g
   Dissolve urea and dilute to 100 mL with distilled water. Stable at room temperature for several months.
2. Calcium chloride, 0.025 M.
3. Normal control plasma.
4. Test tubes, 13 × 100 mm.
5. Pipets, 0.2 and 5.0 mL.
6. Water bath, 37°C.

Specimen

Citrated plasma: 1 part 0.109 M sodium citrate to 9 parts whole blood.

Principle

The patient's plasma is clotted by the addition of calcium chloride. Urea (5 M) is added to the clot. If factor XIII is absent in the patient's plasma, the clot is dissolved in less than 24 hours by the urea.

Procedure

1. Centrifuge the specimen as soon as possible after collection to obtain platelet-poor plasma.
2. Label two tubes for each patient and control.
3. Pipet 0.2 mL of patient's plasma into each of two test tubes. Repeat, pipetting 0.2 mL of normal control plasma into each of two additional test tubes.
4. Add 0.2 mL of 0.025 M calcium chloride to each tube. Mix. A clot should form in each tube.

5. Incubate the fibrin clots at 37°C for 30 minutes.
6. Loosen the clots from the sides of the test tubes by gently tapping the tube.
7. Transfer one of the patient's clots and one of the normal control clots to respectively labeled test tubes containing 5 mL of 5 M urea. To a third tube labeled 'patient/control', and containing 5 mL of 5 M urea, transfer both the remaining patient clot and the normal control clot.
8. Allow all tubes to incubate at room temperature for the next 24 hours. Examine the tubes at 1, 2, 3, and 24 hours and note if the clots have dissolved.
9. Report the length of time it took for the patient's clot to dissolve after urea was added. If the clot is still present at the end of 24 hours, report that the clot was insoluble after 24 hours.
10. If the patient's clot dissolves within the 24-hour period, this is indicative of a factor XIII level of less than 1 to 2%. In this instance, the patient/control clot should not dissolve. If this clot does dissolve, this may indicate the presence of a fibrinolytic process rather than a factor XIII deficiency.

Discussion

1. As an alternate procedure, 2% acetic acid or 1% monochloroacetic acid may be used in place of 5 M urea. These reagents may, however, give an occasional false result.
2. A positive control (a clot that will dissolve in 5 M urea) may also be tested along with the patient, using thrombin and EDTA plasma: Add 10 NIH units of thrombin (0.5 mL of 20 NIH units/mL of thrombin) to 0.5 mL of EDTA plasma. Place the resultant clot in 5 mL of 5 M urea. This clot should be dissolved within 24 hours, due to the lack of calcium which is necessary for the action of factor XIII.

FACTOR IDENTIFICATION (PT AND APTT SUBSTITUTION TEST)

A specific factor deficiency may be identified by mixing correction reagents with a patient's plasma and then performing the prothrombin time (PT) and/or the activated partial thromboplastin time (APTT).

References

Baxter Healthcare Corp.: Dade® adsorbed plasma and serum reagents, pkg. insert, Dade Division, Miami, FL, 1988.

Proctor, R.R., and Rapaport, S.I.: The partial thromboplastin time with kaolin, Am. J. Clin. Path., *36*, 212, 1961.

Reagents and Equipment

1. Water bath, 37°C.
2. Reagents for the APTT.
   a. Calcium chloride, 0.025 M.
   b. Partial thromboplastin with activator.
3. Reagent for the PT.
   a. Tissue thromboplastin reagent.
4. Normal control plasma.
5. Sodium chloride, 0.85% (w/v).
6. Test tubes, 12 × 75 mm.
7. Pipets, 1.0, 0.1, and 0.2 mL.
8. Stopwatch.
9. Adsorbed plasma (rich in factors V, VIII, XI, and XII). Obtainable commercially.
10. Aged serum (rich in factors VII, IX, X, XI, and XII). Obtainable commercially.

Specimen

Citrated plasma: 1 part 0.109 M sodium citrate to 9 parts whole blood.

Principle

An APTT and/or a PT is performed on the patient's plasma diluted 1:1 with:

1. Adsorbed plasma (factors V, VIII, XI, and XII).
2. Aged serum (Factors VII, IX, X, XI, and XII).
3. Sodium chloride, 0.85%.
4. Normal control plasma.

The patient's undiluted plasma is also tested in the same manner. The specific coagulation defect may be detected by noting which reagent, adsorbed plasma, or aged serum corrects the APTT and/or the PT.

Procedure

1. Centrifuge the specimen as soon as possible after collection to obtain platelet-poor plasma.

2. Remove the plasma from the cells, place in a tube and cap. Complete the following procedure within 2 hours of specimen collection.

3. Perform the substitution test on the procedure (PT and/or APTT) that gave abnormal results. (The test for circulating anticoagulants should have been previously performed to rule out the presence of an inhibitor.)

4. Reconstitute the aged serum and adsorbed plasma according to manufacturer's directions. Keep these reagents in crushed ice.

5. Perform an APTT and/or PT, in duplicate, on the following mixtures:
   a. 0.1 mL patient plasma + 0.1 mL adsorbed plasma.
   b. 0.1 mL patient plasma + 0.1 mL aged serum.
   c. 0.1 mL patient plasma + 0.1 mL normal control plasma.
   d. 0.1 mL patient plasma + 0.1 mL 0.85% sodium chloride.

6. Average results and record.

7. For interpretation of results, see Table 5–3.

Discussion

1. If a factor deficiency is noted, the PT or APTT may be performed, using the specific factor-deficient plasma indicated, in a 1:1 dilution with the patient's plasma. The factor deficient plasma unable to correct the PT/APTT is a further check as to the exact coagulation deficiency. When the deficient factor(s) has been positively identified, appropriate specific factor assays should then be performed.

2. In order for the patient's PT or APTT to be considered as corrected, the difference between the original (uncorrected) result and the result obtained with the adsorbed plasma or aged serum, should be 90% or greater than the difference between the original (uncorrected) result and the established upper limit of normal for the PT and/or APTT. The corrected results will not necessarily be within the normal range (because the plasma containing the factor has been diluted with the patient's factor deficient plasma). The specimen diluted with sodium chloride will give an example of uncorrected test results.

3. A factor identification may be difficult to determine in cases of a mild deficiency, since this is a qualitative test and a significant correction (by adsorbed plasma or aged serum) is needed for interpretation of the results.

4. Adsorbed plasma and aged serum reagents are used for qualitative identification of single factor deficiencies. Multiple factor deficiencies may be identified using 1:1 dilutions of the patient's plasma and a battery of specific factor deficient plasmas.

QUANTITATIVE FIBRINOGEN

Decreased concentrations of fibrinogen will be found in congenital afibrinogenemia and hypofibrinogenemia. In dysfibrinogenemia there may be adequate amounts of fibrinogen present, but it does not function correctly. As a result, tests for functional (clottable) fibrinogen will be decreased. Acquired deficiencies of fibrinogen occur in disseminated intravascular coagulation, systemic fibrinolysis, pancreatitis, and severe liver disease. Abnormally high levels of some proteins may interfere with polymerization of the fibrin monomers and therefore give erroneous results. Elevated fibrinogen levels are normally found in pregnancy, near term or after delivery, and have also been associated with a prethrombotic or hypercoagulable state in patients with thrombosis. Fibrinogen is an acute phase reactant, and high levels may be seen in inflammation, states of acute infections, and malignancy. Normally, spontaneous bleeding does not occur in patients with fibrinogen levels above 50 mg/dL, but under traumatic conditions such as surgery, a level of 100 mg/dL may be necessary to prevent bleeding.

The Clauss procedure for measuring clottable fibrinogen is the recommended method (NCCLS, 1991) and is described below. This test is based on the fact that changes in the concentration of fibrinogen are very sensitive to high concentrations of thrombin, when the fibrinogen level is low (e.g., 5 to 50 mg/dL). The clotting time of this test is sensitive to small changes in the fibrinogen concentration but relatively unaffected by changes in the thrombin concentration.

Normal values for this procedure are approximately 150 to 400 mg/dL (1.5 to 4.0 g/L), but each laboratory should determine its own normal range.

Reference

Organon Teknika Corp., *Fibriquik®*, pkg. insert, Organon Teknika Corp., Durham, NC, 1989.

Reagents and Equipment

1. The following reagents are obtainable from Organon Teknika Corp.:
   a. Thrombin reagent, 100 NIH units/mL. Available in a 1.0 or 3.0 mL size. Reconstitute with distilled water. Mix gently. Once reconstituted, the thrombin reagent may be stored in the refrigerator for up to 3 days.
   b. Owren's veronal buffer, pH 7.35, contains sodium barbital (0.028 M). Store in the refrigerator. Discard if the solution becomes cloudy.
   c. Fibrinogen calibration reference plasma, 1.0 mL, for use in preparing the fibrinogen calibration curve. Reconstitute with 1.0 mL of distilled water, allow to stand for 30 minutes, and gently mix. Once reconstituted this reagent may be stored in the refrigerator for up to 24 hours. (A reference plasma is also available from the College of American Pathologists.)
2. Pipets, plastic, 0.1, 0.5, 1.0, and 2.0 mL.
3. Test tubes, plastic, 10 × 75 mm.
4. 2 × 2 cycle logarithmic graph paper.
5. Fibrometer. (Manual methods or any clot detecting instrument may be used.)
6. Normal and abnormal control plasma. The abnormal control plasma should have an assay value between 80 and 120 mg/dL (0.8 to 1.2 g/L).

Specimen

Citrated plasma: 1 part 0.109 M sodium citrate to 9 parts whole blood. Plasma should be placed in crushed ice (2 to 8°C) and tested within 4 hours of specimen collection.

Principle

An excess amount of thrombin is added to a specimen of diluted plasma and the clotting time noted. The concentration of fibrinogen in the unknown sample is determined by comparing results with clotting times of standard reference plasma dilutions containing known amounts of fibrinogen. The clotting time of the plasma is inversely proportional to the concentration of fibrinogen in the specimen (i.e., the higher the clotting time, the lower the fibrinogen concentration).

Procedure

1. Preparation of calibration curve. When procedure is first set up, whenever a new lot number of thrombin is used, or any time changes are made that affect test results a new calibration curve must be set up.
   a. Reconstitute the fibrinogen calibration standard and thrombin reagent.
   b. Label 10 × 75 mm test tubes #1 through #5 (triplicate testing is recommended for preparation of the calibration curve).
   c. Pipet the appropriate amount of buffer (at room temperature) into each tube as indicated in Table 5–2.
   d. Add calibration standard to tube #1 (see Table 5–2). Mix tube well (gently), and transfer 0.5 mL to tube #2 and #4 as indicated. Transfer the appropriate dilutions to each tube as indicated in Table 5–2, being careful to mix each tube well after the addition of calibration standard.
   e. Perform the quantitative fibrinogen procedure on each dilution as described below (steps 5 through 8). Average results of the three dilutions prepared for each standard.
   f. Using 2 × 2 cycle logarithmic graph paper draw a fibrinogen curve by plotting the clotting time (in seconds) on the Y (vertical) axis and the fibrinogen concentration in mg/dL (assay value × the dilution factor from Table 5–2) on the X (horizontal) axis. Draw a straight line that best fits all five data points (Fig. 5–5).
   g. Check the validity of the fibrinogen curve by running normal and abnormal fibrinogen controls. Results should check within ±10% of the assay value of the controls. If they do

TABLE 5–2.   DILUTIONS FOR FIBRINOGEN CALIBRATION CURVE

Tube No.	Fibrinogen Calibration Reference	Owren's Veronal Buffer	Dilution	Dilution Factor
1	0.5 mL	2.0 mL	1:5	2
2	0.5 mL of mixture from tube #1	0.5 mL	1:10	1
3	0.5 mL of mixture from tube #2	0.5 mL	1:20	0.5
4	0.5 mL of mixture from tube #1	2.5 mL	1:30	0.33
5	0.5 mL of mixture from tube #3	0.5 mL	1:40	0.25

TABLE 5–3.   PROBABLE COAGULATION DEFICIENCIES BASED ON THE APTT AND PT SUBSTITUTION TEST RESULTS

APTT	PT	Adsorbed Plasma		Aged Serum		Probable Deficiency
		APTT	PT	APTT	PT	
N	N	—	—	—	—	No deficiency
A	N	C	—	C	—	XI or XII
A	N	NC	—	C	—	IX
A	A	NC	NC	C	C	X
A	A	C	C	NC	NC	V
N	A	—	NC	—	C	VII
A	N	C	—	NC	—	VIII
A	A	NC	NC	NC	NC	II

N = Normal result. A = Abnormal (prolonged result). C = Corrected result. NC = Not corrected.

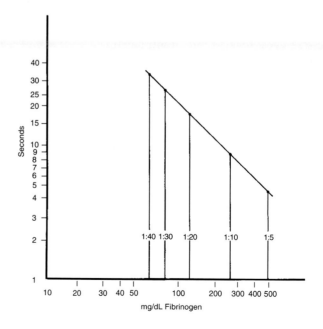

FIG. 5–5. Curve for quantitative fibrinogen procedure.

not, the fibrinogen curve should be repeated.

2. Centrifuge the blood specimens to obtain platelet-poor plasma.
3. Remove Owren's veronal buffer from the refrigerator and allow to warm to room temperature.
4. Reconstitute thrombin with the appropriate amount of distilled water. Mix gently and label bottle with the time and date of reconstitution.
5. Make a 1:10 dilution of each plasma specimen and control (duplicate dilutions are recommended): place 0.9 mL of Owren's veronal buffer into two appropriately labeled 10 × 75 mm test tubes (two tubes for each plasma and control specimen). Add 0.1 mL of plasma to each of the appropriately labeled test tubes. Mix carefully.
6. Pipet 0.2 mL of the first two plasma dilutions to be tested into each of 2 Fibrometer cups. Allow plasma to reach 37°C (3 minutes). Set a clock for 6 minutes. At 30-second intervals, pipet 0.2 mL of diluted plasma into each of two (more) Fibrometer cups.
7. When there is exactly 3 minutes left on the clock, place the first plasma dilution in the Fibrometer test well. Add 0.1 mL of thrombin reagent (unheated) to the test cup and start the timer. When clotting has occurred, record the results. Repeat this step for each diluted plasma or control, beginning the test 3 minutes after incubation was started.
8. Duplicate results should agree within a C.V. of <7%.
9. Average the duplicate results and determine the fibrinogen concentration for each control and patient specimen by referring to the previously prepared fibrinogen curve.

Discussion

1. When the fibrinogen value is below 50 mg/dL, the plasma should be diluted 1:5 (0.2 mL of plasma added to 0.8 mL of buffer) or 1:3 (0.3 mL of plasma added to 0.6 mL of buffer). Perform the fibrinogen in duplicate as outlined above, average results, determine the fibrinogen value from the curve, and divide by 2 (for the 1:5 dilution) or by 3 (for the 1:3 dilution). If no clot forms with the 1:3 dilution, divide the lowest value on the curve by 3 and report a result of less than that value.
2. When the fibrinogen is above 800 mg/dL, (8.0 g/L) the plasma should be diluted 1:20 (0.1 mL of plasma added to 1.9 mL of buffer). Perform the fibrinogen, in duplicate, as outlined above, average the results, determine the fibrinogen value from the curve, and multiply by 2 for the final result.
3. A 1:3 dilution of the plasma is the lowest dilution that may be used in this test. Inaccurate results may occur if a smaller dilution is used because of the presence of interfering substances in the plasma.
4. In the presence of significant levels of fibrin degradation products (above 100 μg/mL) or heparin (above 0.6 USP units/mL), test results will be invalidly decreased.
5. Several manufacturers of coagulation reagents produce a fibrinogen kit similar to the one described above.

FACTOR V (II, VII, X) ASSAY

The prothrombin time (PT) is used to determine the plasma concentration of factors II, V, VII, and X.

The normal plasma concentration of each of these factors is in the range of 50 to 150% activity; however, each laboratory should determine its own normal values.

Reference

Lenahan, J.G., and Smith, K.: *Hemostasis*, Durham, N.C., Organon Teknika Corp., 1986.

Reagents and Equipment

1. Thromboplastin-calcium chloride mixture.
2. Water bath, 37°C.
3. Factor V deficient substrate. Obtainable commercially.
4. Reference plasma with known factor V assay. Obtainable commercially.
5. Normal and abnormal control plasmas assayed for factor V.
6. Owren's veronal buffer, pH 7.40.
7. Ice bath.

TABLE 5–4. DILUTIONS FOR FACTOR ASSAYS

Tube (#)	Buffer (mL)	Plasma (mL)	Activity (%)	Dilution
1	0.9	0.1	100	1:10
2	1.9	0.1	50	1:20
3	0.5	0.5 mL from tube #2	25	1:40
4	0.5	0.5 mL from tube #3	12.5	1:80
5	0.5	0.5 mL from tube #4	6.3	1:160
6	0.5	0.5 mL from tube #5	3.2	1:320

8. Pipets, 1.0, 0.2, and 0.1 mL.
9. Stopwatch.
10. Test tubes, 12 × 75 mm.
11. Two cycle log-log graph paper.

Specimen

Citrated plasma: 1 part 0.109 M sodium citrate to 9 parts whole blood.

Principle

A prothrombin time is performed on factor V-deficient substrates (plasmas) containing varying dilutions of the patient's plasma (Table 5–4), which is used to correct the prothrombin time. The amount of correction by the patient's plasma correlates with its factor activity level and is compared to the results of the prothrombin time performed on varying dilutions of an assayed reference plasma in place of the patient's plasma. The factor V content of the patient's plasma is expressed as the percentage of normal.

Procedure

1. Centrifuge the specimen as soon as possible after collection to obtain platelet poor plasma. Remove the plasma and maintain at room temperature. The test should be completed within 2 hours of specimen collection.
2. Warm sufficient thromboplastin-calcium reagent to 37°C.
3. Reconstitute the factor V-deficient substrate and the reference plasma according to manufacturer's directions and place on ice.
4. Label six 12 × 75 mm test tubes and add

Owren's veronal buffer in the amounts listed in Table 5–4. (At least two separately prepared dilutions [e.g., 1:10 and 1:20] should be made. If this is not done, an error made in the original dilution will affect all of the dilutions and will not be reflected in the results.)
5. Place several 12 × 75 mm empty test tubes in the 37°C water bath. (All testing should be performed in duplicate.)
6. Prepare the dilutions of the reference plasma as indicated in Table 5–4.
7. To one of the 12 × 75 mm test tubes in the water bath, add:
   a. 0.1 mL of factor V-deficient substrate.
   b. 0.1 mL of the first diluted (reference) plasma. Mix and incubate for 2 to 3 minutes until it reaches 37°C.
8. Add 0.2 mL of thromboplastin-calcium reagent to the test tube and simultaneously start a stopwatch.
9. Remove the test tube from the water bath and gently tilt the tube at a rate of about once per second. Stop the watch at the first indication of clot formation. Record results.
10. Repeat steps 7, 8, and 9 for each of the reference plasma dilutions.
11. Prepare 1:10 and 1:20 dilutions of the patient, normal, and abnormal control plasmas (see Table 5–4 for amounts) immediately before use and repeat steps 7 through 9, above, for each of the dilutions. Test each dilution in duplicate.
12. Calculation of results:
   a. Using 2-cycle log-log graph paper and the results obtained on the reference plasma, plot each average clotting time in seconds (on the Y-axis) against the plasma concentration in percent

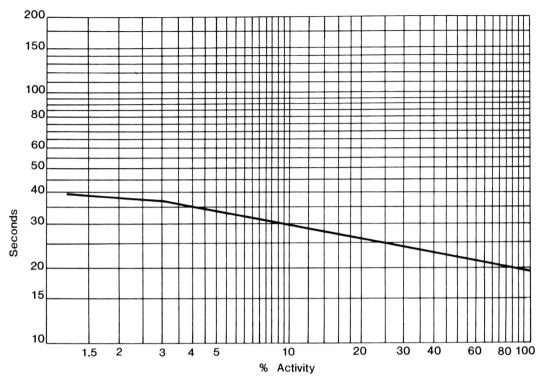

FIG. 5–6. Factor V activity curve.

(on the X-axis). There will be six points plotted (Fig. 5–6).

b. Draw a straight line that best connects the six points of the reference plasma. This represents the normal activity curve.

c. Using the average clotting times of each patient and control plasma dilution, determine from the graph the percent of factor V present in each dilution. The 1:10 dilution represents the percent activity present in undiluted plasma. The results of the 1:20 dilution should be multiplied by 2 in order to arrive at the percent activity present in undiluted plasma. Average these two values for the percent of factor V activity present in the patient and control plasmas. (Duplicate results should agree with each other within 10%.)

Discussion

1. For a factor II, VII, or X assay, substitute factor II, VII, or X deficient substrate in place of factor V deficient substrate and use a factor II, VII, or X assayed reference plasma instead of the factor V reference plasma. Factor V may also be assayed using the Stypven time since Russell's viper venom is quite sensitive to this factor.

2. Factor V-deficient plasma may be used in place of the factor V-deficient substrate. If this is employed, a prothrombin time greater than 60 seconds should be obtained on the factor V-deficient plasma before it is used. (Factor V-deficient plasma may be prepared by incubating normal plasma at 37°C for 24 hours or by refrigerating a normal plasma at 4 to 10°C for 2 weeks.)

3. Samples must be tested immediately after diluting in Owren's veronal buffer, especially when testing for factor VIII. (Premeasure the buffer and add plasma just prior to testing.)

4. A new curve should be prepared each time the assay is performed. As more experience is gained, the curve may be made from tubes #1, 2, 3, and 5.

5. When drawing the factor activity curve, do not extend the curve beyond the upper

and lower concentration limits of the reference plasma. The curve will generally flatten out at a dilution around 5% (most notably factors II and VII), indicating a lack of sensitivity at these concentrations. Results obtained for the patient and control dilutions must fall within the linear (sensitive) part of the reference curve. Do not use extrapolated results. For values outside the linearity range, repeat the test using other dilutions. (Make a 1:2, 1:4, and a 1:8 dilution for results that fall below the lowest value of the reference curve. To obtain the % activity, divide the results by 5, 2.5 and 1.25 respectively. For clotting times above the highest value of the reference curve, make a 1:40, 1:80, and 1:160 dilution and multiply the results by 4, 8, and 16 respectively.)

6. In the presence of nonspecific inhibitors such as "lupus-like" inhibitors or heparin, the results of the more concentrated dilutions (1:10, 1:20) will be lower than the results of the higher dilutions (1:40, 1:80) because the effect of the inhibitor is diminished by dilution. In the presence of a specific inhibitor, such as one directed against factor VIII, there is no correction with dilution. The presence of a specific inhibitor is often picked up in a hemophiliac patient, when a factor assay performed after a therapeutic infusion of factor concentrate does not match expected levels. Spontaneous specific inhibitors are sometimes found in adult or elderly patients with no previous bleeding history who present with unexplained bleeding problems. In either case, the antibody is directed against a specific factor, neutralizing its function.

7. This assay may also be performed on the Fibrometer and on most automated coagulation systems.

FACTOR VIII (VIII:C) (IX, XI, XII) ASSAY

The activated partial thromboplastin time (APTT) is used to determine the plasma concentration of factors VIII, IX, XI, and XII. The normal plasma concentration of each of these factors is in the range of 50 to 150% activity; however, each laboratory should determine its own normal values.

References

Hardisty, R.M., and MacPherson, J.C.: A one-stage factor VIII assay and its use on venous and capillary plasma. Thromb. Diath. Haemorrh., 7, 215, 1962.
Lenahan, J.G., and Smith, K.: Hemostasis, Durham, N.C., Organon Teknika Corp., 1986.

Reagents and Equipment

1. Partial thromboplastin containing an activator (platelet substitute with activator). Obtainable commercially.
2. Water bath, 37°C.
3. Calcium chloride, 0.025 M.
4. Factor VIII deficient substrate. Obtainable commercially.
5. Reference plasma with known factor VIII assay. Obtainable commercially.
6. Normal and abnormal control plasmas assayed for factor VIII.
7. Owren's veronal buffer, pH 7.40 (± 0.1).
8. Ice bath.
9. Pipets, 1.0, 0.2, and 0.1 mL.
10. Stopwatch.
11. Timers, 2.
12. Test tubes, 12 × 75 mm.
13. Two-cycle log-log graph paper.

Specimen

Citrated plasma: 1 part 0.109 M sodium citrate to 9 parts whole blood. Place specimen in a cup of ice immediately after collection.

Principle

An APTT is performed on factor VIII-deficient substrates (plasmas) containing varying dilutions of the patient's plasma (Table 5–4). The patient's plasma is used to correct the APTT. The amount of correction by the patient's plasma correlates with its factor activity level and is compared to results of the APTT using varying dilutions of an assayed reference plasma in place of the patient's plasma. The factor VIII content of the patient's plasma is expressed as the percentage of normal.

Procedure

1. Centrifuge the specimen as soon as possible after collection to obtain platelet-poor plasma. Remove the plasma and

place on ice. Proceed with the test immediately.

2. Maintain the partial thromboplastin at room temperature.

3. Incubate sufficient 0.025 M calcium chloride at 37°C.

4. Reconstitute factor VIII-deficient substrate and the reference plasma according to manufacturer's directions and place on ice.

5. Label seven 12 × 75 mm test tubes and add Owren's veronal buffer in the amounts listed in Table 5–4. (At least two separately prepared dilutions [e.g., 1:10 and 1:20] should be made. If this is not done, an error made in the original dilution will affect the serial dilutions and will not be reflected in the results.)

6. Place several 12 × 75 mm test tubes in the 37°C water bath. (All testing should be performed in duplicate.)

7. Prepare the dilutions of the reference plasma as indicated in Table 5–4.

8. To one of the 12 × 75 mm test tubes in the water bath add:
   a. 0.1 mL of partial thromboplastin.
   b. 0.1 mL of factor-VIII deficient substrate.
   c. 0.1 mL of the first dilution of (reference) plasma.

9. Quickly mix the contents of the test tube and set clock #1 for 5 minutes.

10. When 2 minutes have elapsed on clock #1, repeat steps 8 and 9 for the duplicate sample, setting clock #2.

11. When 5 minutes have elapsed on clock #1, quickly pipet 0.1 mL of 0.025 M calcium chloride into the first test tube, simultaneously starting a stopwatch. Gently mix the contents of the tube and leave it in the 37°C water bath for 30 seconds.

12. After 30 seconds have elapsed on the stopwatch, remove the test tube from the water bath and gently tilt the tube at a rate no faster than once per second.

13. When clotting occurs, stop the watch. This is the end point.

14. Repeat steps 11, 12, and 13 for clock #2 and the duplicate specimen.

15. Average the preceding two results and record the clotting time for that dilution.

16. Repeat steps 8 through 15 for each of the reference plasma dilutions.

17. Prepare 1:10 and 1:20 dilutions of the patient, normal, and abnormal control plasmas (see Table 5–4 for amounts) immediately before use and repeat steps 8 through 15 for each of the dilutions. Test each dilution in duplicate.

18. Calculation of results.
   a. Using 2-cycle log-log graph paper and the results obtained on the reference plasma, plot each average clotting time in seconds (on the Y-axis) against the plasma concentration in percent (on the X-axis). There will be 7 points plotted.
   b. Draw a straight line that best connects the 7 points of the reference plasma. This represents the normal activity curve.
   c. Using the average clotting times of each patient and control plasma dilution, determine from the graph the percent of factor VIII present in each dilution. The 1:10 dilution represents the percent activity present in undiluted plasma. The results of the 1:20 dilution should be multiplied by 2 in order to arrive at the percent activity present in undiluted plasma. Average these two values for the percent of factor VIII activity present in the patient and control plasmas.

Discussion

1. See Factor V Assay, Discussion, items #3, 4, 5, 6, and 7.

2. For a factor IX, XI, or XII assay, substitute factor IX, XI, or XII deficient substrate in place of factor VIII deficient substrate and use a factor IX, XI, or XII assayed reference plasma instead of the factor VIII reference plasma. Assays for prekallikrein and high molecular weight kininogen (HMWK) may also be performed by this procedure if the respective factor deficient substrates and assayed reference plasmas are available.

3. Factor VIII-deficient substrate may be replaced by plasma known to be deficient in factor VIII. This plasma may be stored at −20°C and thawed immediately before use. A plasma to be used as factor VIII-deficient, however, must have a concentration no higher than 0 to 1% of normal

activity of the factor before it is acceptable. Also, even though the plasma is stored at $-20°C$, it may gradually become deficient in additional clotting factors, particularly factor V.

4. The 5 minute activation time in this procedure is critical for accurate results.

5. Excessive mixing of the tubes during the procedure may cause prolonged clotting times.

6. Due to the slope of the curve, a 1-second variation in clotting time will cause a relatively large difference in percent activity. Therefore, a CV of 10 to 15% is not unusual for this procedure.

VONWILLEBRAND FACTOR ANTIGEN (vWF:Ag)

Factor VIII and vonWillebrand factor circulate together in a complex consisting of two antigenically separate components: the procoagulant or factor VIII portion (VIII:C) and the vonWillebrand factor (vWF). The vWF has a specific antigenic determinant on its surface known as vonWillebrand factor antigen (vWF:Ag), which was previously termed factor VIII related antigen (VIII:RAg). Patients with classic hemophilia (hemophilia A) have decreased levels of factor VIII:C, but normal to increased levels of the vWF:Ag, whereas patients with vonWillebrand disease may have decreased to normal levels of both factor VIII:C and vWF:Ag. Elevated levels of vWF:Ag are associated with vascular endothelium injury (such as occurs in cancer, fever, hepatic or renal disorders) the postoperative period, thrombosis, myocardial infarction, pregnancy, oral contraceptive therapy, exercise, stress, and increasing age.

vWF:Ag may be measured by electroimmunoassay, radioimmunoassay, and by enzyme linked immunosorbent assay (ELISA) described below. The normal range for this procedure is 60 to 150%, but each laboratory should determine its own normal values.

References

Diagnostica Stago: Asserachrom® vWF enzyme immunoassay of vonWillebrand factor, pkg. insert, Diagnostica Stago, Seine, France, 1992.

Davis, G.L.: Technical aspects of enzyme immunosorbent assays, Clin. Lab. Sci., 4, 338, 1991.

Reagents and Equipment

1. The following reagents and supplies are available from American Bioproducts Co., Parsippany, NJ (distributor for Diagnostica Stago). Store all reagents at 2 to 8°C when not in use.

   a. Reagent 1: two strips of 16 wells each coated with specific rabbit anti-human vWF F(ab')$_2$ fragments sealed in an aluminum pouch. Stable until the expiration date of the kit, or 15 days after opening.

   b. Reagent 2: a specific rabbit anti-human vWF antibody attached to peroxidase. Prepare just before use: reconstitute one vial with 8 mL of diluted buffer. Reconstituted reagent is stable for 24 hours at 2 to 8°C.

   c. Reagent 3: OPD (ortho-phenylenediamine) substrate. Prepare just before use: place two tablets in a test tube. Add 8 mL of distilled water. Allow the tablets to completely dissolve. Add 5 μL of 30% hydrogen peroxide directly into the solution and mix well. The OPD/H_2O_2 mixture is stable for 1 hour at room temperature.

   d. Reagent 4: concentrated phosphate buffer. Dilute 1:10 with distilled water for working buffer solution: add 6 mL of reagent 4 to 54 mL of distilled water. The diluted buffer is stable for 15 days at 2 to 8°C.

   e. Reagent 5: concentrated washing solution. Dilute 1:20 with distilled water for working wash solution: add 16 mL of reagent 5 to 304 mL of distilled water. The diluted wash solution is stable for 15 days at 2 to 8°C.

   f. Reagent 6: lypholized reference plasma. Reconstitute one vial with 0.5 mL of distilled water. Reconstituted reagent is stable for 4 hours at 20°C and 12 hours at 2 to 8°C.

   g. Asserachrom plate work sheet.

   h. Plate frame and cover.

   i. Plastic reservoir trays.

2. Normal and abnormal control plasmas.

3. Sulfuric acid, 3 M.

4. Adjustable multichannel pipet and tips (0.3, 0.2, and 0.05 mL) (see Fig. 5–7).

5. Pipets, 10, 5, 2, 1, and 0.005 mL.

6. Hydrogen peroxide, 30%.

FIG. 5–7. Plate reader with Asserachrom plate (in frame).

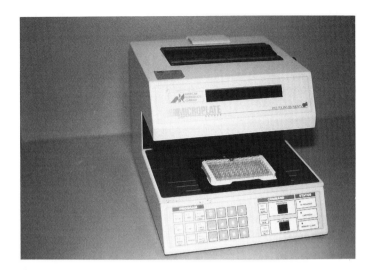

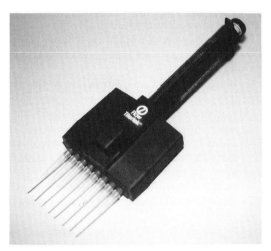

FIG. 5–8. Multichannel pipet.

7. Plate reader set at a wavelength of 492
   nm. (See Fig. 5–8.)
8. Timer.
9. Stopwatch.
10. Distilled water.
11. Test tubes, 10 × 75 mm and 12 × 100
    mm.
12. Log-log graph paper.
13. Variable speed mixer (optional) (Fig.
    5–9).

Specimen

Citrated plasma, 1 part 0.109 M sodium citrate to 9 parts whole blood. Centrifuge specimen at 2500 × g for 10 minutes. Plasma may

be stored at 20°C for 8 hours or for 1 month
at −20°C or below.

Principle

Plasma dilutions containing the vWF antigen
are incubated in microwells coated with rabbit anti-vWF antibody. During incubation,
the plasma vWF antigen binds to the anti-
vWF antibody by one of its antigenic determinants. The anti vWF peroxidase conjugate
(reagent 2) is added, which binds to the free
antigenic determinants of vWF antigen forming a "sandwich." The bound enzyme peroxidase, acts on the substrate ortho-phenylenediamine (OPD) in the presence of
hydrogen peroxide to produce a color change
that is directly proportional to the concentration of vWF antigen present in the plasma.

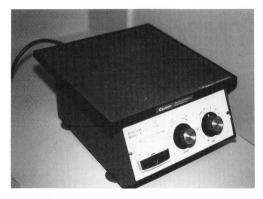

FIG. 5–9. Variable speed mixer.

TABLE 5–5.   vWF:Ag TEST DILUTIONS

vWF level (%)	100	50	25	12.5	6.25	0
vWF:Ag reference plasma 1:50 dilution (mL)	1.0	0.5	0.2	0.1	0.1	—
Diluted buffer (mL)	—	0.5	0.6	0.7	1.15	1.0
Dilution factor	—	2	4	8	16	—

Procedure

1. Preparation of the reference plasma dilution.
   a. Reconstitute vWF:Ag reference plasma (reagent 6) according to directions.
   b. Prepare a 1:50 dilution of the reference plasma (represents 100% vWF:Ag activity): add 50 μL of plasma to 2.45 mL of diluted buffer.
   c. Prepare additional dilutions of the diluted reference plasma as shown in Table 5–5.
2. Preparation of the patient and control plasma.
   a. Prepare an initial dilution (1:50) of each plasma to be tested. (Pipet 50 μL of each plasma into an appropriately labeled tube. Add 2.45 μL of diluted buffer to each tube and mix well.)
   b. Prepare a 1:2 dilution of each initial dilution in step 2a above. (Pipet 0.5 mL of the 1:50 dilution into an appropriately labeled tube. Add 0.5 mL of diluted buffer. This constitutes a 1:100 dilution.)
3. Place the precoated strips from the pouch on a plate frame and label the top row #1 through #4. Label the asserachrom plate worksheet for duplicate testing (label the first two positions as the blanks).
4. Leaving the first two wells empty, pipet 0.2 mL of the 100% reference dilution into each of two consecutive wells. Pipet 0.2 mL of the 50% reference dilution into the next set of wells. Continue adding the remaining reference, patient, and control dilutions in duplicate to the wells as labeled on the worksheet.
5. Cover the plate tightly with parafilm and incubate in the dark for 2 hours at room temperature.
6. Fill a plastic reservoir tray with diluted

washing solution. Decant the strips completely by inverting the plate over a sink. Using a multichannel pipet set at 0.3 mL fill the wells of the strips with washing solution. Empty the wells completely and pat the inverted plate on a pad of absorbent paper. Repeat this step four times, leaving the wash solution in the wells after the fifth wash.
7. Prepare the anti-vWF-peroxidase conjugate (reagent 2) according to directions. Pour the solution into a clean reservoir tray.
8. Decant the last wash from the wells, pat the plate on absorbent paper and immediately add 0.2 mL of the diluted conjugate into each well using the multichannel pipet. Cover tightly with parafilm and incubate in the dark for 2 hours at room temperature.
9. At the end of the 2-hour incubation, decant the plate and wash five times (repeat step 6 above).
10. Prepare the OPD/H_2O_2 solution (reagent 3) according to directions. Pour the solution into a clean reservoir tray.
11. Decant the last wash from the wells, pat the plate on absorbent paper, and immediately add 0.2 mL of the OPD/H_2O_2 solution into each well (including the first two "blank" wells) using the multichannel pipet. Immediately start a stopwatch. Incubate for exactly 3 minutes.
12. At the end of three minutes, add 50 μL of 3M sulfuric acid to each well (including the "blank" wells) with the multichannel pipet in order to stop the reaction.
13. Cover the plate with parafilm and let stand for 10 minutes at room temperature. The color is stable for 2 hours when protected from bright light.
14. Read the absorbance of the wells on a

plate reader set at 492 nm. Use the first two wells as the blanks. Average the absorbance readings for the duplicate samples.

15. To determine the percentage of activity of the reference dilution multiply the percentage (1.0, 0.5, 0.25, 0.125, and 0.0625) by the assigned assay value for that lot of reference plasma. Plot the six points on log-log paper (absorbance vs. percentage of vWF:Ag) and draw a line that best fits all points.

16. To determine the percentage of activity of the vWF:Ag of each plasma, refer to the calibration curve. Read the 1:50 dilution directly from the curve and multiply the results of the 1:100 dilution by 2.

Discussion

1. For accurate and reproducible results, use of a variable speed rotator is recommended. The strip is placed on the mixer and the mixer turned on for several seconds immediately following each addition of reagent. This is not necessary when wash solutions are added.

2. The microwell plates should be incubated in the dark because light reaches the wells at different intensities and will cause an "edge effect" (a condition in which the inner wells read differently from the outer wells).

3. Inconsistent results may be due to poor pipetting techniques. When using a multichannel pipet, tighten each tip individually to ensure that the tips are securely seated on the pipet. Rinse the tips in the solution before pipetting and check the height of the solution in each tip. The pipet tip should be held at the same angle whenever pipetting.

4. A stopwatch must be used to time the addition of the OPD/H_2O_2 and 3 M sulfuric acid reagents to each group of wells, so that the timing is exact for each set of wells pipetted.

5. Hydrochloric acid, 1 M, 0.1 mL, may be substituted for the 3 M sulfuric acid used to stop the reaction.

6. The plate reader should be prewarmed before use. The bottom of the microwell plate must be treated as a cuvet: check for moisture, fingerprints, etc. and wipe if necessary.

7. For vWF:Ag levels <10%, prepare a 1:5 dilution (0.1 mL plasma + 0.4 mL diluted buffer) and a 1:10 dilution (0.1 mL plasma + 0.9 mL diluted buffer). To obtain the percentage of activity, divide the values read from the calibration curve by 10 and 5 respectively.

8. For results higher than the curve (extrapolated values), prepare a 1:4 and 1:8 dilution of the 1:50 initial dilution (see Table 5–5). To obtain the percentage of activity, multiply the values read from the calibration curve by 4 and 8 respectively.

RISTOCETIN COFACTOR ASSAY

Ristocetin cofactor activity is that property of the plasma von Willebrand factor, which is responsible for in vitro platelet agglutination in the presence of ristocetin. Decreased amounts or abnormalities of this factor are associated with the von Willebrand syndrome.

Normally, ristocetin cofactor activity should be above 40% and is generally in the range of 60 to 180%. A normal range should be determined by each laboratory.

References

Bio/Data Corporation, vW Factor Assay™ for the Quantitation of von Willebrand Factor, pkg. insert, Hatboro, Pa., Bio/Data Corporation, 1986.

Helena Laboratories, Ristocetin cofactor assay., pkg. insert, Helena Laboratories, Beaumont, Texas, 1985.

Reagents and Equipment

1. Tris buffered saline, pH 7.3 to 7.5.
   Sodium chloride 8.766 g
   Tris (hydroxymethyl)
   aminomethane 6.055 g
   Dilute to 1 L with distilled water. Store in the refrigerator. (Commercially available.)

2. Lypholized platelets (Helena Laboratories). Reconstitute with 5.0 mL of Tris buffered saline. Let stand for 20 minutes before use. Once reconstituted the platelets may be refrigerated up to 30 days. Resuspend platelets gently by mixing, immediately before use.

3. Ristocetin reagent (Bio/Data Corp.). Reconstitute with diluent to give a final concentration of 12 mg/mL. Invert vial gently and allow to stand at room temperature for 10 minutes prior to use. Once reconstituted this reagent is stable for 7 days stored in the refrigerator.
4. Normal reference plasma for preparation of standard curve.
5. Normal and abnormal control plasma.
6. Platelet aggregometer capable of stir speeds between 900 and 1200 rpm.
7. Platelet aggregometer cuvets.
8. Stir bars.
9. Pipets, 5.0, 1.0, 0.5, 0.2, 0.1, and 0.05 mL.
10. Plastic test tubes, 10 × 75 mm.
11. Distilled water.
12. Log-log graph paper.
13. Slope reader.

Specimen

Citrated plasma: 1 part 0.109 M sodium citrate to 9 parts whole blood. Plasma may be refrigerated for up to 8 hours prior to testing, or frozen at −20°C or lower for up to 8 weeks.

Principle

Patient's plasma (source of ristocetin cofactor) is added to a standardized mixture of platelets and ristocetin reagent. The degree of resultant platelet aggregation is measured using the platelet aggregometer. This result is then compared to a curve prepared from a normal reference plasma, and the % concentration of ristocetin cofactor determined.

Procedure

1. Turn the platelet aggregometer on and allow it to reach 37°C.
2. Centrifuge the specimen as soon as possible after collection to obtain platelet-poor plasma.
3. Preparation of normal reference plasma dilutions (1:2, 1:4, and 1:8).
   a. Label three 10 × 75 mm test tubes: 100%, 50%, and 25%.
   b. Pipet 0.1 mL of tris buffered saline solution into the tube labeled 100%, 0.3 mL of tris buffered saline solution into the 50% tube, and 0.2 mL into the 25% tube.
   c. Pipet 0.1 mL of the normal reference plasma into the 100% and 50% tubes. Mix each tube thoroughly. Transfer 0.2 mL of the mixture from the 50% tube to the 25% tube and mix well.
4. Preparation of patient and control dilutions (1:2, 1:4, and 1:8). For each plasma to be tested, pipet 0.1 mL, 0.3 mL, and 0.7 mL of tris buffered saline solution into appropriately labeled 10 × 75 mm test tubes. Add 0.1 mL of each patient's plasma to each tube. Mix well.
5. Preparation of the aggregometer blank. Pipet 0.25 mL of reconstituted platelets into an aggregometer cuvet and add 0.25 mL of tris buffered saline solution. Mix well. This blank is used to set the baseline in the aggregometer.
6. Place a stir bar into an aggregometer cuvet and pipet 0.4 mL of reconstituted platelets into the cuvet. Add 0.05 mL of ristocetin to the tube (allow no formation of air bubbles) and mix by tapping the cuvet gently. Allow the mixture to equilibrate at room temperature for 2 minutes.
7. Set the baseline using the aggregometer blank prepared in step 5 above.
8. As soon as the 0% baseline is stable, add 0.05 mL of the first reference plasma dilution directly into the test mixture in the cuvet. (Do not allow the reagent to touch the sides of the cuvet.)
9. Watch the pattern of aggregation as it prints out on the chart recorder. Stop the instrument when the reaction is complete.
10. Repeat steps 6 through 9 above for each dilution of the reference plasma and for each patient and control dilution.
11. Determine the slope value for each aggregation curve.
    a. Draw a straight line along the steepest portion of the curve that is linear (immediately following the lag phase resulting from the addition of the diluted plasma). Extend the line to the bottom of the graph paper.
    b. Line up the slope reader so that the slope line bisects the slope reader scale at the bottom right of the base line.

c. Read the slope value at the point on the left scale of the reader where the slope line intersects it.

d. If the slope line is printed in the opposite direction, reverse the above procedure, lining up the baseline of the reader on the left side and reading the slope value from the right side.

12. Preparation of standard curve. Using log-log graph paper, plot the slope values for the reference plasma dilutions on the vertical axis against the percent activity on the horizontal axis. Draw a straight line which best fits these 3 points. If the points do not approximate a straight line, the test should be repeated.

13. Determine the percentage of ristocetin cofactor activity for each plasma and control dilution by looking up the slope value on the reference curve and reading the corresponding percent ristocetin cofactor activity from the horizontal axis. Multiply the results of the 1:4 dilutions by 2 and the 1:8 dilutions by 4 in order to obtain the correct test result. The 1:2, 1:4, and 1:8 dilutions should give results which agree closely. If the 1:2 dilution is above 100%, obtain the results from the 1:4 and 1:8 dilutions.

Discussion

1. If the test results show less than 25% ristocetin cofactor activity, repeat the test using undiluted plasma. The final result would then be divided by 2.

2. Each time this test procedure is performed a standard curve should be prepared.

3. In order to conserve reagents, the above procedure may be performed using micro methods if micro cuvets are available. In this modification, the test mixture should contain 0.2 mL of platelet suspension, 0.02 mL of ristocetin, and 0.02 mL of diluted plasma.

4. This test may also be performed on platelet aggregometers that will automatically determine the slope and activity curve, and calculate the control and patient results.

HEPARIN (ANTI-Xa) ASSAY

Heparin binds with antithrombin III. When this occurs there is an immediate anticoagulant effect. The procedure described below is a chromogenic method for assaying the amount of heparin present in plasma.

Reference

Organon Teknika Corp.: Chromostrate™ Heparin Anti-Xa Assay, pkg. insert, Organon Teknika Corp., Durham, NC, 1988.

Reagents and Equipment

1. Chromostrate™ heparin anti-Xa assay kit (obtainable from Organon Teknika Corp.).

a. Substrate reagent (CH_3OCO-D-valyl-glycyl-arginin-paranitroanilide). Reconstitute according to directions. May be stored in the refrigerator for 30 days after reconstitution. This reagent will be preincubated and kept at 37°C during testing.

b. Factor Xa reagent. Reconstitute according to directions. May be stored in refrigerator for up to 4 days after reconstitution.

c. Antithrombin III reagent. Reconstitute as directed. May be stored in the refrigerator for 7 days after reconstitution.

d. Buffer concentrate (substrate specific), pH 8.4 (caution: contains sodium azide). Dilute 1:10 with distilled water for working buffer solution. Store in refrigerator for up to 30 days after dilution.

2. Acetic acid, 50% (v/v).

3. Heparin (same source as used in the patient's therapy).

4. Plastic test tubes, 12 × 75 mm.

5. Plastic pipets, 5.0, 1.0, 0.1, and 0.2 mL.

6. Stopwatch.

7. Verify H control plasma (Organon Teknika).

8. Normal (platelet poor) plasma pool.

9. Linear graph paper.

10. Water bath, 37°C.

11. Spectrophotometer, wavelength of 405 nm.

12. Sodium chloride, 0.85% w/v.

Specimen

Citrated plasma: 1 part 0.109 M sodium citrate to 9 parts whole blood. The blood specimen should be centrifuged at 10 to 20°C within 1 hour of collection and should not sit for more than 2 hours at 2° to 8°C. The plasma may be frozen rapidly and stored for up to 30 days.

Principle

The patient's plasma (containing heparin) is incubated with a measured amount of antithrombin III and factor Xa (in excess). A complex of heparin, antithrombin III, and factor Xa is formed. Substrate reagent is added to the mixture and during incubation the remaining factor Xa (not complexed) catalyzes the release of paranitroanilide from the chromogenic substrate. The amount of paranitroanilide (pNA) released is then measured spectrophotometrically. It is inversely proportional to the amount of heparin in the plasma. The O.D. of each plasma is read from a reference curve to determine the concentration of heparin present.

Procedure

1. Centrifuge the patient specimen within 1 hour after collection at 10 to 20°C to obtain platelet-poor plasma.
2. Incubate a sufficient quantity of the substrate at 37°C.
3. Preparation of calibration curve.
   a. Prepare a stock solution of heparin, 5 U/mL in sodium chloride. Dilute the stock solution 1:50 with working buffer solution (0.1 mL of stock heparin + 4.9 mL of working buffer) for a concentration of 0.1 U/mL.
   b. Prepare standards for the calibration curve using the volumes shown in Table 5–6. (Equivalent heparin levels correspond to the patient and control samples being diluted 1:10 for testing.) (Antithrombin III is added in case there is any deficiency of this factor in the normal pooled plasma.)
4. Prepare a 1:10 dilution of the patient and control plasmas: 0.1 mL of plasma to be tested + 0.8 mL working buffer + 0.1 mL of antithrombin III reagent. Mix.

5. Test each standard, patient, and control plasma in duplicate and continue with the procedure as described in the Antithrombin III assay (steps 5 through 12) with the following exceptions:
   a. Substitute factor Xa for thrombin reagent in step 7 and incubate for 60 seconds.
   b. Use heparin substrate instead of antithrombin III substrate in step 8.
6. Plot the 4 points of the heparin standards on linear graph paper (O.D. vs. heparin concentration [U/mL]) and connect the points by a straight line which best fits all points.
7. To determine the U/mL of heparin in each plasma and control, refer to the calibration curve.

Discussion

1. To measure the actual heparin effect in the patient's plasma, substitute 0.1 mL of working buffer for the 0.1 mL of antithrombin III reagent in the plasma dilution. (Patient's plasma would be diluted: 0.1 mL patient's plasma + 0.9 mL working buffer.)
2. See the Antithrombin III procedure discussion points 1 and 2.

FIBRINOGEN DEGRADATION PRODUCTS

Fibrinogen degradation products (FDP) may be demonstrated in the blood of patients with primary fibrinolysis and during the process of disseminated intravascular coagulation with secondary fibrinolysis. This test will also be elevated in any kind of a thrombotic state including postoperative deep vein thrombosis, myocardial infarction, and in certain disorders of pregnancy. Slight to moderate increases of FDP will be seen in alcoholic cirrhosis of the liver and during late pregnancy.

The Thrombo-Wellcotest procedure described here is a rapid, sensitive test for fibrinogen degradation products present in the blood. The normal level of serum FDP in the adult is less than 8 μg/mL.

TABLE 5–6. DILUTIONS FOR HEPARIN ANTI-Xa ASSAY CURVE

Equivalent Heparin Level (U/mL)	PPP Pool (mL)	Heparin Solution (0.1 U/mL) (mL)	Working Buffer (mL)	Antithrombin III Reagent (mL)
0.1	0.1	0.1	0.7	0.1
0.2	0.1	0.2	0.6	0.1
0.4	0.1	0.4	0.4	0.1
0.6	0.1	0.6	0.2	0.1

Thrombo-Wellcotest Procedure

Reference

Wellcome Diagnostics: Thrombo-Wellcotest. Rapid latex test for detection of fibrinogen degradation products, Dartford, England, The Wellcome Foundation Ltd., 1986.

Reagents and Equipment

1. The following reagents are available from Burroughs Wellcome Co., Research Triangle Park, N.C. All reagents must be refrigerated when not in use.
   a. Sample collection tubes (contain thrombin to cause rapid and complete clotting and soya bean enzyme inhibitors to prevent the breakdown of fibrin).
   b. Glycine saline buffer.
   c. Latex suspension. (The latex particles have been sensitized with anti-fibrinogen fragments D and E antibodies.)
   d. Positive and negative control serums.
   e. Glass test slide.
   f. Disposable pipet droppers.
   g. Disposable mixing rods.
2. Test tubes, 10 × 75 mm.
3. Timer.

Specimen

Using a clean, dry syringe, obtain 2.0 mL of blood from the patient and transfer immediately to the sample collection tube. These tubes may also be used with a Vacutainer system and will draw 2 mL of blood. As soon as the blood is in the tube, mix well by inverting several times. (A minimum of 0.5 mL of whole blood must be added to the collection tube.)

Principle

Whole blood is added to thrombin (to ensure complete clotting) and soya bean enzyme inhibitors (to prevent breakdown of fibrin). After complete clotting, the patient's serum is diluted and mixed with latex particles coated with anti-FDP (fibrinogen fragments D and E). If fibrinogen degradation products are present, agglutination of the latex particles will occur.

Procedure

1. As soon as the blood sample arrives in the laboratory, ring the clot with an applicator stick to allow for clot retraction. Incubate the tube at room temperature or at 37°C for 30 to 60 minutes. (If the patient is receiving heparin, Reptilase-R should be added to the patient's blood in the sample collection tube in order for complete clotting to occur. Reconstitute the Reptilase-R with 1.0 mL of distilled water. Add 0.1 mL of the reconstituted Reptilase-R for each 1.0 mL of whole blood in the tube.) While the tube is incubating, remove the reagents and controls from the refrigerator and allow to warm to room temperature.
2. At the end of the incubation period, centrifuge the specimen for 5 minutes at 1500 × g. (The blood must be completely clotted before centrifuging.)
3. Carefully remove the serum and place in 10 × 75 mm test tube. No red blood cells should be present.
4. Label two 10 × 75 mm test tubes 1:5 and 1:10 for each specimen to be tested. Using the graduated dropper from the test kit, place 0.75 mL of the glycine buffer

into the test tube labeled 1:5. Using a disposable dropper from the test kit, add 5 drops of the patient's serum to this test tube. Mix. Using a disposable dropper from the test kit, place 4 drops of glycine buffer into the test tube labeled 1:10. Transfer 4 drops of diluted serum from the test tube labeled 1:5 to the test tube labeled 1:10.

5. Label rings on the glass slide: positive, negative, 1:5, and 1:10.

6. Place 1 drop of each control serum in the appropriate ring. Transfer 1 drop of the 1:5 dilution and 1 drop of the 1:10 dilution to the appropriate rings on the glass slide. (Allow all drops to fall freely from the pipet. Do not touch the pipet to the glass slide during this process.)

7. Mix the latex suspension vigorously. Immediately add 1 drop to each of the serum dilutions and control specimens.

8. Using a separate applicator stick for each sample, quickly stir each mixture, spreading over the entire area of the ring. Immediately set a clock for 2 minutes.

9. Rotate the slide for exactly 2 minutes, using a backward and forward motion or place the slide on a rotator for exactly 2 minutes. Examine each mixture for macroscopic agglutination. Determine the presence or absence of agglutination immediately after the 2-minute mixing period. False positive results may occur after the 2-minute period because of drying effects. The appearance of graininess must not be interpreted as macroscopic agglutination.

10. Interpretation of results (see Table 5–7). The negative and positive control specimens must show no agglutination and agglutination, respectively.

11. If the 1:10 dilution of the patient's plasma shows agglutination, further dilutions of the patient's plasma should be made as described below. If qualitative results only are desired, the result may be reported as >20 μg/mL. If semiquantitative results are desired, continue with this procedure.

12. Label four 10×75 mm test tubes 1:20, 1:40, 1:80, and 1:160. Using the disposable pipet, place 4 drops of glycine buffer into each of the test tubes. Transfer 4 drops of the patient's 1:10 dilution into the test tube labeled 1:20. Mix and transfer 4 drops of the 1:20 dilution to the test tube labeled 1:40. Mix and transfer 4 drops of the 1:40 mixture to the test tube labeled 1:80. Mix and transfer 4 drops of the 1:80 dilution to the test tube labeled 1:160.

13. Label the rings on the glass slide for each of the above dilutions and for the negative and positive control specimens.

14. Place 1 drop of each control serum and 1 drop from each patient dilution onto the appropriate ring on the glass slide. Repeat steps 7, 8, and 9 above and interpret the results as shown in Table 5–7.

Discussion

1. This procedure may also be performed using a urine sample. For the exact procedure, the reader is referred to the Thrombo-Wellcotest package insert.

2. The centrifuged serum sample may be refrigerated for up to 1 week or stored at $-20°C$ for longer periods before performing the test.

3. False-positive results may occur in patients with rheumatoid arthritis (patients positive for the rheumatoid factor).

4. It is suggested that a positive and negative control be run on each slide. When interpreting the results, compare the patient's sample with the positive and negative controls to determine the presence of agglutination.

5. The latex suspension is also capable of cross-reacting with fibrinogen, fibrin monomers, or fibrin polymers that are not completely clotted during the serum preparation step.

6. In the presence of non-clottable fibrinogen (as in dysfibrinogenemia) or inhibitors of fibrin, the test results will be invalidly high.

D-DIMER TEST FOR FIBRIN DEGRADATION PRODUCTS

During intravascular coagulation, thrombin converts fibrinogen to fibrin and activates factor XIII, which stabilizes the fibrin clot

TABLE 5–7.   FIBRINOGEN-DEGRADATION PRODUCTS (Interpretation of Results)

Plasma Dilution	Patient Results (− = no agglutination, + = agglutination)						
1:5	−	+	+	+	+	+	+
1:10	−	−	+	+	+	+	+
1:20			−	+	+	+	+
1:40			−	−	+	+	+
1:80			−	−	−	+	+
1:160			−	−	−	−	+
Results (μg/mL)	<10	10– 20	20– 40	40– 80	80– 160	160– 320	>320

formed. Thrombin also activates the fibrinolytic system with the production of plasmin at the site of the clot. The fibrinolytic action of plasmin lyses the factor XIIIa crosslinked fibrin and produces fibrin degradation products that contain the crosslinked portion called D-dimer. Plasmin will also lyse fibrinogen, which will not, however, produce the crosslinked D-dimer portion.

The presence of crosslinked D-dimer indicates that a stable fibrin clot has been lysed and will be found in pulmonary embolism, deep vein thrombosis, disseminated intravascular coagulation with secondary fibrinolysis, arterial thromboembolism, and sickle cell disease.

The Fibrinosticon procedure described here is a rapid, specific test for the detection of fibrin degradation products (D-dimer portion) in plasma. The normal level of D-dimer in the adult is less than 0.5 μg/mL.

Reference

Organon Teknika Corp.: Fibrinosticon, latex agglutination immunoassay, pkg. insert, Organon Teknika, Durham, NC, 1990.

Reagents and Equipment

1. The following reagents are available from Organon Teknika Corp. All reagents must be refrigerated when not in use.
   a. Latex suspension. Latex particles have been sensitized with anti-D-dimer antibodies.
   b. Buffer solution (glycine buffer).
   c. Positive and negative controls. Reconstitute with 0.5 mL distilled water.

Swirl to mix. Do not shake. Allow to stand for 10 minutes at room temperature. Mix gently before use. Stable for 8 hours at room temperature or for four weeks at 2 to 8°C.
   d. Disposable testing slides.
   e. Disposable mixing rods.
   f. Plastic slide holder.
2. Pipets, 20 and 100 μL.
3. 10 × 75 mm test tubes.
4. Timer.

Specimen

Citrated plasma: 1 part 0.109 M sodium citrate to 9 parts whole blood. This tube should be drawn last during phlebotomy. However, if the D-dimer is the only test being drawn, two tubes should be obtained and the first tube discarded. The plasma is stable for 4 hours at room temperature, 8 hours at 2 to 8°C or for 1 month at −20°C. (Specimens collected in EDTA, heparin, and potassium oxalate may also be used.)

Principle

A dilution of the patient's plasma is mixed with latex particles coated with monoclonal antibodies to the D-dimer (portion of fibrin). If fibrin degradation products containing the D-dimer portion are present, agglutination of the latex particles will occur.

Procedure

1. Centrifuge the specimen as soon as possible after collection to obtain platelet-poor plasma.

or place the slide on a rotator for exactly 6 minutes. Examine each ring for macroscopic agglutination immediately after the 6 minute mixing period. Compare the patient's sample to the positive and negative controls.

10. Interpretation of results: A negative test result will show no macroscopic agglutination. The appearance of very fine brownish specks must not be interpreted as macroscopic agglutination. These are red blood cells. A positive test result will show macroscopic agglutination. The intensity of the agglutination will depend on the amount of SFMC present in the plasma. The following agglutination patterns may be found:
    a. Small agglutinates (clumps) that are evenly distributed.
    b. Large agglutinates that are sparsely distributed.
    c. A large massive clump.

The positive and negative controls must show agglutination and no agglutination respectively.

Discussion

1. Agglutination may occur very quickly in plasma containing high concentrations of SFMC, sometimes immediately after mixing in the tube or immediately after transferring the mixture to the card.
2. Borderline test results showing a faint blotchy appearance should be repeated.
3. The F.S. test may be performed with the positive control tested undiluted, and diluted 1:2 and 1:4 (in distilled water), to demonstrate various agglutination patterns and as an aid in interpretation.
4. Concentration of early fibrin degradation products (fragments X and Y) up to 160 μg/mL and late fibrin degradation products (fragments Y, D, and E) up to 1 mg/mL will not affect this test.
5. Heparin concentrations up to 12.5 NIH units/mL will not affect test results.

ETHANOL GELATION TEST

The ethanol gelation test is designed to detect the presence of fibrin monomers in the plasma. It is a screening procedure to be utilized as an aid in the diagnosis of disseminated intravascular coagulation and in distinguishing this condition from primary fibrinolysis.

Reference

Breen, F.A., Jr., and Tullis, J.L.: Ethanol gelation: A rapid screening test for intravascular coagulation, Ann. Intern. Med., 69, 1197, 1968.

Reagents and Equipment

1. Buffered sodium citrate
   Sodium citrate, 0.11 M, 3 parts
   Citric acid, 0.109 M, 2 parts
   (19.2 g dissolved in
   1 liter of distilled water.)
2. Plastic test tubes, 10 × 75 mm.
3. Disposable dropper pipets.
4. Sodium hydroxide, 0.1 N.
5. Ethyl alcohol, 50%, v/v.
6. Plastic dropper pipets.

Specimen

Citrated plasma: 1 part 0.109 M buffered sodium citrate to 9 parts whole blood. Obtain blood for a normal control at the same time the patient's specimen is drawn.

Principle

During the process of disseminated intravascular coagulation, the level of fibrin monomer (intermediate product of fibrinogen conversion to fibrin) in the blood increases. Sodium hydroxide is added to the plasma to increase the pH to above 7.70. Ethyl alcohol, added to the plasma, will cause precipitation of any fibrin monomers which may be present.

Procedure

1. Centrifuge the specimen as soon as possible after collection to obtain platelet-poor plasma.
2. Into two appropriately labeled 10 × 75 mm test tubes, place 9 drops of patient's plasma and normal control plasma.
3. Add 1 drop of 0.1 N sodium hydroxide and mix tubes gently.
4. Add 3 drops of 50% ethyl alcohol to each

tube. Mix gently and place in a test tube rack at room temperature.

5. At the end of 1 minute, inspect tubes for the presence of a precipitate. Precipitation or gel formation, at this time, generally constitutes a positive test.

6. If the test is negative after 1 minute, allow the test tubes to sit for an additional 9 minutes. At the end of this time, if a precipitate or gel forms, add 1 more drop of 0.1 N sodium hydroxide to the tube and gently mix. If the precipitate formed is nonspecific, it will disappear. Persistence of the precipitate or gel constitutes a positive test.

Discussion

1. A positive control may be prepared and used with this test: Dilute 1,000 NIH units of thrombin (Parke, Davis, and Co. may be used) with 10.0 mL of 0.85% sodium chloride (100 NIH units/mL). Add 1.2 μL of diluted thrombin to 4.0 mL of normal plasma for a final concentration of thrombin (in the plasma-thrombin mixture) of 0.03 NIH units/mL. Incubate mixture at 37°C for 30 minutes. After incubation, carefully remove the fibrin strands present in the mixture, using two applicator sticks. (If there are no fibrin strands present, this most probably indicates that the concentration of the thrombin was not sufficient to begin clotting the fibrinogen and there will, therefore, be no fibrin monomers present.) The resultant plasma should test positive for fibrin monomers according to the above procedure.

2. This test must be performed at room temperature. Temperatures of 37°C inhibit gel formation.

3. The final concentration of ethyl alcohol in the final test mixture should be between 10 and 15%.

4. If the pH of the plasma is below 7.70, precipitation of fibrinogen may occur when the ethyl alcohol is added.

5. Perform test as soon as possible after collection of blood at 4°C for 24 hours does not appear to affect results.

6. The presence of heparin, or contamination with red blood cells, does not alter the results of this test.

PROTAMINE SULFATE

The protamine sulfate procedure is used to detect the presence of fibrin monomers. During the process of coagulation, when thrombin acts on fibrinogen, fibrinopeptides A and B are removed from the fibrinogen molecule, leaving fibrin monomers (which are then free to polymerize and form fibrin). Protamine sulfate detects the presence of fibrin monomers by causing the formation of fibrin strands or gel-like clots (this process is also termed *paracoagulation*). Early fibrin(ogen) degradation products (fragments X and Y) will also form fibrin strands and/or a gel clot in the presence of protamine sulfate.

Under certain pathologic conditions, intravascular coagulation may be stimulated and there will be widespread appearance of fibrin clots in the blood vessels of the microcirculation. Fibrin monomers are, therefore, present in the plasma. Because of the presence of coagulation, there is stimulation of the fibrinolytic system and the formation of fibrin(ogen) split products. Rapid detection of the presence of fibrin monomers is an important aid in the diagnosis of disseminated intravascular coagulation. The presence of fibrin monomers is also associated with pulmonary embolism, cirrhosis of the liver, deep vein thrombosis, and acute thromboembolism.

Normally, there should be no fibrin monomers present in the plasma.

References

Baxter Healthcare Corp.: Data-Fi protamine sulfate reagents, pkg. insert, Dade Division, Miami, FL, 1985.

Niewiarowski, S., and Gurewich, V.: Laboratory identification of intravascular coagulation, J. Lab. Clin. Med., 77, 665, 1971.

Reagents and Equipment

1. The following reagents are available from Baxter Healthcare Corp., Dade Division:
   a. Data-Fi protamine sulfate reagent 0.2% (w/v). Store at 2° to 8°C. Reconstitute with 3.0 mL of distilled water. Once reconstituted, this reagent is stable for 8 hours at 2° to 8°C.
   b. Data-Fi positive monomer control plasma. Store at 2° to 8°C. Reconstitute with 1.5 mL of distilled water

while constantly agitating the vial. If the control is not correctly reconstituted, the fibrin monomers may polymerize and form fibrin strands. If no more than one or two strands form, they may be removed with applicator sticks and the control should not be affected. Reconstituted reagent is stable for 4 hours at 2° to 8°C.

2. Test tubes, 13 × 100 mm and 10 × 75 mm.
3. Pipets, 1.0 and 0.2 mL.
4. Timer.
5. Sodium chloride, 0.85% (w/v).
6. Ice bath.

Specimen

Citrated plasma: 1 part 0.109 M sodium citrate to 9 parts whole blood. Obtain a normal control plasma at the same time the patient sample is obtained. The test should be set up immediately after collection.

Principle

Patient and control plasmas are mixed with varying dilutions of protamine sulfate. Each tube is incubated at room temperature for 30 minutes and then observed for fibrin strand or gel formation. The protamine sulfate causes gel formation of fibrin monomers and/or early fibrin split products when they are present in the plasma.

Procedure

1. Centrifuge the specimen as soon as possible after collection to obtain platelet-poor plasma.
2. Label five 13 × 100 mm test tubes 1:5, 1:10, 1:20, 1:40, and 1:80. Add 1.0 mL of 0.85% sodium chloride to each tube except the tube labeled 1:5.
3. Reconstitute the Data-Fi protamine sulfate reagent and the Data-Fi positive monomer control as outlined previously.
4. Pour the entire contents of the protamine sulfate reagent vial into the tube labeled 1:5. Transfer 1.0 mL of protamine sulfate from the 1:5 tube into the tube labeled 1:10. Mix contents of tube well and transfer 1.0 mL of the diluted reagent to the next tube (1:20). Continue

to dilute the protamine sulfate reagent in this manner (transfer 1 mL of mixture from 1:20 tube to the 1:40 tube, mix, etc.) in order to obtain the 1:40 and 1:80 dilutions. Use a clean pipet for each dilution.

5. Label one set of 10 × 75 mm test tubes 1:5, 1:10, 1:20, 1:40, and 1:80 for each patient and control to be tested. Label each set with the patient's name and/or control type.
6. Pipet 0.2 mL of patient plasma into each tube in the appropriately labeled set. Repeat for the normal and abnormal control.
7. Add 0.2 mL of the appropriate protamine sulfate reagent dilution to each tube of the patient, normal control, and abnormal control. Use a clean pipet for each tube, and mix by forcefully expelling the reagent into the plasma. Do not agitate or mix the tubes any further.
8. Incubate all tubes at room temperature for 30 minutes. Do not disturb the tubes during this period.
9. At the end of 30 minutes, tilt each tube several times and observe for fibrin strands or gel formation. Use of a bright light against a dark background is helpful for reading the results. Report the test as positive or negative for fibrin monomers.
10. The positive fibrin monomer control should show clot or strand formation in the tubes labeled 1:5, 1:10, and 1:20. If it does not, repeat the test, reconstituting another vial of fibrin monomer control and another vial of protamine sulfate.
11. The normal control should show no fibrin strands or gel formation.

Discussion

1. Fibrinogen may at times be precipitated by the protamine sulfate especially in the 1:5 and 1:10 dilutions. This shows up as an amorphous, whitish precipitate which will usually clear upon shaking the tube. Continued tilting of the tubes will cause the precipitate to break up. This should not be interpreted as clot or fibrin strand formation.
2. With positive results, continued tilting of the tubes with fibrin strand formation will

cause the strands to accumulate into larger fibrin clots, while the plasma becomes clear.

3. Due to the sensitivity of this test, a positive result should be evaluated in light of other clinical findings. However, a negative result for this test does not automatically rule out intravascular coagulation since fibrin monomers and early fibrin(ogen) split products may not always be present at all stages of the process.

4. This test procedure is not affected by therapeutic levels of heparin.

5. The ethanol gelation test is easier to perform than the protamine sulfate procedure but may not be quite as sensitive to small quantities of fibrin monomers and early fibrin(ogen) split products. The protamine sulfate test is somewhat quantitative in that the more dilute the protamine sulfate tube showing positive results, the higher the concentration of fibrin monomers and/or early fibrin(ogen) split products.

CLOT LYSIS

The whole blood clot lysis time (WBCLT) tests for increased fibrinolysis. It is used infrequently because of its replacement by more sophisticated procedures able to more accurately evaluate fibrinolysis. This test is only able to detect large amounts of fibrinolytic activity.

The tubes used for the Lee and White clotting time may be used for this test. One of the tubes from the clotting time is left in the 37°C incubator and inspected at the end of 8, 24, and 48 hours for disappearance or degeneration of the clot. A second tube used in the clotting time is placed in the refrigerator as soon as it has clotted, to serve as a control. If the incubated clot becomes fluid in less than 48 hours, the blood is poured out onto a piece of filter paper to be certain the clot has disappeared. If the refrigerated clot is still intact, it may be assumed that clot lysis has taken place in the incubated tube. If the refrigerated clot has also disappeared, the absence of a clot in both tubes may have been due to a fibrinogen deficiency rather than clot lysis. If no lysis occurred in either tube, the results are reported as "no clot lysis after 48 hours."

EUGLOBULIN CLOT LYSIS TIME

The euglobulin clot lysis time is a screening procedure for the measurement of fibrinolytic activity. It is a more sensitive test than the clot lysis time. The euglobulin fraction of plasma contains plasminogen, plasminogen activator, and fibrinogen. Once a clot is formed in the euglobulin portion of the plasma, clot lysis occurs more quickly than in whole blood. Increased fibrinolytic activity has been associated with circulatory collapse, adrenalin injections, sudden death, pulmonary surgery, pyrogen reactions, obstetric complications, and extreme stress (e.g., prolonged exercise).

Normally, clot lysis does not occur in less than 1 hour using the following procedure. Clot lysis in less time is indicative of abnormal fibrinolytic activity.

References

Chakrabarti, M., Bielawiec, J.F., Evans, J.F., and Fearnley, G.R.: Methodological study and a recommended technique for determining the euglobulin lysis time, J. Clin. Path., *21*, 698, 1968.

Baxter Healthcare Corp.: Data-Fi euglobulin lysis reagents, pkg. insert, Dade Division, Miami, FL, 1989.

Reagents and Equipment

1. The following reagents are available from Baxter Healthcare Corp., Dade Division:
   a. Phosphate buffered saline, pH 7.2. Store at 2 to 8°C.
   b. Acetic acid, 1% (v/v). Store at 2 to 8°C.
   c. Buffered bovine thrombin, 100 NIH units/vial. Store at 2 to 8°C. Reconstitute with 2.0 mL distilled water. Solution is stable at 2° to 8°C for 8 hours once it is reconstituted.
   d. Pipets, 25 µL, disposable.
   e. Positive control. Store both reagents at 2° to 8°C. Very unstable once prepared. Reconstitute and prepare immediately before use.
      (1) Plasminogen activator. Approximately 12 USP units of streptokinase/vial. Reconstitute with 1.0

mL of distilled water immediately before use.

   (2) Plasmin control plasma. Reconstitute with 1.0 mL of plasminogen activator immediately before use.

2. Test tubes, 12 × 100 mm.
3. Pipets, 0.1, 1.0, and 10 mL.
4. Water bath, 37°C.
5. Ice bath.
6. Distilled water, 2 to 8°C.
7. Stopwatch.

Specimen

Citrated plasma: 1 part 0.109 M sodium citrate to 9 parts whole blood. Place specimen in crushed ice as soon as it is collected. Obtain a normal control plasma at the same time the patient sample is collected.

Principle

Addition of 1% acetic acid to diluted plasma causes the euglobulin portion of the plasma to precipitate. After removing the supernatant, the euglobulins are dissolved in a buffer solution. Thrombin is added in order to clot the euglobulins. The clot is incubated at 37°C and the time of complete clot lysis is noted.

Procedure

1. Centrifuge the specimen as soon as possible after collection to obtain platelet-poor plasma. The test must be set up within 30 minutes after collection.
2. Prepare sufficient distilled water (6 mL/sample) at a temperature of 2° to 8°C.
3. Label one 12 × 100 mm test tube for each patient specimen and control to be tested.
4. Add 0.5 mL of patient sample, normal control, and positive control to the appropriately labeled tube. Proceed to step 5 immediately.
5. Add 6 mL of cold (2° to 8°C) distilled water to each of the above tubes. Add 0.1 mL of 1% acetic acid to each tube. Mix each tube well, by inversion.
6. Place all tubes in the refrigerator (2° to 8°C) for 10 minutes to allow for complete precipitation of the euglobulins.
7. Centrifuge tubes at 1600 g for 3 minutes.

Do not over-centrifuge. Excessive packing of the euglobulin precipitate makes it difficult to dissolve (step 9) and may prolong the lysis time.

8. Carefully pour off the supernatant from each tube and discard. Invert tubes onto filter paper in a test tube rack. Working with one tube at a time, blot the excess supernatant on gauze several times. Remove all liquid from the inside walls of the test tube with cotton tipped applicators. (The supernatant contains inhibitors to fibrinolysis so it is important to remove all traces of the supernatant.)
9. Add 0.35 mL of phosphate buffered saline solution to each tube. Mix each tube gently. All precipitate must go into solution.
10. Reconstitute the thrombin with 2.0 mL of distilled water. Mix gently.
11. Add 25 µL of thrombin reagent to each tube. Mix the tubes immediately by gentle shaking and place in the 37°C water bath, simultaneously starting a stopwatch. After 30 seconds, verify clot formation by gently tilting the tubes.
12. Check each tube in the incubator at 10-minute intervals for lysis of the clot. When clot lysis begins, check the tube every 5 minutes until lysis is complete.
13. Report results as the time for complete lysis to occur. If the clot has not lysed within 1 hour, report results as greater than 60 minutes. The positive control will completely lyse within about 35 minutes. The normal control should not lyse until after 60 minutes.

Discussion

1. If the patient sample has a fibrinogen concentration of less than 80 mg/dL, fibrinolytic activity will be difficult to measure due to the small size of the clot. In this instance, perform the test making a 1:1 dilution with normal plasma (step #4).
2. When removing plasma from the top of the red cell layer, do not pipet too close to the buffy coat. The presence of platelets will prolong the lysis time due to the antiplasmin activity of the platelets.
3. This test should be set up immediately after collection. The plasma should be kept

on ice at all indicated times in the procedure. Plasminogen activator is very labile, and at room temperature, will decrease in concentration quite rapidly.

4. Fibrinolytic activity will be difficult to measure if the patient has an abnormally low plasminogen level.

CIRCULATING ANTICOAGULANTS (INHIBITORS)

Some coagulation disorders are caused by inhibition of the coagulation mechanism rather than by a deficiency of one of its components. These inhibitors are called circulating anticoagulants and they occur when antibodies are produced against specific components of coagulation as a result of replacement therapy in patients with factor deficiencies. They may also occur in a wide variety of conditions, as a result of administration of certain drugs or spontaneously in the absence or presence of disease.

Inhibitors are usually classified into two categories: *specific* and *nonspecific inhibitors.* Specific inhibitors are antibodies that are directed against specific coagulation factors; they are frequently associated with bleeding. Nonspecific inhibitors include lupus anticoagulants, paraproteins, and fibrinogen degradation products. They are not directed against any single coagulation factor. Lupus anticoagulants are directed against phospholipids and are generally not associated with bleeding.

The two most common inhibitors are those specific for factor VIII and the lupus inhibitor. Circulating anticoagulants are usually detected by the prolongation of the APTT (or PT) test, which is not corrected by the addition of normal plasma.

References

Hardisty, R.M., and Ingram, C.I.C.: *Bleeding Disorders, Investigation and Management,* Oxford, Blackwell Scientific Publications, 1965.

Lenahan, J.G., and Smith, K.: *Hemostasis,* Durham, N.C., Organon Teknika Corp., 1986.

Reagents and Equipment

1. Water bath, 37°C.
2. If the APTT procedure is performed:
   a. Calcium chloride, 0.025 M.
   b. Partial thromboplastin with activator.
3. If the PT procedure is performed:
   a. Tissue thromboplastin reagent.
4. Factor deficient plasma. Factor VIII deficient plasma (if APTT prolonged), factor VII deficient plasma (prolonged PT), or factor X deficient plasma (prolonged PT and APTT). Factor deficient plasma is optional but may be used to serve as an example (control) in cases where a factor deficiency (and not an inhibitor) is present.
5. Owren's veronal buffer.
6. Normal control plasma (must be platelet-poor).
7. Test tubes, 12 × 100 mm.
8. Pipets, 1.0 and 0.1 mL.
9. Stopwatch.

Specimen

Citrated plasma: 1 part 0.109 M sodium citrate to 9 parts whole blood.

Principle

Circulating anticoagulants are usually detected by performing the APTT procedure on different ratios of patient and normal control plasma, at specifically timed intervals. (If the routine APTT is normal and the PT is abnormal, this test is performed using the PT procedure. If both the APTT and PT are abnormal, the test is performed using both procedures.) All results are recorded as indicated on a worksheet similar to the format shown in Table 5–9. In the presence of an inhibitor, there will be little to no correction of the clotting time when the patient's plasma is mixed with normal plasma. If a factor deficiency exists, since only 50% of plasma factors are necessary for normal coagulation times, the clotting time of the patient's plasma will show significant correction when mixed with normal plasma.

Procedure

1. Centrifuge the specimen as soon as possible after collection to obtain platelet-poor plasma. Immediately remove the plasma and proceed to step 2.
2. Perform an APTT (or PT) on the patient's plasma and on a normal control plasma.

TABLE 5–9. EXAMPLES OF A CIRCULATING ANTICOAGULANT AND A [FACTOR DEFICIENCY] USING THE APTT PROCEDURE

Time (min)	8:2 Pt. plasma + nl. ctrl. (sec.)	1:1 Pt. plasma + nl. ctrl. (sec.)	8:2 Factor deficient + nl. ctrl. (sec.)	1:1 Factor deficient + nl. ctrl. (sec.)	Normal Control Plasma (sec.)	Patient's Plasma (sec.)
0	52 [40]	43 [34]	34 [34]	30 [30]	29 [30]	60 [44]
60	60 [41]	49 [35]	38 [37]	33 [33]	30 [31]	
120	70 [45]	54 [38]	41 [38]	36 [35]	32 [32]	

If either or both test results are prolonged, proceed with testing.

3. Label five 10 × 75 mm test tubes and prepare the following mixtures (keep tubes covered when not in use):
   a. 0.8 mL patient plasma + 0.2 mL normal control plasma.
   b. 0.5 mL patient plasma + 0.5 mL normal control plasma.
   c. 0.8 mL factor deficient plasma + 0.2 mL normal control plasma.
   d. 0.5 mL factor deficient plasma + 0.5 mL normal control plasma.
   e. 1.0 mL normal control plasma to serve as the control.
4. Mix tubes gently and immediately perform an APTT (or PT) in duplicate, on the five tubes. Average result and record.
5. Place the 5 tubes in step 4 above, in a 37°C water bath and note the beginning time of incubation.
6. Perform an APTT (or PT), in duplicate, on the 5 tubes after 60, and 120 minutes of incubation. Average results and record.
7. Interpretation of results. To interpret the results of this procedure, compare the clotting times at the different time intervals. It must be kept in mind, however, that as the plasmas incubate, there is normally a slight increase in the clotting times because of some loss of labile components in the plasma. For this reason, attention must be paid to the clotting times of the normal control plasma. Before the clotting times of the patient-control mixture are considered prolonged, the degree of prolongation from the previously run test must be greater than that shown by the normal control plasma. See Table 5–9 for an example of a circulating anticoagulant and a factor deficiency.

   a. Circulating anticoagulant. If an inhibitor is present, the clotting times of the patient's plasma will not be corrected (shortened) appreciably by the addition of normal plasma. Generally, in the presence of an inhibitor, the 8:2 mixture of the patient's plasma and normal control shows no significant correction of the clotting time; the 1:1 mixture may show slight correction. It must be kept in mind, however, that some inhibitors act progressively (factor VIII inhibitors and occasionally lupus inhibitors), and it may be a while before the clotting time of the patient plasma-normal control mixtures show the effects of the inhibitor (a prolonged clotting time). It is, therefore, important to incubate the plasma samples for 60 and 120 minutes and note these results.
   b. Factor deficiency. In the presence of a factor deficiency, the clotting time of the patient plasma samples should be corrected by the addition of normal control plasma.
8. Report results as positive or negative for circulating anticoagulants.

Discussion

1. If the patient's APTT is within 5 to 10 seconds of normal (or the PT within 3 seconds of normal) the results of the test may be difficult to interpret.
2. In cases where the circulating anticoagulant increases with time, the APTT coagulation time may show normal or near normal results on a fresh blood specimen.

PLATELET NEUTRALIZATION PROCEDURE

The platelet neutralization procedure is one of a group of assays used for the detection of the lupus anticoagulant. An increased amount of phospholipid is added to the test system to minimize the effect of the phospholipid-dependent anticoagulant, which then produces a shortened clotting time.

References

Triplett, D.A., Brandt, J.T., Kaczor, D., and Schaeffer, J.: Laboratory diagnosis of lupus inhibitors: A comparison of the tissue thromboplastin inhibition procedure with a new platelet neutralization procedure, Am. J. Clin. Path., 79, 678, 1983.

Lenahan, J., and Smith, K., (eds): Clotters' Corner, Durham, N.C., Organon Teknika Corp., 43, 1986.

Reagents and Equipment

1. Expired platelet concentrate (obtain from the blood bank).
2. Tris buffered saline solution, pH 7.3–7.5.
   Sodium chloride 8.766 g
   Tris(hydroxymethyl) 6.055 g
   aminomethane
   Dilute to 1 liter with distilled water. (Obtainable from Sigma Chemical Co.) Store in refrigerator.
3. Calcium chloride, 0.025 M.
4. APTT reagent (partial thromboplastin reagent containing activator).
5. Sodium chloride, 0.85%, w/v.
6. Normal control plasma.
7. Abnormal control plasma (positive for a lupus inhibitor).
8. Centrifuge tubes, plastic, 50 mL and 15 mL.
9. Test tubes, 12 × 75 mm.
10. Pipets, 0.1 mL.
11. Stopwatch.
12. Waterbath, 37°C.

Specimen

Citrated plasma: 1 part 0.109 M sodium citrate to 9 parts whole blood.

Principle

The patient's platelet poor plasma is mixed with a suspension of ruptured platelets (source of phospholipid), APTT reagent, and calcium chloride. The clotting time is noted and compared with the clotting times of: (1) a similar mixture substituting sodium chloride for the platelets, and (2) an APTT performed on the same plasma sample. If a lupus inhibitor is present, the effects of the anticoagulant will be decreased or bypassed by the freeze-thawed platelets and the clotting time of the patient's mixture (containing the platelet suspension) will be shorter than the clotting times of both the mixture containing the saline and the original APTT.

Procedure

1. Preparation of the platelet concentrate.
   a. Obtain a newly expired unit of platelet concentrate from the blood bank.
   b. Place 15 mL aliquots of the platelet concentrate into 50 mL plastic centrifuge tubes.
   c. Add 15 mL of cold tris buffered saline solution to each tube. Mix.
   d. Centrifuge each tube at 197 × g for 15 minutes to remove any red blood cells present.
   e. Remove the supernatant platelet rich plasma from each tube and transfer to 15 mL plastic centrifuge tubes. Centrifuge at 2500 × g for 10 minutes.
   f. Discard supernatant and resuspend platelets in 5 to 10 mL of tris buffered saline solution.
   g. Centrifuge at 2500 × g for 10 minutes.
   h. Repeat steps f and g above 2 more times so that the platelets have been washed three times.
   i. Remove the supernatant from the final wash and resuspend the platelets in an amount of tris buffered saline sufficient to give a platelet count between 200,000 and 300,000/µL.
   j. Place 1 mL aliquots of the platelet suspension into test tubes, stopper, and place in a freezer at a temperature of −20°C or below. (These platelet suspensions are stable for approximately 1 year stored at this temperature.)
2. Centrifuge patient's plasma as soon as possible after collection to obtain platelet-poor plasma.
3. Remove one tube of the frozen platelet

suspension from the freezer and allow to thaw at room temperature.

4. Perform a routine APTT on the patient's plasma. It should be at least 5 to 10 seconds above the normal range.

5. Prewarm a sufficient volume of 0.025 M calcium chloride at 37°C.

6. Pipet 0.1 mL of APTT reagent into a 12 × 75 mm test tube and place in the 37°C water bath. Add 0.1 mL of patient plasma to the tube. Mix. Add 0.1 mL of the thawed platelet suspension and start a stopwatch. Mix the contents of the tube well and allow to incubate for 5 minutes at 37°C.

7. At the end of exactly 5 minutes, add 0.1 mL of calcium chloride to the tube, simultaneously starting a stopwatch. Tilt the tube back and forth and stop the watch as soon as clotting is detected.

8. Perform the test in duplicate.

9. Repeat steps 6, 7, and 8, for the patient control, substituting 0.1 mL of sodium chloride for the 0.1 mL of thawed platelet suspension.

10. A positive and negative control should also be run with this test. Pooled normal plasma may be used as the normal control.

11. Interpretation of results. In the presence of a lupus inhibitor, the clotting time of the patient's plasma mixed with the thawed platelet suspension should be at least 5 seconds shorter than the patient's control mixture (containing the saline solution in place of the thawed platelet suspension) and also shorter than the original APTT. It may not necessarily correct the APTT completely, however. Generally, the more prolonged the original APTT is, the greater will be the shortening of the clotting time with the thawed platelet suspension. False-positive results may be encountered in patients who are receiving heparin and in patients with factor V inhibitors and factor V deficiency.

Discussion

1. If the patient's plasma is frozen prior to performing this test, it is imperative that there be no platelets present in the plasma. It is advisable to perform a platelet count on the plasma prior to freezing.

2. The prepared platelet suspension must be frozen before use. The freezing and thawing of the platelet suspension causes the platelets to rupture, freeing the phospholipid from the platelet.

3. If a lupus inhibitor is present, it can interfere with the action of heparin in open heart surgery.

4. Use of a positive control is necessary in order to monitor the effectiveness of the thawed platelet suspension.

5. This test may be performed manually, on the Fibrometer or by use of a photo-optical detection instrument. For interpretation of results all tests (including the APTT) should be performed using the same clot detection method.

DILUTE RUSSELL VIPER VENOM TEST

Nonspecific inhibitors of the coagulation mechanism include lupus anticoagulants (LA), which are a member of a family of antibodies directed against phospholipids. The major type of these antiphospholipids is the cardiolipin antibody. LA are usually IgG, IgM, IgA, or a mixture of antibodies that inhibit in-vitro assembly of the prothrombinase complex (factors Xa, Va, Ca^{++}, phospholipids). They inhibit the activation of prothrombin to thrombin, thus interfering with phospholipid dependent coagulation tests (PT, APTT, and dRVVT).

The clinical conditions associated with LA include systemic lupus erythematosis, rheumatoid arthritis, exposure to certain drugs, infections, carcinoma, myeloma, and gynecologic disorders. They may also occur spontaneously in persons with no underlying disease. LA have no anticoagulant effect in vivo and are generally not associated with bleeding (bleeding may occur in patients with other underlying problems). Clinical complications associated with LA include venous and arterial thrombosis, recurrent spontaneous abortions, thrombocytopenia, and dermatologic and neurologic complications.

The presence of LA is confirmed through a variety of test methods. The DVVtest™ procedure described here is one of a group of methods characterized by a decreased amount of phospholipid in the test system (which is sensitive to the effect of the phospholipid-dependent anticoagulant and causes a prolonged clotting time in the test sample). The normal range for this procedure is 30 to 35 seconds, but each laboratory should determine its own normal values.

References

Exner, T., Papadopoulos, G., and Koutts, J.: Use of a simplified dilute Russell's viper venom time (dRVVT) confirms heterogeneity among "lupus anticoagulants," Blood Coagulation and Fibrinolysis, 1, 259, 1990.

American Diagnostica, Inc.: DVVtest™, pkg. insert, American Diagnostica, Inc., Greenwich, CT, 1991.

Reagents and Equipment

1. DVVtest reagent (2.0 mL). Obtainable from American Diagnostica, Inc. Reconstitute with 2.0 mL of distilled water and mix well. Reconstituted reagent is stable for 8 hours at 2 to 8°C or 1 year at −20°C if frozen in plastic tubes immediately after reconstitution. The frozen reagent should be thawed at 37°C. (Repeated freezing and thawing is not recommended.) Different lots of the reagent should not be pooled.
2. Normal plasma control.
3. Abnormal plasma (positive for LA).
4. 12 × 75 mm test tubes.
5. Pipets, 2.0, 0.2, and 0.1 mL.
6. 37°C water bath.
7. Stopwatch.

Specimen

Citrated plasma: 1 part 0.109 M sodium citrate to 9 parts whole blood. Do not use excessively hemolyzed plasma, heparinized plasma or samples with small clots. Adjust the anticoagulant to blood ratio if the patient's hematocrit is <20% or >60%.

Principle

The DVVtest™ reagent is a single vial test reagent containing Russell's viper venom, calcium, and a limited concentration of phospholipid. Russell viper venom in the presence of factor V, phospholipid and calcium will activate factor X and begin the coagulation

mechanism at the point of conversion of prothrombin to thrombin. When this reagent is added to plasma containing a lupus anticoagulant, some of the phospholipid in the test system will be neutralized by the LA, thus limiting the amount of phospholipid available for coagulation and causing a prolongation of the clotting time (compared to normal plasma).

Procedure

1. Centrifuge the specimen as soon as possible after collection to obtain platelet-poor plasma.
2. Remove the plasma from the cells and place in capped plastic tubes within an hour after collection.
3. Pipet 0.2 mL of DVVtest reagent into the appropriate number of 12 × 75 mm test tubes (two tubes for each specimen to be tested) and prewarm for 2 minutes at 37°C.
4. Incubate the patient's plasma for 2 minutes until it reaches 37°C.
5. Add 0.2 mL of prewarmed patient's plasma to the tube containing DVVtest reagent and immediately start a stopwatch.
6. Mix the contents of the tube. Gently tilt the tube back and forth and stop the watch as soon as a clot is detected.
7. Perform each test in duplicate. Paired results should agree within ± 1.5 seconds. Average the two clotting times.
8. Interpretation of results.
   a. If the patient's result is within the established normal range, the patient is negative for LA.
   b. If the patient's result is longer than the established normal range, LA may be present. To confirm the presence of LA, perform the following mixing procedure.
9. Confirmation of LA.
   a. Label two 12 × 75 mm test tubes for each patient specimen.
   b. Prepare a 1:1 mixture of the patient's plasma with a normal control plasma (0.3 mL patient plasma + 0.3 normal control plasma). Mix.
   c. Repeat steps 3 through 7 above testing the patient plasma:normal control mixture.
   d. If the clotting time of the mixture is

not corrected (shortened), a lupus-like inhibitor is most likely present. Calculate the DVVtest ratio to confirm this result:

$$\frac{\text{Clotting time of patient:control mixture}}{\text{Clotting time of control}}$$

e. The DVVtest ratio confirms the presence or absence of LA as follows:
1) A ratio > or = 1.20 is positive for LA.
2) A ratio < 1.20 is negative for LA.

Discussion

1. Prior to freezing, the patient's plasma must be platelet-poor, otherwise some shortening of the DVVtest may occur and produce false negative results. (The lupus inhibitor will be neutralized by the phospholipid [platelets].)
2. Patients with factors II, V, or X deficiencies, or those on oral anticoagulant therapy may show prolonged results that will correct with the mixing procedure.
3. The presence of heparin (> 1 U/mL) in the plasma will interfere with the interpretation of the test because it will yield a positive result.
4. The DVVtest reagent is not sensitive to some lupus-like IgM antibodies. Patients with factor VIII inhibitors >1000 Bethesda units may show slight prolongation of the DVVtest ratio.
5. The DVVtest may also be performed on semi-automated or automated coagulation instruments, however, plasmas tested on these instruments must not be icteric or lipemic.
6. The diagnosis of LA should not be made solely on the basis of the DVVtest results. Several different methods may be used to confirm the presence of lupus-like inhibitors.

INHIBITOR ASSAY

Specific inhibitors of the coagulation mechanism are antibodies that are directed against coagulation factors. They are usually classified under two categories: *Neutralizing* and *non-neutralizing inhibitors*. Neutralizing inhibitors include antibodies to factors V, VIII, IX, XI, and XIII, fibrinogen, and vonWillebrand factor (vWF). They inhibit fibrin formation by attacking the active sites of enzymes or cofactors. Non-neutralizing inhibitors include antibodies to factors VIII and X, prothrombin, and vWF. These bind to the non-active sites of the enzymes or cofactors and form complexes that are rapidly cleared by the body. The clearance of these complexes causes a factor deficiency. The most common specific inhibitors are antibodies to factors V, VIII, and IX. Factor VIII inhibitors are frequently associated with bleeding and are commonly found in some cases of classic hemophilia, immunologic disorders, during and following pregnancy, as an allergic reaction to drugs (penicillin), and in the elderly in whom there is no underlying disease.

The factor VIII inhibitor assay described here may be modified to quantitate inhibitors to factors V and IX. The normal range for this method is <0.5 Bethesda units.

Factor VIII Inhibitor Assay (Bethesda Method)

References

Triplett, D.A., and Harms, C.S.: *Procedures for the Coagulation Laboratory,* American Society of Clinical Pathologists, Chicago, 1981.

Kasper, C.K.: *Progress in Clinical Biological Research,* Alan R. Liss, Inc., New York, 87–98, 1984.

Reagents and Equipment

1. Sodium citrated saline (1 mL of 0.109 M sodium citrate [obtained from several blue top tubes] + 9 mL of saline).
2. Normal pooled plasma (lypholized plasma may not be used).
3. APTT reagents (0.025 M calcium chloride and partial thromboplastin with activator).
4. Factor VIII deficient plasma.
5. Normal and abnormal plasma controls.
6. Owren's veronal buffer.
7. Pipets, 2.0, 1.0, 0.2, and 0.1 mL.
8. Test tubes, 12 × 75 mm.
9. Stopwatch.
10. Water bath, 37°C.

Specimen

Citrated plasma: 1 part 0.109 M sodium citrate to 9 parts whole blood.

Principle

Factor VIII inhibitors may be quantitated by mixing varying dilutions of patient plasma with normal pool plasma (NPP) containing a known amount of factor VIII and then determining how much factor VIII activity was not destroyed by the inhibitor. In the presence of an inhibitor, some or all of the factor VIII activity in the normal pooled plasma of the mixture (patient:NPP) will be inhibited. The mixtures are incubated at 37°C for 2 hours because factor VIII inhibitors are time and temperature dependent. At the end of the incubation period, a factor VIII level is measured in all tubes (patient dilutions and NPP). The "residual" factor VIII activity (that factor VIII activity not destroyed or neutralized by the inhibitor) is determined by comparing the difference between the factor activity of the patient:NPP mixture with that of the NPP. Residual factor VIII activity is converted to Bethesda units based on the definition of: one Bethesda unit of inhibitor inactivates 50% of the factor VIII activity present in 1 mL of normal plasma in two hours at 37°C.

Procedure

1. Centrifuge the specimen as soon as possible after collection to obtain platelet-poor plasma.
2. Label three 12 × 75 mm test tubes 1:2, 1:5, and 1:10 and prepare the following dilutions.
   a. 1:2 to 0.2 mL patient's plasma + 0.2 mL citrated saline.
   b. 1:5 to 0.1 mL patient's plasma + 0.4 mL citrated saline.
   c. 1:10 to 0.1 mL patient's plasma + 0.9 mL citrated saline.
3. Label four 12 × 75 mm test tubes #1 through #4 and prepare the following mixtures using the patient's plasma dilutions from step 2 above.
   a. #1: 0.2 mL patient's 1:2 dilution + 0.2 mL normal pooled plasma.
   b. #2: 0.2 mL patient's 1:5 dilution + 0.2 mL normal pooled plasma.
   c. #3: 0.2 mL patient's 1:10 dilution + 0.2 mL normal pooled plasma.
   d. #4: 0.2 mL citrated saline + 0.2 mL normal pooled plasma. This tube serves as the control.

4. Cap each tube and mix well.
5. Place the four tubes in step 4 above, in a 37°C water bath and immediately set a clock for 2 hours.
6. At the end of 2 hours, prepare a 1:10 dilution of tubes #1 through #4 in Owren's buffer and perform a factor VIII assay in duplicate on these dilutions.
7. Perform a factor VIII assay on the normal and abnormal controls. These controls are used to check the reference curve.
8. Interpretation of results.
   a. Determine the factor VIII activity level of tubes #1 through #4 from the reference curve.
   b. Calculate the residual factor activity for each of the patient:NPP dilutions:

   Residual factor activity (%) =
   $$\frac{\text{Factor activity (Patient tubes \#1/2/3)}}{\text{Factor activity (Control tube \#4)}} \times 100$$

   c. The residual factor activity of the dilution(s) chosen to determine the results must be between 25 and 75% (as close to 50% as possible) in order to calculate the inhibitor concentration. If the residual activity is <25%, repeat the test using a greater dilution of the patient's plasma, i.e., prepare 1:20, 1:40, 1:80 dilutions of the patient plasma:NPP mixture with citrated saline. Perform further serial dilutions as necessary until the inhibitor level is constant. The control tube (#4) must be repeated with each batch of dilutions.
   d. Convert the residual factor activity of each patient:NPP dilution (between 25 and 75%) to a Bethesda unit using Table 5–10.
   e. Calculate the factor inhibitor (in Bethesda units) for each incubation mixture as follows: Dilution correction factor for the patient:NPP mixture of patient's plasma used to determine the residual factor activity (e.g., 1:5 dilution = a factor of 5) × (multiplied by) Bethesda units from Table 5–10 (step c) = Bethesda units of factor inhibitor per mL of plasma.
   f. If there is no inhibitor present, the residual factor activity will be 100%. In the presence of an inhibitor, the residual factor activity is <100%.

TABLE 5–10.   BETHESDA UNIT FACTOR CHART

Residual Factor %	Bethesda Units Factor	Residual Factor %	Bethesda Units Factor	Residual Factor %	Bethesda Units Factor
93	0.10	61	0.70	38	1.40
87	0.20	57	0.80	35	1.50
81	0.30	53	0.90	33	1.60
75	0.40	50	1.00	30	1.70
70	0.50	46	1.10	28	1.80
66	0.60	43	1.20	26	1.90
		41	1.30	25	2.00

Discussion

1. Some inhibitors with complex reactive kinetics appear to contain increasing units of inhibitor when tested at increasing dilutions. If a plasma sample has more than one unit of inhibitor per mL, the sample should be retested until the percent residual factor activity is close to 50. The Bethesda unit for the lowest dilution that gives a residual factor level closest to 50% should be used to calculate the result (Bethesda units).

2. The Bethesda unit may also be used to describe inhibitor activity to porcine factor VIII. The assay is performed as described above with the substitution of porcine factor VIII for normal pooled plasma.

3. The Bethesda assay was primarily intended to be used for the measurement of inhibitors developed in hemophiliacs. It may be modified to titer inhibitors to factors V and IX. When performing a factor V inhibitor assay, incubate the tubes in step 4 for 30 minutes and determine the residual factor V activity. No incubation (or, at most, a 5 minute incubation at 37°C) is needed for factor IX inhibitors. Other types of inhibitors, such as the lupus type, may give erratic results.

5. This method may not detect very weak inhibitors. To detect weak inhibitors, the incubation period should be prolonged at lower temperatures (4°C).

6. The inhibitor unit does not necessarily correlate with, or predict bleeding, because inhibitors vary from patient to patient.

ANTITHROMBIN III

The antithrombin III test presented here is a chromogenic assay. The procedure is outlined here in detail and will be used as a reference for other chromogenic assays presented in this chapter.

Antithrombin III slowly and progressively destroys the activated forms of factors XI, XII, IX and X, kallikrein, and most importantly, thrombin. It is also thought of as a heparin cofactor in that heparin, when present, forms a complex with antithrombin III. The anticoagulant effect of heparin is catalytic, dramatically increasing the inhibitory effects of the antithrombin III. A deficiency may be inherited or acquired. It will be decreased in thrombotic disease, disseminated intravascular coagulation, and liver disease (cirrhosis), and in women taking oral contraceptives or on estrogen therapy. Antigenic levels of antithrombin III may be measured by electroimmunoassay, radial immunodiffusion, and by enzyme linked immunosorbent assay. Functional assays include a neutralization of thrombin method, clotting assays, and chromogenic assays (described below).

The normal range for this method is 85 to 111%, but each laboratory should determine its own normal values.

Reference

Organon Teknika Corp.: Chromostrate™ Antithrombin III Assay, pkg. insert, Durham, N.C., Organon Teknika Corp., 1987.

Reagents and Equipment

1. Chromostrate™ assay kit (Organon Teknika Corp.).
   a. Substrate reagent (H-D-cyclohexyl tyrosyl-L-alpha amino butyryl-L-arginine-paranitroanilide). Reconstitute according to directions. May be stored in the refrigerator for 30 days after reconstitution. This reagent will be preincubated and kept at 37°C during testing.
   b. Thrombin reagent. Reconstitute according to directions. May be stored in the refrigerator for 7 days after reconstitution.
   c. Buffer concentrate (substrate specific), pH 8.7 (caution: contains sodium azide). Dilute 1:10 with distilled water for working buffer solution. Store in refrigerator for up to 30 days after dilution.
2. Chromostrate reference plasma (Organon Teknika Corp.). Reconstitute according to directions.
3. Acetic acid, 50% (v/v).
4. Plastic test tubes, 12 × 75 mm.
5. Plastic pipets, 2.0, 1.0, 0.05, and 0.2 mL.
6. Stopwatch.
7. Normal and abnormal control plasmas.
8. Linear graph paper.
9. Water bath, 37°C.
10. Spectrophotometer, wavelength of 405 nm.

Specimen

Citrated plasma: 1 part 0.109 M sodium citrate or buffered sodium citrate to 9 parts whole blood. As soon as the blood specimen is obtained, the plasma should be removed and placed at refrigerator temperatures. Testing should be performed within 4 hours of sample collection. The plasma may be frozen rapidly and stored for up to 30 days without loss of antithrombin III activity.

Principle

The test plasma containing antithrombin III is diluted in the presence of heparin and incubated with an excess amount of thrombin. During this time, the antithrombin III present in the plasma will neutralize the thrombin by forming an antithrombin III-thrombin-heparin complex. Upon addition of the substrate, the remaining thrombin will catalyze the release of paranitroanilide from the substrate. The amount of paranitroanilide released is then measured spectrophotometrically. It is inversely proportional to the amount of antithrombin III present in the plasma. The optical density of each plasma is read from a reference/calibration curve to determine the concentration of antithrombin III present.

Procedure

1. Centrifuge the patient specimen as soon as possible after collection to obtain platelet poor plasma.
2. Incubate a sufficient quantity of the substrate at 37°C.
3. Preparation of the calibration curve.
   a. Reconstitute Chromostrate reference plasma according to directions on the vial.
   b. Prepare a 1:40 dilution (100%) by adding 0.05 mL of reference plasma to 1.95 mL of working buffer. Prepare a 1:80 dilution (50%) by mixing 1.0 mL of the 1:40 dilution with 1.0 mL of working buffer. Prepare a 1:160 dilution (25%) by adding 1.0 mL of the 1:80 dilution to 1.0 mL of working buffer.
4. Prepare 1:40 dilutions (in duplicate) of the patient and control plasmas: Add 0.05 mL of each plasma to 1.95 mL of working buffer solution.
5. Label three 12 × 75 mm test tubes for each plasma dilution. Two tubes will be used for the test (to be performed in duplicate) and the third tube will be used as the blank.
6. Add 0.2 mL of the plasma dilution to the first test tube and incubate at 37°C for 3 to 5 minutes.
7. Add 0.2 mL of thrombin to the tube, mix, and incubate at 37°C for exactly 60 seconds.
8. Add 0.2 mL of prewarmed substrate reagent, mix, and incubate at 37°C for exactly 30 seconds.
9. Add 0.2 mL of 50% acetic acid to the tube and immediately mix well.
10. Repeat steps 6 through 9 above for each plasma dilution.
11. Prepare the blank for each dilution by

mixing together 0.2 mL of the plasma dilution, 0.4 mL distilled water, and 0.2 mL of 50% acetic acid.

12. Read the absorbance of all samples in the spectrophotometer at a wavelength of 405 nm, against a water blank, using a semi-micro cuvet with a 1-cm light path. Average the absorbance readings for the duplicate samples and subtract the reading of the blank.

13. To determine the percentage of activity of the reference dilution, multiply the percent (1.0, 0.50, or 0.25) by the assay value as assigned for that lot of reference plasma. Plot the 3 points on linear graph paper (O.D. vs. % activity) and draw a straight line which best fits all 3 points.

14. To determine the % activity of antithrombin III for each plasma, refer to the calibration curve.

Discussion

1. Addition of the 50% acetic acid stops the reaction. It is therefore imperative that the tube be mixed well as soon as the acetic acid is added. Once added, the color remains stable for several hours.

2. This procedure may be adapted to kinetic analysis. See the package insert for an outline of this method.

PLASMINOGEN ASSAY

Plasminogen is the precursor of plasmin in the fibrinolytic system. Plasminogen deficiencies may be inherited or acquired. It is decreased during thrombolytic therapy (streptokinase, urokinase, and TPA), fibrinolytic disorders, and liver disease (cirrhosis), and may be decreased in disseminated intravascular coagulation (DIC) when fibrinolysis occurs.

Antigenic levels of plasminogen may be measured by electroimmunoassay and radioimmunoassay. Functional assays include fibrin plate and chromogenic (described below) assays.

The normal range for this procedure is 75 to 128%, but each laboratory should determine its own normal values.

Reference

Organon Teknika Corp.: Chromostrate™ Plasminogen Assay, pkg. insert, Durham, N.C., Organon Teknika Corp., 1987.

Reagents and Equipment

1. Chromostrate™ plasminogen assay kit (obtainable from Organon Teknika Corp.) contains the following reagents.
   a. Substrate reagent, 8 μmoles/vial (H-D-valyl-L-cyclohexyl tyrosyl-L-lysine-paranitroanilide). Reconstitute according to directions. Once prepared the reagent may be refrigerated for up to 30 days at 2 to 6°C. This reagent is preincubated and kept at 37°C during testing.
   b. Streptokinase reagent, approximately 10,000 IU/vial. Reconstitute according to directions. Once prepared the reagent may be stored at 2 to 6°C for 7 days.
   c. Buffer concentrate (substrate specific), pH 7.4. (Caution: contains sodium azide.) Dilute 1:10 with distilled water for working buffer solution. Store in refrigerator for up to 30 days after dilution.

2. Chromostrate reference plasma (obtainable from Organon Teknika Corp.).

3. Acetic acid, 50% (v/v).

4. Verify normal citrate control plasma (Organon Teknika Corp.).

5. Stopwatch.

6. Plastic test tubes, 12 × 75 mm.

7. Pipets, 0.4 and 0.2 mL.

8. Water bath, 37°C.

9. Spectrophotometer (wavelength of 405 nm).

10. Linear graph paper.

Specimen

Citrated plasma: 1 part 0.109 M sodium citrate to 9 parts whole blood. Deliver to laboratory immediately. Testing should be performed within 4 hours of obtaining the specimen. The plasma may also be frozen rapidly and stored for up to 30 days without loss of plasminogen activity.

Principle

The patient's plasma is incubated with an excess of streptokinase reagent. The plasminogen present in the plasma specimen forms a plasminogen-streptokinase complex which possesses plasmin-like activity. When the substrate is added to the plasma-streptokinase mixture, the plasmin-like activity present will release paranitroanilide (pNA) from the substrate. The pNA released is measured spectrophotometrically and is directly proportional to the amount of plasminogen present in the plasma. The concentration of the patient's plasminogen is read from a reference curve.

Procedure

1. Centrifuge the patient specimen as soon as possible after collection to obtain platelet-poor plasma. Place the sample in a capped test tube and place at 2 to 8°C until the test is to be performed.
2. Incubate a sufficient quantity of the substrate at 37°C.
3. Preparation of the reference curve.
   a. Reconstitute Chromostrate reference plasma according to directions on the vial.
   b. Prepare a 1:20 dilution (100% activity) by adding 0.1 mL of the reference plasma to 1.9 mL of working buffer. Prepare a 1:40 dilution (50%) by mixing 0.05 mL of the reference plasma with 1.95 mL of working buffer. Prepare a 1:80 dilution (25%) by adding 1.0 mL of the 1:40 dilution to 1.0 mL of working buffer.
4. Prepare 1:20 dilutions (in duplicate) of the patient and control plasmas: Add 0.1 mL of the plasma to be tested to 1.9 mL of working buffer solution.
5. Test each standard, patient, and control plasma in duplicate, and continue with the procedure as described for the Antithrombin III assay (steps 5 through 13, with the following exceptions:
   a. Substitute streptokinase reagent for thrombin in step 7 and incubate for 3 minutes.
   b. Use the plasminogen substrate instead of the antithrombin III substrate in step 8 and incubate for 1 minute.

Discussion

1. See Antithrombin III procedure discussion points 1 and 2.

PROTEIN C

Protein C is a vitamin-K dependent protein synthesized in the liver. It is present in the plasma in the inactive state as a proenzyme. The activation of protein C is initiated by thrombin bound to thrombomodulin (present on the surface of endothelial cells) in the presence of calcium ions. Thrombomodulin modifies thrombin so that its capacity to catalyze clot formation is inhibited while increasing its capacity to activate protein C. Activated protein C forms a complex with free protein S on the surface of platelets or endothelium. This complex regulates the coagulation processes by neutralizing the coagulation effects of activated factors V and VIII, thus preventing further thrombin formation. Activated protein C will also stimulate fibrinolysis by inactivating plasminogen activator I.

A protein C deficiency may be acquired or inherited, and is associated with an increased risk for recurrent venous thrombosis. Acquired deficiencies are associated with DIC, liver disease, post surgery, oral anticoagulant therapy, vitamin K deficiency, adult respiratory distress syndrome, L-asparaginase therapy, and newborns (especially premature infants). Elevated levels are found in patients with nephrotic syndrome. Protein C levels in adults are independent of age and sex.

Antigenic levels of protein C may be measured by electroimmunoassay, radioimmunoassay, and enzyme linked immunosorbant assay. Functional assays include the chromogenic and clotting assays (described below).

Protein C Chromagenic Method

Reference

Kabi Diagnostica, Coatest® Protein C Assay, pkg. insert, Kabi Diagnostica, Sweden, 1988.

Reagents and Equipment

1. The following reagents are available from Helena Laboratories (distributor for Kabi Diagnostica), Beaumont, Texas.

a. Protein C activator (lypholized venom enzyme from Agkistrodon Contortrix). Reconstitute according to directions. Reconstituted reagent is stable for 1 month at 2 to 8°C or 6 months at −20°C.

b. Chromogenic substrate (pyro-glu-pro-arg-pna HCl). Reconstitute according to directions. This reagent will be pre-incubated and kept at 37°C during the test. Reconstituted reagent is stable for 3 months at 2 to 8°C.

2. Protein C calibrator (American Bioproducts Co.). Reconstitute according to directions. Reconstituted reagent is stable for 4 hours at 20°C and 8 hours at 2 to 8°C.
3. Distilled water.
4. Acetic acid, 20% (v/v) or citric acid 2%.
5. Plastic test tubes, 12 × 75 mm.
6. Pipets 1.0, 0.2, and 0.025 mL.
7. Stopwatch.
8. Normal and abnormal control plasmas.
9. Linear graph paper.
10. Water bath, 37°C.
11. Spectrophotometer, wavelength of 405 nm.

Specimen

Citrated plasma: 1 part 0.109 M sodium citrate to 9 parts whole blood. Plasma is stable for 8 hours at room temperature or 3 months at −20°C.

Principle

Plasma is incubated with the protein C activator. Upon addition of the substrate, activated protein C will catalyze the release of paranitroanilide (pNA) from the substrate. The amount of pNA released is measured by the spectrophotometer and is directly proportional to the concentration of protein C in the plasma. The concentration of the test plasma is read from a reference curve.

Procedure

1. Centrifuge the patient specimen as soon as possible after collection to obtain platelet-poor plasma.

2. Incubate a sufficient quantity of the substrate at 37°C.
3. Preparation of the calibrator.
   a. Reconstitute the protein C calibrator according to directions on the vial.
   b. The undiluted calibrator represents 100% activity. Prepare the 50% standard by adding 0.2 mL of protein C calibrator to 0.2 mL of sterile water (1:2 dilution). The 0% standard is water.
4. Prepare a 1:2 dilution of the patient and control plasmas: Add 0.2 mL of the test plasma to 0.2 mL of sterile water.
5. Label two 12 × 75 mm test tubes for each plasma dilution. One tube will be used for the test and the other tube will be used as the blank.
6. Add 0.025 mL of the plasma dilution to the first test tube and place the tube in the 37°C water bath.
7. Add 0.2 mL of protein C activator and immediately start a stopwatch. Mix tube gently and incubate at 37°C for exactly 5 minutes.
8. Add 0.2 mL of the prewarmed substrate reagent and incubate for exactly 5 minutes.
9. Add 0.2 mL of 20% acetic acid to the tube and immediately mix well.
10. Repeat steps 6 through 9 above for each plasma dilution and blank. To prepare the blank, mix 0.025 mL of the plasma dilution, 0.2 mL distilled water (in place of the protein C activator), 0.2 mL substrate, and 0.2 mL of 20% acetic acid.
11. Read the absorbance of all samples in the spectrophotometer at a wavelength of 405 nm, against a water blank, using a 1 cm semi-micro cuvet. Subtract the reading of each test blank from the absorbance reading of the corresponding test sample. To determine the percentage activity of the reference dilution, multiply the percentage (1.0, 0.50, or 0.0) by the assay value assigned for the lot of protein C calibrator used. Plot the three points on linear graph paper (O.D. vs. percentage activity) and draw a straight line that best fits all points.
12. To determine the percentage activity of protein C for each plasma, refer to the calibration curve. Multiply the values obtained for the 1:2 dilutions by 2.

Discussion

1. Addition of the 20% acetic acid stops the reaction. It is therefore imperative that the tube be mixed well as soon as the acetic acid is added. Once added, the color remains stable for 4 hours.
2. The normal range for this method is 70 to 148% activity, but each laboratory should determine its own normal values.

Protein C Clotting Assay

Reference

Diagnostica Stago: Staclot® protein C, pkg. insert, Diagnostica Stago, Seine, France, 1990.

Reagents and Equipment

1. The following reagents are available from American Bioproducts Co. (distributor for Diagnostica Stago), Parsippany, NJ. Store all reagents at 2 to 8°C when not in use. Reconstitute reagents according to manufacturer's directions. Once made the reagents are stable for 8 hours at 20°C and at 2 to 8°C. The reagents must not be frozen.
   a. Protein C deficient plasma (lypholyzed human plasma without protein C).
   b. Protein C activator (extract of Agkistrodon C. contortrix venom).
   c. Protein C calibrator.
2. Owren-Koller buffer (obtainable from American Bioproducts Co.).
3. Calcium chloride, 0.025 M.
4. Normal and abnormal control plasma.
5. Distilled water.
6. Pipets, 2.0, 1.0, and 0.1 mL.
7. Plastic test tubes, 12 × 75 mm.
8. Stopwatch.
9. Linear graph paper.
10. Water bath, 37°C.

Specimen

Citrated plasma: 1 part 0.109 M sodium citrate to 9 parts whole blood. Plasma may be stored at 20°C for 8 hours, at 2 to 8°C for 2 days, and at −20°C for 1 month. Protein C levels will be decreased in patients receiving oral anticoagulant therapy.

Principle

The amount of protein C present in plasma is related to the degree of correction obtained when diluted plasma is incubated with protein C deficient plasma in the presence of protein C activator. The activated protein C inhibits factors V and VIII, thus prolonging the APTT. The clotting time obtained for each plasma dilution is inversely proportional to the percentage of protein C activity read from a calibration curve (prepared using dilutions of a reference plasma with a known percentage of activity).

Procedure

1. Centrifuge the specimen as soon as possible after collection to obtain platelet-poor plasma.
2. Incubate a sufficient quantity of 0.025 M calcium chloride at 37°C.
3. Preparation of the calibrator.
   a. Reconstitute the protein C calibrator according to directions on the vial.
   b. Prepare a 1:10 dilution (100%) by adding 0.1 mL of calibration plasma to 0.9 mL of Owren-Koller buffer. Prepare a 1:20 dilution (50%) by adding 0.1 mL of calibrator plasma to 1.9 mL of buffer. Prepare a 1:40 dilution (25%) by mixing 1.0 mL of the 1:20 dilution with 1.0 mL of buffer.
4. Prepare 1:10 dilutions of the patient and control plasmas: Add 0.1 mL of the test plasma to 0.9 mL of buffer.
5. Label two 12 × 75 mm test tubes for each plasma dilution (test will be performed in duplicate).
6. Add 0.1 mL of the plasma dilution, 0.1 mL of protein C deficient plasma and 0.1 mL of protein C activator to the first tube. Mix well and incubate for exactly 3 minutes.
7. Add 0.1 mL of prewarmed calcium chloride and immediately start a stopwatch.
8. Gently tilt the tube back and forth and note the time of clot formation.
9. Repeat steps 5 through 8 above for each plasma dilution.
10. Average the results of the duplicate tests.
11. To determine the percentage activity of the calibrator dilutions, multiply the percentage (1.0, 0.50, or 0.25) by the assay

value assigned for the lot of protein C calibrator used.

12. Reference curve: Plot the three points on linear graph paper (clotting time vs. percentage activity) and draw a straight line that best fits all points.

13. Using the average clotting time results, determine the percentage activity of protein C for each plasma from the reference curve.

Discussion

1. The assay linearity range for protein C level by this method is between 10 and 120%. If the protein C level of the patient is expected to be very low, or when a severe deficiency is known to exist, the patient's plasma should be tested using a 1:5 dilution (0.4 mL plasma + 0.4 mL buffer). To obtain the percentage activity, divide the test results read from the reference curve by 2.

2. If the protein C level of the patient is greater than 120%, or greater than the assay value of the 100% standard, the patient's plasma should be tested using a 1:20 dilution (0.1 mL plasma + 1.9 mL buffer). To obtain the percentage activity, multiply the test result read from the reference curve by 2.

3. Heparin in concentrations up to 1 U/mL of plasma will not affect results.

4. Factor VIII levels greater than 250% will cause a falsely decreased protein C level.

5. The normal range for this method is 70 to 140%, but each laboratory should determine its own normal values.

PROTEIN S

Protein S is a vitamin K dependent protein that is found in two forms in plasma. Normally, 60% of the total protein S antigen in plasma is bound to C4b binding protein (C4b BP) (an inhibitor of the complement system). The remaining 40% is found as free protein S, which serves as a cofactor for the anticoagulant effects of activated protein C.

A protein S deficiency may be acquired or inherited and is associated with an increased risk for recurrent venous thrombosis. Acquired deficiencies are associated with oral contraceptives, pregnancy, oral anticoagulants, DIC, liver disease, and diabetes type 1, and in newborns and L-asparaginase therapy. The decreased levels of protein S activity that occur in acute inflammatory disorders are due to increased levels of C4b BP, as an acute phase reactant. Elevations of C4b binding protein will shift the protein S from the free form to the bound form. This shift therefore results in a decrease in both the free protein S antigen and the protein S functional activity. Elevated levels of protein S are found in patients with nephrotic syndrome. Protein S levels in adults increase with age and are lower and more variable in females than males.

Antigenic levels of protein S may be measured by electroimmunoassay, radioimmunoassay, and enzyme linked immunosorbent assay (ELISA) (described below). Functional protein S activity is measured by a clotting assay (also described below). Because of the nature of the protein S system, a deficient state should be determined by assays for total protein S, free protein S, functional protein S and C4b binding protein levels.

The normal range for this method is 70 to 140%, but each laboratory should establish its own normal values.

ELISA Method

References

Diagnostica Stago: Asserachrom® protein S enzyme immunoassay of protein S, pkg. insert, Diagnostica Stago, Seine, France, 1991.

Comp, P.C.: Laboratory evaluation of protein S status, Semin. Thrombosis Hemostasis, *16*, 177, 1990.

Reagents and Equipment

1. The following reagents and supplies are available from American Bioproducts Co., Parsippany, NJ (distributor for Diagnostica Stago). Store all reagents at 2 to 8°C when not in use.

   a. Reagent 1: two strips of 16 wells each coated with specific rabbit antihuman proteins S F (ab')$_2$ fragments sealed in an aluminum pouch. Stable until the expiration date of the kit or 15 days after opening.

b. Reagent 2: a specific rabbit anti-human protein S antibody attached to peroxidase. Prepare just before use. Reconstitute one vial with 8 mL of diluted buffer. Reconstituted reagent is stable for 24 hours at 2 to 8°C.

c. Reagent 3: OPD (ortho-phenylenediamine) substrate. Prepare just before use. Place two tablets in a test tube. Add 8 mL of distilled water. Allow the tablets to completely dissolve. Add 5 μL of 30% hydrogen peroxide directly into the solution and mix well. The OPD/H_2O_2 mixture is stable for 1 hour at room temperature.

d. Reagent 4: concentrated phosphate buffer. Dilute 1:10 with distilled water for working buffer solution: add 6 mL of reagent 4 to 54 mL of distilled water. The diluted buffer is stable for 15 days at 2 to 8°C.

e. Reagent 5: concentrated washing solution. Dilute 1:20 with distilled water for working wash solution: add 16 mL of reagent 5 to 304 mL of distilled water. The diluted wash solution is stable for 15 days at 2 to 8°C.

f. Reagent 6: lyophilized reference plasma. Reconstitute one vial with 0.5 mL distilled water. Reconstituted reagent is stable for 4 hours at 20°C and 12 hours at 2 to 8°C.

g. Reagent 7: 25% polyethylene glycol (also contains sodium azide).

h. Plastic reservoir trays.

i. Asserachrom plate sheet.

j. Asserachrom plate (with wells) and frame (Fig. 5–8).

2. Abnormal and normal control plasma.
3. Sulfuric acid, 3 M.
4. Adjustable multichannel pipet and tips (0.3, 0.2, and 0.05 mL) (Fig. 5–7).
5. Pipets, 10, 5, 2, 1, and 0.005 mL.
6. Hydrogen peroxide, 30%.
7. Plate reader set at 494 nm (Fig. 5–8).
8. Timer.
9. Stopwatch.
10. Distilled water.
11. Test tubes, 10 × 75 mm and 12 × 100 mm.
12. Log-log graph paper.
13. Variable speed mixer (optional) (Fig. 5–9).

Specimen

Citrated plasma, 1 part 0.109 M sodium citrate to 9 parts whole blood. Centrifuge specimen at 2500 × g for 10 minutes. Plasma may be stored at 20°C for 8 hours or for 1 month at −20°C.

Principle

Plasma dilutions containing protein S antigen are incubated in microwells coated with anti-protein S antibody. During incubation, the plasma protein S antigen binds to the anti-protein S antibody by one of its antigenic determinants. The anti-protein S peroxidase conjugate (reagent 2) is added which will bind to the free antigenic determinants of protein S, forming a "sandwich." The bound enzyme peroxidase acts on the substrate, ortho-phenylenediamine (OPD), in the presence of hydrogen peroxide to produce a color change that is directly proportional to the concentration of the protein S antigen present in the plasma.

Procedure

1. Preparation of the calibration curve.
    a. Reconstitute the protein S reference plasma (reagent 6) according to directions.
    b. Prepare a 1:100 dilution of the protein S reference plasma to represent 100% activity: add 50 μL of plasma to 4.95 mL of diluted buffer.
    c. Prepare additional dilutions of the initial 1:100 dilution as shown in Table 5–11.
2. Preparation of the patient and control plasmas.
    a. Prepare the initial 1:100 dilution of each plasma to be tested. (Pipet 50 μL of each plasma into an appropriately labeled tube. Add 4.95 mL of diluted buffer and mix well.)
    b. Prepare a 1:2 dilution of each of the initial dilutions in step 2a above. (Pipet 0.5 mL of each 1:100 dilution into an appropriately labeled tube. Add 0.5 mL of diluted buffer. This constitutes a 1:200 dilution.)
3. Continue with the procedure as outlined for the vWF:Ag, steps 3 through 15 using

TABLE 5–11.   PROTEIN S ELISA DILUTIONS

Protein S level, %	100	50	25	12.5	6.25	0
Protein S reference plasma 1:100 dilution (mL)	1.0	0.5	0.2	0.1	0.1	—
Diluted buffer (mL)	—	0.5	0.6	0.7	1.15	1.0
Dilution factor	—	2	4	8	16	—

anti-protein S peroxidase conjugate in place of anti-vWF-peroxidase conjugate in steps 7 and 8.
4. To determine the percentage activity of the protein S of each plasma, refer to the calibration curve. Read the 1:100 dilution directly from the curve, and multiply the results of the 1:200 dilution by 2.

Discussion

1. See discussion points 1 through 6 in the vWF:Ag procedure.
2. For protein S levels <10%, prepare a 1:20 dilution (0.1 mL plasma + 1.9 mL diluted buffer) and a 1:50 dilution (0.1 mL plasma + 4.9 mL diluted buffer). To obtain the percentage activity, divide the values read from the calibration curve by 5 and 2 respectively.
3. For results higher than the curve (extrapolated values) prepare a 1:4 and 1:8 dilution of the 1:100 initial dilution (Table 5–11). To obtain the percentage activity, multiply the values read from the calibration curve by 4 and 8 respectively.
4. This assay measures the amount of total protein S present in the plasma. To determine the amount of free protein S, follow the procedure outlined below.

Free Protein S

Principle

The protein S bound to C4b BP is removed from the plasma by precipitating with polyethylene glycol. Following incubation with this chemical, the supernatant plasma contains only free protein S, which is then assayed using the same procedure described for the total protein S.

Procedure

1. Obtain an aliquot of the test plasma and use only a frozen normal control plasma assayed for free protein S. (Free protein S does not survive the lyophilization process.)
2. Label three tubes for each plasma and control to be tested.
3. Add 0.3 mL of plasma to each appropriately labeled tube.
4. Add 50 μL of polyethylene glycol (PEG) (reagent 7) to each tube. Mix well on a vortex mixer.
5. Incubate for 30 minutes in a melting ice bath.
6. Centrifuge all tubes at 3,000 × g for 10 minutes.
7. Remove the supernatant plasma and place into appropriately labeled tubes. The supernatant plasma contains the free protein S. Discard the precipitate that contains the C4b BP bound protein S.
8. Using the supernatant plasma, perform the ELISA procedure beginning with step 1 b (preparation of the 1:100 reference dilution).

Discussion

1. Two different lots of control plasmas may be used, one lot as the reference plasma for the calibration curve and the other as the control plasma.

Protein S Clotting Assay

The normal range for this method is 65 to 140%, but each laboratory should determine its own normal values.

Reference

Diagnostica Stago: Staclot® protein S clotting assay of protein S, pkg. insert, Diagnostica Stago, Seine, France, 1991.

Reagents and Equipment

1. The following reagents are available from American Bioproducts Co. Store all reagents at 2 to 8°C when not in use.
   a. Reagent 1: human protein S deficient plasma.
   b. Reagent 2: human activated protein C.
   c. Reagent 3: bovine activated factor V. Reconstitute one vial of each of the above reagents with 1 mL distilled water. Allow to stand at 18 to 25°C for 30 minutes. Mix before use. Reagents are stable for 4 hours at 20°C or 2 to 8°C after reconstitution. Do not freeze.
   d. Thrombo calibrator; reconstitute one vial with 1 mL distilled water. Swirl gently until dissolved and let stand at room temperature for 15 minutes before use. Stable for 4 hours at 2 to 8°C or 20°C after reconstitution. Do not freeze. This plasma is used as the reference plasma for the calibration curve.
   e. Owren Koller buffer.
2. Calcium chloride, 0.025 M.
3. Normal control plasma.
4. Distilled water.
5. Pipets, 2, 1, and 0.1 mL.
6. Plastic test tubes, 12 × 75 mm.
7. Stopwatch.
8. Linear graph paper.
9. Water bath, 37°C.

Specimen

Citrated plasma, 1 part 0.109 M sodium citrate to 9 parts whole blood. Plasma may be stored at 20°C for 8 hours, 2 to 8°C for 2 days, and −20°C for 1 month. Functional protein S levels will be decreased in patients receiving oral anticoagulant therapy.

Principle

The percentage of functional protein S present in plasma is determined by the degree of prolongation of the clotting time obtained when diluted plasma is incubated with protein S deficient plasma in the presence of activated protein C and factor Va. Free protein S in the patient's plasma acts as the cofactor of activated protein C, thus enhancing the anticoagulant effect of protein C on factor Va. The clotting time obtained for each plasma dilution is inversely proportional to the percentage of protein S activity read from a calibration curve (prepared using dilutions of a reference plasma with a known percentage of protein S activity).

Procedure

1. Follow the procedure outlined for the protein C clotting assay with the following exceptions:
   a. Preparation of the Thrombo calibrator (step 3b). Prepare a 1:10 dilution (100%), 1:15 dilution (66.6%) (0.1 mL calibration plasma to 1.4 mL buffer), 1:30 dilution (33.3%) (0.5 mL of the 1:15 dilution + 0.5 mL of buffer).
   b. In step 6, add 0.1 mL of the plasma dilution, 0.1 mL of protein S deficient plasma (reagent 1), 0.1 mL of activated protein C (reagent 2), and 0.1 mL of factor Va (reagent 3) to the first tube. Mix well and incubate for exactly 2 minutes.
   c. In step 11, to determine the percentage activity of the reference dilutions, multiply the percentage (1.0, 0.666, or 0.333) by the assay value assigned for the lot of Thrombo calibrator.

Discussion

1. See Discussion points #1 through #4 in the protein C clotting assay procedure.

BLEEDING TIME

The bleeding time is a screening test for detecting disorders of platelet function and von Willebrand's disease, and is directly affected by the platelet count and the ability of platelets to form a plug. The thickness and vascularity of the skin and the ability of the blood vessels to constrict and retract may also affect test results. The coagulation mechanism, however, does not influence the bleeding time unless there is a severe deficiency present. Prolonged bleeding times will result when the platelet count is lower than 30,000 to 50,000/uL, when the platelets are dysfunctional, in von Willebrand's disease, and following ingestion of aspirin, aspirin-containing compounds, anti-inflammatory drugs, anticoagulants, some antibiotics, and certain other drugs. These medications should not be taken for a minimum of 1 week prior to performance of this test. Drug therapy is the most common cause of a prolonged bleeding time.

Historically, bleeding times were performed using the *Duke method*. In this procedure, the earlobe or fingertip was punctured using a sterile blood lancet. The wound was blotted every 30 seconds until bleeding ceased. This method was not precise or very accurate. The *Ivy method* was an improvement over the Duke procedure and introduced some standardization into the procedure. A blood pressure cuff (inflated to 40 mm Hg) was used to exert a uniform pressure on the blood vessels. Two standardized punctures of the forearm were made using disposable blood lancets. The wound was blotted every 30 seconds until bleeding ceased. This procedure was modified by C.H. Mielke, Jr., who introduced the *template bleeding time*, which utilized a template containing a standardized slit in place of the disposable lancets. A Bard-Parker, or similar disposable, blade was placed in a special handle such that when the template was placed on the forearm, the blade would make an incision having a standardized depth and length. Today, the template has been replaced by several commercially manufactured devices: Simplate (Organon Teknika Corp.) and Surgicutt (International Technidyne Corp.), among others. The Simplate contains a spring-loaded blade within a plastic case (Simplastin II holds a double blade). When activated, the blade springs forward from the housing and makes a guillotine-like cut in the skin. Surgicutt utilizes a slicing action using a surgical blade. It is spring-loaded, and when activated the blade moves forward to the outside of the unit and sweeps across the opening in the bottom of the housing. The blade automatically retracts into the housing after it has made a standardized cut. (There are several different Surgicutts (see Table 5–12).

The normal range for the bleeding time will depend on the device and method used and the angle of the incision (perpendicular or horizontal to the bend of the elbow) and must be determined by each laboratory.

References

Organon Teknika Corp.: Simplate, pkg. insert, Organon Teknika Corp., Durham, NC, 1989.

International Technidyne Corp., Surgicutt, pkg. insert, International Technidyne Corp., Edison, NJ, 1988.

Reagents and Equipment

1. Blood pressure cuff.
2. Bleeding time device. (See Figs. 5–10 and 5–11.)
3. Stopwatch.
4. Circular filter paper.
5. Alcohol prep pads.
6. Butterfly bandage.

Principle

A blood pressure cuff is placed on the patient's arm above the elbow, inflated, and maintained at a constant pressure throughout the procedure. One (or two) standardized incisions are made on the volar surface of the forearm. The length of time required for bleeding to stop is recorded as the bleeding time.

Procedure

1. Locate the area for the bleeding time: The patient's arm should be extended with the volar surface facing upward. Beginning at the middle finger move up the arm in a straight line to 5 cm below the fold of the elbow. This area, in the muscular portion of the volar surface of the forearm, 5 cm below the fold in the elbow, is the standardized test site for the puncture. The area should be free of surface veins, bruises, scars, and swelling. (Shave the area if excessive hair is present.)
2. Cleanse the site with an alcohol sponge and allow to dry.
3. Place a blood pressure cuff on the patient's arm above the elbow. Increase the pressure to 40 mm Hg (or lower for newborns—see #3 under Discussion) and hold

TABLE 5–12.   BLEEDING TIME DEVICES

Device	No. of Incisions	Length/Depth of Incision (mm)	Position of Choice	Age	Example of Normal Range
Simplate Pediatric	1	3.0 × 0.5	Perpend./ Parallel	Pediatric	1.6–6.8 min.
Simplate	1	5.0 × 1.0	Parallel		2.3–9.5 min.
Simplate II	2	5.0 × 1.0	Parallel		2.3–9.5 min.
Surgicutt	1	5.0 × 1.0	Parallel	>15 years	1.6–8.0 min.
Surgicutt 2	2	5.0 × 1.0	Parallel	>15 years	1.6–8.0 min.
Surgicutt Newborn	1	2.5 × 0.5	Perpend.	Newborn to 4 mo.	51–99 sec.
Surgicutt Jr.	1	3.5 × 1.0	Parallel	5 mo. to 15 yrs.	1.3–9.0 min.

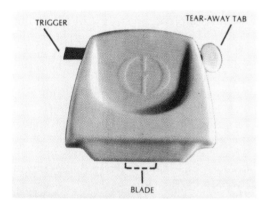

FIG. 5–10. Simplate bleeding time device.

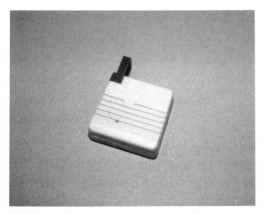

FIG. 5–11. Surgicutt bleeding time device.

this exact pressure for the entire procedure. The incision must be made and the bleeding time started within 30 to 60 seconds (within 30 seconds for infants) after the blood pressure cuff has been inflated.

4. Prepare the bleeding time device. Position it in the correct direction and appropriate area on the arm, using only that amount of downward pressure so that both ends are touching the skin and the device does not cause an indentation. (If too much pressure is applied and the device depresses the skin, the incision will be too deep.)

5. Activate the trigger and start the stopwatch. Remove the device approximately 1 second after making the incision.

6. Blot the blood from the puncture site on a clean section of circular filter paper every 30 seconds. The filter paper must not touch the wound at any time.

7. When bleeding ceases, stop the watch and release the blood pressure cuff. Record the results.

8. Place a butterfly bandage over the puncture site, and advise the patient to keep the bandage in place for 24 hours.

Discussion

1. There is minimal to no scarring at the incision site using the above described devices and procedure.

2. The *aspirin tolerance test* may be useful in

helping to distinguish functionally abnormal platelets from normal platelets: Bleeding times are performed before and 2 hours following the ingestion of 650 mg of aspirin. The bleeding time after aspirin ingestion is usually slightly longer. In von Willebrand's disease, however, the bleeding time after aspirin ingestion will be more markedly prolonged.

3. When performing a bleeding time on infants using Surgicutt Newborn, the blood pressure cuff should be maintained at 20 mm Hg for children weighing less than 2 pounds, at 25 mm Hg for body weights between 2 and 4 pounds, and at 30 mm Hg when the infant weighs over 4 pounds.

4. The incision must be made consistently in the same direction, either parallel or perpendicular to the elbow. A horizontal incision may give a longer bleeding time, although it is considered to be more sensitive in detecting abnormalities, and is, therefore, the method of choice. When performing a bleeding time on infants of 4 months and younger, the incision should be perpendicular to the elbow crease because of the size and vasculature of the arm.

TOURNIQUET TEST (CAPILLARY FRAGILITY TEST)

The tourniquet test is a crude measure of capillary fragility. Because platelets function to maintain capillary integrity, the degree of thrombocytopenia will correlate with the tourniquet test, as will the bleeding time. In normal patients, none to very few petechiae are formed during this test. (Petechiae are minute hemorrhages under the skin and appear as small bruises.) A positive tourniquet test (presence of numerous petechiae) will be found in thrombocytopenia, decreased fibrinogen and in vascular purpura.

References

Cartwright, G.E.: *Diagnostic Laboratory Hematology,* New York, Grune & Stratton, Inc., 1963.

Sirridge, M.S., and Shannon, R.: *Laboratory Evaluation of Hemostasis,* 3rd Ed., Philadelphia, Lea & Febiger, 1983.

Reagents and Equipment

1. Stethoscope.
2. Blood pressure cuff.

Principle

An inflated blood pressure cuff on the upper arm is used to apply pressure to the capillaries for 5 minutes. The arm is then examined for petechiae.

Procedure

1. Examine the forearm, hand, and fingers to make certain no petechiae are present. Apply a blood pressure cuff on the upper arm above the elbow, and take a blood pressure reading.

2. Inflate the blood pressure cuff to a point halfway between the systolic and diastolic pressures. (However, never exceed a pressure of 100 mm Hg.) Maintain this pressure for 5 minutes.

3. Remove the blood pressure cuff and wait 5 to 10 minutes before proceeding.

4. Examine the forearm, hands, and fingers for petechiae. Disregard any petechiae within $\frac{1}{2}$ inch of the blood pressure cuff because this may be due to pinching of the skin by the cuff.

5. The test results may be graded roughly as follows:
   1+ = A few petechiae on the anterior part of the forearm.
   2+ = Many petechiae on the anterior part of the forearm.
   3+ = Multiple petechiae over the whole arm and back of the hand.
   4+ = Confluent petechiae on the arm and back of the hand.

Discussion

1. An alternative procedure uses the inflated blood pressure cuff at a pressure of 80 mm Hg, regardless of the patient's blood pressure.

2. The test should not be repeated on the same arm within 7 days.

3. Normally, there will be 0 to occasional petechiae present.

CLOT RETRACTION

When blood coagulation is complete, the clot normally undergoes retraction (serum is expressed from the clot, and the clot becomes denser). In the past, this procedure has been used as a screening test for platelet function. With the advent of more sophisticated tests for platelet function, however, this test is used infrequently. Normal clot retraction requires a normal number of functioning platelets, calcium, ATP, and a normal fibrinogen level. There must also be normal interaction of the platelets with fibrinogen and fibrin.

An abnormal clot retraction time is found in Glanzmann's thrombasthenia and thrombocytopenia (platelet count less than 100,000/μL). In dysfibrinogenemia or hypofibrinogenemia the formed clot will be small and there will be increased amounts of red blood cells expressed from the clot (*RBC fallout*). Clot retraction may also be abnormal in paraproteinemias (e.g., multiple myeloma) where the proteins interfere with fibrin formation. In disseminated intravascular coagulation, the formed clot will appear small and ragged, and there will be increased RBC fallout. In blood containing a high red cell count, the degree of retraction is limited because of the large volume of red blood cells within the clot. In anemic states, the reverse occurs, and the degree of clot retraction is increased.

Normally, clot retraction begins within 30 seconds after the blood has clotted. At the end of 1 hour, there should be appreciable clot retraction with most retraction occurring within the first 4 hours. Clot retraction should be complete within 24 hours.

Reference

Cartwright, G.E.: *Diagnostic Laboratory Hematology,* New York, Grune & Stratton, Inc., 1963.

Reagents and Equipment

1. Water bath, 37°C.
2. Glass test tubes, 13 × 100 mm.

Specimen

One of the tubes containing 1 mL of whole blood, used in the Lee and White clotting time, or 3 mL of whole fresh blood, placed in a 13 × 100 mm glass test tube.

Principle

Fresh whole clotted blood is placed in a 37°C water bath and inspected at 1, 2, 4, and 24 hours for the presence of a retracted clot.

Procedure

1. If a Lee and White clotting time was not performed, obtain 3 mL of blood and dispense carefully into a 13 × 100 mm glass test tube.
2. Place the test tube of blood in the 37°C water bath and allow the blood to clot. If a Lee and White clotting time was performed, use one of the three tubes of blood.
3. As soon as the blood has clotted, inspect the clot at 1, 2, 4, and 24 hours for the formation of a retracted clot. Generally, there is a small amount of red blood cell fallout during clot retraction. This is seen as a few red blood cells at the bottom of the tube that have fallen from the clot. Normally, the clot will retract from the walls of the test tube until the red blood cell mass occupies approximately 50% of the total volume of blood in the tube. In abnormal states, there may be variable degrees of retraction or no retraction at all.
4. Results are reported as the length of time it took for the clotted blood to retract. As an alternative method, the results may be reported as normal, if clot retraction has occurred at 2 to 4 hours; poor, if retraction occurs after 4 hours and within 24 hours; and none, if no retraction occurs after 24 hours.

PLATELET AGGREGATION

During primary hemostasis platelets clump (aggregate) at the site of injury. Adenosine diphosphate (ADP), derived from injured tissues, red blood cells, or the platelets themselves are responsible for platelet aggregation. There are various reagents which will normally cause the platelets to aggregate and/or release ADP. When platelet dysfunction is suspected, platelet aggregation studies should be performed in which the platelets are exposed to various aggregating reagents and the platelet response noted.

Reference

Bio/Data Corp.: *Operating Instructions and Methods Manual, Platelet Aggregation Profiler® Model PAP-4*, Hatboro, Pa., Bio/Data Corp., 1985.

Reagents and Equipment

1. Platelet aggregation reagents: ADP, epinephrine, collagen, arachidonic acid, and ristocetin. (Available from Bio/Data Corp. individually, or, as Par/Pak II [contains only ADP, epinephrine, and collagen].) Reconstitute vials according to manufacturer's directions.
2. Bio/Data Platelet Aggregation Profiler Model PAP-4.
3. Cuvets, 8.75 mm × 50 mm (Bio/Data Corp.).
4. Plastic pipets, 1.0, 0.5, and 0.05 mL.
5. Plastic test tubes, 12 × 75 mm with caps.
6. Magnetic stir rods (Bio/Data Corp.).

Specimen

All specimens must be drawn using a plastic syringe. Obtain 9 mL of whole blood and immediately transfer to a plastic test tube containing 1.0 mL of 0.109 M sodium citrate. Mix contents of tube well. Collect a specimen of blood from a normal control in the same manner and at the same time the patient's blood is obtained.

Principle

Platelet rich plasma (PRP) is placed in the test well of the platelet aggregometer. An aggregating reagent is added to the PRP and, at the same time, the optical density of the sample is monitored. As the platelets in the plasma clump (aggregate) the plasma becomes more clear and light transmittance through the specimen increases. These changes in optical density are recorded by the instrument in the form of a graph. The aggregometer also calculates the slope of the aggregation curve and the amount (%) of platelet aggregation.

Procedure

1. Turn the instrument on. When the instrument is first turned on, the display will read INSTRUMENT NOT READY. In 8 to 10 minutes the incubation block will reach 37°C, and the temperature indicator will light. The display will then read READY for each of the four channels.
2. Preparation of the platelet rich plasma (PRP) and platelet poor plasma (PPP) specimens.
   a. Prepare the patient and control plasmas in the same manner.
   b. Centrifuge each specimen at 150 × g for 5 minutes (at room temperature). Examine the platelet rich plasma. If any red blood cells are present, recentrifuge the specimen at the same speed for an additional 5 minutes.
   c. Remove the supernatant PRP and place in a covered plastic tube at room temperature. (Specimens should be capped at all times to prevent pH changes due to loss of CO_2.)
   d. Centrifuge the original blood specimen at 1500 × g for 15 minutes. Transfer the PPP to a test tube and cover.
   e. Perform a platelet count on the PRP. The count should be between 200,000 and 300,000/μL. Using the PPP adjust the platelet count of the PRP to this level.
   f. The PRP specimen should be at room temperature for at least 30 minutes prior to testing.
3. Prepare the aggregating reagents (ADP, epinephrine, collagen, ristocetin, and/or arachidonic acid) according to the manufacturer's directions.
4. Pipet 0.5 mL of PPP into a 8.75 × 50 mm aggregometer cuvet. Place a magnetic stir bar into 1 to 4 aggregometer cuvets, depending on how many channels and aggregation reagents are to be utilized for testing. Pipet 0.45 mL of PRP into each cuvet.
5. Place one or more of the PRP cuvets into the wells of the incubation block for approximately 2 minutes.
6. Set the 100% baseline: Place the PPP cuvet into the first test well. Depress the appropriate channel operation switch one time. When the display reads PPP SET, remove the cuvet. Repeat this procedure for the other three channels if they are to be used.
7. Set the 0% baseline: Insert the patient's PRP cuvet into each test well to be used.

Depress each channel operation switch one time. The display should read 0%. (If the display reads LO RANGE or HI RANGE, however, this indicates that the difference in the optical densities of the PRP and PPP are not greater than 5% and/ or less than 95%, respectively. The platelet count on the plasma specimens should be rechecked and/or the specimens reprepared. The procedure must then be repeated beginning with step 4 above.) (If the display reads STIR BAR, after the channel operation switch was pressed, add the stir bar and repeat the procedure beginning with step 4 above.) Wait 1 minute before adding reagents in order to detect spontaneous aggregation.

8. Perform the platelet aggregation test: Add 0.05 mL of the reagent directly into the PRP cuvet in the first test well. At the termination of the test, press the appropriate channel operation switch. Repeat this step for each channel being used. When testing has been terminated in each channel, the printer will print the percent aggregation and slope for each channel.

9. Interpretation of results.
   a. Description of printout from aggregometer.
      (1) One-minute intervals are printed along the bottom of the paper. Each 1 minute is divided into 15-second intervals by dotted lines. Each dot represents 5 seconds.
      (2) Every 30 seconds the appropriate test channel number is printed out on the form.
      (3) Every 4 minutes the 0 to 100% aggregation scale is printed. Each dotted line represents 10% while each dot represents 2%.
      (4) At the conclusion of each test, the percent aggregation and slope are calculated by the instrument and printed out as part of the report. A section is also made available for comments.
   b. *Primary phase aggregation* is the initial response of the platelets to the aggregation reagent. *Secondary phase aggregation* is additional platelet aggregation caused by the release of ADP from the platelets themselves. The *slope* is a number which represents the rate at which platelet aggregation occurs. The *percent aggregation* is a measurement of the extent of platelet aggregation.

   c. Patterns of platelet aggregation (Figs. 7–62 and 7–63).
      (1) Using optimal concentrations of ADP (between 2×10^{-5} M and 5×10^{-6} M), normal platelet aggregation occurs in two waves. The primary wave is caused by the addition of the ADP reagent and the secondary wave by ADP released from the platelets themselves. The secondary wave, however, begins prior to completion of the first wave and the resultant pattern appears as one large wave of aggregation. Abnormalities in ADP induced platelet aggregation will be found in the presence of aspirin, in aspirin-like release defects, afibrinogenemia, uremia, storage pool disease, and thrombasthenia.
      (2) Epinephrine normally causes two waves of irreversible platelet aggregation. However, a small percent of normal people will show only a single wave of aggregation with this reagent. Abnormalities in platelet response to epinephrine will be found in patients with thrombasthenia, uremia, and storage pool disease.
      (3) Collagen will normally cause a single wave of aggregation following a short lag and shape change period (as the platelets adhere to the soluble collagen fibrils). Abnormal collagen induced aggregation is found in aspirin-like release defects, storage pool disease, thrombasthenia, and uremia.
      (4) Arachidonic acid will normally produce a single wave of platelet aggregation. Aspirin is a strong inhibitor of this reagent and its effects on platelet aggregation will last up to 8 days after ingestion. If a patient's platelets show no aggregation with this reagent, the drug status of the patient should be closely examined. In the absence of aspirin effects, abnormal

platelet aggregation with this reagent will be found in thrombasthenia.

(5) Ristocetin induced platelet aggregation normally occurs rapidly with no visible distinction shown between primary and secondary waves. (This is the basis of the von Willebrand Factor Assay procedure [Bio/Data Corp.].) Large platelet clumps are generally formed during the aggregation process. Platelet aggregation with ristocetin is decreased in patients with von Willebrand's syndrome and Bernard-Soulier syndrome.

Discussion

1. To stop a test before its conclusion, press the channel operation switch. Only that channel will be affected.
2. For micro volume testing, 0.2 mL PPP and PRP samples are used in place of the routine 0.5 and 0.45 mL volumes and 0.02 mL of reagent is utilized (instead of the 0.05 mL volume). The test is performed in the same manner as previously described, except that a micro volume adapter is used in the test well, 7.5 × 55 mm cuvets are needed, a micro magnetic stir bar is used, and the micro-volume switch on the aggregometer is activated.
3. To recall the previously run results from the instrument's memory, all channels must be in the READY position, as shown on the display. Press the memory switch. NO PRINT should appear on the display in each channel. Press the channel operation switch for each channel to be recalled. PRINT should appear on each channel's display. (If the oscillations are to be filtered out, press the appropriate trace filter switches.) Press the memory switch a second time. The printer will automatically begin printing and will label the form PRINT FROM MEMORY. The percent aggregation and slope will be printed for each channel activated.
4. This instrument has a diagnostic mode, which is used to determine proper functioning of the instrument. The procedure for entering this mode and performing the tests is clearly outlined in the instrument's operations manual.
5. The magnetic stir motor in each channel turns on when PPP SET appears on the display. It shuts off at the end of the aggregation step. If the test is left unattended for a period of time, the stir bar motor will automatically shut off after 2 hours.
6. The normal range for platelet aggregation should be established by each laboratory. Studies have shown that ADP, arachidonic acid, epinephrine, collagen, and ristocetin normally cause 60 to 90% platelet aggregation in normal donors. The lag phase using collagen is about 1 minute, but when arachidonic acid is used, platelet aggregation should begin within the first 30 seconds.
7. The platelet aggregation procedure should not be performed on any patient who has ingested aspirin within 8 days prior to the test. Aspirin inhibits platelet aggregation and would, therefore, mask any qualitative platelet defect present. Other compounds which inhibit platelet aggregation are antihistamines, alcohol, cocaine, tricyclic antidepressants, dipyridamole, and nonsteroidal anti-inflammatory agents.
8. In most cases of von Willebrand's disease, the platelets fail to show aggregation with ristocetin but do aggregate with the other reagents.
9. Testing must be complete within 3 hours of blood collection. Hemolysis or excessive lipemia will interfere with test results.

PLATELET ADHESIVENESS TEST

One of the functions of platelets is their participation in hemostasis, where they adhere to each other and to the walls of damaged blood vessels to form a hemostatic plug. The adhesiveness of blood platelets may be measured in vitro by their ability to adhere to glass surfaces. Decreased test results are found in Glanzman's thrombasthenia, von Willebrand's disease, Chediak-Higashi syndrome, in some cases of myeloproliferative disorders, uremia, and following ingestion of aspirin and other drugs. Increased platelet adhesiveness has been reported in venous thrombosis, pulmonary embolism, carcinoma, during pregnancy, following splenectomy, and in patients taking oral contraceptives.

The normal values for the test as described below is 26 to 60% platelet adhesiveness. However, it is important that each laboratory determine its own normal range because of the number of variables in the procedure, and the fact that small differences in technique affect test results.

Salzman Method

References

Lenahan, J.G., and Smith, K.: *Hemostasis,* Durham, N.C., Organon Teknika Corp., 1985.

Salzman, E.W.: Measurement of platelet adhesiveness, a simple in vitro technique demonstrating an abnormality in von Willebrand's disease, J. Lab. Clin. Med., *62,* 724, 1963.

Reagents and Equipment

1. A double ended, 20 gauge, Vacutainer needle.
2. Hypodermic needle, 20 gauge.
3. Vacutainer holder.
4. Vacutainer tubes (2) containing EDTA anticoagulant.
5. Siliconized ML-ML adapter, obtainable from Becton-Dickinson Co. (#3113).
6. Siliconized 3200 A adapter, obtainable from Becton-Dickinson Co.
7. Polyvinyl tubing (inner diameter of 0.113 inch). (Obtainable from Insultab, Inc., 252 Mishawuum Rd., Woburn, Ma., 01802.)
8. Glass beads, obtainable from Potter's Industries, Hasbrouck Heights, N. J. (#P-0170).
9. Siliconized nylon mesh, with openings of 0.002 inch. (Nylon stocking material may be used, but must first be washed in 10% silicone solution and allowed to dry.)
10. Duco cement.
11. Materials necessary for two platelet counts.
12. Glass bead filter.
    a. Cut two pieces of siliconized nylon mesh to fit exactly over the ends of the two siliconized adapters.
    b. Using Duco cement, glue a piece of the nylon mesh to one end of each of the adapters.
    c. Attach one end of the polyvinyl tubing to that end of the adapter to which the nylon mesh is glued (Fig. 5–12).
    d. Fill the polyvinyl tubing with 3.3 g of glass beads.
    e. After packing the glass beads into the tube, cut the tubing. Allow a little extra unfilled tubing to remain to fit over that end of the second adapter which contains the nylon mesh. (The degree of packing of the glass beads and, therefore, the length of the polyvinyl tubing should be such that it takes 40 to 50 seconds for the blood to be collected through this system. It is advisable to pack the glass beads by passing an electric vibrator one time along the plastic column as soon as it is filled with beads.)

Specimen

One tube of whole blood collected by routine procedure, using the Vacutainer assembly with a 20-gauge needle and drawing the blood directly into an EDTA vacuum tube. A second specimen of blood is collected through the glass bead collecting system directly into an EDTA vacuum tube.

Principle

A platelet count is performed on both specimens of blood. The number of platelets in the blood, collected through the glass bead collecting system, will be lower than the number obtained by routine venipuncture. This is because platelets have adhered to the column of glass beads due to their adhesive characteristics. The results of this procedure are expressed as the percentage of platelets retained in the glass bead column.

Procedure

1. Perform two clean venipunctures at separate sites, with and without the use of the glass bead collecting system. (The blood collection rate through the glass

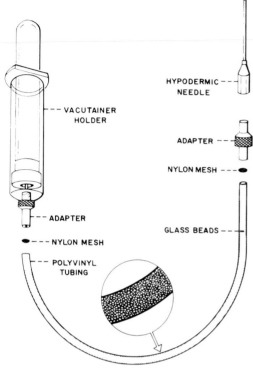

FIG. 5-12. Salzman glass bead collecting system.

bead column should be 6 to 10 mL/minute.)

2. Perform a platelet count on both blood samples.
3. Calculate the percent of platelet adhesiveness as shown below:

% Platelet adhesiveness =

$$\frac{\text{Plt. count without glass beads} - \text{Plt. count with glass beads}}{\text{Plt. count without glass beads}} \times 100$$

Discussion

1. If the glass beads are siliconized, there will be no platelet adhesion.
2. Heparin therapy does not interfere with platelet adhesiveness.
3. It is felt that calcium ions are necessary for platelet adhesion under the conditions of this test. For this reason, the blood passes through the filter system prior to being anticoagulated.
4. This test is difficult to standardize and the results are affected by the rate at which the blood flows through the glass bead column, the length of this column, the size of the glass beads, the hematocrit, and the fragility of the red blood cells.
5. A modification of this procedure may be utilized to produce more standardized and reproducible results. Use of a constant flow syringe pump provides a constant rate of blood flow through the column. Whole blood is collected and anticoagulated with heparin. Part of this whole blood is then drawn through the glass bead column at a constant preset rate by means of an infusion pump and is collected in a tube containing EDTA. Platelet counts are then determined on the whole blood sample drawn through the glass bead column and on the blood sample not drawn through the column. The percent of platelet adhesiveness is calculated as previously outlined. (An infusion pump, Model #901, is obtainable from Harvard Apparatus Company, South Natick, Ma.)

HEPARIN ASSOCIATED THROMBOCYTOPENIA TEST (HATT Test)

The intravenous or subcutaneous administration of heparin may induce thrombocytopenia in some patients. A mild form of thrombocytopenia may be observed in most patients immediately after heparin infusion. The reduction in the platelet count is believed to be due to a non-immune mechanism and has little clinical significance. The thrombocytopenia usually resolves itself spontaneously even in the presence of continued heparin therapy.

A more severe form of thrombocytopenia may be observed in some patients as a delayed, persistent reduction in the platelet count (dropping less than 100,000/μL). This form of thrombocytopenia is believed to be immune mediated and is associated with arterial and venous thrombosis. The thrombocytopenia is resolved only with the discontinuation of heparin. Heparin induced thrombocytopenia has been observed with bovine lung, porcine intestinal, and low molecular weight heparins. It may be demonstrated in the laboratory by the detection of a heparin-dependent platelet aggregating factor in the patient's plasma. This factor is absent in normal blood.

References

Hermelin, L.I.: Heparin-induced thrombocytopenia. Diagnosis and confirmation, Am. Clin. Products Review, 1984.

Feffer, S.E., Carmosino, L.S., Lin, J.H., and Fox, R.S.: In-vitro detection of heparin-induced humoral antiplatelet activity. Southern Med. J., 79, 315, 1986.

Reagents and Equipment

1. Platelet aggregometer and cuvets.
2. Heparin (same type the patient has been receiving).
3. Sodium chloride, 0.85% w/v.
4. ADP (2×10^{-4} M). Prepare according to manufacturer's directions.
5. Plastic pipets, 1.0, 0.2, 0.1, and 0.05 mL.
6. Plastic test tubes, 10 × 75 mm.

Specimen

Citrated plasma: 1 part 0.109 M sodium citrate to 9 parts whole blood. Obtain a 10 mL specimen. Blood must be collected after the discontinuation of heparin (preferrably 24 hours after the last administration of heparin). Obtain a specimen of blood from a type O donor who has not had aspirin or aspirin containing compounds within 8 days, in the same manner and at the same time the patient's blood is collected.

Principle

Patient's plasma is incubated with platelet rich plasma from a normal control in the presence of heparin. The degree of platelet aggregation observed is measured by an aggregometer and compared to the aggregation obtained in the absence of heparin (saline substitution). If the heparin induced antibody is present, platelet aggregation will occur in the presence of heparin.

Procedure

1. Turn the platelet aggregometer on and allow it to reach 37°C.
2. For preparation of the platelet rich plasma (PRP) and platelet poor plasma (PPP) specimens, see the platelet aggregation procedure, step 2 (a through f).
3. Prepare the aggregating reagents:
   a. Heparin working solution (10 U/mL).
   Dilute the appropriate type of heparin to a concentration of 10 U/mL using 0.85% sodium chloride.
   b. Prepare ADP (2×10^{-4}) according to manufacturer's directions.
4. Confirm the activity of the donor platelets with ADP.
   a. Preparation of the aggregometer blank: Pipet 0.5 mL of control PPP into an aggregometer cuvet. This blank may be used throughout the procedure.
   b. Place a stir bar into a second aggregometer cuvet and pipet 0.45 mL of normal control PRP into the cuvet.
   c. Place the cuvet (in step b above) into the well of the incubation block for approximately 2 minutes.
   d. Set the 100% baseline using the aggregometer blank prepared in step a above.
   e. Set the 0% baseline using the donor PRP prepared in step b above. As soon as the 0% baseline is stable, add 0.05 mL of ADP directly into the cuvet. Do not allow the reagent to touch the sides of the cuvet.
   f. Stop the instrument when the reaction is complete. Aggregation for the donor PRP must be between 60 and 100% using ADP.
5. Preparation of plasma dilutions for testing.
   a. Label four cuvets #1 through #4. Place a magnetic stir bar in each cuvet and prepare the following test mixtures:
      1) #1—0.2 mL control PPP + 0.3 mL control PRP.
      2) #2—0.2 mL control PPP + 0.3 mL control PRP.
      3) #3—0.2 mL patient PPP + 0.3 mL control PRP.
      4) #4—0.2 mL patient PPP + 0.3 mL control PRP.
6. Perform the platelet aggregation test.
   a. Repeat step 4c and 4d above for each cuvet, adding 0.05 mL of the heparin working solution (10 U/mL) to cuvets #1 and #3, and 0.5 mL of saline to cuvets #2 and #4.
   b. Allow the aggregation to proceed for 30 minutes.
7. Interpretation of results.

a. > 20% aggregation in cuvet #3 is considered positive for the heparin-dependent aggregating factor. There should be no aggregation in cuvets #1, 2, and 4.

b. Aggregation in cuvets #1, 2, and/or 4 indicates spontaneous aggregation of donor platelets. Repeat the test using PRP from a different donor.

8. If the test is negative using the donor platelets, perform the test in the same manner using the patient's own platelet-rich plasma instead of the donor PRP.

a. Prepare the plasma dilutions as follows:

Cuvet #1—0.2 mL patient PPP + 0.3 mL patient PRP.

Cuvet #2—0.2 mL patient PPP + 0.3 mL patient PRP.

b. Perform the platelet aggregation test as outlined above (step 6) and add 0.05 mL heparin to cuvet #1 and 0.05 mL 0.85% sodium chloride to cuvet #2.

Discussion

1. All testing should be complete within 4 hours of obtaining the specimen.

2. Use of the patient's PRP is thought to increase the sensitivity of the test. However, this may not be possible if the patient's platelet count is too low to obtain adequate platelets for the PRP.

3. Further proof of HAT is the demonstration of platelet aggregation in the presence of 2 U/mL of heparin instead of 10 U/mL.

4. Plasmas must be kept capped and at room temperature.

5. Only plastic/siliconized pipets and cuvets should be used because platelets adhere to, and may become activated when in contact with glass.

REAGENTS

Adsorbed Plasma (Rich in Factors V, VIII, XI, and XII)

1. Add 100 mg of barium sulfate to each 1 mL of fresh oxalated (sodium oxalate) normal plasma.

2. Stir this mixture for 10 minutes at room temperature and refrigerate (or place on ice) for an additional 10 minutes.

3. Centrifuge at 2500 RPM for 10 minutes and remove the supernatant plasma.

4. Dilute the adsorbed plasma 1:5 with 0.85% sodium chloride (1 part adsorbed plasma to 4 parts 0.85% sodium chloride).

Aged Serum (Rich in Factors VII, IX, X, XI, and XII)

1. Incubate a tube of clotted normal blood at 37°C for 3 hours.

2. Add 1 part 0.109 M sodium citrate to 9 parts whole blood to the preceding test tube.

3. Allow the test tube to incubate for 2 additional hours at 37°C.

4. Centrifuge for 10 minutes and remove the serum.

5. The serum may be used immediately, or stored at −20°C.

6. Prior to use, dilute the aged serum 1:5 with 0.85% sodium chloride (1 part aged serum to 4 parts 0.85% sodium chloride).

Calcium Chloride, 0.025 M

Anhydrous calcium chloride, 1.38 g
Dilute to 500 mL with distilled water.

Owren's Veronal Buffer, pH 7.40

Sodium barbital, 5.9 g
Sodium chloride, 7.1 g
Hydrochloric acid, 215 mL
Dilute to 1 liter with distilled water.

DISEASES

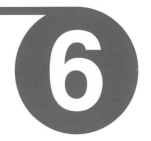

RED BLOOD CELL DISORDERS

Introduction to the Anemias

Anemia signifies a decreased amount of hemoglobin in the blood and, therefore, a decreased amount of oxygen reaching the tissues and organs of the body. This is responsible for many of the symptoms in an anemic person. Anemia has many different causes, and before effective treatment can be initiated, the exact cause must be found. Numerous laboratory procedures are used, in conjunction with clinical findings, to differentiate the various types of anemia.

The medical history of the patient is a source of information and can give important clues which may assist in the diagnosis: an anemia of long duration may indicate an inherited disorder, the racial origin or ethnic background may be of assistance in pointing to red cell enzyme deficiencies or abnormal hemoglobins, and exposure to toxic chemicals or the use of various medications should be noted.

To detect anemia in the laboratory, the two most widely used tests are the hemoglobin and hematocrit. An accurate red blood cell count is also most helpful in calculating the red blood cell indices. The anemia may then be classified as normocytic, microcytic, or macrocytic, depending on the values obtained for the mean corpuscular volume (MCV). The presence or absence of hypochromia, as shown by the mean corpuscular hemoglobin concentration (MCHC), is also valuable in diagnosis. The MCH closely parallels the MCV and generally increases or decreases with the MCV. Most anemias are normocytic-normochromic, macrocytic-normochromic, or microcytic-hypochromic, depending on the cause. The red cell distribution width (RDW) is also useful: this test is increased in iron deficiency anemia and is normal in the microcytic thalassemias.

Examination of the red blood cell morphology on a stained blood smear is a basic tool in evaluating anemia. The shape of the red blood cell may be studied and the presence or absence of nucleated red blood cells, schistocytes, sickle cells, spherocytes, target cells, and inclusion bodies noted. In addition, white blood cell and platelet numbers and morphology should be examined. In certain cases, a clue to the cause of the anemia may rest with these cells, as in the case of leukemia. In some anemias, there are specific abnormalities present in the white blood cells or platelets in addition to those found in the red blood cells.

The reticulocyte count, or the reticulocyte production index, is a test performed routinely for anemia diagnosis. It is a relatively accurate reflection of the amount of effective red blood cell production taking place in the bone marrow. In cases where the reticulocyte count is decreased, there may be defective hemoglobin synthesis, replacement of the normal marrow by tumor cells, or failure of the bone marrow to produce the normal number of cells. On the other hand, increased reticulocyte counts in the presence of anemia may indicate such conditions as increased red blood cell destruction or blood loss. It must be remembered, however, that if effective erythropoiesis is taking place, the reticulocyte count is slightly elevated in proportion to the degree of anemia present.

Examination of bone marrow smears may prove helpful in estimating the relative number and morphology of red blood cells and their precursors being produced by the marrow. Normally, 20 to 35% of the nucleated cells present in the marrow are erythroid cells. This figure may be written as the myeloid:erythroid ratio (M/E), which normally is 3:1, or as the erythroid:granulocyte ratio (E/G), which is, therefore, 1:3 in a normal marrow. This figure may then be studied in conjunction with the reticulocyte count. For example, if the relative number of erythroid cells in the marrow is increased, but the reticulocyte count is normal or decreased, there may be a defect in the maturation of the erythroid cells (since the red blood cells are obviously not reaching the peripheral blood). Ineffective erythropoiesis may be said to be occurring. It is also important to note the morphology of the erythroid cells (as well as other cellular elements) and the presence of any tumor cells.

When a bone marrow biopsy is performed in cases of anemia, an iron stain should be done on a marrow concentrate smear to determine the percentage of sideroblasts. The presence or absence of ringed sideroblasts should also be noted. An estimation of the marrow iron stores may be determined from a marrow particle smear stained with the Prussian-blue iron stain.

The serum lactic dehydrogenase (LDH) test is less specific than the previously discussed procedures but may be of some help. Increased levels are present in hemolytic anemias especially when there is intravascular hemolysis, and also in some cases of ineffective erythropoiesis (such as megaloblastic anemias).

The serum iron and iron binding capacity (tests usually performed by the chemistry department) are helpful aids in differentiating anemias. The high incidence of iron deficiency anemia increases the usefulness of these procedures. The serum ferritin level may be measured by various immunoassay techniques. Generally, the amount of circulating ferritin is proportional to the amount of storage iron so that the body iron stores may be evaluated with this procedure.

A test for the determination of fecal urobilinogen (usually performed by the urinalysis or chemistry department) measures the total excretion of the breakdown products of heme. Increased amounts of urobilinogen are generally found in hemolytic anemias and in those anemias in which ineffective red blood cell production is present.

The zinc erythrocyte protoporphyrin test may be performed to determine the amount of protoporphyrin not used for hemoglobin synthesis. Elevated levels are seen in iron deficient erythropoiesis, lead poisoning, and rare disorders of porphyrin metabolism.

The serum bilirubin (performed in the chemistry department) indicates increased destruction of red blood cells, as found in hemolytic anemias.

In addition to the aforementioned laboratory procedures, other tests concerned with red blood cell production, although not employed routinely, deserve mention here. The plasma iron turnover is a procedure employing the use of radioactive iron (^{59}Fe). A known amount of this isotope is injected into the patient intravenously and its rate of disappearance from the blood is measured. In anemias in which total red blood cell production is decreased, the ^{59}Fe remains in the blood longer. The red cell turnover (or red blood cell utilization of iron) is a measure of effective erythropoiesis. After injection of the ^{59}Fe (as described above), blood samples are collected for a period of 2 to 3 weeks and the radioactivity in the samples is measured to determine how much of the ^{59}Fe was incorporated into the red cells. The life span of the red blood cell may also be determined by the use of radioisotopes. The patient's red blood cells may be tagged with radioactive chromium (^{51}Cr). Blood samples are then measured for radioactivity over a period of time and a red blood cell survival curve plotted.

In summary, *total erythropoiesis* refers to the total production of red blood cells and is measured by the myeloid:erythroid ratio, the fecal urobilinogen, and the plasma iron turnover. *Effective erythropoiesis* is the production of red blood cells that reach the circulation or peripheral blood and is measured by the red blood cell iron turnover (utilization of iron), the reticulocyte count, and the red blood cell life span. In addition, more specific tests have been devised for diagnosing anemias. Many of these procedures have been outlined in Chapter 4, Special Hematology Procedures, and include, among others, hemoglobin electrophoresis, osmotic fragility, autohemolysis, acid serum test, and Heinz body preparation.

Anemia basically results from 1 of 2 causes: (1) decreased red blood cell production or (2) increased red blood cell destruction. In addition, in circumstances where there is an increased plasma volume, laboratory test results (hemoglobin, hematocrit, and red blood cell count) may also show a state of anemia even though the red blood cell mass is normal.

Several classifications of anemia have been devised. None of these is completely satisfactory but they are of some help in learning the basics of anemia. A brief outline of the anemias classified according to morphology and according to cause are given in the following section. These are not complete lists and contain only the more common anemias and causes discussed in this chapter.

Morphologic Classification of Anemias

1. Macrocytic, normochromic red blood cells.
    A. Vitamin B_{12} deficiency, folic acid deficiency.
        (1) Pernicious anemia
        (2) Sprue
        (3) Following gastrectomy
        (4) Dietary
        (5) Abnormal intrinsic factor
        (6) Tapeworm infection
    B. Disease of the liver.
2. Normocytic, normochromic red blood cells.
    A. Defective formation of the blood cells or the presence of tumor cells in the bone marrow.
        (1) Aplastic anemia
        (2) Leukemia
        (3) Hodgkin's disease
        (4) Multiple myeloma
        (5) Leukoerythroblastosis
        (6) Metastatic cancer
        (7) Anemia associated with renal and endocrine disease
        (8) Anemia associated with inflammatory disease (chronic disorders)
    B. Abnormal hemoglobin, increased destruction of red blood cells.
        (1) Certain acquired hemolytic anemias

        (2) Paroxysmal nocturnal hemoglobinuria
        (3) Sickle cell anemia
        (4) Hemolytic disease of the newborn
        (5) Anemia of chronic renal insufficiency
3. Microcytic, hypochromic red blood cells.
    A. Iron deficiency anemia.
    B. Thalassemia.
    C. Sideroblastic anemias.
    D. Chronic blood loss.

Classification of Anemias According to Cause

1. Decreased or impaired production of red blood cells.
    A. Bone marrow damage, infiltration, atrophy.
        (1) Leukemia
        (2) Leukoerythroblastosis
        (3) Aplastic anemia
        (4) Lymphoma
        (5) Multiple myeloma
        (6) Myelofibrosis
        (7) Pure red cell aplasia
    B. Decreased erythropoietin.
        (1) Inflammatory process—anemia of chronic disorders
        (2) Chronic renal disease
        (3) Hypothyroidism
    C. Vitamin and mineral deficiencies.
        (1) Iron deficiency
        (2) Vitamin B_{12} deficiency, folic acid deficiency
    D. Defect in globin synthesis.
        (1) α and β Thalassemia minor
        (2) μ Thalassemia trait
    E. Iron overload.
        (1) Sideroblastic anemia
        (2) Hemochromatosis
    F. Ineffective erythropoiesis.
        (1) Congenital dyserythropoietic anemia
2. Increased red blood cell destruction (hemolytic anemias).
    A. Intrinsic defects within the red blood cell.
        (1) Hereditary—membrane defects
            a. Spherocytosis
            b. Elliptocytosis
            c. Abetalipoproteinemia
            d. Stomatocytosis

e. Rh$_{null}$ disease
(2) Hereditary—enzyme defects
   a. Glucose-6-phosphate dehydrogenase
   b. Pyruvate kinase
(3) Hereditary—hemoglobinopathies
   a. Sickle cell disease
   b. Hemoglobin C disease
   c. Unstable hemoglobin disease
   d. Hemoglobin E disease
(4) Hereditary—defective globin synthesis
   a. β thalassemia major
   b. Sickle β-thalassemia
   c. E-β thalassemia
   d. Hemoglobin H disease
(5) Acquired
   a. Paroxysmal nocturnal hemoglobinuria
B. Extracorpuscular causes: nonimmune acquired hemolytic anemias.
   (1) Chemicals, toxins, venoms
   (2) Physical trauma—disorders causing fragmentation.
      a. Burns
      b. Cardiac replacement valves
      c. Microangiopathic hemolytic anemia
      d. Hemolytic uremic syndrome (HUS)
   (3) Infections
      a. Parasitic (malaria and babesia)
C. Extracorpuscular causes: immune hemolytic anemias.
   (1) Isoimmune antibodies
      a. Incompatible blood transfusion
      b. Hemolytic disease of the newborn (HDN)
   (2) Autoimmune antibodies
      a. Warm reacting
      b. Cold reacting
      c. Drug (antibiotic) induced
D. Miscellaneous
   1. Anemia of liver disease
   2. Sulfhemoglobinemia
   3. The porphyrias
   4. Methemoglobinemia
3. Acute blood loss.

Disorders Related to Iron and Heme Metabolism

Iron-Deficiency Anemia

Iron-deficiency anemia results when the iron stores of the body have been depleted, and there is no longer sufficient iron available for normal hemoglobin production. The iron stores become depleted over time when iron utilization or loss exceeds iron intake.

The normal adult body contains approximately 4,000 mg of iron. About 60% of this total iron is present in the circulating blood, where 1 mL of red blood cells contains approximately 1 mg of iron. The remaining iron is stored as ferritin or hemosiderin, mainly in the liver and reticuloendothelial cells of the bone marrow. Each day, 20 to 25 mL of red blood cells are broken down as a result of normal red blood cell aging. During this process, approximately 1 mg of iron is lost and excreted through the urine, bile, and other secretions. The remaining 19 to 24 mg of iron are reutilized for production of more hemoglobin in the formation of new red blood cells. The normal adult absorbs 5 to 10% of the iron in his diet. This provides 1 to 2 mg per day and compensates for the normal daily losses due to red cell turnover. From this discussion, it can be seen that unless there is an increased need for iron, as in childhood, pregnancy, or excessive blood loss, iron-deficiency anemia will not occur. The commonest cause of iron deficiency is blood loss from gastrointestinal bleeding or excessive menstrual blood loss. Antacids and tetracycline can also block the absorption of iron. When iron deficiency does occur, it develops in three stages: (1) In the first step, there is iron depletion, where iron is being utilized by the red blood cells at a faster rate (as during infancy or bleeding) and the dietary intake of iron is not sufficient to keep up with the increased use. The iron stores will then be utilized. At this time the anemia is normochromic and normocytic. (2) Iron deficient erythropoiesis then takes place, where the iron stores become exhausted and anemia may not yet be present. The anemia is now becoming microcytic. (3) Iron deficiency anemia then results, where intake does not meet demand, stores are depleted and anemia is detectable. This results in the characteristic microcytic, hypochromic blood picture.

An increased amount of dietary iron is needed during infancy, childhood, pregnancy, and in women during the childbearing years. The adult male has no increased demands for iron and could live without dietary iron for approximately 3 to 4 years before iron-deficiency anemia developed.

Therefore, when this anemia is found in men, it is almost always due to chronic blood loss. Iron deficiency is the most common cause of anemia from 6 months to 24 months of age, at which time iron stores present at birth are exhausted. It is usually caused by insufficient dietary iron.

Iron-deficiency anemia is characterized by microcytosis, hypochromia, and poikilocytosis of the red blood cells, as seen on the stained blood smear. The reticulocyte count is within the normal range, except following hemorrhage or iron therapy, when it is increased. The free erythrocyte protoporphyrin level is increased. The platelet count is normal, but it may be increased. Frequently, the platelets may appear smaller in size than usual. When the iron stain is employed on bone marrow concentrate smears, the number of sideroblasts is decreased and storage iron is absent. The serum iron is decreased, whereas the total iron binding capacity is increased.

Treatment for iron deficiency involves replacement therapy with amounts of iron sufficient to correct the anemia and replenish the iron stores. Ferrous iron is given orally as ferrous sulfate to provide 20 to 40 mg per day. Reticulocytosis will develop within 1 to 2 weeks and the hemoglobin usually increases by 1 to 2 g per week. After the hemoglobin returns to normal, treatment should continue for several weeks in order to replace the iron stores.

Sideroblastic Anemia

The sideroblastic anemias are a group of disorders characterized by iron loading and its accumulation in the mitochondria of the erythroid precursors due to a defect in heme synthesis. These disorders may be classified as inherited or acquired. The defect in heme synthesis may occur as a result of decreased activity of the enzyme ALA synthetase.

Hereditary sideroblastic anemia is inherited as a sex linked recessive trait, and it occurs primarily in males. This rare type of anemia usually manifests itself in adolescence, although it may be present at birth or during infancy. The anemia is generally severe, with hematocrit levels of approximately 20%. The blood smear shows a dimorphic population of normochromic-normocytic and hypochromic-microcytic red blood cells. These latter cells

show moderate anisocytosis and poikilocytosis. Also, target cells and basophilic stippling are usually present. The white blood cell and platelet counts are generally normal. There is a marked increase of storage iron in the bone marrow, and the serum iron and the % transferrin saturation are increased. The bone marrow generally shows erythroid hyperplasia, with evidence of inadequate or defective hemoglobin synthesis. The erythroid precursors have pale or decreased amounts of cytoplasm, and 10 to 40% of the late normoblasts are *ringed sideroblasts* (immature red blood cells in which a ring of iron granules surrounds the nucleus).

Primary idiopathic sideroblastic anemia is more common than hereditary sideroblastic anemia and is an acquired disease found in adults above 50 years of age. There is moderate anemia, with hematocrit levels of approximately 25 to 30%. In contrast to the dimorphic population of hereditary sideroblastic anemia, the red blood cells in primary sideroblastic anemia are generally normocytic to slightly macrocytic. A small group of hypochromic-microcytic red blood cells may be found. The white blood cell and platelet counts are normal, and the bone marrow generally shows erythroid hyperplasia along with the presence of large numbers of ringed sideroblasts in all stages of development. Treatment involves the use of transfusions, but only if the anemia is severe, because this contributes to iron overload. Approximately 10% of the patients with this form of sideroblastic anemia develop acute leukemia.

A sideroblastic anemia may also develop in association with other diseases such as leukemia, hemolytic anemia, neoplastic and inflammatory disease, and uremia. In these circumstances, there will be anemia, some hypochromic red blood cells in the peripheral blood, and a few ringed sideroblasts in the bone marrow.

Secondary sideroblastic anemia may be caused by certain agents, toxins, or drugs that interfere with heme synthesis. This anemia may be found in alcoholism, lead poisoning, tuberculosis therapy (antituberculosis drugs), and as a result of receiving large doses of chloramphenicol. Drug induced sideroblastic anemia is reversible, in that withdrawal of the drug results in correction of the anemia. Some patients with sideroblastic anemia

abdominal pain from the accumulation of porphyrin precursors in the liver. Psychologic disturbances and neurologic symptoms may occur because of central nervous system involvement. During the active phase, the white blood cell count is usually elevated, and the urine will contain increased amounts of delta-aminolevulinic acid and porphobilinogen. The acute attacks of this disorder have been successfully treated with large amounts of glucose, hematin, and sodium benzoate.

Hereditary coproporphyria resembles acute intermittent hepatic porphyria in its clinical picture. It is caused by a decrease in coproporphyrinogen oxidase, which results in increased amounts of coproporphyrin III in the urine and feces and accumulation in the liver. Acute attacks of this disease have been successfully treated with hematin.

Variegate porphyria is inherited as an autosomal dominant trait. It has a high incidence in South Africa in descendants of a particular Dutch family. The clinical symptoms are those similar to porphyria cutanea tarda, with accompanying neurological involvement. Acute attacks of this disorder are generally precipitated by exposure to such drugs as sulfonamides, barbiturates, anesthetics, and alcohol. This disease is caused by a deficiency in protoporphyrinogen oxidase. The feces contain large amounts of protoporphyrinogen and coproporphyrin. During acute attacks, the urine will contain increased amounts of porphobilinogen and delta-aminolevulinic acid. This disorder is generally treated in the same way as acute intermittent porphyria.

In the *acquired porphyrias,* several of the enzymes controlling heme synthesis are inhibited. In lead poisoning, delta aminolevulinic acid dehydrase and ferrochelatase are inhibited, resulting in increases in excreted delta aminolevulinic acid and coproporphyrin III. Erythrocyte protoporphyrin IX levels are increased. Anemia associated with lead poisoning is mild, with basophilic stippling on the blood smear. Symptoms include abdominal pain, vomiting, and, in advanced cases, neurologic complications such as seizures, coma, and cerebral edema.

Toxic exposure to hexachlorobenzene, a chemical used to prevent mold in wheat, results in inhibition of the enzyme uroporphyrinogen decarboxylase. Uroporphyrin I

levels are increased, individuals are photosensitive and have reddish urine.

Aplastic Anemia

The basic defect in aplastic anemia is the failure to produce red blood cells, white blood cells, and platelets. Another term used to describe this condition is *pancytopenia,* which is a reduction in all of the formed elements of the blood. Most evidence suggests that this is due to a depletion in the production of the cell precursors as a result of damage to the hematopoietic stem cells. In some unknown way, this alters the stem cell's ability to proliferate or differentiate. Aplastic anemia may be acquired as a result of exposure to chemicals, drugs, and radiation, from infections and autoimmune causes, in association with other diseases, or as a result of an unknown cause (idiopathic). It may also occur as a congenital defect. To a lesser degree, aplastic anemia may occur as the result of an autoimmune mechanism or marrow microenvironment that cannot support stem cell growth.

Acquired aplastic anemia occurs as the result of exposure to certain physical and chemical agents. These include ionizing radiation, benzene and its derivatives, heavy metals, and certain chemotherapeutic agents. Other substances may produce a pancytopenia in some persons due to individual sensitivities. Among these agents are anticonvulsants, sedatives and tranquilizers, insecticides, and certain antimicrobials (particularly chloramphenicol). The clinical course of the disease may show a rapid onset and a rapid progression to death, or it may have a slow onset and a chronic course. Laboratory tests generally show pancytopenia with low white blood cell, red blood cell, and platelet counts. The red blood cells are usually normocytic and normochromic. In rare cases, the red blood cells may be macrocytic. Varying degrees of anisocytosis and poikilocytosis may be present. Basophilic stippling, polychromatophilia, and nucleated red blood cells are absent from the peripheral blood. Reticulocytes are decreased to absent. There is generally a neutropenia along with a relative lymphocytosis. The bone marrow is hypocellular, with an increase in fat. Relative lymphocytosis may also be present in the bone marrow. Occasionally, biopsies show a normal marrow. This is misleading because there may be small areas in the marrow in which there is residual blood cell producing activity. A repeat marrow biopsy at another location gives the typical hypocellular picture. The bleeding time and clot retraction are usually abnormal because of the absence of platelets. The serum iron level is increased, and the iron binding protein is saturated. Erythropoietin levels are greatly increased. Treatment of aplastic anemia involves: (1) removal of the causative agent, if known, (2) red blood cell transfusions to maintain a minimum hemoglobin level, (3) platelet transfusions if necessary, and (4) antibiotics to prevent infection. Previously used corticosteroids and androgens are of limited value and have highly toxic side effects. Complications that develop are due to infection and bleeding, and the prognosis depends on the severity of the marrow damage. Bone marrow transplantation in patients under 50 years of age is the treatment of choice today. Also, immunosuppressive therapy has been used in cases of aplastic anemia from autoimmune causes.

Aplastic anemia may also develop several months following the onset of viral hepatitis. The prognosis in these cases is not good and may result in death. Aplastic anemia has also been found as a complication of tuberculosis, following pregnancy, in autoimmune diseases, and in paroxysmal nocturnal hemoglobinuria.

Idiopathic aplastic anemia is an acquired condition of unknown cause which accounts for about 50% of the cases of aplastic anemia. The symptoms and laboratory tests are similar to those of the other acquired aplastic anemias.

Fanconi's anemia (familial aplastic anemia) is a congenital form of pancytopenia which occurs in children. Some chromosomal defects have been described, and the inheritance pattern is autosomal recessive. Mental and physical developmental abnormalities are present. Deposits of melanin are common, which show up as patches of brown pigmentation of the skin. There is generally a normocytic to slightly macrocytic anemia. Target cells may be present, along with nucleated red blood cells and immature white blood cells. The bone marrow may be normocellular to

hypercellular in the beginning but will become hypocellular as the disease progresses. Hemoglobin F is generally increased.

Pure Red Blood Cell Aplasia

Pure red blood cell aplasia is a term given to a category of diseases in which red blood cell production is suppressed, with little or no abnormalities found in the white blood cells or platelets.

Congenital erythroid hypoplasia (Diamond-Blackfan syndrome) is a rare disorder that is characterized by a moderate to severe anemia. This disorder appears to be the result of defective or reduced numbers of CFU-E (erythroid colony forming units) in the stem cell pool of the bone marrow. It generally manifests itself during the first 2 to 3 months of life. Infants with this disorder generally show pallor and may or may not have splenomegaly and/or hepatomegaly. At diagnosis, the hemoglobin is quite low, 2 to 10 g/dL, and the anemia is normochromic and may be slightly macrocytic. Reticulocytes in the peripheral blood are decreased to absent. The bone marrow is generally normal except for a marked decrease in erythroid cells. Corticosteroid therapy is used in the treatment of this disorder. When patients do not respond to this treatment, blood transfusions are used. Hemochromatosis and severe liver damage may develop, however, as a complication of transfusion therapy.

Acute acquired pure red blood cell aplasia (acute acquired erythropoietic hypoplasia) may suddenly occur for a short period during the course of a hemolytic anemia, certain infections, malnutrition, or with various kinds of drug therapy. The erythroblasts in the bone marrow will suddenly disappear (aplastic crisis), and an anemia soon develops if this condition persists for any length of time. When this condition occurs during drug therapy, removal of the drug is generally followed by a return to normal erythropoiesis.

Chronic acquired pure red blood cell aplasia (chronic acquired erythrocytic hypoplasia) occurs in adults. About one half of the cases of this disorder have been found in patients with a thymoma (thymic tumor). Removal of the tumor, when present, is followed by an improvement in erythropoiesis more than 25%

of the time. Studies have shown that some patients have autoantibodies that react with and inhibit erythroid stem cells. The anemia of this disorder is generally severe and is normocytic to slightly macrocytic. The white blood cells and platelets are usually normal. Reticulocytes are decreased to absent. The bone marrow shows normal white blood cell and platelet development and a marked decrease in maturing red blood cells. The serum iron level is usually increased, and the iron binding capacity is saturated. Some patients have been treated successfully with corticosteroids and immunosuppressive drugs. Patients with systemic lupus erythematosus and with lymphomas may also develop an acquired pure red cell aplasia.

Congenital Dyserythropoietic Anemias

The congenital dyserythropoietic anemias are so named because the normoblasts in the bone marrow show multinuclearity, karyorrhexis, and bizarre malformations as a result of dyserythropoiesis (asynchrony of nuclear and cytoplasmic maturation). These anemias are divided into 3 groups: Type I, Type II (also termed HEMPAS), and Type III. All types are characterized by ineffective erythropoiesis and hyperbilirubinemia.

Type I is rare and thought to be inherited as an autosomal recessive trait. It is a mildly macrocytic anemia and shows marked anisocytosis and poikilocytosis. Cabot rings and basophilic stippling are often present in the red blood cells of the peripheral blood. The bone marrow shows megaloblastic characteristics in the developing red blood cells, along with binucleated and incompletely separated or multilobed cells. Splenomegaly is often present.

Type II is also termed HEMPAS (hereditary erythroblast multinuclearity with positive acidified serum test) and is the most common form of this anemia. It is inherited as an autosomal recessive trait. Hepatosplenomegaly is generally present, and jaundice may or may not occur. There is usually a normocytic anemia, along with anisocytosis, poikilocytosis, and basophilic stippling. The bone marrow shows multinuclearity of the normoblasts but with no megaloblastic changes. The red blood cells display hemolysis in the acid serum test but do not hemolyze in the sugar water test. The red cells in this disorder contain the blood group antigen, i, on them, termed the *HEMPAS antigen.* This disorder generally runs a benign course. A splenectomy is only rarely performed.

Type III is rare and is thought to be inherited as an autosomal dominant trait. It is a normocytic to slightly macrocytic anemia and shows as many as 30% multinucleated red blood cells in the bone marrow.

Megaloblastic Anemias

There are a variety of megaloblastic anemias that result from deficiencies of vitamin B_{12} and folic acid, and from drugs that interfere with DNA metabolism. The major abnormality is the decreased synthesis of DNA due to depleted stores of the DNA precursor thymidine triphosphate. Megaloblastic marrow cells have both a prolonged intermitotic resting phase and a block in early mitosis. This results in enlarged (macrocytic) red cells, granulocytes, and megakaryocytes. Pernicious anemia is a classic example of this form of anemia.

Pernicious Anemia

Pernicious anemia is most often found in people above 60 years of age and rarely in patients below 40 years of age. This disease is caused by a deficiency in vitamin B_{12} resulting from an inability of the gastric mucosa to secrete the intrinsic factor necessary for the absorption of vitamin B_{12}. There is strong evidence at present that this disorder may be an inherited autoimmune disease. Antibodies to intrinsic factor have been found in over half of the cases of pernicious anemia, and antibodies to the parietal cells of the stomach (which produce intrinsic factor) have been found to be present in over 85% of the patients having pernicious anemia. The clinical symptoms evolve slowly over a period of several months. Generally, the person shows weakness and shortness of breath, and the skin takes on a lemon yellow pallor. Characteristically, the tongue may be raw and red or, more commonly, may be sore, pale and smooth. Gastrointestinal symptoms are usually present in the form of abdominal pain, diarrhea, nausea, and vomiting. There are central nervous system disorders in the degeneration of the white matter in parts of the spinal cord. This is the cause of several neurologic symptoms such as numbness and tingling of the extremities, loss of position sense, muscle weakness, and decreased tendon reflexes. In more advanced cases, the brain may be affected, and the patient may become emotionally unstable or show personality changes, commonly known as "megaloblastic madness."

The peripheral blood smear shows characteristic changes. Pancytopenia is the usual finding, with white blood cell counts usually in the range of 4000 to 5000/μL. The majority of red blood cells are macrocytic-normochromic, with some oval macrocytes present. There may be a few microcytes and teardrop-shaped red blood cells, and moderate to marked anisocytosis and poikilocytosis is commonly found. Basophilic stippling, Howell-Jolly bodies, and nucleated red blood cells exhibiting karyorrhexis are usually seen. Neutrophils showing hypersegmentation are commonly encountered, many with 6 to 10 lobes. These cells may be larger in size than the normal neutrophil. The nuclear chromatin pattern of the erythrocytic and granulocytic cells often gives a much looser or more open appearance than normal. A patient with severe, untreated anemia usually shows thrombocytopenia, with giant platelets found on the blood smear. The bone marrow contains an increased number of erythroid cells that are characteristically megaloblastic, and the developing granulocytic cells are often larger in size than normal. The marrow also is hypercellular with erythroid hyperplasia and a M:E (myeloid: erythroid) ratio of 1:1 to 1:3 (normal is 3:1). This is due to increased production of red cells in response to the anemia. Iron laden macrophages may also be seen. The giant metamyelocyte is a characteristic cell present. The absolute reticulocyte count is low, but there are an increased number of reticulocytes in the bone marrow.

One of the more consistent findings in pernicious anemia is the lack of free hydrochloric acid in the gastric secretions (achlorhydria) after histamine stimulation. The Schilling test (usually performed by the radiology department) is used to diagnose pernicious anemia. This procedure involves giving a standard dose of radioactive vitamin B_{12} orally with a concurrent dose of intrinsic factor (IF) and measuring the amount of radioactive B_{12} excreted in the urine. If the Schilling test corrects to normal with the addition of IF, the patient has pernicious anemia. The serum vitamin B_{12} level is decreased. The serum iron level may be normal to elevated (because of the accelerated death of erythroid precursors in the bone marrow), and the serum bilirubin level may show a slight increase due to decreased erythrocyte survival. Treatment involves the use of lifelong injections of vitamin B_{12}.

Other Conditions Caused by Vitamin B_{12} Deficiency

A megaloblastic anemia will result following a total *gastrectomy* because all of the intrinsic factor-secreting cells have been removed. Vitamin B_{12} therapy is used to treat this condition. A partial gastrectomy or surgery for a gastric ulcer may or may not leave the patient with a megaloblastic anemia, which, again, is treatable with vitamin therapy.

A *dietary deficiency of vitamin B_{12}* is rare but may be found in vegetarians who also avoid consuming milk and egg products.

One case of megaloblastic anemia has been reported in a patient who was found to have an *abnormal intrinsic factor.*

Various *diseases of the small intestine,* such as the 'blind loop syndrome', may cause a megaloblastic anemia. Normally, vitamin B_{12} is absorbed in the lower ileum, which contains little or no bacteria. When bacteria are present, they compete for the vitamin B_{12} thus making it unavailable for absorption. Treatment involves aggressive administration of broad spectrum antibiotics.

Reversible malabsorption of vitamin B_{12} has occurred in patients taking para-aminosalicylic acid (PAS), colchicine, neomycin, and a few other drugs.

Imerslund's syndrome is inherited as an autosomal recessive trait and manifests itself during the first 2 years of life. These patients are not able to absorb vitamin B_{12}, regardless of whether it is bound to intrinsic factor, since there is a deficiency of the receptor site in the terminal ileum. They also have persistent proteinuria. The megaloblastic anemia is treated with vitamin B_{12}.

In *Zollinger-Ellison syndrome,* there is impaired vitamin B_{12} absorption but no megaloblastic anemia. This disease is characterized by the hypersecretion of gastric juice, which results in a low intestinal pH. This interferes with the binding of vitamin B_{12} to intrinsic factor.

Patients on *hemodialysis* will have decreased vitamin B_{12} concentrations that are treatable with the administration of vitamin B_{12}.

In *Crohn's disease,* also called regional enteritis or inflammatory bowel disease, there is a vitamin B_{12} deficiency and megaloblastic anemia since the disease affects the terminal ileum where vitamin B_{12} absorption normally occurs.

Vitamin B_{12} deficiency will also be found in carriers of the fish tapeworm, *Diphyllobothrium latum,* because the organism lodges in the ileum and takes up the host's vitamin B_{12}. Treatment consists of expulsion of the organism and vitamin B_{12} therapy. This disorder is common in Finland.

A megaloblastic anemia can also result from an abnormality in the production of *transcobalamin II,* the major protein that transports vitamin B_{12} to the bone marrow for utilization.

Folate Deficiency

Folic acid deficiency manifests itself in a manner similar to vitamin B_{12} deficiency, except that neurologic symptoms are absent.

Dietary deficiencies of folic acid are relatively rare in this country and are found primarily in chronic alcoholics and people with poor dietary habits, where relatively few fresh green vegetables or little animal protein is consumed.

The most common cause of folate deficiency occurs during pregnancy, due to increased fetal requirements for folate. The laboratory findings are generally less abnormal than those found in pernicious anemia, and this condition is treated with folic acid.

Megaloblastic anemia may be found during infancy, occurring most often between 6 and 12 months of age, and is caused by a folic acid deficiency that may be accompanied by a vitamin C deficiency. Laboratory test results

show macrocytosis, anisocytosis, and poikilocytosis but in a less severe state than is found in pernicious anemia. The bone marrow shows mild to severe megaloblastic changes and includes the granulocytic alterations. Treatment consists of administration of vitamin C and folic acid.

Megaloblastic anemia is also found in patients with alcoholic cirrhosis of the liver and is almost always due to folic acid deficiency. This is due in part to lack of dietary folic acid and also to abnormal folate metabolism.

Some contraceptive drugs and anticonvulsants such as phenobarbital, diphenylhydantoin (Dilantin), and primidone (Mysoline) will cause a folate deficiency and mild hematologic changes.

Disorders Affecting DNA Synthesis

A number of disorders affect DNA synthesis and produce a megaloblastic anemia. Transcobalamin II deficiency, foramino-transferase deficiency, N-methyl tetrahydrofolate transferase deficiency, and dihydrofolate reductase deficiency are all inherited disorders, in addition to orotic aciduria (disorder of pyrimidine metabolism) and Lesch-Nyhan syndrome (disorder of purine metabolism). There are also acquired drug induced disorders caused by a variety of drugs, including those used in chemotherapy which act by inhibiting DNA synthesis.

Steatorrheas

Three malabsorption disorders have been classified as steatorrheas: *tropical sprue, nontropical sprue (idiopathic steatorrhea),* and *celiac disease.* The last two disorders are now called *gluten-sensitive enteropathies* because they are caused by an abnormal reaction to gluten.

The exact cause of tropical sprue is unknown. At the onset of the disease, there is diarrhea, anorexia, and marked weakness. After several weeks to months, there is a depletion of nutrients, and malabsorption takes place. Following this phase a macrocytic anemia develops, most likely caused by a lack of absorption of folic acid in the beginning and an ensuing lack of vitamin B_{12} as the disease becomes more chronic. Administration of folic acid is used for treatment of the anemia and also appears to improve the intestinal problems.

The gluten-sensitive enteropathies may be inherited and represent an abnormal reaction to gluten, a component of wheat and other grains. In these enteropathies, there is an abnormal small bowel mucosa with a resultant malabsorption of vitamin B_{12}. These patients show chronic diarrhea and weight loss, with possible hypocalcemia, demineralization of bones, and possible deficiency of vitamin K dependent coagulation factors. Children with celiac disease generally show an iron deficiency anemia, with about 30% having a folic acid deficiency. Adults usually have a folic acid deficiency. About 40% of adults will also show malabsorption of vitamin B_{12}. Iron absorption is decreased, and iron stores may be low. Treatment includes folate and/or vitamin B_{12}, in addition to iron therapy and a gluten free diet.

ANEMIAS RELATED TO OTHER (PRIMARY) DISORDERS

Anemia of Chronic Renal Insufficiency

Patients with chronic renal insufficiency generally show anemia due to failure of the kidneys to produce erythropoietin and to a decreased bone marrow response to erythropoietin. Many times, there is a direct relationship between the blood urea nitrogen levels and the severity of the anemia. Generally, the higher the blood urea nitrogen, the more severe the anemia.

In anemia of chronic renal insufficiency, the red blood cells are normocytic-normochromic, and the hematocrit level is generally 15 to 30%. Hemolysis may be present due to mechanical trauma or to the adverse metabolic environment of the red blood cells in uremic plasma that is highly toxic. Burr cells and irregularly contracted and fragmented red blood cells are seen on the peripheral blood smear. The reticulocyte count may be normal but often is decreased. Basophilic stippling is often striking. Some macrocytosis may be present in patients in a dialysis program, due to loss of folic acid during dialysis. The white blood cell count is usually normal, with slight neutrophilia. The platelet count is normal to slightly increased. In many cases, however, platelet function is impaired, resulting in bleeding from the genitourinary or gastrointestinal tracts. When this occurs, iron deficiency anemia may develop. The bone marrow generally shows erythroid hyperplasia. When the renal failure becomes acute, however, the bone marrow may show erythroid hypoplasia. Clinical trials have shown that recombinant human erythropoietin may improve erythropoiesis in patients with anemia of renal failure.

Anemia of Endocrine Diseases

Anemia is frequently associated with diseases of the thyroid, the pituitary, the adrenals, and the gonads. Many hormones are involved in the regulation of erythropoiesis, and deficiencies of such hormones lead to the development of anemia.

In *hypothyroidism*, there is generally a mild to moderate normochromic-normocytic anemia. The reticulocyte count is normal, as is the red blood cell survival time. This anemia is usually a result of decreased bone marrow production of red cells caused by a decrease in the oxygen requirements of the tissues. Hypothyroidism, however, is often complicated by iron deficiency, or a folic acid or vitamin B_{12} deficiency. In such cases, the red blood cells will be microcytic-hypochromic or macrocytic, respectively. Because plasma volume is decreased in hypothyroidism, the degree of anemia may not be reflected in the red cell mass or hematocrit. The hemoglobin concentration may be decreased while the hematocrit is normal. The response of the anemia to therapy is generally slow, and it may take 6 months to 1 year for the hemoglobin to become normal. Anemia is uncommon and does not generally occur in *hyperthyroidism*.

In *Addison's disease* (a disorder of the adrenal gland), a mild normocytic-normochromic anemia may be present. Anemia may not be readily apparent in the presence of the reduced plasma volume which accompanies this condition.

In *hypopituitarism*, there is generally a moderate normocytic-normochromic anemia present. This may be caused by a deficiency of the pituitary hormones or by deficiencies of hormones secreted by glands that are regulated by the pituitary.

Androgens are capable of increasing erythropoietin synthesis. A decrease in testosterone secretion in males will result in decreased red blood cell production, causing a drop in hemoglobin of 1 to 2 g/dL. This is probably due to loss of the erythropoietic effect of the androgen hormone.

A normocytic anemia has been reported in some cases of *hyperparathyroidism.*

Anemia of Chronic Disorders

Anemia associated with chronic disease is present in disorders such as chronic infections, rheumatoid arthritis, and malignancy. It has also been called anemia of inflammation because the immune system becomes involved in the process. Evidence strongly suggests that the cytokine IL-1 produced by activated macrophages during the acute phase of inflammation inhibits erythropoiesis. IL-1 also stimulates neutrophils to release lactoferrin, which binds iron. This complex is phagocytized by marrow macrophages, which makes iron unavailable for hemoglobin synthesis. It is the most common form of anemia among hospitalized patients and is second to iron deficiency as the most common of all the anemias.

Anemia of chronic disorders is generally a mild to moderate anemia that develops during the first or second month of illness. The hematocrit rarely falls below 30%. In severe illness, however, the hematocrit level may decrease further. This usually begins as a normocytic-normochromic anemia. Slight hypochromia may develop, and, more rarely, microcytosis may be found, but not to the degree seen in iron-deficiency anemia. Also, microcytosis occurs after hypochromia is present. In iron-deficiency anemia, microcytosis develops before hypochromia. There may be slight anisocytosis and poikilocytosis. The reticulocyte count is generally normal to decreased and the ESR is elevated. The white blood cell and platelet counts are unaffected by the anemia. The serum iron level is decreased, and the total iron binding capacity (TIBC) is normal to decreased. The percent saturation is usually decreased. Three factors which may contribute to the anemia of chronic disorders are: (1) a reduced red blood cell life span, (2) inability of the bone marrow to increase red blood cell production enough to compensate for the decreased red blood cell life span, and (3) a decrease in the transfer of iron from the storage sites to the bone marrow. The anemia of chronic disorders shows no improvement with iron therapy and only improves with correction of the primary underlying disorder.

Anemia of Liver Diseases

Anemia is a common finding in the presence of cirrhosis of the liver and other liver diseases. There is generally a normocytic to slightly macrocytic anemia present. The MCV is rarely greater than 115 fL. This anemia may be caused by folate deficiency from poor nutrition, a decreased red blood cell survival, an inability of the bone marrow to respond to the anemia, or an increase in the total blood volume that exaggerates the anemia. In some cases, a microcytic, hypochromic, iron deficiency anemia may result from acute and chronic blood loss. A sideroblastic anemia may develop in cases of chronic alcoholism. The anemia, however, is rarely severe. The bone marrow will show normal cellularity or an increased cellularity with erythroid hyperplasia. The reticulocyte count is often increased but can be decreased as a result of alcohol ingestion. The platelet count may be normal or slightly decreased, as found in cirrhosis of the liver. In hepatitis, obstructive jaundice, and cirrhosis of the liver, there may be changes in the red blood cell membrane lipids. An increase in cholesterol and phospholipid levels leads to an increased red blood cell membrane surface, which gives rise to 'thin' macrocytes or target cells. In some instances, there will be an increase in the red blood cell membrane cholesterol level, but not the phospholipid level. In this circumstance, spur cells are formed, which are red blood cells with thorny projections, similar to acanthocytes. This may lead to a hemolytic anemia because of changes in the red cell membrane and a loss of deformability. In acute and chronic alcoholism, ethanol has a direct toxic effect on the red cells and their precursors. This results in a characteristic vacuolization of the erythroblasts in the bone marrow.

Anemia of Blood Loss

The clinical symptoms associated with anemia due to blood loss depend on the severity of the bleeding. The patient's cardiovascular status, age, and emotional and physical health also play a part in the response to bleeding.

In acute blood loss, when there is a sudden loss of 25 to 30% of the total blood volume (1,000 to 1,500 mL), most healthy patients show light headedness, hypotension, and rapid heart rate when they are in an upright position. A loss of 30 to 40% of the blood volume leads to shortness of breath, sweating, loss of consciousness, and decreased blood pressure. The pulse becomes rapid and weak, and urine volume is reduced. With a sudden loss of 40 to 50% of the total blood volume, the patient goes into a severe state of shock, with the possibility of death.

Immediately after an acute major blood loss, the hemoglobin and hematocrit remain normal due to vasoconstriction. After about 3 to 4 hours, fluid enters the circulation in order to restore the plasma volume. This causes dilution of the blood and is the body's initial defense mechanism to compensate for the lost blood. When this occurs, the hemoglobin, hematocrit, and red blood cell count begin to drop and the platelet count and white blood cell count increase. The peripheral blood smear shows a normocytic-normochromic anemia with slight anisocytosis and poikilocytosis. The white cells display a shift to the left. Following severe bleeding, large polychromatophilic red blood cells and nucleated red blood cells are present in the peripheral blood. The reticulocyte count becomes elevated within 2 to 3 days, peaks in about 6 to 10 days, and remains elevated until the hemoglobin returns to the normal level. This usually occurs about 6 weeks after the episode of blood loss. The white blood cell count returns to normal in 2 to 4 days.

In chronic blood loss, when the bleeding occurs in small quantities over a period of time, iron deficiency anemia may develop as a result of the depletion of the iron stores. The white blood cell count is generally low, as is the reticulocyte count, and polychromatophilia is present. (See Iron Deficiency Anemia.)

Leukoerythroblastosis

Leukoerythroblastosis has several synonyms: *leukoerythroblastic anemia, myelophthisic anemia,* and *myelopathic anemia,* to name a few. It is a condition of anemia caused by space occupying malignant tumors of the bone marrow.

The most common cause of leukoerythroblastosis is metastatic carcinoma of the breast, prostate gland, lungs, adrenal gland, or thyroid, due to the tendency of the cancer to spread by vascular channels to the bone marrow. The marrow becomes infiltrated with fibrotic, granulomatous, or neoplastic cells. It is also found secondary to such diseases as Niemann-Pick disease, Gaucher's disease, Schüller-Christian disease, leukemias, and in some cases of Hodgkin's disease and multiple myeloma.

A normochromic-normocytic anemia of varying degrees is present. One distinguishing characteristic of this condition is the increased presence of nucleated red blood cells in the peripheral blood, quite out of proportion to the degree of anemia. Polychromatophilia, basophilic stippling, and reticulocytosis are usually present. The white blood cell count is generally normal to decreased, and frequently a few immature granulocytes may be present. The platelet count is normal to moderately decreased with occasional bizarre forms of the platelet present. Examination of the bone marrow usually shows the cause of leukoerythroblastosis.

Hemolytic Anemias

The hemolytic anemias are characterized by an increased destruction of red blood cells. In this condition, the bone marrow is able to respond to the red blood cell destruction. These anemias may be divided into those that are inherited and those that are acquired. Generally speaking, the red blood cells in inherited hemolytic anemias have intracorpuscular or intrinsic defects within the red blood cell itself. These intrinsic defects involve membrane disorders, defects in hemoglobin synthesis, and enzyme disorders within the red cell. The acquired hemolytic anemias usually have normal red blood cells that are destroyed by extrinsic, extracorpuscular factors or agents outside of the red blood cell. Intravascular hemolysis and extravascular hemolysis refer to the site of red blood cell breakdown: within the bloodstream or outside the blood in other organs.

Hereditary Spherocytosis

Hereditary spherocytosis, also known as *congenital hemolytic anemia* and *congenital hemolytic jaundice,* is inherited as a non-sex-linked dominant trait. However, in about 25% of the cases, there is no abnormality found in either parent. The symptoms of this condition are variable, depending on the severity of the disease. As a general rule, those cases recognized early in the life of the patient are likely to be more severe than those cases in which the symptoms appear later in life. Most often, hereditary spherocytosis is diagnosed in childhood, adolescence, or early adult life. The disorder is caused by a defect in the red blood cell membrane. Evidence suggests the primary defect involves the structure of spectrin, a skeletal protein on the internal surface of the red blood cell membrane. The exact defect present seems to involve a quantitative decrease in spectrin that correlates with the degree of spherocytosis and severity of the disorder. The red cells become hyperpermeable to sodium because of the weakened membrane structure. Normally, the osmotic balance of the red cell is maintained with sufficient glucose and ATP to expel sodium at a rate equal to its influx. However, spherocytes consume glucose at a rapid rate. When the amount of glucose is low, there is an increased rate of destruction of the red cells. The water content of the red cell increases and as a result, swelling and hemolysis of the red blood cells occur, and the cells are less deformable than normal. As the name of the disease implies, the red cells are spherocytic. The exact defect present, however, is not known.

The most consistent physical finding is splenomegaly. Jaundice is commonly present and increases during hemolytic episodes. The liver is usually enlarged, and the patient may also exhibit pallor, depending on the degree of anemia present.

This disease is usually accompanied by a moderate anemia. The most consistent finding in the peripheral blood is spherocytes. These cells have a decreased diameter and an increased concentration of hemoglobin. The number of spherocytes varies from a few to many. Polychromatophilia is present, and the reticulocyte count may be increased to 20% or higher. There are usually a few nucleated red blood cells present in the peripheral blood. This number increases, however, as the bone marrow responds during hemolytic episodes. The white blood cell and platelet counts are usually normal, except during periods of hemolysis, when there is thrombocytosis and a slight leukocytosis with a left shift. The MCHC is >36% in over 50% of the patients with hereditary spherocytosis. The osmotic fragility test is increased, and the autohemolysis test usually shows greater than 20% hemolysis after 48 hours' incubation. The serum bilirubin level is elevated, and the urine and stool may contain increased amounts of urobilinogen. Plasma haptoglobin is generally reduced and may be absent. The direct Coombs' test is negative. The bone marrow is hypercellular, with an absolute increase in the erythroid cells. These cells usually constitute 25 to 60% of all the marrow cells.

In severe cases, the treatment for this condition is splenectomy. Spherocytosis continues, but the red blood cell survival time is no longer decreased, because the spleen was the organ responsible for the destruction of the red blood cells (extravascular hemolysis). The red blood cell count (also hemoglobin and hematocrit) increases, and the bilirubin level returns to normal. The reticulocyte count decreases, and increased red blood cell production is no longer present. The osmotic fragility and autohemolysis tests continue to be increased.

Hereditary Elliptocytosis

Hereditary elliptocytosis is a red cell membrane disorder and is transmitted as an autosomal dominant gene. The most common defect involves the impaired association of spectrin dimers, resulting in free, unconnected dimers. This condition is characterized by the presence of variable numbers (30 to 75%) of elliptical, or oval shaped, mature red cells on the blood smear. The nucleated red blood cells and reticulocytes are normal in shape, however.

Approximately 90% of the individuals showing elliptocytosis have no clinical symptoms other than the presence of elliptical red blood cells. The remaining patients with this condition, however, display a hemolytic anemia and splenomegaly similar to hereditary spherocytosis. In this case, the osmotic fragility and autohemolysis of the red blood cells are increased. A splenectomy alleviates the hemolytic condition.

Abetalipoproteinemia

Abetalipoproteinemia is a rare disorder characterized by the absence of beta-lipoprotein in the blood. Normally, beta-lipoproteins are major components of the red cell membrane. This disorder manifests itself during the first few months of life with growth failure, abdominal distention, and steatorrhea. Acanthocytosis of the red blood cells, retinitis pigmentosa, and neurologic damage are also present. Laboratory tests show a decreased cholesterol level (usually less than 50 mg/dL) and the absence of beta-lipoprotein and triglycerides in the plasma. The blood smear exhibits large numbers of acanthocytes. The reticulocyte count is normal to increased, and if anemia is present, it is mild. The red blood cell life span may or may not be shortened. There is no definite treatment for this disorder.

Stomatocytosis (Hydrocytosis)

Several causes of stomatocytosis have been described: (1) because of increased permeability of the membrane, red blood cells contain an increased amount of sodium and a decreased amount of potassium, (2) red blood cells lack the Rh blood group antigens (Rh_{NULL} phenotype), or (3) red blood cells have neither of the above characteristics. Stomatocytes may also be found in acute alcoholism, liver disorders, cardiovascular disease, and in a small percentage of normal individuals.

Stomatocytosis caused by increased sodium and decreased potassium is inherited as a rare autosomal dominant trait. There is a marked increase in the passive permeability of the red cell membrane to sodium and potassium ions. As a result, the red cells accumulate sodium, and potassium leaks out of the cell at a greater rate. This irreversible ion exchange results in an influx of water and the formation of stomatocytes. The hemolytic anemia may be mild to severe. The reticulocyte count may be normal to moderately elevated and is usually 10 to 20%. Approximately 10 to

50% of the red blood cells will appear as stomatocytes. The serum bilirubin level will be increased and the haptoglobin decreased, depending on the amount of hemolysis present. The osmotic fragility may be decreased, normal, or increased. Autohemolysis is increased and is partially corrected with glucose and ATP. Red blood cell survival is generally slightly shortened. Splenectomy may or may not aid in the treatment of this disorder.

Rh$_{NULL}$ Disease

Rh$_{NULL}$ disease is inherited as a result of gene suppression or the presence of a silent Rh gene (X^0). It represents an absence of all Rh-Hr antigens on the red blood cell which results in red cell membrane abnormalities. It is characterized by a mild, chronic normocytic-normochromic hemolytic anemia. The blood smear shows both stomatocytes and spherocytes. The reticulocyte count is generally slightly elevated. The autohemolysis and osmotic fragility are both increased.

High Phosphatidylcholine Hemolytic Anemia

High phosphatidylcholine hemolytic anemia is inherited and represents an imbalance in the membrane phospholipid content of the red blood cell. It usually causes a mild anemia with morphologically normal red blood cells. The anemia may increase in the presence of infection or under conditions of stress.

Paroxysmal Nocturnal Hemoglobinuria. Paroxysmal nocturnal hemoglobinuria (PNH) is a rare, chronic, acquired, hemolytic disease found in young to middle-aged adults. There appears to be an acquired intrinsic defect in the red blood cells that makes the cell more sensitive to lysis by heat labile serum factors (complement). This defect is associated with an abnormal clone of hematopoietic stem cells because the platelets and white blood cells are affected also. (The exact nature of this defect is unknown.) However, the defective membrane may be due to a deficiency of decay-accelerating factor (DAF) that normally inhibits complement mediated lysis. Infections and physical stress may result in complement activation and subsequent hemolytic episodes. The severity of the disorder varies from patient to patient and from time to time in the same patient depending on the degree of sensitivity to complement. In cases of severe hemolytic episodes, blood transfusion may be necessary. The transfused red blood cells have normal survival rates. Thrombotic complications are common in these patients because of the overactivation of complement sensitive platelets.

This disorder is characterized by intravascular hemolysis and hemoglobinuria during and following sleep in the classic case. However, typical sleep related hemoglobinuria is seen in less than 25% of the patients. The peripheral blood shows normocytic-normochromic anemia. The platelet and white blood cell counts are usually decreased. The reticulocyte count is elevated. The bone marrow may be hypercellular with erythroid hyperplasia, or, as occurs in some patients, it may be hypocellular. The leukocyte alkaline phosphatase is decreased, the direct Coombs' test is negative, and the serum haptoglobin is decreased. Diagnosis of this condition may be confirmed by the acid serum test and sugar water test. There is no specific treatment for PNH; steroids have been used to control the hemolytic episodes, anticoagulants are given to those forming venous thromboses, and antibiotics to combat infections. Washed or deglycerolyzed red cells are given for severely anemic conditions.

Sulfhemoglobinemia

Sulfhemoglobinemia, when present, is generally the result of exposure to sulfonamides, acetanilid, or phenacetin but may accompany methemoglobinemia. Sulfhemoglobin is incapable of transporting oxygen, and once formed is very stable and remains for the life of the red blood cell. Sulfhemoglobinemia is generally a benign disorder, and about the only symptom it causes is cyanosis. Treatment consists of removing the offending drug.

Methemoglobinemia

Methemoglobinemia may be inherited as an autosomal recessive trait caused by a deficiency in NADH methemoglobin reductase, it may be acquired as a result of exposure to various chemical compounds, or it may be caused by any one of five hemoglobin M variants. Methemoglobin differs from normal oxyhemoglobin in that the iron in the heme molecule is in the ferric (Fe^{3+}) state rather than the ferrous (Fe^{2+}) state. Ferric hemoglobin (methemoglobin) is unable to transport oxygen, and normally less than 1% is present. Due to decreased affinity of methemoglobin for oxygen, one of the primary characteristics of these disorders is cyanosis, which gives a bluish color to the skin and mucous membranes. The blood is chocolate brown in color.

In *hereditary methemoglobinemia,* infants are cyanotic at birth. NADH methemoglobin reductase is the deficient enzyme that normally reduces cytochrome b5, which then converts ferric iron back to the ferrous state. Mental retardation may be present, but otherwise the disease is usually benign. A mild polycythemia may sometimes occur. The cyanosis is generally only of importance cosmetically. This disease may be treated with methylene blue taken orally to maintain the methemoglobin concentration below 10%. Ascorbic acid is also used in treatment.

Acquired methemoglobinemia is the most common type of this disorder and is usually due to the toxic effect of such drugs as aniline dyes and derivatives, sulfonamides, nitrates and nitrites, chlorates, nitroglycerin, and some benzenes, among others. The concentration of methemoglobin in the blood will depend on the degree of exposure to the drug. Cyanosis generally appears when the methemoglobin reaches a level of 15%. Concentrations exceeding 60 to 70% are generally associated with coma and even death. Treatment consists of withdrawal of the offending drug, and when symptoms are present, methylene blue or ascorbic acid may be given.

Hemoglobin M disease is characterized by an amino acid substitution in the alpha or beta globin chain that stabilizes iron in the ferric form. It is genetically inherited as an autosomal dominant trait. Cyanosis is the only clinical symptom present and is generally not apparent until the infant is 3 to 6 months of age if the substitution is in the β chain. However, if the disorder is an α chain variant, cyanosis will be present at birth. These individuals lead normal lives and do not respond to methylene blue or ascorbic acid therapy.

Enzyme Deficiencies

Glucose-6-Phosphate Dehydrogenase Deficiency. Glucose-6-phosphate dehydrogenase (*G-6-PD*) deficiency is inherited. It is sex linked, being carried on the X chromosome. The disease becomes fully expressed in the hemizygous male and the homozygous female. The heterozygous female has two populations of cells, one with normal enzyme activity and the other deficient in G-6-PD. It is the most common red cell enzyme abnormality, and it affects about 10% of American black males.

G-6-PD is an enzyme present in the red blood cell. Its activity is highest in young red cells and decreases as the cell ages. It plays a major role in the hexose monophosphate shunt. It is concerned with the regeneration of NADPH, necessary for the reduction of oxidized glutathione, a mechanism by which hemoglobin is protected from oxidation. The absence of this enzyme is usually harmless unless the red blood cell is exposed to redox compounds (the antimalarial drug primaquine, sulfonamides, nitrofurans, sulfones, analgesics, and antipyretics). When there is a deficiency of G-6-PD, the red blood cell is unable to generate reduced nicotinamide-adenine dinucleotide phosphate (NADPH) rapidly enough to combat the effects of oxidizing drugs. Hemoglobin is oxidized to methemoglobin which denatures and precipitates as Heinz bodies. Red cell hemolysis occurs as a result of the increased rigidity of the red cell caused by Heinz body inclusions and membrane damage from the oxidants.

There are both quantitatively and qualitatively abnormal forms of the enzyme, which may be due to a decrease in the enzyme activity or to a qualitative abnormality of the enzyme itself. Certain individuals have a type of the deficiency which renders them sensitive to fava beans, resulting in severe hemolytic episodes.

Upon continual ingestion of a redox compound by a patient deficient in G-6-PD, a hemolytic episode will occur. This condition may be divided into three phases: (1) During the acute hemolytic phase, there is destruction of 30 to 50% of the red blood cells. There is Heinz body formation, and basophilic stippling and polychromatophilia are present on the peripheral blood smear. The serum bilirubin is elevated, as is the reticulocyte count.

(2) During the recovery phase (tenth to fortieth day), the reticulocyte count reaches a peak of 8 to 12%. Macrocytes are present on the peripheral blood smear, and the hemoglobin and hematocrit levels begin to increase to normal. Haptoglobin is absent in the blood, and methemalbumin is present. Plasma hemoglobin is increased during the first two stages. (3) The resistant phase begins when the anemia disappears and continues as long as the same dose of the drug is administered. If the drug dosage is increased, another hemolytic episode will occur. Usually the hemolytic episodes are self limiting because young cells released from the bone marrow in response to the anemia have higher levels of G-6-PD.

A few patients continually show chronic anemia, but the majority are not anemic except during a hemolytic episode after exposure to certain drugs. The autohemolysis test shows increased hemolysis of red blood cells after 48-hour incubation in patients with glucose-6-phosphate dehydrogenase deficiency. The autohemolysis, however, is partially corrected by the addition of glucose or ATP. The ascorbate-cyanide test is positive for patients with this deficiency. Heinz body formation is increased when blood from G-6-PD deficient individuals is incubated with acetylphenylhydrazine. Treatment involves the avoidance of drugs known to induce hemolysis.

Pyruvate Kinase Deficiency. Pyruvate kinase is an enzyme in the Embden-Meyerhof pathway and may be the most common cause of hereditary nonspherocytic hemolytic anemia involving this pathway. Pyruvate kinase catalyzes the formation of pyruvate from phosphoenolpyruvate (PEP) with subsequent conversion of ADP to ATP. ATP provides the energy required for normal red cell membrane function and other glycolytic reactions. Pyruvate kinase deficient red cells have a decreased life span due to the lack of ATP and their inability to utilize glucose. The red blood cells are removed from the circulation extravascularly by the spleen and liver.

Pyruvate kinase deficiency is inherited as an autosomal recessive trait, with members of both sexes being equally affected. Heterozygous individuals manifest no symptoms (as there is sufficient pyruvate kinase activity to support normal red cell survival), whereas homozygous individuals have the clinical disease. If the disorder is present at birth, the newborn is jaundiced and may require transfusions or exchange transfusions. In most instances of pyruvate kinase deficiency, however, the disease is first found in infancy or childhood, with some cases not appearing until adulthood. Characteristics of this disorder are jaundice, splenomegaly, anemia of varying severity, and occasional dark urine.

The laboratory findings in this disorder show mild to severe anemia with hematocrit levels of approximately 18 to 36%. The red blood cells are normochromic and may be slightly macrocytic. The reticulocyte count is moderately to markedly increased, and the peripheral blood smear shows polychromatophilia and the presence of nucleated red blood cells. There may be slight anisocytosis, and there are generally irregularly contracted red blood cells present. Unlike G-6-PD deficiency, Heinz bodies are not formed. The white blood cell and platelet counts are usually normal. The autohemolysis test is abnormal except in mildly affected patients, in whom the results may be normal. The bone marrow shows erythroid hyperplasia. The serum bilirubin and fecal urobilinogen levels are increased. The serum haptoglobin is decreased to absent. The red blood cell pyruvate kinase activity is in the range of 5 to 25% of normal.

There is no exact treatment for pyruvate kinase deficiency. Limited use of blood transfusions and splenectomy have been utilized to raise the blood hemoglobin levels.

Other Red Blood Cell Enzyme Deficiencies.

Other red blood cell enzyme deficiencies, not as common as G-6-PD and pyruvate kinase deficiencies, can also cause a hemolytic anemia.

Pyrimidine-5-nucleotidase (PN) deficiency causes an abnormality in nucleotide metabolism. Pyrimidine-5-nucleotidase deficiency is inherited as autosomal recessive and is characterized by mild to moderate chronic hemolytic anemia, reticulocytosis of greater than 10%, and splenomegaly. Pyrimidine nucleotides from degraded RNA in the reticulocyte normally cross the red cell membrane and leave the cell aided by pyrimidine-5-nucleotidase. A deficiency results in an accumulation of these pyrimidines in the red cell,

impaired degradation of RNA, and pronounced basophilic stippling. The red blood cell autohemolysis is increased and only poorly corrected with glucose.

Glucosephosphate isomerase deficiency causes an abnormality in anaerobic glycolysis and is the third most common red blood cell enzyme deficiency. It causes a moderately severe anemia. The stained blood smear shows anisocytosis, poikilocytosis, marked polychromatophilia, and nucleated red blood cells may also be present. The reticulocyte count may be significantly increased, and the autohemolysis test is increased with only partial correction by glucose and ATP. *Triosephosphate isomerase, hexokinase,* and *diphosphoglycerate mutase* are other enzyme deficiencies that have been found to occur and are involved in anaerobic glycolysis.

Several deficiencies (in addition to G-6-PD) have been found in enzymes required in the hexose monophosphate shunt. These deficiencies are rare and have been reported only in a few families, but do cause a hemolytic anemia. These deficiencies include *glutathione synthetase, glutathione peroxidase,* and *glutathione reductase.* As with G-6-PD deficiency, hemolysis increases with oxidant drug exposure or infection.

Immune Hemolytic Anemias

The immune hemolytic anemias result from the removal from the circulation of red cells sensitized by antibody with or without complement. There is direct lysis of the cells within the vascular system. The immune hemolytic anemias may either be isoimmune, autoimmune, or drug induced.

Isoantibodies are antibodies formed by a person in response to foreign red cell antigens. The antibodies coat the red cells resulting in hemolysis. An example of this would occur if an Rh negative person were transfused with Rh positive blood causing a hemolytic transfusion reaction, characterized by acute intravascular hemolysis. Isoimmune hemolytic anemia will occur as a result of pregnancy, as foreign antigens on fetal cells cross into the maternal circulation resulting in antibody production and hemolytic disease of the newborn.

Hemolytic Disease of the Newborn. Hemolytic

disease of the newborn, (previously termed *erythroblastosis fetalis*) is a disorder found in the fetus that manifests itself in the infant during the first several days of life. This disease is usually associated with cases of Rh incompatibility where the mother is Rh negative, and the newborn is Rh positive. It is found, with more frequency and less severity, when there is incompatibility within the mother and child's ABO groups. Usually, the mother is type O, and the fetus is type A or B. This disorder may also be caused by other blood group systems such as Kell and Duffy. Transplacental hemorrhage of fetal erythrocytes containing an antigen absent on maternal red blood cells results in antibody production by the mother. Since transplacental hemorrhage usually occurs at the time of delivery, first born infants are usually asymptomatic. In ABO hemolytic disease, first born infants can be affected. IgG antibodies with subsequent pregnancies cross the placental barrier from the maternal to fetal circulation, where they combine with the antigens on fetal erythrocytes to destroy them by extravascular hemolysis.

In hemolytic disease of the newborn, the infant's peripheral blood shows a large increase in nucleated red blood cells, usually present in all stages of development. Fetal erythropoietic tissues increases red cell production in response to increased destruction. There is very little anisocytosis; however, a marked polychromatophilia is present. The reticulocyte count is increased and may even be as high as 60%. The red blood cells are usually normochromic and macrocytic. When the hemolytic anemia is due to an ABO incompatibility, there may be marked spherocytosis (accompanied by an increase in the osmotic fragility of the red blood cells). The main clinical manifestation is jaundice, and is milder than in Rh incompatibility. The hemoglobin level at birth is generally slightly lower than normal, decreasing rapidly as the disease progresses. At the same time, the nucleated red blood cells decrease in number and may disappear from the peripheral blood. The white blood cell count is generally elevated, and immature forms of the granulocytic cells are usually present. Platelets are normal to decreased in number. If decreased, there may be a prolonged bleeding time, poor clot retraction, and petechiae. The serum bilirubin level of umbilical cord blood will be

above 3 mg/dL. After birth, the bilirubin level (indirect fraction) rises rapidly and may reach 40 to 50 mg/dL by the third day in cases where no treatment has been given. Lipid soluble unconjugated bilirubin may be taken up by nervous tissue causing toxic damage (kernicterus). The direct Coombs' test on the baby's red blood cells is positive in all cases except in ABO incompatibility, where the direct Coombs' test is generally negative or weakly positive, becoming negative within 12 hours after birth. The infant with this disorder has an enlarged spleen and liver as a result of extramedullary hematopoiesis.

The most common treatment for hemolytic disease of the newborn is the exchange transfusion. If the cord blood bilirubin level at birth is above 4.5 mg/dL, an exchange transfusion is usually carried out immediately. Albumin infusions are also used to bind unconjugated bilirubin, and light treatments are used in milder cases to convert bilirubin to less toxic derivatives. During the first few days of life, the bilirubin level is allowed to rise to 20 mg/dL before an exchange transfusion is performed. More than one exchange transfusion may or may not be required, depending on the severity of the disease.

Autoimmune Hemolytic Anemia. *Autoantibodies* are antibodies produced by individuals that react with specific antigens on their own red blood cells. Therefore, in autoimmune hemolytic anemia, the antibodies are produced by the patient's immune system. These anemias may be classified as (1) warm reactive, (2) cold reactive, or (3) drug induced.

Autoimmune hemolytic anemia caused by warm reactive antibodies may occur without any obvious cause. They may be secondary to or associated with trauma, surgery, and pregnancy, or various disease states such as viral infections, malignant tumors, systemic lupus erythematosus, and other autoimmune disorders. They account for about 70% of all cases of autoimmune hemolytic anemia. These warm-reactive IgG antibodies bind optimally at 37°C and the red cell-antibody complexes are cleared by the spleen. The clinical symptoms will include weakness and dizziness. Fever may be present, and jaundice is a fairly common finding. This anemia may be variable in its severity, ranging from mild to very severe. The blood smear generally shows anisocytosis, polychromatophilia, spherocytosis, some macrocytosis, and nucleated red blood cells may also be present. The reticulocyte count is variable and may show a marked increase. Siderocytes will be increased. The white blood cell count may be increased during the acute phase of the disease. Generally, the platelet count is normal. The autohemolysis test is increased, and the osmotic fragility will be increased during the acute phase but may be normal during periods of remission. The direct antiglobulin test is generally positive but may be negative in cases of weak red blood cell sensitization. Several methods of treatment are used for this disorder. If the hemolytic anemia is secondary to another disorder, treatment of the primary condition may alleviate the hemolytic anemia. Blood transfusions are used only in life threatening circumstances because this may accelerate hemolysis. Steroids are the therapy of choice, with good results. When steroid therapy is ineffective, a splenectomy may be performed to decrease antibody production and removal of sensitized red cells. Cytotoxic drugs have also been used as a last resort.

Autoimmune hemolytic anemia due to IgM cold reactive antibodies is caused by antibodies most reactive at temperatures below 32°C. This disease occurs most often in people over 50 years of age and may occur in association with infection, lymphoproliferative disorders, malignancy, or autoimmune disorders. Cold winter months usually bring on the symptoms of cold autoimmune hemolytic anemia because there is agglutination of the patient's red cells in the skin capillaries, mainly in the extremities. It is also commonly found as a complication of Mycoplasma pneumoniae, respiratory infections, and infectious mononucleosis. The two most common cold agglutinins are IgM immunoglobulins with anti-I and anti-i specificity. A stained blood film generally shows polychromatophilia, possibly some spherocytosis, and agglutination of the red blood cells (unless measures were taken to maintain the blood and equipment at 37°C during smear preparation). The white blood cell count may or may not be elevated. The direct antiglobulin test will be positive if the reagents used contain anticomplement activity. The cold agglutinin titer is increased. Treatment of the patient includes keeping body temperature above the temperature at which the antibody reacts. Plasmapheresis and transfusions have been used for the acutely ill patient. Also, treatment of the primary illness may lessen the hemolytic disorder.

Drug-induced autoimmune hemolytic anemia may result from penicillin, stibophen, or an alpha-methyldopa type of drug. The mechanism by which the drug causes hemolysis depends on the type of drug involved. Penicillin and cephalosporin combine with proteins on the red cell membrane and provoke an immune response by the formation of antibodies to these drugs. Stibophen, quinidine, and sulfonamides cause an antibody response with subsequent absorption of the complex to the red cell membrane. α-Methyl dopa (aldomet) induces the formation of an antibody (exact mechanism is unknown) specifically directed against normal red blood cell antigens, and is the most common drug-induced immune hemolytic anemia. About 15% of the patients develop a positive direct Coombs test. Discontinuation of the offending drug is the treatment of choice.

Paroxysmal Cold Hemoglobinuria. Paroxysmal cold hemoglobinuria is a rare disorder caused by a complement dependent hemolytic antibody described by Donath and Landsteiner, which has thus been named the *Donath-Landsteiner antibody*. It has classically been found secondary to syphilis but has also been seen in viral infections with no apparent cause. The Donath-Landsteiner antibody is an IgG immunoglobulin. The hemolytic reaction occurs as the antibody is bound to the red blood cell in the presence of complement at low temperatures, followed by hemolysis at body temperature.

This disorder manifests itself following exposure to cold, and the patient will exhibit fever, chills, and back and leg pain, along with hemoglobinuria. The patient generally recovers from the attack quickly and may have no symptoms in between attacks.

Laboratory tests show an anemia, the severity of which depends on the severity of the attacks. The reticulocyte count is usually increased. During attacks, the plasma shows marked hemolysis and will contain methemalbumin. The urine contains hemoglobin and methemoglobin, and the serum bilirubin level is elevated. Treatment consists of improving the primary infection, when present, or having the patient avoid cold temperatures.

Nonimmune (Acquired) Hemolytic Anemias

A nonimmune hemolytic anemia may develop as a result of exposure to various physical agents such as heat. A substantial amount of third degree burns to the body will damage red blood cells. The blood smear in these cases will show schistocytes, microspherocytes, and irregularly contracted red blood cells. The red cells also show increased osmotic fragility. In cardiac valve disease where the diseased valve has been surgically replaced, mechanical damage to the red blood cells may occur.

Infectious agents, such as Clostridium perfringens, Bartonella bacilliformis, and some staphylococcal and other bacterial infections, have been known to produce a hemolytic anemia by producing toxins. Intracellular organisms such as babesia and the plasmodium species (malaria) can also result in a hemolytic anemia.

Some compounds such as arsenic, lead, and copper, and strong oxidizing drugs are capable of denaturing hemoglobin or causing a hemolytic response. Venom from some spiders and snakes may also cause intravascular hemolysis of the red blood cells.

Disorders Causing Fragmentation of the Red Blood Cells. There are numerous circumstances during which the red blood cells are subjected to physical and mechanical trauma, causing fragmentation and lysis.

Replacement of cardiac valves by artificial plastic *prosthetic devices* may result in enough damage and destruction to the red blood cell (by the prosthetic device itself) to cause anemia of varying severity. This has been aptly called the 'Waring blender syndrome'. In this situation, the stained blood smear characteristically shows schistocytes. Polychromatophilia and some macrocytosis may also be present. The reticulocyte count will be increased. The bilirubin and plasma hemoglobin may be elevated, depending on the severity of the anemia. Cases where the anemia is severe may indicate a malfunction of the replaced valve, and repeat surgery may be necessary.

Microangiopathic hemolytic anemia is generally a result of fibrin deposits within the small blood vessels, as found in association with thrombotic thrombocytopenia purpura and intravascular coagulation. Blood flowing through fibrin strands from the intravascular activation of the coagulation system (DIC) results in "clothesline-like" shearing of the red blood cells. The peripheral blood shows a large number of schistocytes and a decreased to low normal platelet count. It is also present in malignant hypertension, disseminated carcinoma, and hemolytic uremic syndrome (HUS) in children. The common denominator in these diseases is the presence of small blood vessel diseases or pathologic lesions of the small blood vessels. Red cell contact with damaged endothelial cells of the blood vessels results in fragmentation. In this anemia, red blood cell fragmentation (schistocytes) and irregular contraction of the red blood cells are characteristic findings on the blood smear. Microspherocytes may also be present. The reticulocyte count is generally elevated, and the white blood cell count may be slightly to moderately increased. The platelet count may be normal or decreased, largely depending on the primary disorder. The bone marrow usually shows increased red blood cell hyperplasia and megakaryocyte hyperplasia. The plasma hemoglobin is generally increased, urine hemoglobin is present, and hemosiderin can most often be demonstrated in the urine. Therapy usually consists of treating the primary disease. Blood transfusions have been used to treat the anemia when necessary.

Malaria. Parasites that cause malaria in man and other animals belong to the class Sporozoa, suborder Haemosporidia, genus *Plasmodium*. The four species most commonly found in man are *Plasmodium vivax, malariae, falciparum,* and *ovale.*

Malaria is mainly transmitted from person to person through the bite of the female *Anopheles* mosquito. Other means of transmission are through the use of contaminated needles, by congenital means, and through blood transfusions.

The life cycle of the malaria parasite requires two types of hosts: the invertebrate (female Anopheles mosquito), where the parasite reaches maturity and the sexual cycle occurs (*sporogony*), and the vertebrate (e.g., the human), where the immature stages occur and asexual multiplication takes place (*schizogony*). When the infected Anopheles mosquito bites a human, sporozoites are injected into the peripheral blood of the individual. The sporozoites then invade the parenchymal cells of the liver, where preerythrocytic development takes place, ending with the schizont phase. At this time, the parasites rupture the cells, and the merozoites from the schizont penetrate the red blood cells or continue the exoerythrocytic phase by penetrating other liver cells and repeating the cycle, again developing into schizonts.

When the red blood cell has been penetrated by the merozoite, the parasite develops into the trophozoite ring form and thence to a mature schizont. This process takes 48 hours in P. falciparum, P. ovale, and P. vivax infections and 72 hours in P. malariae, and is called *schizogony.* The merozoites rupture from the mature schizonts and penetrate other red blood cells. Fever and chills are associated with the rupture of the red blood cells. The merozoites entering the red blood cell then repeat the process of schizogony, forming mature schizonts from which more merozoites emerge. When several of the preceding asexual cycles have occurred, some of the merozoites enter red blood cells and become sexually differentiated into the male microgametocyte or the female macrogametocyte. In this circumstance, the gametocyte remains in the red blood cell as long as the red blood cell lives and does not influence the patient's symptoms.

The gametocyte is the only form of the parasite that is now infective to the Anopheles mosquito. When the mosquito bites the infected person, the gametocytes enter the mosquito and mature in its stomach. The zygote is formed when the male microgamete exflagellates and fertilizes the female macrogamete. The zygote matures, becoming actively motile, to form an *ookinete,* which penetrates the stomach wall of the mosquito. It moves to the outside of the stomach wall and becomes an oocyst. The oocyst matures to a sporocyst, which ruptures and gives rise to sporozoites. These sporozoites migrate to the salivary glands of the female Anopheles mosquito, where they remain until a person is

bitten by this mosquito. At this time, the sporozoites enter the peripheral blood and the cycle is repeated (Fig. 6–2).

It is important, when diagnosing malaria, to be able to identify the infecting species. Occasionally, mixed infections occur, the most common being P. falciparum and P. vivax. This may be accomplished by microscopic examination of thick and thin blood smears stained with Giemsa stain. Care should be taken not to confuse blood platelets with various stages of malarial parasites. Blood films several hours apart may be required to demonstrate the infection or diagnose the species.

Malaria may occur in the chronic, recurrent, or acute form. Parasites of P. vivax and P. ovale can persist within hepatic cells, resulting in relapses from activation of these parasites. The patient has sudden onsets of severe chills, along with fever, weakness, and often, splenomegaly. Generally, mild anemia is present as a result of shortened red blood cell life span due to the parasite invading the red blood cell. The osmotic fragility of the red blood cells is increased, and due to the hemolysis present, the haptoglobin is decreased to absent. The white cell count is usually normal or elevated with developing neutropenia. Thrombocytopenia can result as platelets are removed by the spleen.

Blackwater fever, although rarely seen, may occur in P. falciparum infections. As many as 50% of the red blood cells can be parasitized. This condition is characterized by severe, acute intravascular hemolysis, severe anemia, chills, weakness, fever, and vomiting. It has sometimes been found in patients who have been treated for malaria with quinine.

Babesiosis. The causative agent of babesiosis in man is a sporozoan parasite spread by the bite of infected ticks. In North America, and particularly in the endemic regions of Cape Cod, MA (Martha's Vineyard and Nantucket) and Long Island, NY, most infections are caused by the species Babesia microti. The peak incidence of babesiosis is in early August, and the symptoms appear 1 to 4 weeks following the tick bite. Upon entering the circulation, the sporozoite penetrates the red cell where the organism transforms into a ring-shaped merozoite. The babesia organism divides by budding (rather than schizogony)

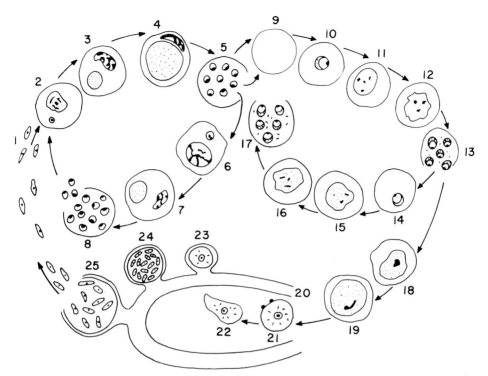

FIG. 6–2. Life cycle of the malaria parasite. 1, Sporozoites from mosquito. 2, 3, 4, Primary exoerythrocytic parasite in liver cells. 5, Merozoites being released from the ruptured exoerythrocytic schizont. 6, 7, Merozoite of the secondary exoerythrocytic cycle in liver cells. 8, Second generation of merozoites being released from the exoerythrocytic schizont. 9, Red blood cell in peripheral blood. 10, 11, 12, Erythrocytic schizogony in peripheral blood. 13, Erythrocytic merozoites and gametocytes being released from the ruptured erythrocytic schizont. 14, 15, 16, 17, Erythrocytic schizogony. 18, 19, Development of female gametocyte (macrogametocyte) in peripheral blood. 20, Stomach wall of mosquito. 21, Macrogamete. 22, Ookinete. 23, Oocyst. 24, Development of oocyst and production of sporozoites. 25, Sporozoites leaving the ruptured oocyst.

entirely within the red cell; a sexual stage of reproduction is not evident.

Mild and subclinical cases occur, although babesiosis can present as an acute febrile illness characterized by fever, chills, malaise, and anemia from hemolytic episodes. In older, splenectomized individuals the disease can become life-threatening and fatal as a result of fulminant intravascular hemolysis with subsequent renal failure.

The babesia organism is about 1.0 to 2.0 μm in size and infects the red blood cells, appearing pleomorphic and ring-shaped with a prominent vacuole that can enlarge up to 2 to 4 μm. These trophozoites closely resemble the ring forms found in Plasmodium falciparum, although babesia can be differentiated from malaria by the absence of gametocytes and enlarged red cells.

As the organism undergoes schizogeny, the organism enlarges displaying a prominent red-staining nucleus and blue cytoplasm. The red chromatin dot eventually becomes fragmented into multiple organisms or rings, four of which may be connected by strands of blue cytoplasm into the characteristic "tetrad" formation.

Clinically, parasitemia may persist for several months after the symptoms abate, and the degree of parasitemia does not closely parallel the severity of the symptoms. Babesiosis is usually treated with quinine and the antibiotic clindamycin.

Hemoglobinopathies

The globin portion of the hemoglobin molecule is composed of two pairs of polypeptide chains, each with a specific amino acid sequence. This is the *primary structure.* Each polypeptide chain has a single heme group, consisting of an atom of iron bound within a protoporphyrin-IX ring. The chains are twisted around on an axis in a helical arrangement (the *secondary structure*), are bent into a three-dimensional shape (the *tertiary structure*), and are bound together to form the hemoglobin tetramer.

Different types of normal hemoglobins have been described and given specific names based on the number and sequence of amino acids composing each polypeptide chain. On the following pages, the normal and more common abnormal hemoglobin forms are discussed.

Normal Hemoglobins. The major portion of normal hemoglobin in adult blood is termed *hemoglobin A.* The globin portion of each hemoglobin A molecule is composed of two alpha chains, containing 141 amino acids, and two beta chains, made up of 146 amino acids. The molecule is ellipsoidal, with the four heme groups (responsible for oxygen transport) at the surface. The formula for hemoglobin A is: $\alpha_2^A\beta_2^A$, indicating that the molecule is made up of two normal hemoglobin A, alpha chains, and two normal hemoglobin A, beta chains. The concentration of hemoglobin A is 95% or more of the total adult hemoglobin.

A second type of hemoglobin, hemoglobin A_2, is normally found in the adult in a concentration of 1.5 to 3%. Iron deficiency can cause decreased hemoglobin A_2 synthesis. Hemoglobin A_2 consists of two alpha^A chains, and two other chains that differ from the beta^A chains by the substitution of 10 amino acids. These two chains, since they differ so greatly from beta^A chains, are termed delta, thus giving hemoglobin A_2 the formula: $\alpha_2^A\delta_2^{A2}$.

Fetal hemoglobin, hemoglobin F, is normally present in high concentrations during fetal life. At birth, at least half of the hemoglobin present in the newborn is hemoglobin F. The concentration then falls rapidly and assumes the normal adult level of 2% or less by 1 or 2 years of age. Hemoglobin F is composed of two alpha chains and two other chains that differ from the beta^A chains and are termed gamma. The formula for hemoglobin F is $\alpha_2^A\gamma_2^F$.

In early fetal life, three primitive or embryonal hemoglobins are found, namely, *hemoglobin Gower 1, hemoglobin Gower 2,* and *hemoglobin Portland.* These three hemoglobins persist for only a short time in the embryo. Hemoglobin Gower 1 is composed of 2ζ (zeta) and 2ϵ (epsilon) chains, hemoglobin Gower 2 contains 2α and 2ϵ chains, and hemoglobin Portland, 2ζ and 2γ chains.

Abnormal Hemoglobins. The structure of abnormal hemoglobins is based on at least four kinds of polypeptide chains, alpha, beta, delta, and gamma, and possibly a fifth chain, epsilon. The synthesis of any given type of chain is under genetic control. The structurally abnormal hemoglobins usually consist of polypeptide chains with a normal number of amino acids but with a single amino acid substitution. For example, if a normal pair of chains has glutamic acid at the sixth position, the abnormal form may have a valine molecule in place of the glutamic acid. In clinically significant disease, either the alpha or beta chains are affected. The majority of hemoglobinopathies result from β chain abnormalities, either inherited or as a result of genetic mutations. A large number of hemoglobin variants involving the gamma or delta chains are not clinically significant because of the small amount of hemoglobin involved. Alterations in the amino acid composition of the polypeptide chain usually cause a change in the net charge of the molecule. This property is then employed to detect the presence of different hemoglobins. Using the techniques of electrophoresis, blood is placed on a medium in an electric field in a buffer with a specific pH. The difference in the net charge of the hemoglobin molecule determines its mobility and the speed with which it migrates. Many of the abnormal hemoglobins are detected by this method.

Hemoglobin S is an abnormal hemoglobin that causes sickling of the red blood cells under conditions of reduced oxygen concentration. It shows an amino acid substitution in the beta chains and is written as $\alpha_2^A\beta_2^{6\ val}$, indicating a substitution of valine for glutamic acid at the sixth position in the normal beta chain. Hemoglobin S is confined to blacks and, in the homozygous state, causes sickle cell anemia. An individual heterozygous for hemoglobin S shows the sickle cell trait.

Hemoglobin C ($\alpha_2{}^A\beta_2{}^{6\ lys}$) is found primarily in blacks and only rarely in whites and occurs as a result of the substitution of the amino acid lysine for glutamic acid on the sixth position of the beta chain. It is, many times, inherited in combination with hemoglobin S and may also be found in the homozygous or heterozygous state. When hemoglobin C is present, the red blood cells appear as target cells, or, less often, precipitated hemoglobin C crystals may be demonstrated within the red blood cell.

Hemoglobin D shows several varieties of abnormal hemoglobin that are indistinguishable from each other by electrophoretic methods using cellulose acetate at a pH of 8.4. The variants with the highest frequency are hemoglobin D Punjab and hemoglobin D-Los Angeles. Both alpha and beta chain abnormalities have been reported. The electrophoretic mobility of hemoglobin D is the same as hemoglobin S, although red blood cells containing hemoglobin D show no sickling at a reduced oxygen concentration.

Hemoglobin E ($\alpha_2{}^A\beta_2{}^{26\ lys}$) shows the same electrophoretic mobility on cellulose acetate at a pH of 8.4, as hemoglobin A_2 and is sometimes associated with thalassemia.

Hemoglobins have also been found that contain no alpha chains. For example: *hemoglobin H* consists of four beta chains: $\beta_4{}^A$; and *hemoglobin Bart's* is composed of four gamma chains: $\gamma_4{}^F$.

Sickle Cell Anemia.

A person homozygous for hemoglobin S is said to have sickle cell anemia. This disorder occurs chiefly in blacks or persons of black ancestry. Its incidence in the United States is 2.5 to 3.5%. The red blood cells contains 90 to 100% hemoglobin S, with the remainder being hemoglobin F and hemoglobin A_2. There is normal synthesis of the α, γ, and δ chains, but only the characteristic β^s chains are synthesized. The symptoms of sickle cell anemia rarely occur prior to about 6 months of age, because hemoglobin F predominates at birth and for a short time thereafter. This disease is usually fatal by the age of 30. The physical properties of the red blood

cells have much to do with the clinical manifestations of the disease. Under decreased oxygen tension, hemoglobin S is much less soluble than hemoglobin A. Hemoglobin S polymerizes to form tactoids, which force the red blood cell into a rigid sickle-shape when the oxygen concentration is reduced. As a result, painful vaso-occlusive crises occur. There is severe abdominal, bone, and joint pain due to the plugging up of some of the small blood vessels by masses of the sickled red blood cells. This results in tissue death and necrosis (e.g., leg ulcers). There may be local thrombus formation as platelets adhere to damaged endothelium, factor XII is activated, and tissue thromboplastin is released. This, in turn, causes infarcts in different organs of the body. The spleen, enlarged during infancy, eventually shrivels up and becomes fibrotic in the adult (autosplenectomy) because of these numerous infarcts. Irreversibly sickled red blood cells also have an increased mechanical fragility from permanent membrane damage that results in a decreased survival time. There is severe marrow hyperplasia, and changes such as necrosis and lesions are produced in the bones. Serious bacterial infections are a major cause of death.

On a stained smear, the red blood cells show moderate anisocytosis, poikilocytosis, and hypochromia. Some sickle cells are generally present. Target cells, Howell-Jolly bodies, and nucleated red blood cells are usually seen. Polychromatophilia is generally present, and an elevated reticulocyte count is found. The platelets are usually increased, and there may be moderate neutrophilia. The osmotic fragility test is decreased, and the erythrocyte sedimentation rate is low. Sickle cell preparations are quickly and strongly positive. Hemoglobin electrophoresis shows a single abnormal band, hemoglobin S, which migrates more slowly than hemoglobin A. Hemoglobin F, if present in concentrations over 20%, has a mediating effect on the severity of the disease (as in hgb S/hereditary persistence of fetal hemoglobin [HPFH]). The hemoglobin A_2 levels may be slightly increased. The bone marrow is hypercellular due to an increase in the erythroid cells. Cell maturation and morphology in the bone marrow are normal.

Treatment involves the use of antibiotics to combat infections and analgesics for pain, during crises. Hydration to maintain normal electrolyte balance is important. There are a number of antisickling agents under trial (such as hydroxyurea), and nifedipine as a vasodilator has been used with good success. Exchange transfusion has been used in severe cases to reduce the hemoglobin S concentration in the blood.

Sickle Cell Trait. The sickle cell trait is found in approximately 10% of American blacks. In this condition, the patient is heterozygous for hemoglobin S. The red blood cells contain about 40% hemoglobin S and approximately 60% hemoglobin A. The hemoglobin A_2 level is usually slightly elevated. Under normal conditions, sickling of the red blood cells does not occur, there are no clinical symptoms of the disease, and the patient lives a normal life span. There is no anemia present, and the red blood cell morphology is normal. An occasional target cell may be found, but no sickle cells are demonstrable in the stained blood smear. The reticulocyte count is normal, and there is no polychromatophilia on the stained blood smear. The sickle cell preparation is always positive, and hemoglobin electrophoresis shows a band of hemoglobin S. Over 50% of the patients with sickle cell trait do not have the ability to concentrate urine (hyposthenuria).

Under certain conditions, such as a respiratory infection, administration of anesthesia, or airplane flight in a nonpressurized cabin, there may be some sickling of the red blood cells with accompanying clinical manifestations.

Persons with sickle cell trait seem resistant to infection with P. falciparum malaria. Various hypotheses have been suggested about why cells containing hemoglobin S are not parasitized, but none are definite.

Hemoglobin C Disease and Trait. In the homozygous condition, there is almost 100% hemoglobin C present in the red blood cells. In some patients, there may also be an increased concentration of hemoglobin F. *Homozygous hemoglobin C disease* is characterized by a mild to moderate microcytic (average MCV is 72 fL), normocytic-normochromic, hemolytic anemia with splenomegaly. The stained blood smear shows 40 to 90% target cells, a

few spherocytes, and slight polychromatophilia. The reticulocyte count is slightly increased. In some instances, rod-shaped crystals (termed *hemoglobin C crystals*) may be seen within the red blood cell in the Wright-stained blood smear, or the crystals may be demonstrated by incubating the red blood cells at 37°C in 3% (w/v) sodium citrate. Hemoglobin electrophoresis shows 90 to 100% hemoglobin C and less than 7% hemoglobin F. Most patients with hemoglobin C disease live a normal life span. The incidence of hemoglobin C disease is rare in the United States with only about 0.02% of blacks having the disease.

In the heterozygous condition (hemoglobin C trait), there are no clinical symptoms. The blood smear shows about 40% target cells and mild hypochromia. About 2 to 3% of American blacks have hemoglobin C trait. Hemoglobin electrophoresis shows 35 to 45% hemoglobin C and 55 to 65% hemoglobin A.

Hemoglobin D Disease and Trait. Hemoglobin D is rare in the United States, with the highest incidence in India or in British people with Indian ancestry. The trait is asymptomatic, with no anemia and a normal blood smear. The homozygous condition is extremely rare, but still asymptomatic with no hemolytic anemia. Hemoglobin D migrates with hemoglobin S on cellulose acetate at pH 8.6.

Hemoglobin E Disease and Trait. Hemoglobin E is rare in the United States, but is a common abnormal hemoglobin in southeast Asia. It is seen with increasing frequency in the United States as southeast Asians emigrate to this country.

The homozygous state is characterized by mild hemolytic anemia and the peripheral smear shows marked hypochromia, many target cells, and microcytosis. Hemoglobin E is slightly unstable. The heterozygous state is asymptomatic with slight microcytosis on the blood smear, and approximately 70% hemoglobin A and 30% hemoglobin E on cellulose acetate electrophoresis. Hemoglobin E migrates with hemoglobins A_2 and C on cellulose acetate at pH 8.6, but with hemoglobin A on citrate agar gel at pH 6.2.

Hemoglobin SC Disease. The combination of two abnormal β chain hemoglobins (S and C) leads to a disease only slightly less severe than the homozygous state of hemoglobin S. There is a high incidence in blacks of hemoglobin SC. This disease shows bone necrosis, splenomegaly, muscular pain, and complications during pregnancy in which crises are more frequent and can lead to fatal infarctions.

The peripheral blood smear shows up to 85% target cells, slight to marked anisocytosis and poikilocytosis, with sickle cells and hemoglobin C crystals often present. The anemia may be mild to moderate. Alkaline hemoglobin electrophoresis (pH 8.6) shows the presence of two bands, hemoglobin S and C, in approximately equal concentrations.

Hemoglobin SD Disease. The combination of hemoglobins S and D is uncommon, but resembles hemoglobin SC disease in severity when found. Only the combination of hemoglobins S and D Punjab shows moderate hemolytic anemia.

Unstable Hemoglobin Disease. Unstable hemoglobin disease is rare and may be caused by any one of a large number of hemoglobin variants, all of which are less stable than normal hemoglobin. Unstable hemoglobins occur as a result of amino acid substitutions, deletions, or cross-overs in one or several of the four polypeptide chains, which weakens the structure of the hemoglobin molecule. They are inherited as autosomal dominant traits and all of the known cases are heterozygous. It has been suggested that homozygosity is incompatible with life. The severity of the disease varies according to the hemoglobin variant, and there may be no clinical symptoms or the disease may produce a mild, moderate, or severe hemolytic anemia. Jaundice is common if the hemolysis is severe. Cyanosis may be present in certain unstable hemoglobin diseases due to the formation of methemoglobin or sulfhemoglobin, or due to a decreased affinity of the hemoglobin molecule for oxygen. Hemoglobins H, Köln, and Zurich are examples of unstable hemoglobins causing hemolysis. Many unstable hemoglobins have a high affinity for oxygen, and therefore there is no anemia.

The degree of anemia and reticulocytosis present will depend on the severity of the disease. Heinz bodies are characteristically present in the red blood cells because of the instability of the hemoglobin. These may cause a lower than normal MCHC because the hemoglobin present in Heinz bodies is not measured. The stained blood smear generally shows anisocytosis, poikilocytosis, basophilic stippling, polychromatophilia, and sometimes hypochromia. If the anemia is severe, spherocytes and schistocytes may also be present. If the spleen is enlarged, there may be a thrombocytopenia caused by sequestering of the platelets in the spleen. The reticulocyte count will generally be increased. Much care must be taken when performing the reticulocyte count to distinguish the Heinz bodies from true reticulocytes. The heat denaturation test and the isopropanol precipitation test are both positive. Citrate agar gel electrophoresis at pH 6.2 and cellulose acetate hemoglobin electrophoresis at pH 8.6 are not useful for isolating unstable hemoglobins as most variants migrate with other major hemoglobins. Therapy is generally not necessary in cases of mild anemia. When the anemia is more severe, a splenectomy may be performed.

Hereditary Persistence of Fetal Hemoglobin (HPFH). Hereditary persistence of fetal hemoglobin is characterized by the persistence of fetal hemoglobin in adult life and is a benign condition with no hematologic abnormalities. There is a suppression of β chain synthesis in a heterozygous state, with 15 to 30% hemoglobin F. The rarer homozygous state (found only in blacks) with 100% hemoglobin F has a complete absence of β and δ chain synthesis. These patients have mild hypochromia and microcytosis but no anemia. When combined with hemoglobin S, persons exhibit no symptoms or anemia of the sickle cell disease. The presence of hemoglobin F in red cells inhibits in-vivo sickling. Using the acid elution (Kleihauer-Betke) test, HPFH can be categorized as *pancellular* (pan = all) where hemoglobin F is uniformly distributed among all of the red cells, or *heterocellular*, in which hemoglobin F is unevenly distributed.

Thalassemia. Thalassemia is an hereditary disease found in people of Mediterranean, Asian, and African ancestry. It is caused by impaired production of one of the polypeptide chains of the hemoglobin molecule, as well as excess production of the other globin chains. The structural formation of the chains is normal, but the rate of formation is decreased, or the chains may not be synthesized at all. Defects have been discovered at various stages of globin synthesis and include gene deletions, transcription errors, and mutations. Impaired synthesis of the beta chain is the most common, and the term applied to this abnormality is *beta thalassemia*. Decreased production of alpha chains and delta chains may also be found.

Thalassemia Major. Thalassemia major, or *Cooley's anemia*, is a homozygous beta thalassemia. (In β^0 thalassemia, β chain synthesis is absent. In β^+ thalassemia, β chain synthesis is reduced.) Despite impaired or absent synthesis of the β chains, synthesis of α chains continues at a normal rate. This imbalance results in precipitation of excess α chains in the erythrocyte and membrane damage to the red blood cell resulting in hemolysis. This disease generally has its onset during infancy. The most common physical findings are marked pallor and moderate to marked splenomegaly. Enlargement of the liver is also frequently present. Most of these patients exhibit retarded growth, and their facial features show a mongoloid appearance. Patients with Cooley's anemia rarely live beyond the second decade.

Severe hemolytic anemia is present with hemoglobin levels below 7 g/dL. The peripheral blood smear shows microcytic, hypochromic red blood cells, probably due to the decreased synthesis of globin. There is marked anisocytosis and poikilocytosis. Basophilic stippling, increased polychromatophilia, numerous target cells, Howell-Jolly bodies, and siderocytes are commonly found in the blood smear. Nucleated red blood cells are present in the peripheral blood and may be as numerous as 200 or more per 100 white blood cells. The reticulocyte count is increased. The white blood cell count may be slightly increased, with occasional immature granulocytes present. A slight increase in platelets may also be found. The osmotic fragility test is decreased. The bone marrow shows an erythroid hyperplasia. Due to chronic hemolysis and frequent blood transfusions, excess iron accumulates in the spleen

and liver. The plasma haptoglobin level is generally markedly decreased to absent and serum bilirubin is elevated. Hemoglobin electrophoresis most often shows 40 to 60% hemoglobin F, and hemoglobin A_2 is also increased. This is due to a compensatory increase in γ and δ chain production as β chain production is decreased. In the homozygous β^+ thalassemias there is a variation in the severity of the disease, depending on the degree of production of the β chains. Type I produces about 10% normal β chains, type II about 50%, type III is the mildest form of β thalassemia. The mild types do not require transfusion therapy and have been called *thalassemia intermedia*.

Thalassemia Minor. Thalassemia minor is a heterozygous beta thalassemia that is also known as Cooley's trait. This condition is characterized by slight splenomegaly and mild anemia. Patients with this trait generally live a normal life span.

The peripheral blood usually shows a hemoglobin of 10 to 11 g/dL. Microcytic, hypochromic red blood cells are found on the blood smear. Target cells, increased polychromatophilia, basophilic stippling, and an occasional nucleated red blood cell are found on the Wright stained smear, which distinguishes thalassemia minor from iron deficiency anemia. The reticulocyte count is slightly elevated. The white blood cell count is normal. The bone marrow shows slight erythroid hyperplasia and increased storage iron. Hemoglobin electrophoresis shows 2 to 6% hemoglobin F and 3 to 7% hemoglobin A_2, with the remainder being hemoglobin A.

Alpha (α) Thalassemias. An α thalassemia of varying severity results from reduced or absent α-chain synthesis affecting the two pairs of α globin genes (one pair in each chromosome). The degree of abnormality and the amount of excess β chain production varies in proportion to the number of genes affected. As the capacity to produce α chains decreases, this results in an accumulation of excess γ chains in fetal life to form hemoglobin Bart's (γ_4) and an excess of β chains to form hemoglobin H (β_4) later on.

When there is deletion of only one gene, the resultant microcytosis is slight with no anemia. This is the "silent carrier" state. In a two gene deletion, there is a moderate microcytosis with mild anemia, and it is termed α thalassemia trait. In Asians, both deletions are on the same chromosome, whereas in blacks a single gene is deleted from each of the two chromosomes. A three gene deletion causes hemoglobin H disease with MCVs less than 70 fL and mild to severe hemolytic anemia caused by hemoglobin H denaturation and red cell destruction. At birth there is 10 to 40% hemoglobin Bart's and 5 to 30% hemoglobin H in adult life. The peripheral blood smear shows hypochromia, microcytosis, anisocytosis, target cells, and basophilic stippling. The reticulocyte count is between 5 and 10%, and the spleen is enlarged. Hemoglobin H (excess β chain production in which the β chains are arranged in unstable tetramers) readily precipitates in the form of characteristic H bodies when fresh blood is incubated with brilliant cresyl blue. The condition may be exacerbated by exposure to oxidant drugs and during pregnancy. When α chain production is totally absent, there is no hemoglobin A or F production or oxygen transport, which leads to death in utero (hydrops fetalis). Hemoglobin Bart's concentration is greater than 80%.

Sickle Cell-β-Thalassemia Disease. Patients doubly heterozygous for β thalassemia and hemoglobin S show an anemia which may be mild to severe. In severe cases (β^0 thalassemia), the peripheral blood smear shows microcytosis, target cells, hypochromia, anisocytosis and poikilocytosis. Sickle cells are rare in the unsplenectomized patient. The reticulocyte count is about 10 to 20%. Hemoglobin electrophoresis shows hemoglobin S in excess of hemoglobin A (which may be absent in the β^0 type) and increased hemoglobins A_2 and F. Clinical manifestations are similar to sickle cell anemia, and the spleen is enlarged. Mild cases (β^+ thalassemia) have little or no anemia because of the presence of varied amounts of hemoglobin A.

Hemoglobin E-β Thalassemia Disease. This disease is common in Thailand and southeast Asia, and resembles β-thalassemia major in severity. The blood smear shows microcytosis, hypochromia, and target cells. There is a severe anemia requiring blood transfusions, with retarded physical growth. Hemoglobin electrophoresis shows hemoglobins E and F

in equal concentrations, with no hemoglobin A.

WHITE BLOOD CELL DISORDERS

Neutrophil Disorders

Pelger-Huët Anomaly

The Pelger-Huët anomaly is inherited as an autosomal dominant trait and is characterized by decreased segmentation of the nucleus of granulocytes, and coarseness and condensation of the nuclear chromatin in the granulocytes, lymphocytes, and normoblasts. These changes are most evident in the neutrophil, eosinophil, and basophil where the nuclei will appear round, dumbbell shaped ("pince-nez" appearance), or peanut shaped. In the homozygous state, all of the granulocyte nuclei are round or oval with mature, coarsely clumped chromatin. This anomaly, however, is most frequently seen in the heterozygous state, where less than 40% of the neutrophils contain a single-lobed nucleus; the majority (70 to 90%) of neutrophils contain a bilobed nucleus, and a small percentage (<10%) of neutrophils have three lobed nuclei. None of the neutrophils have more than three lobes. Pelger Huët cells appear to function normally. A defect in nucleic acid metabolism is thought to be responsible for the abnormal maturation seen in the nuclei of these cells.

Acquired or *pseudo-Pelger-Huët anomaly* is most often seen in chronic myelogenous leukemia and myeloid metaplasia but may also be seen in patients receiving chemotherapy. Most of these pseudo-Pelger-Huët cells have a round, centrally located nucleus. The acquired form can also be differentiated from the inherited form by the presence of more than 10% of normal three lobed neutrophils.

May-Hegglin Anomaly

The May-Hegglin anomaly is inherited as an autosomal dominant trait. It is characterized by the presence of oblong, or crescent-shaped, pale blue staining inclusions resembling Döhle bodies in the cytoplasm of neutrophils in the absence of toxic granulation, and by thrombocytopenia with giant and abnormal appearing platelets. The inclusion bodies consist of RNA, are larger and more prominent than Döhle bodies, and may also be found in eosinophils, basophils, monocytes, and occasionally, lymphocytes. Approximately 40% of the patients with this anomaly have a mild to severe bleeding disorder which may result from the decreased platelet count or from a functional abnormality of the platelets.

Chédiak-Higashi Anomaly

Chédiak-Higashi syndrome is inherited as an autosomal recessive trait. In this condition there is a defect in the lysosomes (cytoplasmic granules that are involved with the destruction of material ingested by phagocytic cells). Abnormal lysosomes are present in many cells of the body and appear predominately in the white blood cells. The affected patient generally shows albinism, photophobia, and poor resistance to infection. This disorder is generally fatal by early childhood. Death often occurs from recurrent infection or from a lymphoma-like disease. The Wright-stained blood smear is striking in that the granulocytes and monocytes contain large azurophilic or reddish-purple lysosomal granules in the cytoplasm. There are often multiple granules in the same cell. The lymphocytes and, less often, the monocytes may also contain one or more of these granules that stain a reddish-purple. Cytochemical staining of these cells shows the granules to be peroxidase positive.

Alder-Reilly Anomaly

Alder-Reilly anomaly is inherited as an autosomal recessive trait and is characterized by the presence of dense clusters of azurophilic staining granules in the cytoplasm of neutrophils, representing mucopolysaccharide deposits. These granules are similar to those seen in toxic granulation, but they are slightly larger, are unrelated to infection, and are a permanent feature of the cells. The granules may also be seen in the eosinophils, basophils, monocytes, and lymphocytes, totally obscuring the nucleus. These granules most often occur in conjunction with *Hurler's* or *Hunter's syndromes.* The basic defect in these conditions appears to be a metabolic disorder in which there is a deficiency of lysosomal enzymes needed to break down mucopolysaccharides. The end result is a deposition and storage of mucopolysaccharides in multiple organs of the body. The facial and skeletal abnormalities observed have led to the use of the term gargoylism to describe these syndromes. The granules of Alder-Reilly anomaly have also been observed in otherwise healthy individuals.

Chronic Granulomatous Disease

Chronic granulomatous disease is inherited primarily as a rare sex-linked recessive trait and is caused by a defect in white blood cell function. The disease is seen primarily in males and is generally fatal during early childhood because of recurring staphylococcal gram-negative or catalase positive bacterial infections. The development of granulomas (sites of chronic inflammation involving primarily large macrophages) in many organ systems is also a characteristic of this disorder. The white blood cells are morphologically and quantitatively normal. The white blood cell count (primarily neutrophils) does increase during periods of infection. The nitroblue-tetrazolium (NBT) test is used to diagnose this disorder. Failure to reduce the NBT dye is indicative of a lack of the oxidative burst which occurs in normal leukocytes during the process of phagocytosis and bacterial killing. Neutrophils and monocytes from chronic granulomatous patients ingest bacteria normally but are unable to kill catalase positive organisms due to a defect in the oxygen-dependent bacteriocidal mechanism of these cells.

The Leukemias

Introduction to the Leukemias

Leukemia is an abnormal, uncontrolled proliferation and accumulation of one or more of the hematopoietic cells. Usually, there are qualitative changes in the affected cells, but this does not always have to be true. It is a disease of the blood forming tissues and the bone marrow is always involved. The proliferating cells can infiltrate other organs such as the spleen, liver, and lymph nodes.

Many different factors appear to play a role

in the cause of the various leukemias. The ability of ionizing radiation to cause leukemia has been recognized for years; the evidence of this has come from observations regarding nuclear accidents and the atomic explosions in Japan in 1945. An increased frequency of leukemia has been found in patients receiving radiation therapy. It has been shown that chemical agents contribute in a major way to leukemia incidence, with benzene cited most frequently as well as the cytotoxic alkylating agents used to treat other neoplasms. Viruses have also been isolated from patients with T-cell leukemias (lymphomas). The precise mechanisms by which these factors cause leukemia are not known.

It is now clear that hereditary factors and genetic composition are of importance in the occurrence of leukemia. Statistics indicate that there is a significant tendency for leukemia to cluster in families, particularly in childhood twins. Acute leukemia has long been associated with Down's syndrome, and has occurred with increased frequency in persons with chromosomal breakage. The Philadelphia chromosome (Ph[1]), characterized by the shortening of the long arm of chromosome number 22, is seen in the majority of patients with chronic granulocytic leukemia. Chromosomal abnormalities have been found in more than 60% of patients with acute myelogenous leukemia and 65% of those with acute lymphoblastic leukemia.

Leukemia occurs at any age. Chronic lymphocytic leukemia, however, is usually found in patients over 50 years of age, whereas acute leukemia is generally found in persons under 20 years of age. Chronic granulocytic leukemia occurs in the 20- to 50-year age bracket. Cases of acute leukemia are generally more common in males than females, and in whites than blacks.

The major symptoms of leukemia are fever, weight loss, and increased sweating. Enlargement of the liver, spleen, and lymph nodes may occur more predominantly in the chronic leukemias. The basal metabolic rate is often elevated, and there may be hemorrhagic tendencies if marked thrombocytopenia is present. Bone pain from a large leukemic cell mass in the bone marrow is typical in the acute leukemias.

The different types of leukemia may be classified according to the duration of the disease, number of white blood cells present in the peripheral blood, and the type of white blood cell involved.

1. Duration of the untreated disease.
   a. Acute leukemia: rapidly progressive disease that lasts several days to 6 months.
   b. Subacute leukemia: 2 to 6 months.
   c. Chronic leukemia: the length of this disease is somewhat variable, depending on the age of the patient and the type of cell involved. Most patients live a minimum of 1 to 2 years or more.
2. Number of white blood cells present in the peripheral blood.
   a. Leukemic leukemia: white blood cell count greater than $15,000/\mu L$.
   b. Subleukemic leukemia: white blood cell count less than $15,000/\mu L$ with immature or abnormal forms of white blood cells present in the peripheral blood.
   c. Aleukemic leukemia: white blood cell count less than $15,000/\mu L$ with no immature or abnormal white blood cells present in the peripheral blood.
3. Type of white blood cell involved.
   a. Acute leukemia: there is a predominance of immature cell types (blasts and ''pro'' stages).
   b. Chronic leukemia: the cell types are predominantly mature.

The above categories can be further subdivided according to cell lineage. The myeloid leukemias involve the granulocytic, monocytic, erythrocytic, and megakaryocytic cell lines. The lymphocytic leukemias involve the T and B lymphocytes.

In *acute leukemia,* the onset of the disease is sudden, and almost half of all cases occur in children under 14 years of age. There is generally normocytic-normochromic anemia that increases as the disease progresses with resultant fatigue and weakness. The platelet count is low to markedly decreased. The bleeding time is usually prolonged, and there is poor clot retraction. Occasionally, the clotting time is also prolonged. The white blood cell count is variable, usually showing a moderate to marked elevation. White blood cell counts of 50,000 to $100,000/\mu L$ are not uncommon. Frequently, however, the white blood cell count may be normal to decreased. Blasts cells are present on the peripheral blood smear and may predominate. The bone marrow is hypercellular, with blast cells usually predominating, typically over 75% of the marrow cell total.

Acute leukemia is generally treated by *chemotherapy* (the use of chemicals that damage the capacity of the cell for reproduction). Combinations of several different drugs are utilized. These drugs may also destroy some normal cells and have toxic side effects. The primary goal of chemotherapy is to prolong life by eliminating the leukemic cells. When the patient becomes asymptomatic and has only normal cells in the blood and bone marrow, the patient is said to be in complete remission. A patient in partial remission shows improvement, but some leukemic cells remain. The period of time a patient remains in remission is variable, as is the number of remissions possible. In addition, general supportive therapy for bone marrow failure due to replacement by leukemic blasts and cytotoxic therapy includes the administration of packed red blood cells to treat anemia. Platelet concentrates are given in cases of severe thrombocytopenia (less than 20,000/μL). Severely neutropenic patients are given leukocyte concentrates to combat infections. Antibiotic therapy is also used to treat bacterial infections as a result of the neutropenia. The cause of death in patients with acute leukemia is most often infection and/or hemorrhage due to thrombocytopenia. Bone marrow transplantation has also emerged as a viable treatment of patients with acute myelogenous leukemia. This involves the complete eradication of the bone marrow with chemotherapy and total body radiation. Then the patient is "rescued" with bone marrow cells from an HLA compatible donor. The donor cells migrate to the patient's bone marrow, where they grow and repopulate the empty marrow with normal cells.

Subacute leukemias are similar to and are usually treated clinically as acute leukemia. The white blood cell count may show elevations up to 50,000/μL or in some instances may be normal to decreased. The predominant cell present in the peripheral blood is usually the blast, although there are not as many as in acute leukemia. Thrombocytopenia and normocytic-normochromic anemia are also present.

Chronic leukemia has an insidious onset, frequently being asymptomatic for a long time. Anemia is not usually present until late in the disease, and hemolytic anemia may develop as the disease progresses. Platelet counts are usually normal and may frequently be increased in myelogenous leukemia. In the late stages of chronic leukemia, however, thrombocytopenia and anemia usually occur. The white blood cell count is most often markedly increased and may be as high as 900,000/μL. However, it is not unusual for the white blood cell count to be normal to decreased. Less than 10% blast cells are found in chronic myelogenous leukemia, whereas a rare blast cell (or none) is seen in chronic lymphocytic leukemia. Eventually, the majority of these patients go into blast crisis, where they present an acute type of leukemia. Chemotherapy may or may not induce a remission, and, as in acute leukemia, the main cause of death is hemorrhage and/or infection. Chronic lymphocytic leukemia (CLL) generally has a much longer life span than the other types of leukemia. However, complete remission is generally not attained, and treatment may be used only when complications occur. Death is usually caused by infection, or, because this is a disease found in the elderly, the cause of death may be unrelated to CLL.

In 1976, a system for the classification of acute leukemias was developed and is now termed the *French-American-British (FAB)* classification of acute leukemias. It divides the acute leukemias into lymphoblastic or myeloblastic. These two main groups are subdivided according to cellular morphology, cytochemical staining results, cytogenic studies, and T and B lymphocyte marker study (immunologic techniques) results. The lymphoblastic leukemias have been divided into three types (L1, L2, and L3), whereas the myeloblastic leukemias have been separated into seven types (M1, M2, M3, M4, M5, M6, and M7).

The three types, M1, M2, and M3, are predominantly granulocytic in origin. Types M4 and M5 have at least 20% monocytic precursors, and type M6 has a high proportion of erythroblasts. The M6 type may be difficult to distinguish from certain myelodysplastic syndromes. The purpose of the FAB classification is to attain consistency by sorting the morphologic variants of leukemias into types. In general, patients in group M1, M5a, and

M6 do less well than patients classified as M2, M3, M4, and M5b (see Acute Myelomonocytic Leukemia for M5a and M5b). Also, the presence of Auer rods is observed to be an important parameter in prognosis with a complete remission rate of 68% in patients with Auer rods. The FAB classification requires a minimum of 30% blasts for the diagnosis of acute myelogenous leukemia (M1 through M6). Type M7 involves megakaryocytes.

Acute Lymphoblastic Leukemia (ALL)

In the FAB classification, the acute lymphoblastic leukemias have been divided into 3 types: L1, L2, and L3. In type L1, the lymphoblasts are small and homogeneous (vary little in size), and they have scanty cytoplasm and inconspicuous nucleoli; the nucleus is round and regular in shape. The lymphoblasts have a very high N/C ratio. It is the most common type (84%) of childhood ALL (acute lymphoblastic leukemia), and has the best prognosis. In type L2, the lymphoblasts are larger and variable in size with abundant, basophilic cytoplasm, and the nuclei are often clefted with nucleoli present. This type accounts for 14% of the cases of childhood ALL, and includes 64% of the adult type of ALL. In type L3, the Burkitt-type, the lymphoblast is large, but varies little in size. The nucleus is rounded with fine chromatin structure and one to three nucleoli. The cytoplasm is moderate in quantity and deeply basophilic, often with prominent vacuoles. This type accounts for only about 2% of the cases of ALL, and the prognosis is poor.

Acute lymphoblastic leukemia can also be divided into five subtypes, based on the reaction of the blast cells with lymphocyte cell marker assays. These include markers for surface immunoglobulins (sIg), cytoplasmic immunoglobulin (cIg), the HLA surface antigens, and surface markers detected with monoclonal antibodies, as well as the nuclear enzyme TdT (terminal deoxynucleotidyl transferase) and the formation of rosettes with sheep erythrocytes. T-cell leukemias (T cell ALL) account for 10 to 20% of the cases of ALL, usually have a high white blood cell count, a high frequency of mediastinal tumor, central nervous system involvement, and a poor prognosis. It affects males more

than females and generally occurs in older children. Early pre-B-cell or common ALL accounts for 60 to 70% of all cases, and has a good prognosis. Blast cells in this subtype are positive for the CD10 or common ALL (cALLa) antigen. Pre-B-cell leukemias also have a good prognosis and account for about 18% of the cases of ALL. The rarest subclass is B-cell leukemia, and it represents the L3 variant of the FAB classification (Burkitt-type).

At the time of diagnosis, the white blood cell count is generally elevated, with 60% or more lymphoblasts and immature lymphocytes present. Frequently, the white blood cell count may be normal or decreased, in which case there would be relatively fewer lymphoblasts present. Only occasionally are the white cell counts over $100 \times 10^3/\mu L$ (100 $\times 10^9$/L). A normocytic-normochromic anemia is present, which is generally severe. The reticulocyte count is decreased, and moderate to marked thrombocytopenia is present. Approximately 2% of the cases of ALL have central nervous system involvement at presentation, with blast cells present in the cerebrospinal fluid. It is treated with intrathecal methotrexate, cytosine arbinoside, and cranial irradiation if the patient is over 2 years of age. The bone marrow shows a predominance of lymphoblasts. The periodic acid-Schiff stain is variable, and the peroxidase stain is negative. The sudan black B stain is negative in lymphoblasts, and the acid phosphatase is positive in blasts of the T-cell variant of ALL. There are many treatment regimens currently used for ALL. In general, prednisone, vincristine, and asparaginase in combination are used to achieve remissions in over 90% of the cases in 4 to 6 weeks. A maintenance therapy of mercaptopurine daily, and weekly methotrexate is given for 2 to 3 years.

Chronic Lymphocytic Leukemia

The majority of cases of chronic lymphocytic leukemia appear to involve the B lymphocyte. In 50% of the cases of CLL, there are cytogenetic abnormalities involving chromosomes 12 or 14. The T lymphocyte is less often involved. The white blood cell count is usually 20,000 to 200,000/μL, with the peripheral blood smear showing 60 to 95% lymphocytes. These cells are generally the small type of mature lymphocyte that often show a small cleft or indentation in the condensed chromatin of the nucleus. Lymphoblasts are generally absent from the peripheral blood, but a rare prolymphocyte may sometimes be found. These lymphocytes are somewhat more fragile than normal, resulting in many of the cells being ruptured during the preparation of the blood smear. Therefore, large numbers of smudge cells are usually seen on the Wright-stained smear. A normocytic, normochromic anemia generally develops as the disease progresses. The platelet count is usually normal or shows only a slight decrease. The bone marrow is hypercellular, and the predominant cell is the small mature lymphocyte. An autoimmune hemolytic anemia may develop during the course of this disease in about 10% of the cases, and the patient shows a positive direct Coombs' test. Transformation to an acute leukemia is rare in CLL.

Chronic lymphocytic leukemia is more than twice as common in men as in women. Lymphadenopathy, fatigue, weight loss, splenomegaly, and hepatomegaly are common clinical features. A system of five stages (the Rai classification) has been devised to allow clinical categorization of patients into prognostic groups. In stage 0 (zero), there is absolute lymphocytosis (greater than 15,000/μL) in the peripheral blood and bone marrow only. Stage I includes enlargement of the lymph nodes. Stage II also includes an enlarged liver and/or spleen. Stage III includes all of the above clinical symptoms and anemia. In stage IV, there is also thrombocytopenia.

Usually, there is no treatment for the disease in stage 0; however, in the later stages alkylating agents such as chlorambucil are used to reduce the total lymphocyte count. Corticosteroids and radiation of an enlarged spleen are also employed. Patients in stage 0 have a better prognosis (about 10 years) than those in the later stages, with anemia and thrombocytopenia, where the median survival is 1 to 2 years. Unmanageable bacterial infection is the major cause of death.

Prolymphocytic Leukemia (PLL)

Prolymphocytic leukemia is a malignant lymphoproliferative disorder characterized by massive splenomegaly and a marked lymphocytosis usually exceeding $100 \times 10^3/\mu$L

(100×10^9/L). The prolymphocyte is the predominant cell type in the peripheral blood and bone marrow. These cells are larger than a normal lymphocyte with more abundant cytoplasm, condensed nuclear chromatin, and a singular, prominent nucleolus. Anemia and thrombocytopenia are usually present. Most (80%) of the cases of prolymphocytic leukemia are of the B cell type, and 20% are of the T cell type, which has a more aggressive course. The disease has a male predominance; 50% of the patients are over age 70 at the time of diagnosis. PLL has a poor prognosis with an average survival of about 2 years. Splenectomy and chemotherapy have been used with only short term success.

Hairy Cell Leukemia

Hairy cell leukemia (*leukemic reticuloendotheliosis*) is a chronic, malignant lymphoproliferative disorder. It is characterized by the presence of variable numbers of a distinct type of cell called "hairy" cells in the blood and bone marrow. Monoclonal antibody studies show these cells to be of lymphocytic origin and show characteristics of B lymphocytes. They are medium-sized cells with a diameter of 15 to 30 μm. The nucleus is round to oval in shape with fine chromatin and may contain one to five distinct nucleoli. There is a small to moderate amount of grayish cytoplasm that has hairlike projections around the outer border of the cell. The acid phosphatase stain using L(+) tartaric acid will be positive (the hairy cells are resistant to inhibition by tartaric acid).

This disease occurs in males between 40 and 60 years of age. Usually there is a pancytopenia or depression of all cell lines in most patients upon presentation, but the white blood cell count may be increased depending on the number of hairy cells in the peripheral blood. Splenomegaly is a common finding. There is generally a mild normocytic, normochromic anemia. The platelet count is usually decreased below 50,000/μL, and the white blood cell count below 3,000/μL, with no previous therapy. Cell-mediated immunity is impaired because of depressed monocyte production. Splenectomy is normally the first choice of treatment. There has been excellent success with the use of α-interferon and pentostatin to induce remission. Hairy cell leukemia responds well to splenectomy, with a median survival rate between 5 and 6 years. Death usually results from infections due to neutropenia and monocytopenia.

Acute Myeloblastic Leukemia (M1 and M2)

The peripheral white blood cell count usually shows moderate to marked elevation, with 60% or more of the cells being myeloblasts. Auer rods may or may not be present in the cytoplasm of these cells. Some cases of this disease show micromyeloblasts, a much smaller myeloblast than normal. A severe normocytic-normochromic anemia develops, along with thrombocytopenia. Enlargement of the lymph nodes, spleen, and liver is not pronounced. The platelets that are present may be large and bizarre-looking. The bone marrow shows an increased number of myeloblasts. The granulocytes on the blood smear give the following reactions to cytochemical stains: Sudan black B, positive; peroxidase, positive; ASD chloroacetate, positive; leukocyte alkaline phosphatase, decreased; periodic acid-Schiff, faint diffuse granules.

In acute myeloblastic leukemia of the M1 FAB classification (myeloblastic leukemia without maturation), the predominant cell is a poorly differentiated myeloblast without any granulation, or only a few fine azurophilic granules. The nuclear chromatin is fine with one or more distinct nucleoli. The cytoplasm is usually moderate in amount, and Auer rods are rare. About 20% of the cases of AML are of the M1 type. In type M2, (myeloblastic leukemia with maturation) cells differentiate beyond the promyelocytic stage. There are about 50% blasts and promyelocytes. Myelocytes, metamyelocytes, and mature granulocytes have abundant cytoplasm and may be agranular. Increased numbers of eosinophilic precursors can be found. Auer rods are often present, and about 30% of the cases of acute myelogenous leukemia are of the M2 type.

Treatment involves prophylactic platelet transfusions for thrombocytopenia, broad spectrum antibiotics for infection, and chemotherapy. This is an extremely toxic program involving the use of daunorubicin and cytosine arabinoside; however, there is no universally accepted therapeutic program. In both the M1 and M2 types, the use of both drugs can result in a 60% rate of remission.

However, remissions are of short duration and the median survival is 12 to 18 months. Compatible sibling bone marrow transplantation is being used in some cases in patients under 45 years of age in their first remission.

Acute Promyelocytic Leukemia (M3)

In acute promyelocytic leukemia, the predominant cell (>30%) in the bone marrow and blood is the promyelocyte. It accounts for about 10% of the cases of granulocytic leukemias. A significant feature is the occurrence of a translocation involving chromosomes 15 and 17. Often, the nucleus of the promyelocyte is more immature than usual, and the cytoplasmic granules may be large and abnormal appearing. There is also an increased incidence of bleeding disorders in this disease. Disseminated intravascular coagulation may occur, which is thought to be due to the release of thromboplastin-like substances by the abnormal promyelocytes. The DIC may become more severe as the promyelocytes are destroyed by chemotherapy and the granules are released.

The majority of cells have abundant heavy cytoplasmic granulation often obscuring the nucleus; Auer rods are common, often multiple and in bundles. The nucleus varies in size and shape and may be kidney-bean shaped or bi-lobed. A variant of type M3 (M3m) called micro or hypogranular promyelocytic leukemia has similar cell morphology, but only a few granules are present. Morphologically, the microgranular promyelocytes appear monocytoid with bi-lobed nuclei. However, Sudan black B and peroxidase cytochemical stains are strongly positive, and the nonspecific esterase is usually negative.

Treatment involves the same regimen of cytotoxic drugs as types M1 and M2, plus the administration of fresh frozen plasma to provide clotting factors consumed by DIC when present. Heparin is also used to treat DIC during induction therapy.

Acute Myelomonocytic Leukemia (M4)

At diagnosis, the white blood cell count usually shows a moderate to marked elevation. Anemia is commonly found, and thrombocytopenia may also be present. The most common types of abnormal cells found in this disorder are the myeloblast and the mono-cyte. The monocyte nucleus is convoluted or folded with a fine chromatin pattern, and the cytoplasm is abundant. The myeloblasts, pro-myelocytes, myelocytes, and more mature forms represent 30 to 80% of the non-eryth-roid cells. These cells are present in the bone marrow and peripheral blood in all stages of development, from the blast stage to the ma-ture monocyte. Often the monocyte differ-entiation is more prominent in the peripheral blood, with a monocytosis of greater than 5 $\times 10^3/\mu L$ ($5 \times 10^9/L$). The monocytic cells must account for 20% but not more than 80% of the white cells in the bone marrow for the leukemia to be classified as M4. Auer rods may be present in the blast cell. Some im-mature granulocytes are also present in the peripheral blood. In the nonspecific esterase stain, the blasts are negative to weakly pos-itive, whereas the mature monocytoid cells stain positively. (AMML accounts for about 25% of adult acute myelogenous leukemia.)

A small percentage of patients have vari-able numbers of marrow eosinophils (0.5 to 30%). The eosinophils appear immature and may contain large basophilic staining gran-ules. It is also associated with an abnormal chromosome 16. This variant has been called M4E or acute myelomonocytic leukemia with eosinophilia.

Acute Monocytic Leukemia (M5)

Acute monocytic leukemia (AMoL) exists in two forms: differentiated (M5b) and poorly differentiated (M5a). In both forms, the white blood cell count is moderately elevated, with the absolute percentage of granulocyte pre-cursors showing less than 20%. The other 80% consists of monoblasts, promonocytes, and monocytes. The poorly differentiated type is characterized by large (30 μm or larger) blasts in the bone marrow (>80%) and in the peripheral blood. The nuclei of the blasts have delicate, lacy chromatin with three to five nucleoli and are folded or in-dented. The basophilic cytoplasm is abundant with rare granules, and often has pseudopods or buds. The differentiated form has blasts, promonocytes, and monocytes (>80%) in the bone marrow, and the peripheral blood has a high proportion of monocytes. The predom-inant cell type in the bone marrow is the

promonocyte which has less basophilic cy-toplasm with a grayish ground-glass appear-ance, and fine azurophilic granules.

Anemia and thrombocytopenia are usually present, and acute monocytic leukemia shows a high degree of skin and gum in-volvement due to the migration of the mono-cytes. The monocytic cells stain positively in the nonspecific esterase stain. In this disease, however, the staining is inhibited by the ad-dition of fluoride. An abnormal chromosome (11) has been found in about 35% of patients with AMoL. Both types (M5a and M5b) ac-count for 10% of the total cases of acute mye-logenous leukemia.

Di Guglielmo's Syndrome (M6)

Di Guglielmo's syndrome has been referred to as *erythroleukemia* and *erythremic myelosis* and may occur in the acute or, less com-monly, in the chronic form. The white blood cell count may be slightly decreased to mod-erately elevated, and myeloblasts and im-mature granulocytic cells are usually found in the peripheral blood. Immature red blood cells including normoblasts may be present in the blood in few to moderate numbers. These cells may appear megaloblastic-like and show bizarre-shaped, fragmented, and multilobed nuclei. Anemia and thrombocy-topenia are common findings. The bone mar-row is hypercellular and shows a predomi-nance (more than 50%) of erythroid cells, and >30% myeloblasts. The abnormal erythroid cells will show positive staining in the non-specific esterase stain, as well as strong PAS staining.

Abnormal megakaryocytes are present in the bone marrow, including giant forms. Howell-Jolly bodies are present in the pe-ripheral blood. Iron stores of the bone mar-row show ringed sideroblasts. This type of leukemia is rare, constituting only 5% of pa-tients with acute myelogenous leukemia. Pa-tients with erythroleukemia have a poor prognosis.

Acute Megakaryocytic Leukemia (M7)

Acute megakaryocytic leukemia (M7) is a sys-temic and rapidly progressive proliferation of atypical and immature megakaryocytes. Since the proliferation of megakaryocytes is common in the chronic myeloproliferative and myelodysplastic syndromes, only rarely will a patient be diagnosed with true acute megakaryocytic leukemia.

This form of acute leukemia usually presents with pancytopenia (anemia and leukopenia) without lymphadenopathy, splenomegaly, or hepatomegaly. The disease generally occurs in the middle or late years of life, with males affected more than females. The peripheral blood shows undifferentiated blasts and megakaryocytic fragments, and bleeding is a frequent mode of presentation. The bone marrow displays a predominance of atypical megakaryocytes, and >30% of the blasts are megakaryoblasts. The blast cells may be small with a high nuclear to cytoplasmic ratio, cytoplasmic vacuoles, multiple nucleoli, and may actually be seen shedding platelets. There is also an increase in reticulum fibers in the bone marrow.

Cytochemical staining involves the use of the platelet peroxidase enzyme to identify megakaryoblasts, and immunophenotyping utilizes monoclonal antibodies against platelet glycoproteins. The clinical course is very short and the response to therapy is usually poor. Terminally, the patient has an acute leukemic phase with high blast counts and widespread infiltration of the lymph nodes, spleen, liver, and bone marrow.

Eosinophilic Leukemia

Eosinophilic leukemia is rare. Anemia and thrombocytopenia may or may not be present. Large numbers of immature eosinophils are present in the blood and bone marrow, and the maturation of these cells may be abnormal.

It is difficult to differentiate between eosinophilic leukemia and a non-neoplastic eosinophilia. However, there are greater than 5% blasts in the bone marrow and tissue infiltration by immature eosinophils in eosinophilic leukemia.

Plasma Cell Leukemia

Plasma cell leukemia is a rare disorder generally found only as an acute terminal stage in multiple myeloma. The white blood cell count may be slightly to moderately elevated, and the peripheral blood smear shows up to 90% plasma cells. There is bone marrow failure due to infiltration with abnormal plasma cells and splenomegaly. The malignant cells are poorly differentiated, and patients do not respond well to therapeutic drugs used in multiple myeloma.

Plasma cell leukemia is found in more males than females, with a median age of 50 to 60 years. The clinical picture includes general fatigue, weight loss, hemorrhagic tendencies, and hepatomegaly. Moderate to marked anemia and thrombocytopenia are seen in 70% of the cases. There is widespread infiltration of plasmacytoid cells in various organs and tissues of the body. Remissions are of short duration (1 to 3 months) and the mean survival is about 9 months.

Mast Cell Leukemia

Mast cell leukemia is extremely rare. Up to 50% of the cells in the peripheral blood may be mature and immature forms of the tissue mast cell, which is of the monocyte-macrophage lineage, and is difficult to distinguish from the basophil.

Stem Cell Leukemia

In stem cell leukemia, the blast cells present are so immature and undifferentiated that they cannot be identified by cytochemical or immunologic methods. As the disease progresses, these cells may change and become identifiable. This disorder is rare, found mainly in children, and is generally present in the acute form.

The Myeloproliferative Disorders

The chronic myeloproliferative disorders are a group of acquired, malignant disorders that develop from the proliferation of an abnormal pleuripotential stem cell. This stem cell differentiates into the granulocytic, megakaryocytic, and erythroid cell lines. The specific myeloproliferative classification depends on the predominant cell type involved. The disorders include chronic myelogenous leukemia (CML), polycythemia vera, myelofibrosis with myeloid metaplasia, and essential thrombocythemia (to be discussed under platelet disorders).

These diseases share several clinical and hematologic features. They primarily affect middle-aged to older people, and the onset is gradual. Fever, night sweats, weight loss, and general weakness are common complaints upon presentation. Splenomegaly is a typical finding, due to extramedullary hematopoiesis. The bone marrow is hypercellular with increased myelopoiesis and increased numbers of megakaryocytes, and may eventually become fibrotic. An acute leukemia is usually the end stage, and chromosomal abnormalities are common.

Chronic Myelogenous Leukemia

CML is a stem cell disorder affecting the granulocytic, monocytic, erythrocytic, and megakaryocytic cell lines. It is primarily a disease of adults, occurring between the ages of 30 and 50. Rarely does a juvenile form of CML occur. This disorder accounts for about 20% of all leukemias. The white blood cell count is usually 50,000 to 300,000/μL at the time of diagnosis. Less than 10% myeloblasts are present in the peripheral blood, and there is a complete spectrum of granulocytic cells from the myeloblast to the mature neutrophil with a predominance of neutrophils and myelocytes. Eosinophils and basophils are commonly increased, and the percentage of monocytes may also show an increase. Mild normochromic anemia is generally present. The platelet count is usually increased, and large forms of the platelets may be present, as well as megakaryocyte fragments. The bone marrow is hypercellular and usually shows an increased number of myeloid cells, with a slightly higher percentage of immature granulocytes than is present in the peripheral blood, and megakaryocytes are more numerous than usual. The myeloid-to-erythroid (M:E) ratio can be as high as 25:1. Leukocyte alkaline phosphatase is decreased or absent in this disorder. In 90% of the cases of this disease one arm of the chromosome in pair number 22 is found to be translocated to chromosome 9. This chromosome is termed the *Philadelphia chromosome* and occurs in the erythroid, granulocytic, monocytic, and megakaryocytic cells. Patients with this disorder who are negative for the Philadelphia chromosome usually have a poorer prognosis and do not respond particularly well to chemotherapy. Splenomegaly is a fairly consistent finding upon presentation.

The cytotoxic drug, busulphan (myleran), is most commonly used to treat CML to maintain the disease in the chronic phase and to reduce the total granulocytic cell mass. However, the chronic phase is highly unstable and can transform to a drug resistant accelerated phase, usually after 2 to 5 years. Finally, CML converts to a terminal myeloblastic or lymphoblastic acute leukemia. Most patients die within 3 months as a result of complications arising during blast crisis, such as bleeding, infection, and bone marrow aplasia. To date, bone marrow transplantation offers the best hope for a cure for CML.

Myelofibrosis

Myelofibrosis, also called *idiopathic myelofibrosis* or *agnogenic myeloid metaplasia*, is a chronic myeloproliferative disorder that is characterized by fibrosis and granulocytic hyperplasia of the bone marrow, with granulocytic and megakaryocytic proliferation in the liver and spleen. Its basic cause is unknown, although cytogenetic studies do reveal chromosomal abnormalities. The disease has been shown to arise from a defect in a single multipotential stem cell, which explains the abnormal proliferation of granulocytes, erythrocytes, and megakaryocytes. It is generally found in middle aged or elderly people.

At diagnosis, the patient may show an enlarged liver and spleen due to extramedullary hematopoiesis, weight loss, a tendency to bruise easily, fatigue, and a normochromic-normocytic anemia (from ineffective erythropoiesis and shortened red cell survival). The anemia becomes more severe as the disease progresses. The stained blood smear characteristically shows teardrop-shaped red cells that form as erythrocytes pass through the narrow, fibrotic sinusoids of the bone marrow and spleen. There are nucleated red blood cells in numbers out of proportion to the degree of anemia. Polychromatophilia is present, and the reticulocyte count is increased. The white blood cell count is variable but is increased in the majority of patients.

Immature granulocytes are generally present on the stained blood smear and the number of basophils is often increased. Dwarf megakaryocytes or small megakaryoblasts are often present in small numbers in the peripheral blood and, in certain cases, may be present in large numbers. The platelet count is increased in about 50% of the cases at diagnosis but decreases below normal as the disease progresses. Large and bizarre forms of the platelets are usually present on the stained blood smear and most patients demonstrate functional platelet abnormalities. The leukocyte alkaline phosphatase stain is increased in the majority of cases but may be normal or decreased. The bone marrow is usually hypocellular, the collagen content is increased, and it is often impossible to obtain marrow, except by surgical biopsy. In the early stages of the disease, however, the marrow may be hypercellular and contain an increased number of megakaryocytes, some of which are abnormal. The marrow generally becomes fibrotic, with an abundance of reticulum fibers.

The cause of death is variable and may be due to infection, bleeding, cardiac failure, or a conversion to leukemia. Asymptomatic patients may be stable for several years without specific treatment. Chemotherapy with busulfan and other alkylating agents is used to treat myelofibrosis, and splenectomy is an option when the spleen is painfully enlarged and there is severe thrombocytopenia. Transfusions are given for the anemia, as well as androgen and glucocorticoid therapy to normalize the red cell survival. Patients will generally survive for 1 to 5 years or longer following diagnosis.

The Polycythemias

Polycythemia is a term used to signify an above normal hemoglobin, hematocrit (>50%), and red blood cell count. It may also be referred to as *erythrocytosis*. This condition is classified as relative or absolute. Absolute polycythemia is further subdivided into the chronic myeloproliferative disorder, polycythemia vera, and secondary polycythemia.

Absolute Polycythemia

Polycythemia Vera. Polycythemia vera is a chronic myeloproliferative disease of unknown origin that is found most often in patients over 60 years of age. It is a hematopoietic, pleuripotential stem cell disorder characterized by the excessive proliferation of the erythroid, granulocytic, and megakaryocytic cell lines. At onset, this disease is characterized by an absolute increase in red blood cells, white blood cells, and platelets. This gives rise to an increased blood volume that may measure 2 to 3 times normal. The plasma volume shows little or no change. Because of the increased red blood cell concentration, the viscosity of the blood becomes increased, and the patient exhibits a ruddy skin coloration. The blood pressure is usually elevated and headaches, dizziness, and vertigo are common. Increased platelets, along with the increased blood viscosity, may cause the formation of intravascular thrombi. Splenomegaly due to extramedullary hematopoiesis is a relatively common finding, and an enlarged liver is found in some cases. The arterial oxygen saturation is normal, and the erythropoietin level is decreased. There is a marked increase in the incidence of peptic ulcer among patients with this disorder.

The peripheral blood smear shows normocytic-normochromic red blood cells, moderate anisocytosis, and slight polychromatophilia. There may be occasional nucleated red blood cells and immature granulocytes present. Giant and atypical platelets or megakaryocyte fragments may also be seen. The relative and absolute number of eosinophils and basophils may be increased, and neutrophilia is usually present. The red blood cell count, hemoglobin, hematocrit, white blood cell count, and platelet count are increased. The reticulocyte count generally shows a slight elevation, although not usually over 4%. The erythrocyte sedimentation rate is usually decreased. The bone marrow is hypercellular, showing an overall increase in the granulocytic, erythroid, and megakaryocytic cells (*panhyperplasia*). The distribution, morphology, and maturation of the marrow cells are normal. Bone marrow iron stores are decreased or absent from unknown blood losses and excessive erythropoiesis. The leukocyte alkaline phosphatase is usually increased, which aids in distinguishing polycythemia vera from other types of erythrocytosis.

Methods of treatment for polycythemia vera include phlebotomies at regular intervals to reduce hyperviscosity and total red cell mass, and radioactive phosphorus and alkylating agents to control the unregulated production of cell lines in the bone marrow. (Hydroxyurea is a non-alkalylating agent that has been used with good results and a lesser risk of leukemic transformation than with other chemotherapy. If the patient does not die from hemorrhagic complications of the disease, the bone marrow may become fibrotic until it reaches an aplastic stage.) A mild iron deficiency anemia usually develops, which later becomes marked. Hemorrhagic problems may develop because of platelets that are abnormal in function. Hematopoiesis may begin to occur in the liver and spleen. Nucleated red blood cells, myelocytes, and sometimes even myeloblasts may be found in the peripheral blood. Some cases terminate in acute myelogenous leukemia or myelofibrosis with myeloid metaplasia.

Secondary Polycythemia. Secondary polycythemia is caused by an increased level of erythropoietin in the blood. This may occur as a normal response to hypoxia or as the result of inappropriate erythropoietin production. An appropriate response to hypoxia occurs in any disorder or circumstance that decreases the arterial oxygen saturation of the blood or decreases the capacity of the hemoglobin molecule to carry oxygen. Specific causes include: residence at high altitudes, chronic pulmonary disease, chronic congestive heart failure, heavy smoking, abnormal hemoglobins that have a high oxygen affinity, and methemoglobinemia. An inappropriate production of erythropoietin is found in certain tumors of the liver, brain, kidney, and adrenal and pituitary glands. In this type of secondary polycythemia, the erythropoietin level is elevated, but the arterial oxygen saturation of the blood is normal and no conditions of hypoxia are present.

The peripheral blood smear shows normocytic-normochromic red blood cells, and normal white blood cell, red blood cell, and platelet morphology. The hemoglobin, hematocrit, and red blood cell count are elevated. The white blood cell count is normal. The whole blood volume is increased as a result of the increased total red blood cell mass. The bone marrow shows erythroid hyperplasia, and the leukocyte alkaline phosphatase is normal.

Relative Polycythemia. Relative polycythemia is caused by a decrease in the fluid (plasma) portion of the blood. Therefore, the actual number of red blood cells in the blood is not increased, but the number of cells per unit volume of blood is increased.

Relative polycythemia is found in association with acute dehydration and in cases of stress or spurious polycythemia (Gaisböck's syndrome). This latter condition occurs primarily in middle-aged males and may be associated with smoking, cardiovascular problems, hypertension, and diuretic therapy.

The peripheral blood smear shows normocytic-normochromic red blood cells and normal white blood cell, red blood cell, and platelet morphology. The hemoglobin, hematocrit, and red blood cell count are elevated. The white blood cell count may be normal or, in dehydration, slightly elevated. The whole blood volume is decreased, whereas the total red blood cell volume is normal. A normal bone marrow is found in this condition, and the leukocyte alkaline phosphatase is also normal.

The Myelodysplastic Syndromes (MDS)

The myelodysplastic syndromes are a group of disorders that result from clonal abnormalities of hematopoietic pleuripotential stem cells. They are characterized by a hypercellular bone marrow and abnormalities in the cellular maturation of the erythroid cells, granulocytes, and megakaryocytes. Historically, it has been termed 'preleukemia' as patients may progress to an acute nonlymphocytic leukemia. The exact cause is not known, although exposure to hazardous chemicals (benzene and toluene) and the use of alkylating chemotherapeutic agents seem to be common factors. MDS occurs primarily in persons over the age of 50. Clinically, they present with a macrocytic anemia and thrombocytopenia, and neutropenia and/or monocytosis is usually present. The spleen, liver, and lymph nodes are generally not enlarged. The peripheral blood shows anisocytosis, poikilocytosis, nucleated red blood cells, basophilic stippling, Howell-Jolly bodies, and oval macrocytes. In general, in MDS the blast count is less than 30%. It has been shown that the deletion of a large portion of the long arm of chromosome 5 is a consistent finding in MDS (except in CMML).

In the bone marrow and peripheral blood, dyserythropoiesis is indicated by nuclear fragmentation, multinuclearity, lobulated nuclei, basophilic stippling, ringed sideroblasts and megaloblastic maturation of the red cells. Dysgranulopoiesis is indicated by the presence of pseudo-Pelger-Huët forms, retarded nuclear maturation, hypersegmented forms, and abnormal or absent granulation. Dysmegakaryocytopoiesis results in the presence of large megakaryocytes and micromegakaryocytes, decreased numbers of megakaryocytes, giant platelets, and abnormal platelet granulation. Due to abnormal platelet structure and function, hemorrhagic complications are common.

The French-American-British (FAB) group has classified this syndrome into five groups (RA, RARS, RAEB, RAEB-T, and CMML) based on the bone marrow and peripheral blood blast count, and the degree of abnormalities in the three cell lines (erythrocytes, leukocytes, and megakaryocytes). These classifications have proved helpful in diagnosis and treatment; however, not all patients fall neatly into one category.

In *refractory anemia* (RA), there is anemia with a decreased reticulocyte count, less than 1% blasts in the peripheral blood, and less than 5% blasts in the bone marrow. It is the mildest form of MDS. Abnormal erythrocytes are found, but abnormal granulocytes are rare. *Refractory anemia with ringed sideroblasts* (RARS) includes the presence of more than 15% ringed sideroblasts in the bone marrow. In *refractory anemia with excess blasts* (RAEB), the peripheral blood shows less than 5% circulating myeloblasts; however, there are 5 to 20% myeloblasts in the bone marrow. The marrow is hypercellular with abnormalities in the three cell lines. *Refractory anemia with excess blasts in transformation* (RAEB-T) shows more than 5% blasts in the blood and 20 to 30% blasts in the bone marrow. This subgroup has a high risk of evolving into acute myelogenous leukemia. *Chronic myelomonocytic leukemia* (CMML) has 5 to 20% blast cells in the bone marrow, and increased promonocytes. The peripheral blood shows a persistent monocytosis and less than 5% circulating blasts.

Median survival rates range from 6 years for RARS to 5 months for RAEB-T. Low dose cytosine arabinoside has been used to treat MDS with varied success, and supportive therapy involves the use of white cell, red cell, and platelet transfusions and antibiotics to combat infections. Bone marrow transplantation in patients under 50 years of age has been used with success.

Infectious Mononucleosis

Infectious mononucleosis was first described in the 1880s. One of the names ascribed to it at that time was glandular fever, a term no longer in use today. In the early 1900s, several cases of 'cured leukemia' were reported. These cases are now felt to have been examples of infectious mononucleosis.

Infectious mononucleosis is predominantly a disease of children and young adults and occurs in all races in all parts of the world. As a rule, the symptoms include fatigue, sore throat, moderate fever, and enlargement of the lymph nodes. Some patients may show splenomegaly, hepatomegaly, or jaundice. The causative agent for infectious mononucleosis is the Epstein-Barr (EB) virus, a member of the herpes group of viruses.

In patients with infectious mononucleosis, the red blood cell count and platelet count are usually normal, although there may be thrombocytopenia and a variable degree of anemia that is hemolytic in nature due to the presence of a strong autoanti-i antibody. The white blood cell count may be variable but is usually normal to slightly elevated. Generally, the WBC is lowest in the beginning of the disease and increases slowly during the first 2 to 5 days after onset, not usually going over 20,000/μL. There is a relative and absolute increase in lymphocytes, of which 20 to 90% are atypical. These cells are transformed T lymphocytes responding to B lymphocytes which are infected with the EB virus. The cells vary in size but are usually equal to or larger than the normal lymphocyte. They are often irregularly shaped because the cytoplasm is frequently indented by the surrounding red blood cells. The nucleus of the lymphocyte may be round or oval but is often irregularly shaped. The cytoplasm of the cell is often increased in relative size and appears basophilic. This basophilia may appear throughout the entire cytoplasm but more often appears radially or at the peripheral edge of the cell. It is not uncommon to find a few immature lymphocytes as a result of lymphocyte transformation into blast-like cells in response to stimulation by the virus. Lymphocytes with foamy or vacuolated cytoplasm may also be present. The three types of lymphocytes as suggested by Downey are found in this disorder. Usually, the number of atypical lymphocytes increases for several days and reaches a maximum by the fifth to tenth day. From then on, the number decreases, becoming normal within the next 3 weeks. In some instances, however, some atypical lymphocytes persist for 3 months or more. The heterophile antibody test, is positive in 90% or more of the patients with infectious mononucleosis. Generally, relatively high titers are obtained, reaching a peak in the second or third week of the illness and lasting for 2 to 8 weeks. In some cases, a positive test may persist even longer.

The diagnosis of infectious mononucleosis is generally based on the presence of atypical lymphocytes in the peripheral blood, a positive heterophile test, and the patient's clinical symptoms. Other laboratory findings may include abnormal liver enzyme tests (alkaline phosphatase, serum lactic dehydrogenase, and serum glutamic oxaloacetic transaminase levels).

Infectious mononucleosis is a benign, self-limited illness. Treatment is aimed at the symptoms and the condition usually resolves itself over a 4- to 6-week period. Complications occur in a small percentage of patients. These include neurologic, cardiac and liver function abnormalities.

Malignant Lymphomas

The term *lymphoma* represents a group of malignant tumors of the lymphoid tissue (lymph nodes and spleen) that vary greatly in degree of malignancy and response to therapy. Usually the blood and bone marrow are not involved. Various methods for classifying this group of disorders have been suggested. No one classification system, however, has been completely accepted. The malignant lymphomas include the non-Hodgkin's lymphomas, the miscellaneous lymphomas (Sézary syndrome and Burkitt's lymphoma) and Hodgkin's disease.

Non-Hodgkin's Lymphomas

Non-Hodgkin's lymphomas (NHL) are proliferations of malignant lymphocytes that are arrested at certain stages of maturation. They are primarily neoplasms (new or recent growth of cells) of the B-cell lymphocytes and occur predominantly in the middle and older age groups. The exact cause of the non-Hodgkin's lymphomas is not known, but in 60% of the cases there is evidence of chromosomal damage that may account for the unregulated growth of lymphocytes. Chemicals, ionizing radiation, and viruses could all play a role in initiating this damage.

Non-Hodgkin's lymphomas have been classified by the system of Rappaport for the last 20 years. This system separates the non-Hodgkin's lymphomas morphologically by cell type into four categories, each of which shows a nodular or diffuse pattern. (1) In *well-differentiated lymphocytic lymphoma*, the characteristic cell resembles a small lymphocyte. (2) *Poorly-differentiated lymphocytic lymphoma* is characterized by lymphocytic cells that may vary in size. The nuclear chromatin is less clumped than in the mature lymphocyte, may contain a visible nucleolus, and may be indented or clefted. There is little cytoplasm. (3) The cells in *histiocytic lymphoma* are relatively large, with fine nuclear chromatin and variable amounts of cytoplasm. The nucleus may be eccentric and may or may not show a nucleolus. (4) *Mixed histiocytic-lymphocytic lymphoma* shows equal proportions of poorly-differentiated lymphocytes and histiocytes. (The cells in categories 3 and 4 may not be true histiocytes but are, in fact, lymphoid in an active state of proliferation.)

Due to problems with terminology in the Rappaport classification, the NCI (National Cancer Institute) funded a study of 1175 cases of non-Hodgkin's lymphoma to develop the Working Formulation for Clinical Usage in 1982. The Formulation is in widespread use today, and it incorporates the older Rappaport system. The Working Formulation confirms the significance of differentiating the nodular (follicular) from the diffuse pattern.

The Working Formulation bases the categorization of NHL on prognosis and recognizes three major groups: low, intermediate, and high grade malignancies. Patients diagnosed with low grade lymphomas experience longer survival rates than those with the high grade variety. The *low grade malignancies* include three subgroups: (1) malignant lymphoma, small lymphocytic, (2) follicular, small cleaved (indented or clefted nucleus) cell, and (3) follicular, mixed small cleaved and large cell. In the *small lymphocytic type,* the predominant cell is the small lymphocyte with clumped chromatin, inconspicuous nucleoli, and scanty cytoplasm. Marker studies indicate that these well-differentiated cells are mostly B lymphocytes. There is a diffuse pattern of lymph node and marrow involvement with an elevated blood lymphocyte count. This is synonymous with chronic lymphocytic leukemia. In the *follicular, small cleaved cell type* of lymphoma, the lymphocytes are irregularly shaped, small cleaved lymphs of the poorly-differentiated type, and are predominantly B cells. In spite of spleen, liver, and bone marrow involvement, these patients have a survival of 7 years. Over 95% of patients with follicular lymphomas demonstrate a chromosomal transformation involving chromosomes 14 and 18 (t[14;18]). In the *follicular mixed, small cleaved and large cell type,* there are equal numbers of large non-cleaved cells with prominent nucleoli and small cleaved lymphocytes.

The *intermediate grade of malignant lymphomas* include (1) follicular, predominantly large cell, (2) diffuse small cleaved cell, (3) diffuse, mixed small and large cell, and (4) diffuse, large cell. These lymphomas have a more aggressive clinical course than the low grade lymphomas. In the *follicular, predominantly large cell type,* there are predominantly large cleaved cells mixed with non-cleaved cells representing B lymphocytes in a follicular pattern. Many mitotic figures are present. The *diffuse small cleaved cell type* of tumor has small cleaved lymphocytes with scanty cytoplasm. The *diffuse, mixed small and large cell* type has a mixture of small cleaved cells and large cells with prominent nucleoli in a diffuse pattern. They may be either B or T cells. The *diffuse, large cell type* of tumor is composed primarily of large cells with fine chromatin, a large prominent nucleolus, and abundant cytoplasm. These cells may be cleaved or non-cleaved, and may be either B or T lymphocytes.

The *high grade malignancies* represent lymphomas with an aggressive clinical course. The *large cell, immunoblastic type* consists of several types of cells, including those with eccentric nuclei and cells which resemble activated lymphocytes (immunoblasts) which are 4 times the size of normal lymphocytes with large, round nuclei. The *lymphoblastic type* shares many of the same features of T-cell acute lymphoblastic leukemia. The cells are blast-like with fine chromatin. This type of tumor has widespread involvement of the lymph nodes, peripheral blood, and may disseminate to the bone marrow and cerebrospinal fluid. The *small, non-cleaved cell type* includes the Burkitt's lymphomas. These cells have a high proliferation rate, interspersed with isolated macrophages which results in a 'starry sky' appearance in tissue sections of lymphoma tumors. Marker studies show these cells to be of B cell origin.

At the time of diagnosis, most patients have enlarged lymph nodes, where the disease is primarily located. The liver and spleen are often enlarged. Usually the white blood cell count is normal, but there may be some abnormal lymphocytes (lymphoma cells) present in the peripheral blood. The hemoglobin level is generally normal in the early stages of the disease. Diagnosis is generally made by examining a lymph node biopsy. The lymphoma cells, however, may also be present in the bone marrow. Combination chemotherapy (the administration of more than one cytotoxic drug) and radiotherapy are methods of treatment, depending on the stage of the disease. In some patients, malignant lymphoma will change into leukemia.

The majority of patients with low grade malignant disease with a follicular pattern survive for longer than 5 years, with a 10-year survival rate not uncommon. The low grade lymphomas are managed conservatively, often with no treatment at all if there are few symptoms and the clinical course is non-progressive. With intensive chemotherapy, patients with widespread high grade lymphomas have a 40 to 50% survival rate after 2 years. A basic regimen of COP (cyclophosphamide, vincristine, and prednisone) has been used to treat intermediate and high grade non-Hodgkin's lymphomas. Other drugs such as bleomycin, adriamycin, and procarbazine have been added to the basic protocol to treat more resistant cases.

Hodgkin's Disease

Hodgkin's disease is generally regarded as a malignant lymphoma but differs in that the cells reacting to the neoplasm predominate rather than the neoplastic cells themselves. This disorder is distinguished from other lymphomas by the presence of *Reed-Sternberg cells.* This is a large cell, varying in size from 50 to 100 μm or more. There is an abundance of cytoplasm, and the cell usually has irregular margins. The nucleus may be single or multilobed with large nucleoli. These cells are present in the involved tissue.

Hodgkin's disease is most frequent among young and middle-aged adults with a 2:1 male predominance. There is a bimodal distribution representing the 15 to 35 year age group and the over 50 age group. When a patient is diagnosed as having Hodgkin's disease, his disorder is further classified according to the histologic appearance of the involved tissue from a lymph node biopsy. The universally adopted Rye classification subdivides Hodgkin's disease into four types. These are not fixed and rigid categories as the patient who has one type may change to another category in time.

(1) The *lymphocytic predominant* form shows predominantly small mature lymphocytes with a varying number of mature histiocytes. The diagnostic Reed-Sternberg cells are rare and few in number. Prognosis is best in this group where the disease tends to be localized in the cervical lymph nodes in young males. The lymphocyte predominant type accounts for about 7% of the cases of Hodgkin's disease.

(2) In the *lymphocyte depleted* form, there are few lymphocytes, but there may be many histiocytes and varying numbers of eosinophils and atypical Reed-Sternberg cells. This type of Hodgkin's disease is seen as a rapidly progressive disease with fever, pancytopenia, and frequently without lymphadenopathy. There is extensive involvement of the liver, spleen, and bone marrow. This type accounts for about 2% of the cases of Hodgkin's disease.

(3) The *mixed cellularity* type shows eosinophils, lymphocytes, histiocytes, neutrophils, and plasma cells which obliterate the basic structure of the lymph node. Diagnostic Reed-Sternberg cells are frequent. The mixed cellularity type accounts for 23% of the cases of Hodgkin's disease.

(4) In *nodular sclerosis,* bands of collagen are present that divide the tissue into islands. This is the most common type (68%) of Hodgkin's disease, and is often first discovered as a mediastinal mass in young women. Classic Reed-Sternberg cells are difficult to find. Large, atypical histiocytes with abundant pale cytoplasm (*lacunar cells*) are found.

A second classification of the patient's disease may also be made based on the location and extent of the involved tissue. This process is termed *staging.* The most widely used staging scheme is the Ann Arbor Classification. Prognosis for Hodgkin's disease depends on both the histologic type and the extent of tissue involvement, as determined by staging. Staging of the disease is essential in order to initiate an appropriate treatment program, it correlates well with prognosis and helps in deciding whether radiotherapy or chemotherapy should be used.

The staging process involves the following procedures: chest x-ray, bone marrow, and liver biopsy, lymphangiography (x-ray of lymph nodes following the injection of a contrast medium), and laparotomy and splenectomy with accompanying node biopsy. Stage I involves a single lymph node region. The stage II disease involves two or more lymph node areas confined to one side of the diaphragm, and stage III involves lymphatic structures on both sides of the diaphragm which may also involve the spleen. Stage IV is disseminated involvement of the bone marrow, liver, and other extranodal sites in addition to lymph node involvement. Each stage is further divided into A or B categories depending on the absence (A) or presence (B) of unexplained fever, night sweats, and unexplained loss of 10% of total body weight.

At diagnosis, the most common finding is an enlarged, painless, cervical lymph node. Recurring fever is also characteristic, and night sweats are a fairly common symptom. A normocytic-normochromic anemia may be present in 50% of the cases, sometimes severe. Increased eosinophils and monocytes may also be present. The most frequent finding is moderate leukocytosis with white blood cell counts ranging from 12,000 to 25,000/μL, generally due to neutrophilia when the lymph nodes are involved. There is usually neutropenia when the bone marrow is involved. As a rule, lymphopenia, when present, is a poor prognosis. Reed-Sternberg cells have been found in the blood occasionally. The platelet count is usually normal, but may be increased or decreased if the bone marrow is involved. The erythrocyte sedimentation rate is commonly elevated.

Generally, the less extensive the disease, the longer the patient will live. In Hodgkin's disease, survival is significantly better in patients less than 40 years of age, and in the earlier stages of the disease. Also, patients with more mature lymphocytes have a better prognosis. However, many patients with active Hodgkin's disease have a defect in cell-mediated immunity, which makes them susceptible to bacterial, viral, and mycotic infections.

Chemotherapy and irradiation are used to treat patients with Hodgkin's disease. New treatment strategies for Hodgkin's disease, which was fatal 20 years ago, have resulted in an 85% 10 year survival rate for stages I and II, 70% for III and 50% for stage IV. Radiotherapy is the treatment of choice in patients with stage I and II disease to treat all lymph node areas. Chemotherapy is used in patients with stages III and IV Hodgkin's disease and a quadruple therapy with mustine, vincristine, procarbazine and prednisolone (MOPP) has proven superior to single agent therapy. Adriamycin, bleomycin, vinblastine, and dacarbazine (ABVD) chemotherapy has also been used to treat a resistant disease, and is now used alternately with MOPP.

Other Lymphomas

Sézary syndrome and Burkitt's lymphoma are two miscellaneous lymphoma variants. Both are described as lymphomas as they are lymphoproliferative disorders with lymph node infiltration.

Sézary syndrome, a malignant lymphoma, affects the skin and involves primarily the T lymphocytes. Immunologic marker studies of these T lymphocytes are positive with monoclonal antibodies for the CD2, CD3, and CD4 antigens. The tumor cells (Sézary cells) are characteristic. In the peripheral blood they resemble a medium-sized lymphocyte with a convoluted (cerebriform) nucleus, somewhat resembling the monocyte nucleus. (See Plate V, G, H.)

These cells have also been found in skin biopsies of patients with cutaneous mycosis fungoides. The disease usually presents with a skin eczema or dermatitis that progresses to cutaneous plaques and nodules. Sézary syndrome is considered to be the leukemic phase of mycosis fungoides affecting predominantly older males. This disorder may follow a prolonged, chronic course. However, as the disease infiltrates the lymph nodes and disseminates to the liver and spleen, the prognosis becomes worse. The bone marrow is not usually involved until the terminal stages.

Burkitt's lymphoma is found most often in children in Africa and New Guinea and commonly affects the jaw and facial bones. In American children, a similar tumor has been found that affects the lymph nodes in the abdominal and pelvic areas, and those in the neck. This lymphoma is sensitive to chemotherapy, and a complete remission is relatively common. If relapse occurs after a complete remission, this usually indicates a poor prognosis. The cause of Burkitt's lymphoma is unknown; however, evidence suggests that the Epstein-Barr virus (EBV) isolated from the tumor cells plays a role in transforming the B-cell lymphocytes by binding to surface receptors. In about 90% of the patients with Burkitt's lymphoma, there is a translocation of genetic material between chromosomes 8 and 14. Therapy consists of combination chemotherapy. Central nervous system treatment with intrathecal methotrexate and cranial irradiation has been used in more advanced cases.

Plasma Cell Disorders

Multiple Myeloma (Plasma Cell Myeloma)

Multiple myeloma is a malignant proliferation of atypical and immature forms of plasma cells, primarily occurring in the bone marrow. Onset of this disease is usually between the ages of 40 and 70 years, and the incidence is greater in males than females. The mean age at the time of diagnosis is 60 years of age. The exact cause of multiple myeloma is unknown, and there is no evidence that heredity plays a role. Bone pain is the main clinical finding in more than 60% of these patients. Pathologic fractures of the bone are common. Pain in the vertebrae of the back, ribs, and sternum is common, and multiple bone tumors are usually present. Abnormal bleeding may occur from impaired platelet function. Weakness, fever, and weight loss are frequently encountered. Neurologic complications can develop as a result of vertebral plasma cell tumors pressing on spinal nerves and the spinal cord. Gastrointestinal symptoms in the form of nausea, diarrhea, and vomiting are also observed in this disease. Renal failure is a common complication from disseminated intravascular coagulation, obstruction from light chain cast formation, and from the precipitation of monoclonal proteins in renal tissue.

The plasma proteins are increased, notably in the globulin portion. On protein electrophoresis, this generally appears as an increased gamma and less frequently as an increased alpha or beta band. Such abnormal patterns are said to contain an M-spot or M-component. Further testing of these M-components by immunoelectrophoresis shows them to be monoclonal proteins (proteins involved in the production of a single specific class of immunoglobulin). The protein types most often found, in order of their frequency, are IgG in greater than 50% of cases, IgA in approximately 20% of cases, and IgM in about 10% of cases. IgD and IgE myelomas are rare. The Bence Jones urine test (for free immunoglobulin light chains) is positive in approximately 50% of the cases of multiple myeloma. Approximately 20% of the patients produce only these light chain portions of the immunoglobulin molecule.

Moderate normocytic-normochromic anemia almost always develops in this condition. The peripheral blood smear shows marked rouleaux formation. There may be a bluish tinge to the Wright-stained blood smear when it is examined macroscopically. This can be attributed to the increased protein content of the plasma. Occasional nucleated red blood cells may be found in the peripheral blood. Polychromatophilia and reticulocytosis may also be present. The white blood cell count is normal to decreased but is seldom increased. A slight increase in eosinophils and lymphocytes may occur, and a few immature granulocytes may be present. A small number of plasma cells may also be found in the peripheral blood of approximately 15% of myeloma patients. The platelet count is generally normal but may be decreased. Coating of platelets by the myeloma protein may result in functional abnormalities of the platelets. The erythrocyte sedimentation rate is usually elevated. Some coagulation tests may be abnormal due to interference with some of the coagulation factors by the abnormal IgM plasma proteins. The most frequent cause of coagulation abnormalities is defective fibrin polymerization as the IgM proteins bind to fibrin monomers resulting in poor clot formation. Increased serum calcium levels may also be present, and bone radiographs showing punched-out lesions are seen in about 90% of the cases of multiple myeloma. The most characteristic finding in the bone marrow is the myeloma cell (a morphologically abnormal plasma cell), which may account for from 10% to 95% of all the cells. These (mature/immature) cells may be indistinguishable from normal plasma cells but usually show some bizarre abnormalities or variations. Generally, the cell is moderately large and contains an eccentric nucleus with one to two nucleoli. The nuclear chromatin is not as fine as in the myeloblast but not as coarse as that found in the plasma cell. Multinuclear plasma cells are frequently seen. The abundant cytoplasm may be basophilic and bright blue or a little lighter in color and may contain various types of inclusions: red-staining crystalline bodies, Russell bodies (eosinophilic globules), and Mott bodies (colorless vacuoles). In some cases of IgA myeloma, the cytoplasm will be pink to red in color (flame cell).

Chemotherapy with alkylating agents, steroids, and radiation therapy are common treatments in multiple myeloma. Severe anemia is treated with transfusions of packed red cells. Bleeding due to interference with coagulation factors may be treated by plasmapheresis. Recurrent bacterial infections resulting from a deficiency in normal immunoglobulins is the major cause of death.

Heavy Chain Diseases

The heavy chain diseases are a rare group of disorders in which there is malignant proliferation of lymphoid cells which produce incomplete immunoglobulins. These cells produce heavy chain fragments without the associated light chains. This may be caused by the deletion of amino acids which code for the synthesis of the area in the heavy chain that is responsible for attaching to the light chains. Four types of heavy chain disease have been found.

Gamma (γ) heavy chain disease resembles lymphoma with atypical lymphocytes and plasma cells present in the peripheral blood. It is usually a disease of the elderly. Anemia and leukopenia are generally present, and the platelets are decreased in about 50% of the cases. The bone marrow shows increased plasma cells and lymphocytes. These patients are usually susceptible to infection and have enlarged lymph nodes, spleen, and liver. This disorder is diagnosed by detecting the presence of IgG heavy chain fragments in the urine or serum. These chains are reactive on immunoelectrophoresis with antisera to gamma chains but not with antisera to light chains.

Alpha (α) heavy chain disease is the most common form of heavy chain disease, seen frequently in young Mediterraneans, and is commonly known as Mediterranean lymphoma. It usually presents as an abdominal mass with extensive lymphocyte and plasma cell infiltration of the small intestine and the abdominal lymph nodes. These patients have severe malabsorption with weight loss and diarrhea. Small amounts of the alpha chain may be detected by immunoelectrophoresis.

Mu (μ) heavy chain disease is rare and is often found in patients with chronic lymphocytic leukemia. Vacuolated plasma cells are usually found in the bone marrow of these patients. Routine electrophoresis generally shows marked hypogammaglobulinemia. The mu heavy chain is detected by serum immunoelectrophoresis.

Delta (δ) heavy chain disease is rare. It has the same clinical features as myeloma. The abnormal protein has been identified as a tetramer of delta heavy chains.

The clinical course of heavy chain diseases is variable. Most cases are progressive and fatal. Remissions have been obtained in some patients. Melphalan or cyclophosphamide and prednisone are the agents which are used to treat these disorders, although chemotherapy regimens have generally yielded poor results. Death usually follows from infection due to defective immunoglobulin production.

Waldenström's Macroglobulinemia

Waldenström's macroglobulinemia is a disease of the elderly, presenting with weight loss and fatigue, and most often occurring in males between the ages of 60 and 70. It is a low-grade lymphoma-like disorder characterized by infiltration of the bone marrow with small, mature B lymphocytes, many of which have plasmacytoid features. These cells produce macroglobulins (monoclonal IgM immunoglobulins of high molecular weight). These increased macroglobulin levels produce a condition called the *hyperviscosity syndrome*. This causes neurologic symptoms, visual impairment, bleeding from the nose and gums, and congestive heart failure. In contrast to multiple myeloma, bone pain and lesions are not symptoms of this disease, the serum calcium is normal, and malignant plasma cells are not found.

The blood generally shows normocytic-normochromic anemia that may become severe. The white blood cell count is usually normal. In the terminal stages of the disorder, the peripheral blood may contain large numbers of abnormal plasmacytoid lymphocytes. The liver, spleen, and lymph nodes may also be infiltrated with these cells. Thrombocytopenia is present in about 30% of these patients, and abnormal platelet function is a result of the platelet becoming coated with IgM molecules. The production of abnormal fibrin monomers may result in abnormal coagulation studies. Marked rouleaux is seen on the Wright stained smear, and the erythrocyte sedimentation rate and serum viscosity are elevated. The bone marrow usually contains increased numbers of lymphocytes, plasmacytoid lymphocytes, and plasma cells. The periodic acid-Schiff stain is positive and often shows positive inclusions in the cytoplasm and nucleus of the lymphoid cells. This PAS positive material is probably identical with the circulating macroglobulin.

Alkylating agents such as chlorambucil and melphalan have been used to treat this incurable disorder. The hyperviscosity responds to plasmapheresis. The average life span of patients diagnosed with this disorder is 2 to 4 years depending on the degree of bone marrow involvement.

Storage Diseases

The storage diseases outlined here represent a group of disorders in which there are deficiencies in the enzymes responsible for the metabolic breakdown of lipids. All tissues of the body are affected and accumulation of lipid is prominent in the cells of the monocyte-macrophage system.

Gaucher's disease is a rare, chronic disorder caused by an inherited deficiency of the enzyme, beta-glucosidase. As a result, there is an accumulation of glycolipids within the cells of the body. Patients with this disorder generally have splenomegaly, hepatomegaly, some skin pigmentation, mental retardation, and a hypochromic anemia. The WBC and platelet count are generally decreased. When this disease is found in infants, it is generally characterized by retarded growth and neurologic signs. The diagnostic cell, termed the *Gaucher cell*, will be present in the bone marrow and in aspirates from the liver, spleen, and lymph nodes. The Gaucher cell is large, 20 to 80 μm, with a small eccentric nucleus. The markedly abundant cytoplasm is filled with lipid, giving it a fibrillar appearance. The periodic acid Schiff reaction of these cells is positive.

Niemann-Pick disease affects primarily infants and is due to a deficiency in sphingomyelinase that causes an accumulation of sphingomyelin. These patients show enlarged livers and spleens. Accumulation of undegraded sphingomyelin leads to neuron (nerve cell) degeneration and mental retardation. Death usually occurs within a few months of diagnosis, and few patients live beyond the age of 20 years, with most patients dying between 2 and 3 years of age. In the stained blood smear, vacuoles may be present in the cytoplasm of the lymphocytes and monocytes. There is usually a microcytic anemia and thrombocytopenia. Niemann-Pick cells will be found in the bone marrow and spleen.

These cells are similar in size to the Gaucher cell and have an eccentrically placed nucleus. The accumulated sphingomyelin gives the cytoplasm a more globular appearance. These cells are often called foam cells. They stain blue-green with Wright stain and will also stain with sudan black B and oil red O.

Sea-blue histiocytes are found in the bone marrow, spleen, and liver of patients with sea-blue histiocytosis. These cells are large (20 to 60 μm in diameter), with an eccentric nucleus containing one nucleolus. The cytoplasm contains varying numbers of granules, which are blue to blue-green in color when stained with Wright stain. These cells contain an accumulation of lipid and are found in association with increased tissue stores of phospholipids and glycolipids.

Histiocytosis X

Eosinophilic granuloma of the bone, Letterer-Siwe disease, and Hand-Schüller-Christian disease have all been categorized as histiocytosis X by some hematologists because they all show an abnormal proliferation of mature histiocytes or Langerhans cells in various tissues of the body. In the peripheral blood, there are no unusual or diagnostic findings. The cause of this abnormal proliferation is unknown. The process may result in impaired function of certain organs or tissues, or it may result in their destruction.

Eosinophilic granuloma of the bone is a benign disease found primarily in older male children and young adults. Biopsy of the bone shows many eosinophils and histiocytes, particularly in the skull, ribs, and femur. This is a localized process that produces skeletal lesions, treated by surgical removal of the areas.

Letterer-Siwe disease is generally found in young children. It is an acute and disseminated process that is usually fatal. Proliferation of histiocytes is found primarily in the lymph nodes, skin, spleen, liver, lungs, and bone marrow. As the bone marrow becomes involved, anemia and thrombocytopenia can result. At this time, chemotherapy has somewhat improved the prognosis.

Hand-Schüller-Christian disease is a chronic and progressive form of histiocytosis found in older children. It affects primarily the bones, skin, and lymphoid tissue. Some patients also have abnormal hypothalamic-pituitary function. The treatment and prognosis is a function of the age of the patient, the extent of organ involvement, and the degree of organ impairment. Spontaneous recovery can occur or chemotherapy can be used to treat this disorder.

PLATELET DISORDERS

Quantitative Platelet Disorders

Thrombocytopenia

Thrombocytopenia is the most common cause of abnormal bleeding and is generally attributed to the following causes: (1) decreased platelet production, (2) decreased platelet survival time due to increased destruction and/or consumption, (3) increased platelet sequestration by the spleen, and (4) dilution of the platelet count by multiple blood transfusions.

Decreased Platelet Production

Decreased megakaryocytes in the bone marrow. *Congenital hypoplasia of the megakaryocytes* in the bone marrow is found in a number of clinical conditions: (1) Fanconi's syndrome, in which there is pancytopenia and bone marrow hypoplasia, along with various congenital abnormalities. (2) TAR syndrome (thrombocytopenia with absent radii [bone in the arm]) characterized by renal, cardiac, and skeletal malformation. (3) In the newborn as a result of intrauterine exposure to drugs (thiazides) and viral infections (rubella).

Acquired hypoplasia of the megakaryocytes may be a result of the action of chemicals, drugs, radiation, chemotherapy, or infectious agents. Some drugs, such as thiazide diuretics, the estrogen hormone DES (diethylstilbestrol), and alcohol, selectively decrease megakaryocyte production.

Infiltration of the bone marrow by malignant cells will generally result in decreased numbers of megakaryocytes. The thrombocytopenia associated with such conditions as metastatic cancer, myeloma, lymphoma, myelofibrosis, leukemia, and granulomatous diseases may be due to marrow replacement or inhibitors of thrombopoiesis (toxins) produced by the abnormal cells.

Ineffective thrombopoiesis. *Ineffective thrombopoiesis* is characterized by normal to increased marrow megakaryocytes in association with decreased circulating platelets. The disorder may be due to defective platelet formation, abnormal marrow release of platelets, or destruction of platelets in the bone marrow. It is found in patients with megaloblastic anemias due to vitamin B_{12} or folic acid deficiency as a result of impaired DNA synthesis, DiGuglielmo's syndrome, paroxysmal nocturnal hemoglobinuria, myelodysplastic syndromes, and leukemia. Hereditary conditions associated with ineffective platelet production include autosomal dominant thrombocytopenia, May-Hegglin anomaly, and Wiscott-Aldrich syndrome.

Disorders of the control of thrombopoiesis are not very common and result from an impairment in the mechanisms that control platelet production. Cyclic thrombocytopenia has been described as a condition in which thrombocytopenia and normal platelet counts alternate at regular intervals.

Decreased Platelet Survival Time

Increased platelet destruction: immunologic thrombocytopenia. Thrombocytopenia due to increased platelet destruction may occur as a result of immunologic disorders.

Idiopathic thrombocytopenic purpura (ITP) refers to thrombocytopenia that occurs in the absence of any disease associated with decreased platelets or toxin exposure. ITP may occur in the acute, chronic, recurrent, and neonatal form. Acute ITP is found predominantly in children, in the 2 to 6 year age group, and occasionally in young adults. The majority of the cases develop after recovery from a viral infection. The bone marrow contains abundant megakaryocytes; young, large platelets with abnormal shapes are seen on a stained blood smear. The decreased platelet survival time is thought to be due to destruction by immune complexes or foreign antigens adsorbed by platelets as a result of an infection. Acute ITP is self limiting, and spontaneous remissions occur in about 80% of cases. Chronic ITP is found predominantly in adults, and more often occurs in women between the ages of 20 and 40 years. As in the acute form, the bone marrow contains abundant megakaryocytes. Circulating platelets are young with a decreased lifespan. In patients with chronic ITP, platelet associated IgG levels are significantly elevated.

Thrombocytopenia results from the clearing of the antibody coated platelets by the spleen and liver. Spontaneous remission is rare. Effective treatment of this disorder usually consists of corticosteroid therapy or splenectomy. Recurrent ITP is found in patients who do not experience permanent remission following corticosteroid therapy or splenectomy. It is characterized by alternating intervals of thrombocytopenia and normal platelet counts. Immunosuppressive drugs and plasmapheresis are used to treat these patients. Neonatal ITP is found in the newborns of women with ITP. It is caused by transplacental passage of antiplatelet antibodies and occurs most frequently when the mother is thrombocytopenic at the time of delivery. Recovery follows clearance of the antibody from the circulation and treatment, when indicated, involves prenatal use of corticosteroids and intravenous infusion of high-dose gamma globulin (IVIgG).

Drug induced immunologic thrombocytopenia may be caused by any one of many substances such as antibiotics, hypnotics, analgesics, heavy metals, diuretics, chloroquine, digitoxin, quinine, heparin, and tolbutamide, to name a few. Antibody production will occur in only a small number of people exposed to a given drug. Generally both the drug and the antibody must be present in the system at the same time for destruction of platelets to occur. Severe thrombocytopenia may result within 12 hours of ingestion of the drug, or the reaction time may be delayed. Bleeding may be severe and begin abruptly. The megakaryocytes in the bone marrow are generally normal in number. Removal of the offending drug is usually curative, with return of the platelet count to normal.

Immunologic thrombocytopenia, a condition indistinguishable from chronic ITP, is associated with a number of disorders such as autoimmune hemolytic anemias, chronic lymphocytic leukemia, Hodgkin's disease and other lymphomas, systemic lupus erythematosus, rheumatoid arthritis, and acquired immunodeficiency syndrome.

Post transfusion purpura (PTP) occurs 7 to 10 days after transfusion of blood or blood products containing platelets. PTP is thought to result from sensitization of individuals negative for the platelet antigen PIA[1]. PIA[1] is found in approximately 97% of the normal population. The disorder is rare and has most commonly been reported in multiparous women who have been previously transfused. It is believed that primary immunization occurs during pregnancy as a result of PIA[1]-positive fetal platelets sensitizing a PIA[1]-negative mother. PTP has also been found in previously transfused patients. The disorder is generally self limiting, because the patient recovers when the antibody disappears. Bleeding complications associated with PTP are treated with IVIgG and plasma exchange.

Isoimmune neonatal thrombocytopenia is a rare disorder analogous to hemolytic disease of the newborn. It occurs in newborns as a result of transplancental transfer of maternal antiplatelet antibodies produced in response to fetal antigen inherited from the father. It generally affects the first-born child, although subsequent children may also be affected. The platelet antigen PIA[1] has most often been associated with this disorder. In most cases, treatment may not be required. In severe cases, platelets compatible with maternal antibodies are transfused. Corticosteroids and IVIgG have been used prenatally.

Thrombocytopenia due to increased platelet consumption may occur in association with many conditions. Generally, the mechanism of thrombocytopenia in these disorders is nonimmunologic.

Increased platelet consumption: nonimmunologic thrombocytopenia. Thrombotic thrombocytopenic purpura (TTP) is a rare disorder, the exact cause of which is unknown. In addition to thrombocytopenia, it is characterized by hemolytic anemia, changing neurologic symptoms, fever, and renal abnormalities. Most of these findings are caused by the formation of platelet thrombi in capillaries and arterioles throughout the body. The vascular defects also give rise to red blood cell fragments, and peripheral blood smears show poikilocytosis and normoblasts. The hemolytic anemia probably occurs as a result of the trauma to the red blood cells. Patients may develop disseminated intravascular coagulation (DIC) as the disease progresses, although the severity of hemolysis and red cell fragmentation is much greater in TTP. It affects all ages, although it is most commonly found in women (mean age 40). TTP is a serious disease, but at present more than 50% of the patients respond favorably to therapy. Treatment consists of a combination of the administration of antiplatelet agents, high doses of steroids, plasma transfusions, and splenectomy. Plasma exchange and plasma transfusion are the current treatment of choice.

Hemolytic-uremic syndrome resembles TTP. However, it occurs primarily in children, and the intravascular clotting is generally confined to the kidney. Fever, hypertension, and renal failure are common findings, whereas neurologic symptoms are rare. Treatments include dialysis, plasma transfusion or exchange, and antihypertensive therapy.

Nonimmunologic thrombocytopenias are varied and may also be found in DIC, fibrinogenolysis, and other microangiopathic processes. Thrombocytopenia may be present in a number of rickettsial, bacterial, viral, or malarial infections, more commonly as a result of increased consumption of platelets and less commonly as a result of decreased production. Generally, the thrombocytopenias are nonimmunologic, although immune destruction of platelets has been implicated in septicemia, infectious mononucleosis, and malaria. The thrombocytopenia that may occur during pregnancy or obstetric complications may be due to consumption of platelets as occurs in DIC, as well as immunologically mediated platelet destruction. Thrombocytopenia related to cardiopulmonary bypass can result from DIC, dilution, sequestration, platelet destruction in the oxygenator, and increased fibrinolysis. Qualitative platelet defects are also present.

Increased platelet sequestration. An abnormal distribution of platelets may also cause thrombocytopenia. Normally, the spleen pools approximately one-third of the total platelet mass. In patients with an enlarged spleen (splenomegaly), an increased percentage of the platelets will be found in the spleen, thereby producing thrombocytopenia. Increased splenic pooling is differentiated from destruction of platelets by the spleen in that the platelets are essentially normal but transit time through the spleen is prolonged. Splenomegaly is associated with many conditions.

Dilution of the platelet count. Multiple transfusions used to treat massive blood loss cause hemodilution and produce thrombocytopenia because stored blood contains nonviable dysfunctional platelets. The splenic pool is usually insufficient to keep up with losses, and compensation by increased platelet production does not occur as an acute response to hemorrhage. Transfusion with platelet concentrates usually prevents excessive bleeding in patients with dilutional thrombocytopenia.

Thrombocytosis

A platelet count increased above normal will be found as a result of a variety of circumstances. *Reactive thrombocytosis* describes a moderate increase in the platelet count, which is usually short lived and generally asymptomatic. *Autonomous thrombocytosis* refers to a marked increase in the platelet count, which generally persists, and is associated with thrombotic and/or hemorrhagic complications.

Reactive thrombocytosis. Reactive thrombocytosis generally responds when the underlying disorder is treated. Recovery from splenectomy, major surgery, and acute blood loss are commonly associated with reactive thrombocytosis. Following splenectomy, the platelet count will generally rise during the first postoperative week, peak at about 2 to 3 weeks, and return to normal over a period of several months. Thrombocytosis following major surgery usually occurs during the first postoperative week, with the platelet count generally decreasing to normal levels within about 2 weeks. Within about a day or so following acute blood loss, a reactive thrombocytosis may occur as a result of increased bone marrow stimulation. Other conditions associated with reactive thrombocytosis are (1) iron deficiency anemia, (2) malignant diseases such as carcinoma and Hodgkin's disease, (3) following withdrawal of cytotoxic drugs, (4) association with increased hematopoiesis, as in patients with hemolytic anemia or secondary polycythemia, and (5) association with acute and chronic inflammatory diseases. In all of these conditions, the megakaryocytes are increased in number, platelet production is effective, and platelet survival is normal.

Autonomous Thrombocytosis.
Autonomous thrombocytosis is a common feature of the myeloproliferative disorders, which include essential thrombocytosis (thrombocythemia), chronic myelogenous leukemia, polycythemia vera, and myeloid metaplasia.

Thrombocythemia is found most often in middle aged patients of both sexes. Patients with this disorder may have bleeding or thrombosis, with bleeding episodes predominating. Gastrointestinal hemorrhage is the most common form of bleeding. Thrombosis in both the venous and arterial circulation may develop, and involvement of the coronary and cerebral vasculature is common. Splenomegaly is a frequent finding, although platelet life span is generally normal. The platelet count is usually greater than 1 million/fL and may be as high as several million/fL. Because of the extremely high number of platelets, it is frequently difficult to obtain an accurate platelet count, and determination of the packed platelet volume is useful. Stained blood smears often show platelet aggregates as well as abnormal platelet size, shape, and structure. Megakaryocyte fragments are also frequently present. In the bone marrow a marked increase in the size, volume, and number of megakaryocytes is seen, and they often display bizarre morphology. Platelet function tests are usually abnormal. Treatment for this disorder is aimed primarily at controlling the platelet count. In symptomatic patients where the platelet count is elevated above 1 million/fL radioactive phosphorous, hydroxyurea, and plateletpheresis are used. Aspirin is often employed in an attempt to prevent thromboembolic complications.

The other myeloproliferative disorders share the thrombotic and hemorrhagic complications, as well as many of the morphologic features of the platelets and megakaryocytes seen in thrombocythemia.

Qualitative Platelet Disorders

Hereditary Qualitative Platelet Disorders

Qualitative or functional platelet disorders may be attributed to defects of platelet adhesion, platelet aggregation, or the release reaction.

Platelet Adhesion Defects.
The *Bernard-Soulier syndrome* is inherited as an autosomal recessive trait. It is characterized by bruising and moderate to severe bleeding. One of the most striking characteristics of this disorder is the presence of giant platelets, which may range in size up to 20 μm in diameter. The platelets also show coarse granulation and vacuoles. Mild thrombocytopenia is generally present. The megakaryocytes in the bone marrow are normal to slightly increased in number and appear morphologically normal. The platelets lack the glycoprotein 1b (GP1b), which functions as a receptor for the vonWillebrand factor. They are therefore are unable to adhere normally to vascular endothelium. In addition, the platelets lack glycoproteins V and IX, they do not bind coagulation factor XI normally, and bind a decreased amount of thrombin. The bleeding time is prolonged, but clot retraction is normal. Platelet aggregation is normal with ADP, epinephrine, and collagen, but abnormal with ristocetin and thrombin. There is decreased platelet retention in glass bead columns. At present, there is no specific treatment for this disorder. Platelet transfusion is usually avoided because of development of antibodies that interfere with platelet function and cause platelet destruction.

In *vonWillebrand's disease,* an absent or abnormal form of the vonWillebrand factor results in impaired platelet adhesion. Aggregation studies with ADP, epinephrine, and collagen are normal, whereas ristocetin-induced aggregation is usually abnormal.

Platelet Aggregation Defects.
Glanzmann's thrombasthenia is inherited as an autosomal recessive trait. People who are heterozygous for this trait are asymptomatic carriers. In this disorder, bleeding tendencies are variable and range from minor bruising to severe hemorrhages that may begin during infancy. Platelet aggregation studies show a defective primary response in the presence of collagen, epinephrine, ADP, and thrombin, but a normal response with ristocetin. Platelet retention is markedly decreased. The platelet count is generally normal but may occasionally be slightly decreased. Clot retraction is decreased to absent, and the bleeding time is prolonged. When viewed on a Wright stained

blood smear, the platelets appear morphologically normal and show a normal shape change in the presence of aggregating agents. The impaired aggregation seen in Glanzmann's thrombasthenia is due to a decrease or absence of the platelet membrane glycoprotein IIb-IIIa complex, which acts as a fibrinogen binding site on the platelet surface. Few treatment options are currently available for this disorder, except for transfusion of platelet concentrates, which may result in the development of platelet antibodies.

Platelet Secretion Defects. Defects of platelet secretion may be subdivided into two categories: (1) storage pool disorders and (2) "aspirin-like" defects.

The *storage pool disorders* are a group of hereditary conditions in which there is a defective platelet release reaction due to a lack of dense bodies and/or α granules. In these disorders, there is a mild to moderate bleeding tendency, and easy bruising is common. Abnormalities of the dense bodies or α granules (*gray platelet syndrome*) result in reduced concentrations and abnormal release of both α and dense granule components (e.g., ADP, calcium, platelet factor 4). Platelet aggregation studies usually show abnormal aggregation with collagen and an absent or diminished secondary wave with ADP and epinephrine. There is decreased platelet retention using the glass bead column. Storage pool disorders may also be found in association with certain congenital abnormalities such as *Wiskott-Aldrich, TAR,* and *Chediak-Higashi* syndromes. At present, there is no specific treatment for this disorder. All drugs that inhibit platelet aggregation should be witheld from these patients.

Aspirin-like defects. Patients whose platelets have normal granules but defective release have been classified as having an "aspirin-like" defect. A deficiency of the enzyme cyclo-oxygenase or thromboxane synthetase may account for this defect. The clinical features are similar to other platelet function defects. Patients with this disorder have a prolonged bleeding time and abnormal aggregation with ADP, epinephrine, and collagen.

Hereditary Forms of Platelet Dysfunction. Some inherited connective tissue disorders (*Ehlers-Danlos syndrome*) may show very large platelets and abnormalities in platelet adhesion and aggregation. Patients with *hereditary afibrinogenemia* usually have a prolonged bleeding time and abnormal platelet aggregation with ADP. Abnormalities of platelet aggregation and release reaction have also been found in patients with *glycogen storage disease type 1* (glucose-6-phosphate dehydrogenase [G-6-PD] deficiency). The bleeding time is also prolonged. The platelet defects may be secondary to the metabolic defect.

Acquired Qualitative Platelet Disorders

Acquired disorders of platelet function are associated with a number of conditions and with the ingestion of certain drugs.

In *uremia*, metabolites that are toxic to the platelets accumulate in the plasma. These toxins, and possibly platelet metabolites, contribute to the impaired platelet function seen in this disorder. The platelet release reaction, aggregation, and retention are all abnormal, and the bleeding time is prolonged. Platelet dysfunction and abnormal platelet-vessel wall interaction may be the major cause of bleeding, which may be severe at times. Dialysis is of temporary therapeutic value; the administration of cryoprecipitates will aid in controlling major bleeding episodes.

Platelet dysfunction and bleeding disorders will be present in the various *paraproteinemias.* In multiple myeloma and Waldenstrom's macroglobulinemia, abnormalities of platelet aggregation, and reduced platelet retention are thought to be due to the coating of the platelet membrane and vessel walls with the abnormal proteins.

In *acute myeloblastic leukemia,* the megakaryocytes in the bone marrow may be small and somewhat abnormal. The resultant platelets are abnormal, showing defective platelet aggregation and a defective release mechanism.

The *myeloproliferative disorders* (polycythemia vera, chronic myelogenous leukemia, myeloid metaplasia, and essential thrombocythemia) display functional abnormalities in addition to thrombocytosis. Bleeding and/or thrombosis are common complications. In myeloid metaplasia the bleeding time is prolonged and there is defective platelet adhesion, aggregation, and storage pool deficiencies. Abnormal platelet aggregation is seen in polycythemia vera. In thrombocythemia, the platelets appear large and morphologically abnormal. There is defective platelet retention and platelet aggregation. A prolonged bleeding time and defective platelet aggregation are often seen in chronic myelogenous leukemia.

Increased amounts of *fibrinogen degradation products,* which may be present in DIC, fibrinogenolysis, and liver disease, will inhibit ADP induced platelet aggregation. Fragments D and E, which adsorb onto the platelet surface, interfere with platelet function and will inhibit thrombin induced platelet aggregation.

The *platelet associated antibodies* found in idiopathic thrombocytopenia purpura and in certain autoimmune disorders such as systemic lupus erythematosis may cause functional platelet disorders. These antibodies have been shown to cause platelet lysis, platelet aggregation, and serotonin release because of the reaction of the antibody with the platelet membrane.

Many *drugs* have been shown to inhibit platelet function. Aspirin inhibits both the release reaction and the secondary wave of aggregation. This is a direct result of aspirin's ability to inactivate the enzyme cyclo-oxygenase. The effect of the aspirin lasts for the life of the platelet. In the presence of aspirin, there is defective platelet aggregation with ADP, epinephrine, and collagen. Other drugs that induce qualitative platelet abnormalities include some antihistamines, antidepressants and antibiotics, heparin, dextran and other plasma expanders, ethanol, and certain local anesthetics.

VASCULAR DISORDERS

Vascular disorders are characterized by easy bruising or purpura (bleeding into the skin) caused by defects in the structure or function of the walls of the blood vessels. Extravascular or endothelial defects may also lead to vascular disorders.

In *hereditary hemorrhagic telangiectasia (Osler-Weber-Rendu disease),* there is localized dilation of the walls of the small blood vessels of the skin and mucous membranes. These blood vessels form disorganized and tortuous patterns throughout the body. The walls of the affected blood vessels are thin and lack smooth muscle. For this reason they are unable to contract and bleed readily when injured. This disorder is inherited as an autosomal dominant trait and is the most common inherited vascular bleeding disorder.

Extravascular defects result from loss of elasticity of the skin, as in the benign condition *senile purpura* (bruised areas commonly on the forearms of elderly persons), or from more serious *connective tissue abnormalities.* Ehlers-Danlos syndrome and *Marfan's syndrome* are both inherited as autosomal dominant disorders and display abnormal bleeding due to increased vascular fragility. This increased fragility is caused by abnormalities of the collagen and elastin fibers which form the supporting tissues for blood vessels.

Scurvy (deficiency of ascorbic acid) causes acquired defects in the synthesis of collagen and hyaluronic acid, a component of the intercellular cement substance found between endothelial cells. This disorder is eliminated by the administration of ascorbic acid (vitamin C).

Henoch-Schönlein purpura is a disorder in which gastrointestinal hemorrhage and joint swelling occur in association with a purpuric rash. This condition is most common in children and often follows an upper respiratory infection. Immunologic damage to endothelial cells is most probably the cause of the vascular abnormalities seen in this disorder. Certain drugs and infectious agents are also known to cause vascular abnormalities due to endothelial cell damage.

In vascular disorders, there may be spontaneous bleeding or bleeding as a result of minimal trauma. Petechiae (small purpuric spots on the skin) are present, and in some cases, ecchymoses (larger superficial hemorrhages) may appear secondary to mild trauma. Intramuscular bleeding is rare, but nosebleeds are not uncommon. Generally, the platelet count is normal, as are most platelet function tests and coagulation studies. The bleeding time and tourniquet test are usually abnormal.

COAGULATION DISORDERS

Coagulation Factor Deficiencies

Coagulation factor abnormalities may be due to a defect in the synthesis of the factor (leading to a decreased concentration) or may be due to synthesis of a defective factor (leading to normal amounts of an inactive or abnormally functioning factor). Abnormalities may be classified as quantitative or qualitative based on results of immunologic procedures. The results of these tests are expressed as positive (+) or negative (−) for *cross-reacting material (CRM + or CRM −)*. A test that is CRM − indicates that a specific factor is not present. CRM − disorders are quantitative abnormalities. On the other hand, a coagulation disease that is CRM + is considered to have the factor present, but it is thought to be functionally abnormal, and it is, therefore, a qualitative disorder.

Factor I Deficiency

A deficiency in fibrinogen is rare, but when it does occur, severe hemorrhaging may result. Congenital deficiencies of fibrinogen may fall into one of three categories: (1) *Afibrinogenemia,* in which there is no measurable fibrinogen except trace amounts when tested immunologically. (2) *Hypofibrinogenemia,* where the plasma levels of fibrinogen are lower than 100 mg/dL. (3) *Dysfibrinogenemia,* where the fibrinogen present is functionally abnormal.

Hereditary afibrinogenemia is an extremely rare disorder. To date, only about 150 cases have been reported. It is inherited as an autosomal recessive trait and appears to be the result of deficient synthesis of fibrinogen. Patients homozygous for this disorder have low levels of fibrinogen. This hemorrhagic disorder is present from birth, and there may be severe bleeding from the umbilical cord. There may be excessive bleeding following surgery or trauma, as well as gingival (bleeding from the gums) and gastrointestinal bleeding, along with menorrhagia (excessive menstrual bleeding). Subcutaneous hemorrhages and defective wound healing are also seen. These patients may, however, have long periods where they have no bleeding, and the disorder is generally not as debilitating as Hemophilia A. In most cases, the blood will not clot. The PT, APTT, and thrombin time are markedly prolonged, and the bleeding time is abnormal in about 50% of the cases. Because of the total absence of fibrinogen, the erythrocyte sedimentation rate is generally 0.

Hereditary hypofibrinogenemia has been found to be inherited as both an autosomal dominant trait and an autosomal recessive trait. This condition may possibly be the heterozygous expression of afibrinogenemia. Generally the plasma fibrinogen (clottable and immunologic) levels are less than 100 mg/dL, and major bleeding is not seen. The laboratory test results are similar to those described for hereditary afibrinogenemia but are not as markedly abnormal.

Hereditary dysfibrinogenemia is usually inherited as an incompletely dominant autosomal trait. More than 55 different qualitatively abnormal fibrinogens have now been found. These fibrinogens have structural variations which result in abnormalities of all three aspects of the thrombin-fibrinogen reaction (release of fibrinopeptides, polymerization of the fibrin monomers, and stabilization of the fibrin clot). Most patients with this disorder show few symptoms other than a mild hemorrhagic tendency and some problems with wound healing. At birth there may be bleeding from the umbilical cord. The PT and APTT generally show slightly prolonged results, and the thrombin time is prolonged. Chemical or immunologic assays of quantitative fibrinogen levels are generally normal. Procedures testing for clottable fibrinogen (those procedures using a thrombin reagent), however, are abnormal.

Cryoprecipitate, purified fibrinogen, and fresh frozen plasma are used to treat the inherited fibrinogen deficiencies.

An *acquired deficiency of fibrinogen* is more commonly found than a congenital deficiency. The acquired deficiency may be caused by impaired fibrinogen production in conditions such as liver disease. It may occur as a result of excess utilization of fibrinogen, or it may be found as a result of fibrinogen destruction. Both of these processes are present in DIC and liver disease. Acquired deficiencies of fibrinogen are most commonly found in abnormal obstetric cases and may also occur as a complication of surgery.

Factor II Deficiency

A *congenital deficiency of prothrombin* is the rarest of the factor deficiencies and is inherited as an autosomal recessive trait. It is a relatively mild hemorrhagic disorder, and bleeding is most common following trauma. A few cases of dysfunctional prothrombin have also been found. Laboratory tests show both the PT and APTT to be abnormal. The whole blood clotting time may or may not be abnormal, and the Stypven time is abnormal. The most sensitive test for this abnormality is the two-stage prothrombin time, which will show a marked reduction in prothrombin. Levels of prothrombin are usually less than 10% of normal in this disorder. Fresh frozen plasma or Proplex (a purified prothrombin complex) may be administered for treatment.

Prothrombin is produced by the liver and depends on vitamin K for its synthesis. An *acquired deficiency of prothrombin* is commonly found in association with vitamin K deficiency, in which case deficiencies of factors VII, IX, and X are also present. These deficiencies are found in gastrointestinal disease, obstructive jaundice, and coumadin therapy where there is defective absorption or utilization of vitamin K.

Factor V Deficiency

A *congenital deficiency of factor V* has been designated *parahemophilia*. It is inherited as an autosomal recessive trait and manifests itself clinically in those patients who have inherited the defective gene from both parents (homozygotes). This defect is extremely rare. Clinically, these patients may show varying degrees of mucosal membrane bleeding, easy bruising, gastrointestinal bleeding, and excessive bleeding following dental or surgical procedures. The PT, APTT, and Stypven time are abnormal. The whole blood clotting time and the prothrombin consumption may or may not be abnormal. Heterozygous individuals are usually asymptomatic. A factor V assay, based on the prothrombin time, should be performed to determine the extent of the deficiency. Fresh or fresh frozen plasma given once daily is used when treatment of this disorder is necessary. Platelet concentrates have also been used as a source of platelet factor V.

A *combined deficiency of factor V and factor VIII:C* has been described. It is a rare finding and its biochemistry and genetics have not yet been fully described.

Acquired deficiencies of factor V have been found to be associated with DIC, liver disease, and acute leukemia.

Factor VII Deficiency

Congenital factor VII deficiency is a rare disorder and is inherited as an autosomal recessive trait. It produces a severe deficiency in the homozygous (less than 10% of normal concentrations) patient and a moderate deficiency in heterozygous individuals. Patients have also been found with qualitative abnormalities of factor VII. Clinically, homozygous patients show mild mucosal, genitourinary and gastrointestinal bleeding. Easy bruising and prolonged menstrual bleeding may also occur. However, the severity of the clinical bleeding does not always correlate well with assayed factor VII levels in the patient. A high incidence of factor VII deficiency has been found in patients with Dubin-Johnson syndrome (an hereditary disorder of bilirubin metabolism). The PT is significantly prolonged. The APTT, whole blood clotting time, and Stypven time are normal. A prothrombin time with substitutions may be performed to help identify the factor VII deficiency. An assay for factor VII, based on the prothrombin time, may then be performed to determine the level of factor VII present. This disorder may be treated with fresh frozen plasma or Proplex (a purified prothrombin complex). Because of the short half-life of factor VII (6 hours) treatment must be given at least three times daily.

Factor VII is synthesized in the liver and is vitamin K dependent. *Acquired factor VII deficiency* is found in the same conditions that cause acquired deficiency of factor II.

Factor VIII Deficiency

Genetic abnormalities of factor VIII are found in hemophilia A (or *classic hemophilia*) and *von Willebrand's disease*. These are the two most common hereditary coagulation disorders. It is currently accepted that several functions can be attributed to the factor VIII-von Willebrand factor complex: (1) Factor VIII:C refers to the procoagulant portion of the molecule and represents the ability of the factor VIII molecule to correct coagulation abnormalities associated with hemophilia A. This clotting activity is measured in the APTT and the factor VIII assay procedure. (2) Factor VIII:Ag is the factor VIII antigen that is measured immunologically. (3) Factor VIIIR:RCo refers to that part of the molecule which makes possible platelet aggregation in the presence of ristocetin, and is termed the ristocetin cofactor. (4) Factor VIII:vWF is also termed the *von Willebrand factor* and is required for normal platelet adhesion to endothelium in the hemostatic process. (5) vWF:Ag is the antigenic portion of the von Willebrand factor.

Hemophilia A. Hemophilia A is inherited as a sex linked recessive trait and is felt to be the result of a deficiency or dysfunction of the factor VIII:C component of the factor VIII molecule. The condition is transmitted to males by their mothers who have the defective gene on one X chromosome. Hemophilia A affects about 1 in 10,000 males. The female carrier of hemophilia theoretically passes this defect on to half of her sons (who will demonstrate hemophilia A) and half of her daughters (who will be carriers). The affected male transmits the defective gene to all of his daughters but to none of his sons because the sons acquire the X chromosome from their mother. Hemophilia has also been found in females, most commonly seen in the heterozygous carrier, where unusually low levels of factor VIII:C activity may be seen. However, female carriers usually do not have a bleeding tendency. Females who are homozygous for hemophilia have been seen in whom the disorder was passed on from the parents (an affected father and a mother carrying the defective gene). In these cases, the disorder resembles that seen in the affected male. However, in about one-third of newly diagnosed cases, there is no familial history of bleeding that suggests either a high incidence of mutation or a mother who is a "silent carrier."

Except in mild deficiencies, this hemorrhagic disorder appears early in life and remains as a lifelong affliction. The disorder may not be evident in infancy until the child begins to walk and falls, triggering bleeding episodes. Bleeding may occur in the gastrointestinal tract, the renal tract, or from the nose. Dental extractions are often followed by excessive bleeding. Hemarthrosis (hemorrhaging into the joints) is a common finding, particularly in the knees. This causes pain and swelling that may progressively impair joint function and lead to chronic arthritis and joint destruction. Intramuscular bleeding with resultant hematomas is also common. Intracranial bleeding is seen in some patients and is a frequent cause of death.

Patients with severe hemophilia have less than 1% factor VIII:C activity. The laboratory data are usually characteristic. The platelet count, tourniquet test, PT, and bleeding time are normal. The APTT is abnormal. The Lee and White clotting time is most often abnormal. The APTT with substitutions should be performed, followed by a factor VIII:C assay. The clinical severity of the disease correlates well with the level of factor VIII.

Patients with factor VIII:C levels of 2 to 5% are considered to have moderate hemophilia. These individuals will also suffer spontaneous bleeding but less frequently than the more severely deficient patients. Mild hemophilia is characterized by factor VIII:C levels of 5 to 25%. This type is more difficult to diagnose. The patient generally shows a normal Lee and White clotting time but may bleed profusely during or following surgery. As a general rule, spontaneous bleeding does not occur unless the factor VIII:C level falls below 20% of normal.

Approximately 10% of severe hemophiliac patients develop circulating inhibitors, usually in the form of antibodies to factor VIII:C.

Treatment of hemophilia consists of halting any local bleeding by pressure and coagulants and raising the factor VIII:C level in the blood. The level to which the factor VIII:C activity is raised depends on the severity and cause of bleeding. Surgical and post trauma bleeding require that the level be elevated and maintained close to 100% of normal until healing occurs. There are several therapeutic materials now available for raising the factor VIII:C level in the blood, including the cryoprecipitated fraction of plasma and purified factor VIII concentrates. Administration of DDAVP (a drug which releases endogenous factor VIII:C from the endothelium) is used

When treatment is necessary, fresh frozen plasma and cryoprecipitate are administered.

Prekallikrein Deficiency

Prekallikrein (Fletcher factor) deficiency is thought to be inherited as an autosomal dominant trait. This abnormality has been identified as CRM −, and is, therefore, a quantitative defect.

Like those with a factor XII deficiency, people with prekallikrein deficiency show little to no bleeding tendencies.

Laboratory data show a normal PT, thrombin time, and bleeding time. The whole blood clotting time and APTT are usually moderately prolonged due to the slow contact activation time caused by the deficiency of prekallikrein. Repeating the APTT with a prolonged 10 minute incubation will normalize the APTT.

High Molecular Weight Kininogen Deficiency

High molecular weight kininogen (Fitzgerald Factor) deficiency, is thought to be transmitted as an autosomal recessive trait. Patients with this rare deficiency are asymptomatic. This disorder is characterized by a prolonged APTT (which remains prolonged following a 10 minute activation phase incubation) and whole blood clotting time.

Coagulation Disorders Caused by Vitamin K Deficiency

Factors II, VII, IX, and X depend on vitamin K for their synthesis and are produced in the liver. Therefore, a *vitamin K deficiency* or liver dysfunction may produce coagulation disorders. These include gastrointestinal, genitourinary, and gingival bleeding from a combined deficiency of all the above factors. In addition, the oral anticoagulant drug, coumadin, acts as an antagonist which impairs the synthesis of the vitamin K dependent coagulation factors.

Hemorrhagic disease of the newborn results from vitamin K deficiency. Normally, the newborn has a moderate deficiency of these factors at birth and for the following 2 to 5 days. Bleeding from the GI tract, nose, and umbilical cord may be seen. Routine administration of vitamin K however, has made this problem relatively rare. This disorder is prevented by administering vitamin K to the mother before delivery and by giving vitamin K to the infant at birth.

Circulating Anticoagulants and Inhibitors

Acquired circulating anticoagulants or coagulation inhibitors can be divided into two separate classes based on how they affect the coagulation process: (1) those which act immediately to inactivate an activated coagulation factor or block the interaction between coagulation factors and platelets, and (2) a class of inhibitors that progressively inactivates individual coagulation factors. Most circulating anticoagulants are IgG type immunoglobulins. They usually develop in response to replacement therapy in patients with a specific factor deficiency or they may arise spontaneously in the presence or absence of disease.

Inhibitors of most of the coagulation factors have been reported. With the exception of factor VIII and IX inhibitors, these occur rarely. In some patients, inhibitors are associated with the administration of certain drugs. Factor V inhibitors have been found following streptomycin therapy and Factor XIII inhibitors have been found following treatment with isoniazid, an antituberculosis drug.

Inhibitors of factor VIII occur in about 10% of patients with severe hemophilia A. They will also occur in patients with autoimmune disorders such as systemic lupus erythematosus, in rheumatoid arthritis, in pregnancy, in some women within a few weeks or months of giving birth, in association with drugs such as penicillin, and in normal individuals. Bleeding may range from mild to severe. Immunosuppressive therapy may be effective and spontaneous remissions may occur in some patients. Treatment of these patients is difficult because replacement therapy with factor VIII may produce an increased titer of the inhibitor, which neutralizes or inactivates the factor VIII given. Some patients with low titers of inhibitor respond well to transfusion of fresh frozen plasma.

Factor IX inhibitors occur in about 2% of the patients with hemophilia B and are rarely seen in non-hemophiliacs.

Inhibitors of coagulation have also been found in patients with multiple myeloma, Waldenström's macroglobulinemia, and autoimmune disorders. The abnormal proteins present may be absorbed by fibrinogen or fibrin, and they will act as inhibitors of fibrin polymerization, causing structurally abnormal clots.

Lupus Inhibitor

About 10% of the patients with systemic lupus erythematosus (SLE) have been found to have a nonspecific anticoagulant that is termed the lupus inhibitor. This inhibitor is an IgG, IgA, or IgM type immunoglobulin which is thought to interfere with the phospholipid portion of the complex (factor Xa-Va-Ca^{++}-platelet phospholipid) which converts prothrombin to thrombin. In addition to patients with SLE, the lupus inhibitor has been found in patients with other autoimmune disorders, after the administration of certain drugs, following viral infections and in some normal, healthy individuals.

Bleeding is uncommon. It may occur, however, if there is an associated thrombocytopenia, platelet function abnormality, or prothrombin deficiency. Thrombosis occurs in about 30% of the patients. Pregnant women with the lupus inhibitor are at high risk for recurrent intrauterine deaths or spontaneous abortion. The exact nature of the association between the lupus inhibitor and the thrombotic tendency and obstetric complications seen in some patients is not understood.

The lupus inhibitor is the most frequently occurring inhibitor and one of the commonest causes of a prolonged APTT encountered in the laboratory. In the presence of the lupus inhibitor, phospholipid dependent coagulation tests will be abnormal. The PT may be normal or slightly prolonged, the APTT will be prolonged and factor assays based on the APTT (Factors VIII, IX, XI, and XII) will show decreased levels. The test for a circulating anticoagulant (inhibitor) will not show correction when patient plasma is incubated with normal control plasma. The platelet neutralization procedure (PNP) is positive in the presence of the lupus inhibitor, as well as the dilute Russell viper venom test (DRVVT). The anticardiolipin antibody immunoassay is also used to specifically detect the presence of lupus anticoagulants.

Treatment for the lupus inhibitor is usually not indicated. Before a surgical procedure, it is essential to ascertain that the prolonged APTT is not due to a specific factor deficiency, and that the patient is not at risk for bleeding. It is important, however, that an awareness be maintained that these patients are at high risk for thrombotic and obstetric complications.

Liver Disease

A variety of hemostatic defects may be found in liver disease. These include multiple factor deficiencies, abnormalities of fibrinolysis, thrombocytopenia and qualitative platelet abnormalities. Alterations in clearance mechanisms of the liver further compromise the integrity of the hemostatic process. All of the coagulation factors, except factor VIII, are synthesized in the liver. Decreased levels of the vitamin K dependent factors (II, VII, IX, and X) are among the earliest and most important changes seen in liver disease. Factors V and the contact factors (XI, XII, prekallikrein, and Fitzgerald factor) are also decreased; however, the clinical significance of these deficiencies in patients with liver disease is unclear. Quantitative and/or qualitative abnormalities of fibrinogen are found in most cases of liver disease. For an unknown reason, factor VIII levels are generally increased in disorders of the liver. Abnormal fibrinolysis is seen due to decreased synthesis of plasminogen, decreased levels of plasmin inhibitors and impaired clearance from the circulation of plasminogen activators and fibrin split products. The thrombocytopenia seen in liver disease is usually secondary to splenomegaly, while the qualitative abnormalities of platelets may be attributed to increased levels of fibrin split products or to the intake of alcohol.

Patients with liver disease may have severe hemorrhaging. Gastrointestinal bleeding is most common and generally results from an ulcer, esophageal varices, or gastritis.

Laboratory test results will be extremely variable, depending on the severity of the liver disorder. The PT, APTT, bleeding time and platelet count are often abnormal. Fibrinogen levels may be decreased, normal or increased. Functionally abnormal variants of fibrinogen are common and usually account for a prolonged thrombin time. Treatment of liver disease may take the form of administration of vitamin K or antifibrinolytic agents, or, transfusions of fresh frozen plasma (for factor replacement) or platelets, depending on the severity of the disease and the resultant bleeding.

Disseminated Intravascular coagulation

Disseminated intravascular coagulation *(DIC), defibrination syndrome,* and *consumption coagulopathy* are terms used to refer to the generalized over-activation of the coagulation and fibrinolytic systems in the circulating blood. The results of this activation are consumption of coagulation factors and platelets, generation of thrombin, widespread deposition of fibrin in small blood vessels (thrombi) and formation of large amounts of fibrinogen degradation products. Depending on which process predominates (the clotting or the fibrinolysis), symptoms may range from a low grade thrombosis to an acutely severe hemorrhage. All of these contribute to the bleeding, shock, and vascular occlusion that develop.

There are two basic causes of an episode of DIC: (1) the release of tissue thromboplastin or thromboplastin-like substances into the circulation, and (2) the activation of coagulation proteins by exposure to damaged endothelium or in association with the intravascular aggregation of platelets. Clinical conditions associated with the release of thromboplastic material include obstetric complications, acute promyelocytic and monocytic leukemias, intravascular hemolysis of various origins, massive trauma, head injury, burns, major surgical procedures, and malignant tumors. Endothelial damage may occur as a result of infections (viral, bacterial, rickettsial, fungal, and protozoal), heat stroke, or shock. Intravascular platelet aggregation may result from the action of toxins, drugs or antigen-antibody complexes. Venoms from various snakes may produce vascular endothelial damage. They may also contain certain thrombin-like enzymes or substances that may activate prothrombin or factor X.

When thromboplastic material or activated coagulation proteins enter the circulating blood, intravascular coagulation occurs, with a resultant decrease in fibrinogen, prothrombin, factor V, and factor VIII. Factors VII, IX, and X and other coagulation proteins, namely antithrombin III, alpha-2 antiplasmin, and plasminogen, may also be decreased. The platelet count is generally low because the platelets are used in the coagulation process, and they also tend to adhere to the damaged tissues. An immediate reaction in DIC is the formation of small fibrin strands and microclots. This will cause injury to the red blood cells in the area, and schistocytes and microspherocytes will form. Fibrinolysis is almost always present in DIC and may be activated by the thromboplastic substances responsible for the DIC, activated factor XII, or from plasminogen activators present in the vascular endothelium. The resultant fibrin degradation products formed act as antithrombins and inhibit fibrin polymerization. This may be a major cause of hemorrhage. The liver is primarily responsible for removing the procoagulants and coagulation products from the system.

Thrombosis with infarction and necrosis may be the major feature of DIC when fibrinolytic activity is insufficient to remove clots and the coagulant processes predominate. Hemorrhage predominates as coagulation factors are consumed and clotting becomes minimal. In a typical case of DIC, the PT, APTT, and thrombin time are generally prolonged. These tests, however, may be normal for some unknown reason. A normal APTT, however, may reflect the partial coagulation (activated coagulation factors) present in the blood. The platelet count is decreased, as is the fibrinogen. Because of the formation of excess thrombin, soluble fibrin monomers are formed, so the protamine sulfate and ethanol gelation tests are usually positive. This indicates a highly activated coagulation system. Antithrombin III is usually decreased in this disorder. Tests for fibrinogen degradation products may show increased levels of these substances. It is not unusual, however, to find normal results in these tests because these fragments form a complex with fibrinogen during serum preparation. The D-dimer assay, which indicates the presence of fibrin fragments (d-dimer), is usually positive in early DIC. The presence of these fragments indicates that there is accelerated plasmin-induced breakdown of the fibrin clot. The euglobulin clot lysis test may be normal due to depletion of plasminogen.

When DIC occurs, it must be treated as a medical emergency. There may be acute hemorrhage where there is generalized bleeding and oozing from venipuncture sites. Because it occurs secondary to another disorder, the most important aspect of therapy is to treat the primary disorder. To halt the intravascular clotting mechanism, heparin is generally given. Replacement therapy using platelets and/or fresh frozen plasma (for coagulation factors) may sometimes be administered if necessary. If the patient is in shock, this must be treated immediately. Whole blood or packed red blood cells are given when indicated.

Fibrinolysis

Fibrinolysis, without intravascular coagulation, is found as a complication of severe liver disease, as a complication following cardiopulmonary bypass surgery, in metastatic prostate carcinoma and some leukemias, and as a complication of thrombolytic therapy. Generally, bleeding is rare in these patients. However, when it does occur it can be severe and may be fatal.

Fibrinolysis results when excess amounts of plasminogen activators convert plasminogen to plasmin within the circulation. Plasminogen activators may be derived from various tissues, secretions, or the vascular endothelium. The contact factors, XII, Fletcher, and Fitzgerald, are also capable of activating plasminogen. Plasmin digests factors V and VIII and, in addition, breaks down fibrin and fibrinogen to fibrin(ogen) degradation products.

The PT, APTT, and thrombin time are generally prolonged because of the anticoagulant effect of the fibrin(ogen) degradation products and because of decreased amounts of fibrinogen. The euglobulin clot lysis time is abnormally short, unless there is depletion of plasminogen. Factors V and VIII are generally decreased. Factor XIII may also be decreased in some patients. However, in contrast to DIC, the platelet count and the d-dimer test are normal.

Treatment for fibrinolysis usually involves administration of an agent, such as EACA (epsilon aminocaproic acid), which will inhibit the activation of plasminogen.

Hypercoagulable States

Several conditions are associated with an increased tendency to develop thrombosis (formation of intravascular clots). Collectively, they are referred to as hypercoagulable or prethrombotic states and represent changes in the regulatory mechanisms of the coagulation and fibrinolytic systems. This condition may be divided into two categories: (1) primary disorders, in which there is a qualitative or quantitative abnormality of a specific anticoagulant or inhibitor of the hemostatic system and (2) secondary disorders, in which the mechanism of the clot formation is not completely known.

Primary disorders are relatively uncommon and include hereditary deficiencies of antithrombin III and of proteins S and C, as well as abnormalities of plasminogen, plasminogen activators and fibrinogen. The most common of the secondary disorders are stasis (inhibition) of blood flow from vascular disorders, malignant tumors, the postoperative state, pregnancy, and the use of oral contraceptives.

Deficiencies of antithrombin III, protein C, and protein S have an autosomal dominant inheritance pattern. Most patients are heterozygous with levels of 25 to 60% of normal. The homozygous condition is rare and life-threatening, with levels often less than 1%. Two types of *antithrombin III deficiency* exist. In type I, there is reduced synthesis of antithrombin III, whereas in the type II deficiency, antithrombin III quantitative levels are normal, although it is qualitatively (functionally) abnormal. *Protein C deficiency* also exists as type I and type II. In the homozygous condition, newborn infants develop purpura fulminans with resultant cutaneous gangrene from thrombotic occlusion of blood vessels. Deep veins may also be occluded with thrombi, resulting in a critical situation and often death. *Protein S deficiency,* type I individuals have decreased levels of free and total protein S. In type II, total protein S is normal, but levels of free protein S are decreased.

Laboratory evaluation of these patients often shows non-specific elevations of factors V, VII, VIII, and fibrinogen. Elevated levels of fibrin split products and platelet products (beta thromboglobulin, thromboxane B_2 and platelet factor 4) may also be found. In addition, there are increased levels of prothrombin fragments 1 and 2, and fibrinopeptides A and B. Assays for antithrombin III, proteins C and S, and certain components of the fibrinolytic system may reveal abnormalities which indicate a specific primary disorder.

Patients with primary hypercoagulable disorders usually display early onset of thrombotic episodes, have a positive family history of thromboembolism, and do not have any underlying disease. Treatment of these patients is difficult and some may require life long oral anticoagulant therapy. Recurrent deep venous thrombosis in the lower extremities and pulmonary emboli are common and are treated acutely with intravenous heparin.

AUTOMATION

CELL COUNTERS

Sysmex™ E-5000

The TOA Sysmex™ E-5000 series instrument (TOA Medical Electronics Co., Ltd.) analyzes the blood specimen and reports a complete blood count, red blood cell indices, RDW, platelet count, MPV (mean platelet volume), PDW (variation in platelet size), PLCR (platelet large cell ratio, indicates platelet size above 12 μm), and nucleated cells according to size: (1) white small cell ratio (WSCR) and small cell count (WSCC) (normally, lymphocytes), (2) white mixed cell ratio (WMCR) and mixed cell count (WMCC) (normally, monocytes, basophils, and eosinophils), and (3) white large cell ratio (WLCR) and large cell count (WLCC) (normally, neutrophils and bands).

The E-5000 is composed of six separate units. (See Fig. 7–1.) The blood sample is identified, aspirated, diluted, and analyzed by the *main unit*. The *sampler unit* attaches to the front of the main unit and is used to hold and feed samples to the instrument when in the automatic mode. The *data processing unit* (DPU) receives data from the main unit, performs calculations, develops histograms, and displays sample results and error and status messages via the video display. It contains a bubble memory and special functions through which the operator may view results, manipulate discriminators and data, and transmit test data. The *pneumatic unit* supplies the vacuum and pressures to the main unit for operating the valves and pistons, which move the air and fluids through chambers and tubing. The *data printer* receives information from the data processing unit and prints this data on manually inserted report cards. The *serial matrix printer* will automatically print the sample number, date, error codes, flags, histograms, and numerical results or may be used as a line printer.

Aspiration and Dilution of Test Sample

When the *power switch* on the main unit is first pressed to the on position the unit will enter an auto rinse mode in which the instrument is rinsed three to five times, waste is drained, background counts are reviewed, and the electronics, injector piston motors, ROM, RAM, bubble memory, and instrument status are automatically checked. (An *auto rinse switch* is available to the operator for a background check whenever desired.) To operate in the manual mode place the specimen under the *whole blood aspiration tube* and press the *start switch* to aspirate the sample and begin testing. To aspirate a sample in the automatic mode place the bar code labeled tubes in the rack, and place in the right side of the sampler unit. Press the *sampler switch*. (The *sampler operation panel* on the main unit will indicate the status: ready, running, or interrupt.) The rack is automatically forwarded to the *measurement line* where it will be moved to the left, one sample tube distance at a time. The *ID read mechanism* reads the bar code on the first tube and then shifts the rack one space to the left. The bar code is read on the next tube whereas the sample volume is checked on the first tube by the *blood volume sensor*. If the volume is adequate (0.5 to 3.0 mL in a 12 mm test tube, or 0.7 to 5.0 mL in a 16 mm test tube), the *mixer* is lowered into the first tube, where it rotates to mix the

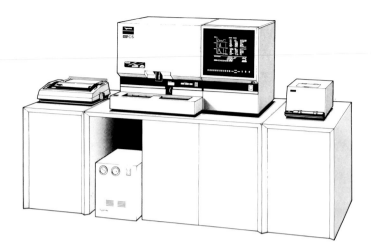

FIG. 7–1. Sysmex™ E-5000. (Courtesy of TOA Medical Electronics Co., Ltd.)

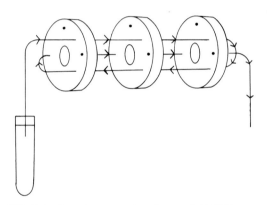

FIG. 7–2. Sample rotor valve, Sysmex™ E-5000.

sample. If the sample volume is insufficient, testing will not be performed on the specimen. After the first sample has been mixed, the rack moves one position to the left. The sample processing continues and the bar code is read on the next sample (#3), the mixer and aspirator are lowered into tubes #2 and #1, where they are mixed and aspirated respectively at a rate of one sample aspiration every 30 seconds. The specimen (0.2 mL) is pulled through the *sample rotor valve* (SRV). There are two *sensors* located along the aspiration tubing (one in front and one behind the SRV) that monitor the presence of the sample as it enters and leaves the SRV for the detection of a problem (e.g., short sample, air bubbles, clots), in which case, an error code is displayed on the DPU. The SRV is composed of three sections (Fig. 7–2): front, back and center (rotating) pieces. Each of the sections

has six connecting holes. As blood is drawn up through the aspiration line it passes through the front sensor, travels into the SRV, out the back, in again through a second port (hole), out the front, and back into the valve through a third port in the front, out again at the back of the valve and through the back sensor. The center section of the SRV then rotates in such a manner that the three ports in the valve that contain sample (in amounts of 2.67 μL, 6 μL, and 12 μL) are lined up with the three empty ports on the outer sections of the SRV.

Cellpak™ diluent (1.988 mL) is dispensed through the port in the SRV where it picks up the 12 μL sample and carries it through the tubing to the *WBC transducer chamber*. Lysing reagent (1 mL) is dispensed into the WBC chamber, giving a final dilution of 1:250. The WBC lyse reagent lyses red cells, shrinks platelets, and pierces the white cell cytoplasmic membranes, leaving only cell nuclei to be counted and sized.

While the blood is diluted for the WBC, 2.0 mL of diluent is dispensed through the SRV where it picks up the 2.67 μL aliquot of sample. This diluted sample then travels to the *RBC sample chamber* for mixing (1:750 dilution). A segment of the 1:750 dilution is later injected into the sheath detector for sample analysis.

Concurrently, the hemoglobin is diluted: 1.994 mL of diluent is dispensed through the SRV where it picks up the 6 μL blood sample on its way to the *hgb flow cell*. At the same time, 1 mL of hgb lyse reagent is added to the diluted sample in the flow cell (dilution of 1:500).

Sample Testing

Each sample cycle takes approximately 53 seconds. However, samples may be introduced into the instrument at 30 second intervals. Thus, in the automatic mode, the instrument can analyze 119 samples per hour.

WBC and three part differential. The *WBC detector unit* contains a nonmercury manometer and is responsible for starting and stopping the WBC count cycle. The top portion of the manometer is connected to the *transducer* in the WBC transducer chamber (containing the diluted WBC sample). The manometer is filled with Cellpak diluent and contains a ball float. On either side of and near the top of the manometer, the start detector is located. There is a similar detector located near the bottom of the manometer. During the count, a vacuum is applied to the bottom end of the manometer. The diluted sample is drawn through the aperture (diameter of 100 μm) in the transducer. At the same time, the ball float falls downward in the manometer. As the ball passes the start detector the count cycle begins. Counting continues until the ball passes the bottom detector, which stops the counting cycle. During the count cycle of 5 to 6 seconds, 0.25 mL of diluted sample is drawn into the transducer through the aperture. There is an electric current passing between the internal electrode in the transducer and the external electrode in the transducer chamber. As each nucleus travels through the aperture, it causes a change in voltage. The size of the voltage change is directly proportional to the volume of the nucleus. During the counting cycle, the count time is monitored, and the count is checked for consistency and recorded every ½ second. These ½ second counts may be displayed on the video screen if desired. If the counts do not agree with each other within pre-set limits an error code will be given. The white cell nuclei are sorted by size, and a distribution curve (histogram) is displayed along with results produced by the DPU. Floating thresholds are used rather than fixed thresholds. For the white count the lower threshold will be set between 30 and 60 fL depending on the

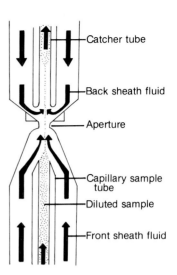

FIG. 7–3. RBC sample flow, Sysmex™ E.5000.

size range of the specimen's cells. At the completion of the count cycle, the white count is corrected for dilution, volume, and coincidence. The histogram is derived, thresholds set, and the number and percentage of each size of white cell is determined.

The *RBC and platelet count* are performed using *hydrodynamic focusing*. Part of the 1:750 red cell dilution (11.7 μL) in the RBC sample chamber is withdrawn and forced up into and through the capillary *sample tube* (Fig. 7–3) in the *RBC detector unit*. As the diluted sample is forced through the sample tube, it is directed at the orifice (diameter of 76 μm). Cellsheath flows (under pressure) toward, and through, the orifice, surrounding the diluted sample, and restricts the sample flow diameter to 10 μL as it passes through the detecting aperture. This causes the particles in the sample to flow in single file through the center of the aperture. As the sample passes through the aperture, it is met by the back sheath fluid, which quickly carries the sample away from the back of the aperture to waste. Because the particles pass through the center of the orifice there should be no distortion of particle size. There is virtually no coincidence error because the cells pass through the aperture and are counted one at a time unless the count is too high (above the upper linearity), on which occasion an alarm will alert the operator. The back sheath flow forces particles away from the aperture as soon as they flow through, thus virtually preventing platelet count errors associated with recirculation. As the particles pass through the orifice they are counted in the same manner as the white cells (by electrical resistance), and their size (volume) is also measured. The red cell count is monitored and checked approximately once per second. Each of these 1 second counts must agree within preset limits in order for the final count to be considered valid by the computer. During the count cycle a red ball in the *sheath fluid flow meter* will descend to monitor the sheath flow. If this ball falls too quickly, it may indicate a clog in the orifice, and an error message will be given. A histogram (distribution curve) is obtained for both the red cells and platelets. Again, floating thresholds are used and are determined for each individual sample based on the particular histogram. The thresholds for the RBC are between 25 and 75 fL at the lower level and between 200 and 250 at the upper level. The platelet threshold is between 2 and 6 fL at the lower end and between 12 and 30 fL at the upper end.

Hematocrit measurement. As the red cells are being counted their size is also determined. This information is digitized. When the red cell histogram is obtained, the upper and lower thresholds are determined and all of the digitized data between these two points are added up and multiplied by a constant factor (accounting for dilution, volume, and calibration) to produce the red blood cell mass in 1 μL of whole blood. This number is then converted to percent for the final hematocrit result.

Hemoglobin measurement. Immediately prior to the preparation of the hemoglobin dilution, rinse diluent from the previous cycle is drained from the hgb flow cell and 2 mL of fresh diluent is dispensed into the chamber. A reading of the absorbance is taken (represents the hemoglobin blank reading). The diluent is drained and a reading is then taken of the empty cuvet, to monitor the mechanical performance of the flow through the cuvet. The hemoglobin dilution is delivered to the hgb flow cell (which also serves as a cuvet). The hemoglobin lyse reagent (1.0 mL) is added to the cuvet. A total of five absorbance readings are taken. The unit will use the

reading that is lowest (the one most likely to be clear and free of bubbles). The blank reading is subtracted from the sample reading for the final hemoglobin result.

The *WBC* and *RBC clog removal switches* may be used for removing a clog from the red or white cell apertures when necessary. There is a *reagent heater* in the main unit that warms the diluent and sheath reagent to preset temperatures prior to use. During the count and testing cycle, if the instrument monitoring system detects an error, the operator will be notified by way of an audible beep and message on the DPU's video display. The ability of the instrument to utilize a floating lower threshold (discriminator) for each patient sample is thought to improve its counting accuracy. The various chambers and flow lines are rinsed during each sample cycle.

Calculated Parameters

The *red blood cell indices* (MCV, MCH, and MCHC) are calculated by the DPU. The *RDW-SD*, a measure of anisocytosis, is the width, in femtoliters (fL), of the red cell distribution curve at a point 20% above the base line. If an abnormal histogram is obtained, an error message is given. The *RDW-CV* is determined by dividing the RDW-SD by the red cell MCV and multiplying the result by a constant factor.

The *WBC size distribution* is determined using the lower floating threshold (or discriminator) set in the range between 30 and 60 fL and the upper threshold set at 300 fL. When the white cell histogram is constructed, two low points (valleys or troughs) within the WBC curve are normally present. The *WBC small cell population* consists of those white cells that fall between the lower threshold and the first trough, and are normally the lymphocytes. Nucleated red blood cells in low numbers will generally fall below the area of the lower threshold but, if present in large numbers, will fall into the WBC population and cause an abnormal curve. The *WBC mixed cell population* consists of those cells that fall between the two troughs within the WBC curve. These cells are considered to be the monocytes, basophils, and eosinophils. The *WBC large cell population* falls between the second (higher) trough and the upper threshold, and are normally the neutrophils. Any time one of the thresholds, or troughs, is not discernible, the instrument will recognize the problem, inform the operator via an error message, and allow the operator to manually set the discriminators (troughs) in order to obtain results. (Caution: This setting should not be made without valid reason.)

The *mean platelet volume* (MPV) is calculated for each sample (plt hct/plt count). The *platelet distribution width* (PDW) is calculated in a manner similar to the RDW-SD. The *platelet large cell ratio* (PLCR) is an indicator of the percentage of platelets larger than 12 fL and is calculated by dividing the number of platelets between the fixed threshold (12 fL) and the upper threshold, by the number of platelets that fall between the lower and upper threshold.

Video Display Screen

The video display screen is divided into five areas separated by lines. (1) The upper screen displays the 18 parameter data and histograms from the last sample analyzed. This area also displays information related to other programs, such as Q.C., stored data, and calibration data according to the menu chosen. (2) The *system area*, located at the bottom line of area 1, displays the numerical entries as well as messages to assist or direct the operator. (3) The *system status area* (bottom right) displays the current date and time, sample identification number for both manual and auto mode, sample number to be transmitted to the data printer, main unit status, bubble memory activity (including the number of samples in stored data), auto erase selection, XM quality control selection, host computer activity, and printer selection. (4) The *system message line* below area 2 provides priority messages relating to the main unit. (5) The eight program *Select Menus* and their subprograms (bottom center and left) allow the operator increased flexibility in operation, data review, data output, quality control assessment, and instrument function. A program and its subprograms are selected by pressing the corresponding numeric key. Programs that contain important data or system settings may require a password for entry. Following is a brief description of the Select Menu programs. *Auto Out* allows operator control of the automatic output of data to

printers and host computer. *Command* program allows operator to review data from the 20 cycles, print STATS, start and stop the XM Q.C. program, access service data, and set ID numbers. *Stored Data* program allows the operator to display, sort, erase, manually discriminate histograms, correct ID numbers, and output data, and also allows access to Q.C. charts and set number. The *Quality Control* program has 10 QC files including the XM program available for storing up to 60 data points for up to 12 user-defined parameters. Features of this program are Levy Jennings graphs, modified Bull's moving average, statistical analysis, calibration history, output of control data and graphs to host computer and printers, and a choice for assaying commercial controls singly or in duplicate. The *Set Number* program is used for setting the sample ID number and tube position. The *Settings* program allows the operator to enter user defined information into the unit. The *Calibration of Hgb/Hct* program allows the operator to calibrate the hemoglobin and hematocrit. The *Service* program contains various tests to check proper operation of the unit for troubleshooting and maintenance.

Reagents

The instrument's *reagent system* is composed of five reagents for testing and cleaning. During each sample cycle *Cellpack* (24 mL) is used for diluting the sample, *Cellsheath* (10 mL) forms a sheath around the RBC dilution (during count phase), STROMATOLYZER-3WP™ (lyse reagent) (1 mL) is added to the WBC dilution, and STROMATOLYZER-C™ (hemoglobin lyse reagent) (1 ml) is added to the hemoglobin dilution. Weekly, *Manoresh* (10 mL) is used to clean the WBC manometer, and daily, 20% Clorox (1 mL) is aspirated through the unit for cleaning. Because of dilution and the characteristics of the Stromatolyzer-C reagent, white counts up to $100,000/\mu L$ do not interfere with the hemoglobin reading.

Sysmex NE-8000

The Sysmex NE-8000 is a 23-parameter closed sampling automated hematology analyzer manufactured by TOA Medical Electronics Co., Ltd. Similar to the Sysmex E-5000, it performs a complete blood count;

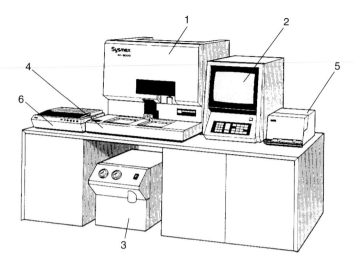

FIG. 7–4. Sysmex NE-8000. (Courtesy of TOA Medical Electronics Co., Ltd.)

calculates red blood cell indices and RDW; performs a platelet count; and calculates an MPV (mean platelet volume), PDW (platelet distribution width), and P-LCR (platelet large cell ratio, a measure of platelets larger than 12 microns). A five-part white blood cell differential includes the percentages and absolute numbers of neutrophils, lymphocytes, monocytes, eosinophils, and basophils. The NE-8000 is capable of testing 120 samples per hour.

The NE-8000 consists of three standard units (Fig. 7–4): The *main unit* (1), *data processing unit* (2), and *pneumatic unit* (3). Optional components are the *sampler unit* (4), *data printer* (5), and *graphic/line printer* (6).

The main unit mixes, aspirates, dilutes, and then counts, measures, and/or computes each parameter. This information is received, displayed, and stored by the data processing unit (DPU). The DPU stores numerical data for up to 500 samples. It also supplies power to the main unit. The pneumatic unit supplies pressures and vacuums to the main unit. Once loaded, the sampler, which holds up to 100 tubes (10 racks of 10 tubes each), feeds the sample tubes to the main unit for automatic mixing and aspiration. The data printer is a ticket-style printer that will give a hard copy of numerical data for each sample. The graphic/line printer prints histograms, scattergrams, numerical data, and flagging information, featuring one sample per page. When the printer is set to line print, a hard copy of numerical results may be printed.

The NE-8000 is designed to mix and aspirate whole blood samples in the automatic, closed-tube sampling mode. As an alternative, samples may be hand mixed and aspirated in the manual, open-tube sampling mode, or prediluted samples (1:5) may be hand mixed and aspirated in the capillary mode. Samples prediluted 1:5 are analyzed and automatically corrected for the dilution factor.

Sample Aspiration

Barcode labeled samples (with tops on) are placed in a rack on the right side of the *sampler tray* (in the sampler unit). Analysis in the automatic mode is begun by pressing the *sample switch* on the sampler unit. The rack is forwarded to the measurement line where it is automatically shifted to the left one sample at a time. A sensor detects the presence of the tube in the rack. The ID read mechanism reads the bar code on the first tube then the rack is shifted one space to the left. A second sensor checks for sufficient sample volume. If adequate (minimum of 1 mL is required), the first mixer hand moves forward, grasps the tube, and lifts and mixes it by inversion five times. (Tubes with an outer diameter ranging from 12 mm to 15 mm may be used.) If less than 1 mL is present, the sample will not be mixed or aspirated. An alarm will sound to indicate that an analysis error has occurred for that sample. The DPU will display a message: "analysis error—low blood volume." After the first tube is mixed, it is returned to the sample rack, the bar code is read on the second tube, and the rack is shifted one further space to the left. The first

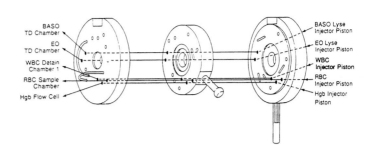

FIG. 7–5. Sample rotor valve, Sysmex NE-8000. (Courtesy of TOA Medical Electronics Co., Ltd.)

and second tubes are then grasped, lifted, and mixed by the second and first mixer hands respectively. The tubes are returned to the sample rack, the bar code is read on the third tube, and the rack is shifted one space to the left. The first tube is grasped by the transfer hand (third hand), which lifts, inverts, and carries it to the cap piercer, located behind the front panel. The sample (approximately 200 μL) is aspirated and diluted while the second and third tubes are grasped, lifted and mixed by the second and first mixer hands, respectively. Each tube is inverted (mixed) a total of 10 times. The transfer hand places the first tube upright and returns it to the rack, while the mixer hands return the second and third tubes to the rack. The bar code is read on the next tube and the rack shifts one position to the left. The process described above continues until each tube in the rack has been mixed and aspirated. The next rack is then moved into place and the above procedure repeated.

Manual sample aspiration is accomplished by placing the specimen under the *whole blood aspiration tube* and pressing the *start switch*, whereas diluted samples are aspirated in the same manner after setting the DPU in the Cap Mode. Approximately 125 μL of sample is aspirated in each mode.

Sample Dilution

The specimen (125 or 200 μL, depending on aspiration method) is drawn up through the sample rotor valve (SRV) (Fig. 7–5). (There are two *sensors* located along the aspiration tubing [one in front of the SRV and one behind] that monitor the presence of the sample as it enters and leaves the SRV, for the detection of the blood sample. The absence of sample at either sensor indicates a short sample, clot, air bubbles, and other problems, in which case an error code is displayed on the DPU.) The SRV is composed of fixed front and back sections and a center section that rotates. Clockwise and counterclockwise rotation of the center section allows ports in this section to be aligned with various ports on the outer sections, depending on the position of the center piece. As the specimen is aspirated, it flows through the SRV, out the back, in again through another port, out the front, and back in again until five of the ports in the center section contain specimen. Each of these holes (center section) is calibrated to contain a specified amount of sample. The center section will then rotate and line up with open ports in the fixed front and back sections, through which diluent will be forced. As reagent flows through the SRV, it picks up the sample and travels out of the SRV to its respective chamber for mixing and subsequent testing as described below. The sample is diluted in this manner.

WBC. Cell Pack Gl diluent is dispensed through the appropriate port in the SRV where it picks up the 12 μL sample (in the center section of the SRV) and carries it through the tubing to the first of two temperature regulated chambers, called *detain chambers*. In the first chamber, the white blood cells are stabilized by the Cell Pack Gl prior to their reaction with 1 mL of WBC Lyse reagent (Stromatolyser-Gl) in the second chamber. The reaction with Stromatolyser-Gl gently shrinks the white cells so that they are decreased in overall size and cellular density. Stromatolyser-Gl lyses the red blood cells. The final WBC sample dilution of 1:250 is transferred from the second WBC detain chamber into the *WBC transducer chamber*, where the white blood cells are counted.

Eosinophil count. In the same manner as described for the WBC above, 12 μL of blood in the SRV is picked up and diluted 1:250 by Eo reagent (Stromatolyser-Eo). This reagent uses an alkaline surfactant (surface tension reducer) (sodium hydroxide) to lyse and eliminate red blood cells and those white blood cells which are not eosinophils. The diluted sample is transferred directly through the SRV to the *Eo transducer chamber*, where the eosinophils are counted.

Basophil count. Stromatolyser-Ba is dispensed through the SRV and picks up the 24 μL sample (1:125 dilution) and carries it to the *baso transducer chamber*. The baso reagent is an acid surfactant (hydrochloric acid) that lyses the red blood cells and all of the white blood cells with the exception of basophils.

RBC/Platelet counts. Cell Pack diluent picks up 4 μL of blood in the SRV, making a 1:500 dilution, and moves to the *RBC sample chamber*.

Hemoglobin. The SRV measures 6 μL of blood, which is diluted with 1.994 mL of Cell Pack as it travels to the *hemoglobin flow cell*. Here 1 mL of hemoglobin lyse reagent (Stromatolyser-C) is added making a final dilution of 1:500.

Sample Testing

The *WBC, Eo,* and *Baso detector units* each use a nonmercury volumetric *manometer*, which is responsible for starting and stopping the count cycle. The functioning of these manometer systems is the same as that described for the Sysmex E-5000. Each manometer is filled with its respective diluent and contains a ball float. On either side of the manometer, near the top and bottom respectively, are the start and stop detectors. During the counts, vacuum is applied to the bottom of each manometer. The diluted sample is drawn through the aperture (diameter of 90 μm for WBC, 100 μm for eo., 100 μm for baso) in the transducer. At the same time, the ball float falls downward in the manometer. As the ball passes the start detector, the count cycle begins. Counting continues until the ball passes the bottom detector, which stops the counting cycle. During the count cycle (approximately 7 seconds for WBC and 5.5 seconds for both eosinophil and basophil

counts), 0.25 mL of diluted sample is drawn into the transducer through the aperture.

The *RBC and platelet counts* are performed using hydrodynamic focusing. Diluted sample (11.7 μL) in the *RBC sample chamber* is forced up into the hydraulic line of the *RBC detector unit* and injected through the *sample tube* by the *sheath flow injector piston* (see Fig. 7–3). The sample tube is mounted in front of the *aperture* and directed at its center. As sample passes from the sample tube to the aperture, front sheath reagent surrounds the diluted sample, thus restricting the sample flow diameter to 10 μL as it passes through the aperture. This causes the particles in the sample to flow in single file through the center of the aperture. After the sample has passed through the aperture, back sheath reagent directs it into the catcher tube. The action of the back sheath fluid prevents recirculation of the sample through the flow cell.

The *WBC, eosinophil, basophil, RBC,* and *platelet counts* are determined by the aperture impedence method using direct current (DC). This method of sizing and counting cells employs an internal electrode in the transducer and an external electrode in the transducer chamber. As a cell passes through the aperture, it causes a voltage change, which is directly proportional to its size. The white blood count (including granulocytes, lymphocytes, and monocytes) also employs radio frequency (RF). Using this method, the internal and external electrodes of the WBC detector unit have an added high frequency current flowing between them. Whereas the DC detection method determines overall cell volume, the RF method provides information on cellular density and intracellular composition.

The *hematocrit* is measured electronically, based on the principle that pulse height (voltage change) produced by cells passing through the aperture of the RBC detector unit is proportional to cell volume. Electrical information from the RBC count is digitized, and a distribution curve (histogram) is then obtained. Floating thresholds are determined between 25 and 75 fL at the lower end, and between 200 and 250 fL at the upper end. The hematocrit is computed by integrating (combining) the pulses between the two threshold levels, multiplying by a constant factor (accounting for dilution, volume, and calibration), and expressing the result as the ratio of the total RBC volume to whole blood. This ratio is expressed as a percentage (%).

The *hemoglobin* is measured by a variation of the internationally standardized cyanmethemoglobin method. When the hemoglobin measurement cycle begins, diluent is drained from the flow cell and fresh diluent is dispensed into the flow cell. An absorbance measurement (hemoglobin blank) is taken on this diluent and the flow cell is drained again. The diluted sample (6 µL of blood + 1.994 mL of Cell Pack) enters the flow cell, along with 1 mL of hemoglobin lyse reagent (final dilution of 1:500). Air bubbles are injected into the flow cell to mix the sample. An absorbance measurement is taken on the sample. The final hemoglobin is determined by subtracting the blank measurement from the sample measurement.

The *red blood cell indices* (MCV, MCH, and MCHC) are calculated from the red blood cell count, hemoglobin, and hematocrit values. Analysis of the RBC histogram determines the RDW values. The RDW-SD is the width (in femtoliters) of the red cell distribution curve at a point 20% above the baseline. The RDW-CV is determined by dividing the RDW-SD by the red cell MCV and multiplying the result by a constant factor.

Histograms of the RBC, platelet, eosinophil, and basophil populations are constructed from direct current and relative frequency data (numbers present). Using floating discriminators, the upper and lower size thresholds are set for each cell type and the histograms are plotted, using both cell numbers and size determinations.

A three dimensional plot (Fig. 7–6) is formed by graphing direct current (DC), radio frequency (RF), and relative frequency (particle numbers) data. Viewing this figure from the top, the *WBC scattergram* (Fig. 7–7) is obtained, on which floating discriminators (a total of eight) are placed at optimum locations for the separation of particles. The main discriminator line is placed at a 45° angle to separate RBC ghosts and extraneous pulses. Seven additional discriminators are placed to separate and identify the lymphocytes, monocytes, and granulocytes. The tri-modal histogram (three peak plot) (Fig. 7–8) is derived by viewing the three dimensional plot from the front and uses both the direct current and

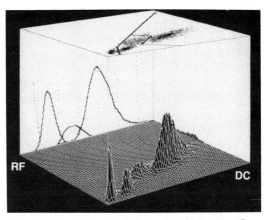

FIG. 7–6. Normal sample isometric histogram, Sysmex NE-8000. (Courtesy of TOA Medical Electronics Co., Ltd.)

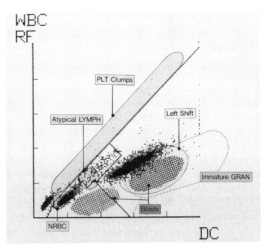

FIG. 7–7. WBC scattergram showing normal WBC scatter (also see top of isometric histogram, Fig. 7–6) and location of abnormal WBC and platelets, Sysmex NE-8000. (Courtesy of TOA Medical Electronics Co., Ltd.)

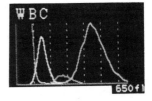

FIG. 7–8. Tri-modal histogram, Sysmex NE-8000. (Courtesy of TOA Medical Electronics Co., Ltd.)

relative frequency data (cell numbers) information. The microcomputer analyzes this histogram plot from 0 to 650 fL and locates troughs (places floating discriminators) between each of the peaks. These troughs represent points of separation between the lymphocyte, monocyte, and granulocyte populations.

The *neutrophil count* is computed by subtracting the eosinophil count and basophil count from the granulocyte count (as determined from the WBC scattergram analysis). Cell percentages for the five part differential are computed from the absolute number of each cell type and the total white blood cell count.

A final report showing all numerical data, scattergram, histograms, and flagging information may be printed for each sample tested using no additional work time.

Discussion

The DPU, in addition to both displaying and storing data, screens the numerical, histogram, and scattergram data and may assign an abnormal or *suspect flag*. These flags suggest, but do not define, cell types or abnormalities that may be present in the sample. Flagging information is an indication to the technologist that the sample requires further investigation before a final report is given. Flags may be grouped as WBC, RBC, or Platelet. WBC flags include the following: Increased and/or decreased cell types (such as neutropenia or neutrophilia), the limits of which are set by the individual laboratory, factory-set flags for WBC abnormal distribution (abnormal histogram), blasts, immature granulocytes, left shift, atypical lymphs, and NRBCs. RBC flags include laboratory set messages indicating anisocytosis, microcytes, macrocytes, hypochromia, anemia, and erythrocytosis. The factory set RBC flags include a dimorphic population, RBC agglutination, turbidity/hemoglobin interference, iron deficiency, hemoglobin defect, fragments, and RBC abnormal distribution (abnormal histogram). Each laboratory may set platelet flags for thrombocytopenia and thrombocytosis. The factory-set flags include those for large platelet, small platelet, platelet clumps, mi-

crocytic RBC/platelet interference, and abnormal platelet distribution (abnormal histogram). All flagged reports will have the message "Positive" printed on the graphic printout. The message "Negative" will appear when no flagging occurs.

Additional features of the DPU include (1) Storage of numerical, histogram and flagging information for up to 500 samples; (2) Seven operator-assigned, quality control files and an XM control file, each capable of storing up to 60 data points; (3) Auto output of data to peripheral printers and to a host computer; (4) A settings program to set operator defined limits and host computer hardware configuration; (5) A Hgb/Hct calibration program that allows for automatic or manual calculation of calibration values; (6) A service program, which may be used to confirm that the instrument is operating properly or to assist the operator in finding the cause of abnormalities detected in the instrument; (7) A display of system status (Ready/Not ready) and analysis, microcomputer, and ID read error messages to alert the operator to problems encountered during the testing sequence.

A new hemoglobin reagent, Sulfolyser, has been introduced by TOA Medical Electronics Co., LTD for use on its cell counters. Sulfolyser is a cyanide-free hemoglobin reagent containing sodium lauryl sulfate, a negatively charged surfactant (lowers surface tension) that has an affinity for binding protein (via its alkyl group, $C_{12}H_{25}^-$). The sodium lauryl sulfate breaks down the red blood cell membrane, freeing hemoglobin. The globin portion of the molecule becomes bound to the alkyl group ($C_{12}H_{25}^-$), which causes a change in the arrangement of the globin chain and resultant oxidation of the iron from the ferrous ($+2$) to the ferric ($+3$) state, to produce methemoglobin (hemiglobin [Hi]). The formed hemiglobin binds to the sulfate group (OSO_3^-) of the sodium lauryl sulfate to form sodium lauryl sulfate hemoglobin, which has a wide absorption peak with maximum absorbance at 535 nm. The Sulfolyser reagent hemolyzes red blood cells rapidly, and the above reactions occur very quickly. Linearity and precision studies have shown the reagent to give similar results to those obtained by the cyanmethemoglobin method (Pearson, Houwen, Mast).

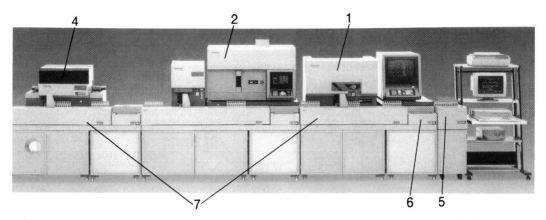

FIG. 7–9. Sysmex Total Hematology System (HS). (Courtesy of TOA Medical Electronics Co., Ltd.)

Sysmex Total Hematology System (HS)

The Sysmex Total Hematology System (HS) (Fig. 7–9), manufactured by TOA Medical Electronics Co, Ltd., is a combination of various hematology instruments connected by a conveyor belt and designed to perform the following procedures via automated closed sampling: CBC, RBC indices, RDW, platelet count, five part differential, reticulocyte count, preparation of a wedge blood smear, and identification of the bar coded patient specimen.

System Components

The *line controller unit* coordinates testing by the HS components. It directs the bar coded samples to be analyzed or bypassed at each unit.

The *Sysmex NE-8000* (1) is a 23 parameter hematology analyzer that performs a CBC, RBC indices, RDW, platelet count, and five part differential. This instrument has been described in more detail previously in this chapter.

The *R-series reticulocyte counter* (2) is described further on in this chapter.

The *Smear Preparation (SP) unit* (4) uses robotics to produce wedge type blood smears on glass slides. This unit contains a bar code reader for sample identification. It mixes samples and aspirates the specimen using a cap piercing mechanism. The hematocrit reading (information provided by the NE-8000 for each individual sample) determines the amount of blood (5 to 10 µL) used for the smear, the angle of the spreader blade, and the speed at which the blood is pulled along the slide by the SP unit. In this manner, relatively uniform wedge-type blood smears are prepared and then dried by a cool air fan. A specimen ID number (read from the bar coded sample tube) is stamped on the slide by the SP unit, and the slide is then placed into a cassette for storage in the SP unit.

Each of the above units is serviced by a specially designed *conveyer belt sample transport system* (7). This mechanism replaces the rack sampler unit of the NE-8000 and R-3000. It consists of two belt-type conveyors placed parallel to each other and attached to the front of each of the instruments. The inner belt next to the instruments carries the sample racks to the testing stations. The outer belt allows the racks to bypass the instrument. The inner conveyor belt contains a tube rotator prior to the test station, which assists in locating the bar code if the label is not facing the instrument. A *rack slider unit* (6) is located before each instrument and attached to the conveyor belt transport system (connects conveyor belts). This mechanism allows a rack to skip the next instrument if no testing is required for any sample. The sample racks are moved between the two conveyor belts by this mechanism. The *starting pool unit* (5) is attached to the conveyor belt system via the rack slider unit, at the beginning of the HS. It holds up to 20 sample racks and is the point of entry into the HS for testing. The *finish pool unit* is attached to the end of the conveyor belt and is the final destination area for the specimen racks at the conclusion of testing. It will hold a maximum of 20 racks (10 tubes per rack).

The *Data Entry Unit* (or an IBM personal computer with appropriate software) allows the operator to create a worklist for the system, and instructs each unit to process or skip the test specimens. This unit is not necessary for operation of the HS. A laboratory host computer will also allow input of the necessary test selection information.

System Operation

Work flow begins with test selection, which may be performed manually via the data entry units keyboard or by downloading from a host computer to the line controller unit. Selections may include any combination of complete blood count with differential, reticulocyte count, and/or blood smear preparation. A maximum of 10,000 samples may be registered in the line controller. A list of samples, tests selected, and the current status of each sample registered may be displayed on the data entry monitor, or it may be printed by a data entry unit printer. Sample analysis begins when loaded sample racks are placed in the starting pool unit and the start switch is pressed. The first sample rack is moved into the rack slider unit. If a CBC, differential, or platelet count is ordered on any one of the specimens, the rack is moved onto the inner conveyor belt and forwarded to the testing station of the NE-8000. A bar code reader scans the bar code for sample identification. The CBC, WBC differential, and platelet count are performed. When all testing is completed for that specimen rack, it is forwarded to the rack slider unit by the conveyor belt. If there are no reticulocyte counts ordered on any specimen in the rack, it is moved to the outer conveyer belt, where it is carried to the next rack slider unit. It is now moved to the inner conveyor belt if smears are to be prepared on any of the specimens. "Positive" samples (those flagged by the NE-8000 for an abnormality) are automatically forwarded to the SP unit even if a smear was not originally selected on the data entry unit/line controller. (This is referred to as *reflexive testing*.) If a reticulocyte count was ordered on one or more of the specimens, at

the completion of NE-8000 testing the rack would remain on the inner conveyor as it passed through the rack slider unit. The R-3000 analyzer would read the barcode, mix the sample(s), and perform the reticulocyte count(s). The sample rack would proceed to the next rack slider unit as described above. When all required testing is complete, the specimen racks are moved into the finish pool unit, where they may be removed by the operator.

Discussion

The HS allows for continuous operation of the system in the event of failure of any of the instruments.

Sample racks can accommodate tubes 13 to 16 mm × 75 mm.

Sample volumes and throughput for the HS are as follows: NE-8000: 200 µL, 120 samples/hour; R-3000: 180 µL, 80 samples/hour; SP unit: 200 µL, 120 samples/hour.

Although consolidated hardcopy reports are not available, all results may be automatically output to a host computer.

The HS may be used with or without the R-3000 instrument. Additional conveyor units are available for insertion into the system, and turn units are also manufactured for a U or L shaped configuration of the HS.

Coulter Counter Analyzers

Principles of Testing

Coulter Corporation has manufactured numerous sophisticated cell counters over the past 20 plus years, beginning with the COULTER COUNTER® Model S. The primary differences between the various models have been a constant upgrading in the form of computerization, streamlining of sample flow, increased automation, and addition of new tests. Methods of testing for each parameter have, in general, remained constant from one model to the next. Rather than explain these theories for each cell counter, an explanation of testing principles will be given below, to which the reader is referred when studying a particular Coulter cell counter.

White Blood Cell Count. The white blood cell

count is determined using the *aperture imped-ence method* (Coulter Principle). The blood sample is diluted in a solution capable of carrying an electrical charge. The diluted specimen is placed in the WBC aperture bath, which contains three apertures. There is one external electrode in the bath, and each aperture contains its own internal electrode. A specific amount of the diluted sample is drawn through the orifice (opening) of each aperture for a predetermined time. During the counting cycle an electric current passes between the internal and external electrodes (through the orifice of each aperture). Each time a cell passes through the orifice it causes a change in voltage that produces a voltage pulse, the magnitude of which is proportional to the size of the particle (cell) causing the voltage change. The number of voltage pulses determine the white blood cell count, while the amount of the voltage change indicates the size of the white cell.

Red Blood Cell Count and MCV. The diluted blood sample in the RBC aperture bath is counted in the same manner as described for the white blood cell count above (aperture impedence method). In addition, the volume of the red blood cells (MCV) is electronically derived from the size of the voltage change. White cells will also be counted along with the red blood cells. Their numbers, however, are usually too small to be of any significance to the red cell count.

Coulter Pulse Editing. The principle of cell counting and volume measurement in the Coulter counters is based on the detection and measurement of voltage pulses created by cells, suspended in a conductive diluent, as they travel through a small orifice. During the counting cycle, the number of voltage pulses corresponds to the cell count, while the size, or amplitude, of the pulse corresponds to the volume of the cell. The amplitude and the shape of the voltage pulse, however, are affected by the pathway the cell takes through the aperture. The speed of the diluent through the aperture is at a maximum in the center of the aperture opening, and the density of the current is the most uniform in this area. On the other hand, the speed of the fluid adjacent to the aperture wall is slower, and the density of the current here is

higher. Refer to Figure 7–10. In this diagram, cell B travels through a uniform current density to give a voltage pulse as shown. Cell A, however, first travels close to the aperture, where there is a higher current density. The resultant pulse begins prior to that from cell B, has a higher amplitude, and is atypical. Cell C travels through the aperture very close to the aperture wall. The voltage pulse contains two peaks because of the higher current density at the two corners of the aperture. The pulse itself is of longer duration because of the slower speed of the cell through the aperture (the flow through the center of the aperture is at a maximum). The Coulter pulse editor is contained in the COULTER COUNTER Model S Plus instruments and functions to recognize and eliminate the atypical pulses such as those described above. Only those pulses obtained from cells passing through the center of the aperture are used in deriving cell volume distribution histograms.

Hemoglobin. The hemoglobin for each test sample is determined spectrophotometrically using the cyanmethemoglobin method. Diluent flows into the hemoglobin cuvet and a blank reading is made. After the white blood cell count has been completed, this dilution moves out of the aperture bath and into the hemoglobin cuvet, where the amount of light passing through the hemoglobin sample is determined.

Hematocrit. The hematocrit is calculated from the values determined for the red cell count and MCV: Hematocrit = Red Blood Cell Count × MCV.

MCH and MCHC. The MCH and MCHC are calculated using the red blood cell count, hemoglobin, and hematocrit.

Platelet Count. During the count cycle, as the platelets and red blood cells pass through the apertures, those particles which are between 2 and 20 fL in size are counted as platelets. In the analyzer unit, as the platelets are counted, they are divided into groups (channels) according to size. This information is then used for plotting the platelet graph. Normal platelets, when graphed according to size and number, are log-normally distributed and

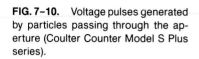

FIG. 7–10. Voltage pulses generated by particles passing through the aperture (Coulter Counter Model S Plus series).

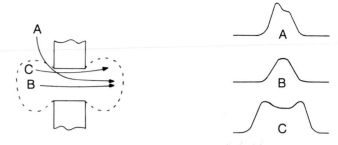

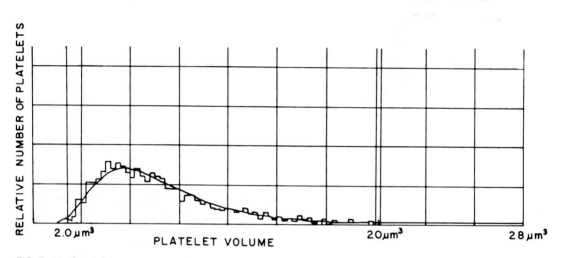

FIG. 7–11. Graph of normal platelet size distribution, Coulter Counter Model S Plus.

yield a log-normal curve (Fig. 7–11). There are platelets smaller than 2 fL and larger than 20 fL. However, red blood cells might be included in the platelet count if the range were expanded. Therefore, a graph is made of the size distribution of the platelets between 2 and 20 µL. If the analyzer recognizes the platelet count as having a log-normal distribution, it chooses the peak of the curve and the lowest point on either side of the peak. Using the two low points, the platelet data are fitted to a log-normal curve and extrapolated to read from 0 to 70 fL; everything within this curve is counted as platelets. The first graph of the platelet count is a plot of the actual count between 2 and 20 fL. If the platelet count shows log-normal distribution, a fitted curve is graphed from 0 to 70 fL over the original curve, and all platelets contained within this curve are counted and reported as the platelet count. If the platelets do not show log-normal size distribution, the curve will only extend from 2 to 20 fL (Fig. 7–12).

A symbol ($) appears on the printout form, signifying a "no-fit" platelet count. This platelet count represents the raw data count for those platelets contained in the curve between the two minimum points (not necessarily between 2 and 20 fL). A fitted curve must be obtained to have a valid platelet count. The criteria for a fitted curve are (1) a platelet count above 20,000/µL, (2) log-normal distribution (positive curve), (3) no platelet count vote out, (4) mode of fitted curve between 3 and 15 fL, and (5) PDW <20.

Red Cell Distribution Width (RDW) (COULTER COUNTER Model S Plus Only). The RDW is an indication of the degree of anisocytosis. The size of red blood cells shows a normal distribution (Gaussian) curve (Fig. 7–13). The RDW is determined and calculated by the analyzer, using the MCV and RBC. The point on the curve (the MCV reading) at which 20% of the red blood cells are larger than the rest is recorded as the 20th percentile, and the

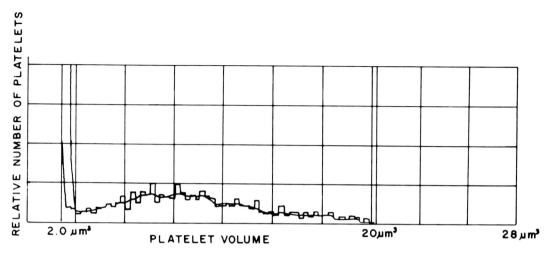

FIG. 7–12. Graph of no-fit platelet size distribution, Coulter Counter Model S Plus.

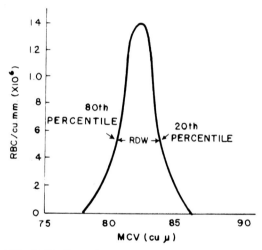

FIG. 7–13. Normal red blood cell size distribution showing RDW.

point (MCV) at which 80% of the red blood cells are smaller is noted as the 80th percentile. The space between these two points represents the RDW. Mathematically, the RDW is determined as follows:

$$RDW = \frac{(20th\ percentile - 80th\ percentile)}{(20th\ percentile + 80th\ percentile)} \times Constant$$

The constant represents the number that is required to give a normal value of 10 to this test. The normal range for the RDW is 8.5 to 11.5.

Red Blood Cell Histogram and Red Cell Distribution Width. The red blood cell dilution contains red blood cells, white blood cells, and platelets. Those particles between 2 and 20 fL in size are categorized as platelets. Particles greater than 36 fL are counted as red blood cells. As the red cells are counted, their size (MCV) is also determined. This information is used to create the red blood cell histogram, where the relative number of red blood cells are plotted on the vertical axis of the graph and the size of the red blood cell is plotted on the horizontal axis. Normally, the red blood cell histogram will be almost symmetric with a single peak (Fig. 7–14A). The tail seen to the left of the curve may represent large or clumped platelets, or electrical interference. The larger tail on the right of the curve is termed the *foot* and may represent doublets and triplets (two or three cells).

The red cell distribution width (RDW) represents the coefficient of variation of the red blood cell size and is determined by the following formula for the Coulter Counter S Plus Models II, III, IV, V, VI, STKR, and STKS:

$$RDW\ (CV\%) = \frac{S.D.\ (of\ RBC\ distribution)}{Mean} \times 100$$

Before the RDW is calculated, the upper and lower portion of the histogram, containing the two tails, is excluded from the calculations. If a relatively large secondary population of red blood cells is present (Fig. 7–14B), this will be detected by the instrument

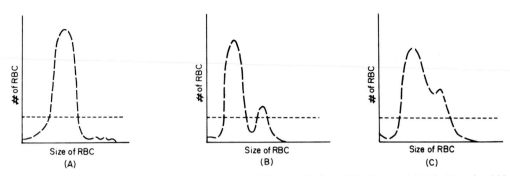

FIG. 7–14. RBC histograms. A. Normal distribution of red blood cells. B and C. Abnormal distribution of red blood cells.

because the two populations are well separated, and the RDW will be flagged as abnormal. If, however, the second population of red blood cells present is not as distinctly different from the other red blood cells present (Fig. 7–14C), the RDW will not be flagged, but should be markedly increased. The recommended normal range for the RDW determined in this manner is 11.5 to 14.5%.

COULTER COUNTER Histogram Differential. The COULTER COUNTER® Model S Plus IV and the ensuing models (Jr, V, VI, STKR, and JT Series) are capable of reporting a white count differential based on the size distribution of the white cells. In addition to counting the white blood cells, the instrument determines the size of these cells. This information is then used to plot the histogram. Using the specific Coulter reagent system, the nucleated cells in the approximate size range of 35 to 90 fL have been found to be normal lymphocytes, those cells ranging in size from 90 to 160 fL are considered mononuclear cells, and the granulocytes are in the range of 160 to 450 fL. The percentage of each of these cell types is calculated by comparing the number of cells present in each size range, with the total number of cells present in all three size categories. The instrument multiplies the percentage of each cell type by the total white count in order to obtain the absolute number of each cell class present. A normal white blood cell histogram (Fig. 7–15) shows three distinct populations of white cells separated at approximately 90 and 160 fL. If nucleated red blood cells are present, these are characteristically indicated by the lack of a valley at 35 fL. In addition, abnormal flags will alert the operator to abnormal cell distribution patterns. The lymphocyte category will contain mature and some atypical lymphocytes; the mononuclear class includes monocytes, promyelocytes, myelocytes, and blasts; eosinophils, basophils, metamyelocytes, bands, and neutrophils are classified as granulocytes.

Five-Part Differential: COULTER™ STKS and COULTER™ MAXM. Classification of the white blood cells is performed using VCS technology flow cytometry. Three measurements (Volume, Conductivity, and light Scatter) are performed simultaneously, yet independently in a single sample analysis chamber. The volume measurements are based on the Coulter principle of cell sizing and aperture impedance. Conductivity measurements use a high frequency electromagnetic probe to examine the cell's internal structure. The last measurement, light scatter, is a function of cell surface features and internal structure. The STKS and MAXM use a helium-neon

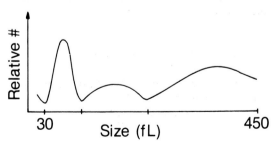

FIG. 7–15. WBC Histogram (Coulter Counter Model S Plus IV).

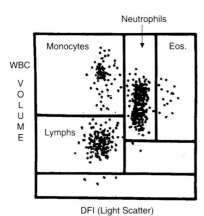

FIG. 7–16. DF1 scatterplot, Coulter STKS.

laser for this measurement. The laser light is passed through a lens block and is focused horizontally and vertically, making the light beam smaller and elliptically shaped. The beam penetrates the sensing zone of the flow cell so that a constant amount of illumination is provided, regardless of the cell's position within the sample stream. Light scatter, from 10° to 70°, is collected by a photodetector. Photocells change the scattered light into electronic pulses, which are analyzed by one of the system's computers. The combined volume, conductivity, and laser light scatter data on each cell are plotted within a three dimensional matrix. The WBCs are classified according to their VCS (volume, conductivity, scatter) properties. These raw signals are sent to the analyzer for processing, computation, and generation of WBC scatter plots. The *DF1* (discriminant function 1) scatterplot is the most routinely displayed and plots light scatter analysis properties on the X axis and cell volume on the Y axis (Fig. 7–16). Monocyte, lymphocyte, neutrophil, and eosinophil populations are shown on this plot. The basophil population will not be seen on this display because of its location behind the lymphs. Two additional scatterplots are derived and are available to the operator: The *DF2* plot shows data derived from volume and conductivity analysis (Fig. 7–17). Although the *DF3* plot also graphs cell volume and conductivity properties, it shows differentiation of the basophil population by gating out the neutrophil and eosinophil populations (Fig. 7–18). See Figure 7–19 for identification (location) of various abnormal cell types on the scatterplot.

$\bar{X}_B$ and Quality Control. The $\bar{X}_B$ (pronounced X bar B) is used as a quality control check for hematology instruments. This mathematical formula was published in 1974 by Dr. Brian Bull. Essentially, it is a weighted moving average of the patient's red blood cell indices (MCV, MCH, and MCHC) and is calculated by the Coulter Counter data terminal using a relatively complex mathematical formula. Studies have shown that the population of patients in medium to large hospitals show relatively stable values for the red blood cell indices. Also, in the calculations used by the Coulter instruments, less weight is given to extremely high and low patient results.

Basically, each successive group of 20 patient results are grouped into a batch. As each patient's blood is tested, the mean ($\bar{X}_B$) value from the previous batch (of 20 patient samples) is subtracted from the respective current

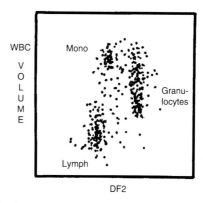

FIG. 7–17. DF2 scatterplot, Coulter STKS.

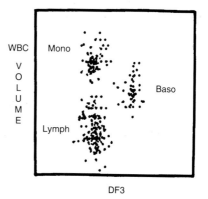

FIG. 7–18. DF3 scatterplot, Coulter STKS.

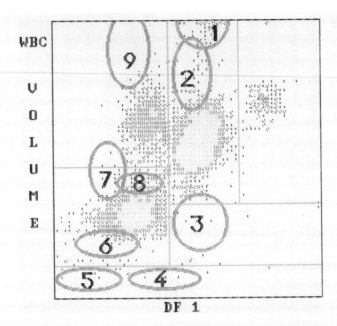

FIG. 7–19. Location of abnormal cell types on the scatterplot, Coulter STKS. (Courtesy of Coulter Corp., Hialeah, FL.)

1. Suspect Blasts	4. Giant Platelets	7. Suspect Blasts
2. Suspect Immature Granulocytes	5. Nucleated Red Blood Cells	8. Variant Lymphocytes
3. Aged and Damaged Neutrophils	6. Variant Lymphocytes	9. Suspect Blasts

red blood cell index (MCV, MCH, or MCHC). The square root of the resultant number is then determined. After 20 patient blood specimens have been analyzed, the sum of the square roots for each of the three indices is added up and divided by the number of patient samples (usually 20). This number is then squared and added to or subtracted from the respective previous $\bar{X}_B$ value obtained in order to derive the $\bar{X}_B$ value for the current batch of patient samples. This new mean value is then used to help determine the $\bar{X}_B$ value for the next batch of 20 blood specimens. Each laboratory should have its own set of target values for each of the indices. Once set, the $\bar{X}_B$ value for each index in each batch should fall within ±3% of the target value. If, however, an instrument or reagent problem exists, this will be indicated by one or more of the red blood cell indices moving consistently in one direction (up or down) or in the $\bar{X}_B$ value falling outside of the allowable laboratory preset range. The recommended target values are ±3% of (1) 89.5 (MCV), (2) 30.5 (MCH), and (3) 34.0 (MCHC).

The hemoglobin bias, RBC percentage difference, and hematocrit percentage difference are further calculations made by the instrument (except the STKS and MAXM) for use in detecting specific instrument problems. The automatic *hemoglobin bias* is defined as the difference between the hemoglobin assay value and the actual hemoglobin reading (average of last five control values in the file). A manual hemoglobin bias is also available.

COULTER COUNTER Model S Plus

The Model S Plus COULTER COUNTER performs a seven parameter CBC (WBC, RBC, hgb., hct., RBC indices), an RDW (red blood cell distribution width, a measure of anisocytosis), and a platelet count. It consists of five connected units: power supply, diluter unit, analyzer unit, printer, and X-Y recorder.

The *power supply* furnishes regulated voltages to run the electronic system and also provides the necessary pressures and vacuum to the diluter unit and reagent system. The *diluter unit* aspirates, pipets, dilutes, mixes the blood, physically moves the blood sample through the unit for testing, and senses the samples in the baths. The *analyzer unit* contains electronic cards that control the sequence of the various operating cycles of the diluter unit. Messages are received from the diluter unit, and the analyzer counts, sizes, measures, and computes this information, which is then sent to the printer unit in the form of test results. Information is also sent from this unit to the X-Y recorder. The *printer unit* gives a printed copy of the test results obtained by the instrument and is connected to the power supply and analyzer unit. The *X-Y recorder* provides a graph of the platelet size distribution and also plots simulated platelet distributions based on test pulses as part of the electronic voltage check.

Sample Aspiration. When the instrument has not been cycled for approximately 15 minutes, the pneumatic system automatically shuts off. To activate the cell counter the *prime button* is pressed; as soon as the pressure and vacuum gauges register correctly, the *Ready light* will be displayed on the *system status indicator*. The tube of well-mixed blood is placed under the *whole blood aspirator tip* (inserted at least 1 inch into the blood), and the *whole blood button* is pressed. When Wipe is displayed on the indicator, the blood sample is removed and the aspirator tube is wiped with a piece of gauze moistened in diluent. Hands or any other objects must not be near the whole blood aspirator tip during the remainder of the cycle. Approximately 1 mL of whole blood is drawn up into the instrument through the *blood sampling valve (BSV)*. The sample is split into two pathways prior to reaching the BSV. One half of the sample enters the back of the valve, where it fills the small metal loop for the WBC dilution (Fig. 7–20). The remaining portion of the sample enters the front of the BSV for the red blood count dilution.

Sample Dilution. The blood sampling valve changes to position 2 and approximately 10 mL of diluent enters the back of the valve, picks up the 42.9 μL of whole blood contained in the small loop, and carries it to the *WBC aperture bath*. At the same time, approximately 10 mL of diluent enters the front of the blood sampling valve and picks up the 1.6 μL of whole blood in the center section. The diluted sample goes directly to the *RBC aperture bath*. At the same time, 0.7734 mL of lyse reagent (containing cyanmethemoglobin reagent) is forced into the WBC aperture bath (1:251 dilution). Bubbles are introduced into each bath through tubing attached at the

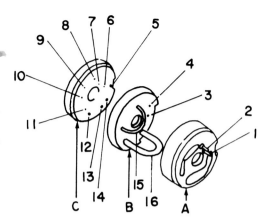

FIG. 7–20. Blood sampling valve, Coulter Counter Model S Plus. Whole-blood aspiration. RBC and WBC dilutions are performed simultaneously. RBC dilution, position 1 (as shown above): Whole blood enters line 1 (section A), goes through passage 4 (section B), and out of sampling valve through passage 6 (section C). Center section rotates counterclockwise to position 2: Diluent enters line 2 (A), goes through passage 4 (B) picking up the blood sample, and out passage 7 (C) to RBC aperture bath. (Remaining whole blood aspirated travels through passage 3 [B] and out passage 6 [C].) WBC dilution, position 1: Whole blood enters back of section C through passage 10 into loop 15 (B) and out line 8 (C). Position 2: Diluent enters section C through back of passage 11, through loop 15 (B), picking up blood sample, and out passage 9 (C) to aperture bath. Microsample aspirations: Diluted sample enters back of section C through passage 12, into loop 16 (B), and out passage 14 (C) to the WBC aperture bath. Midway during the aspiration, the middle section rotates to position 2. The dilution continues to enter the back of passage 12 (C), into an etched-out passageway in the back of section B, and out passage 14 (C) to the WBC aperture bath. At the same time, diluent enters the back of passage 5 (C), through loop 16 (B), picks up the diluted blood, and carries it out passage 13 (C) to the RBC aperture bath.

bottom. These bubbles (between 12 and 16) are utilized to mix the diluted blood samples.

Sample Testing. While the aperture baths are filling, the *hemoglobin cuvet* is being drained into the *waste chamber*. As Wipe is displayed, an internal voltage check is automatically performed (voltage patterns are displayed on the *oscilloscope screens*), and the hemoglobin cuvet is filled with diluent (5 mL) for the hemoglobin blank reading. At this point, the instrument is ready for testing, and Count is displayed. A 4 second counting cycle takes place. At the beginning of the first 4 second count cycle, the voltage reading for the hemoglobin blank is shown on the *DVM/test number display*. This number immediately changes to the number 1 to indicate the first counting cycle. The white blood cells are counted from the WBC aperture bath on the right side. From the RBC aperture bath, the red blood cells and platelets are counted, and the MCV is determined from the size of the voltage pulses. The RBC, WBC, platelet count, and MCV are all measured through three apertures. Up to five 4 second platelet counts are performed during each test cycle, depending on the platelet count of the sample introduced. The instrument automatically counts the platelets for additional cycles, up to five, until the equivalent of a 190,000 to 250,000/μL platelet count is attained. As each platelet count is performed by the instrument, the number corresponding to the platelet count being done (2, 3, 4, or 5) appears on the DVM/test number display. During the first count cycle, three platelet counts, red blood cell counts, white blood cell counts, and MCVs are performed simultaneously (one count through each aperture). When the counting cycle(s) is completed, Analyze appears on the system status indicator, and the analyzer unit compares the counts from each aperture. If all three results for each parameter tested (RBC, WBC, platelet count, and RDW) agree with the others within 4 S.D., Data Accept appears on the system status indicator, and the three counts are averaged for a final result. If one count does not match the other two, the corresponding data rejection lamp lights on the voting matrix, and the other two counts are averaged for the final result. A total vote out for a parameter is obtained when none of the counts agree within 4 S.D. of each other. In such instances, all three data rejection lamps are lit, Data Reject appears on the indicator, and the cycle stops. The *recount* and *count buttons* flash for 30 seconds. If a recount is desired on the rejected parameter, the recount button is pushed. At the completion of the counting cycle, the aperture baths will empty (RBC bath into the waste chamber and the WBC bath into the hemoglobin cuvet) and refill with diluent. Backwash appears on the system status indicator, and 4 mL of diluent is pushed through the blood sampling valve and

out the aspirator tip into the rinse cup (for cleaning), which has moved into a locked position beneath the aspirator. Hgb Read is displayed on the indicator, and the amount of light passing through the diluted hemoglobin sample is read. The voltage reading is displayed on the DVM/test number display. The hematocrit (RBC × MCV), MCH (hemoglobin ÷ RBC), and MCHC (hemoglobin ÷ hematocrit) are calculated in the analyzer unit. The printer unit prints the results of the nine parameters.

Microsample Testing. If 1 mL of whole blood is not available or if fingertip blood is used, 44.7 μL of whole blood is added to one aliquot (approximately 10 mL) of diluent from the diluent dispenser. The well-mixed, bubble-free diluted sample is placed under the microsample aspirator tip. When the *1:224 dilution button* (behind the aspirator) is pressed the instrument aspirates the entire sample, which enters the back of the blood sampling valve and goes into and completely fills the large loop of the center section (Fig. 7–20). It continues through the blood sampling valve and leaves by way of the back, going directly to the WBC aperture bath. During the aspiration of the microsample, the blood sampling valve moves to position 2. The large loop is now completely filled with the original microsample dilution. Diluent then enters the blood sampling valve at the back, picks up the diluted sample in the large loop for the RBC dilution, and carries it to the RBC aperture bath, where it enters the right bottom side of the bath. While this is occurring, the diluted sample continues to be aspirated through the back of the blood sampling valve but now enters the trough in the middle section and continues out the back of the blood sampling valve, where it continues to go directly to the WBC aperture bath, entering through the line at the top of the bath. The cycle continues as described for the whole blood cycle. A vacuum is applied to the microsample aspirator tip for a short period at the end of the cycle, immediately before the Ready light comes on (for cleaning purposes).

Discussion. It is advisable to keep a spare cube of diluent adjacent to the instrument. This prevents unnecessary mixing of the diluent with resultant formation of microscopic air bubbles when it is attached to the instrument.

Build up of protein on the orifices of the apertures will cause an initial increase in the MCV, followed by a decrease in the counts (WBC, RBC, and/or platelet).

Testing time for each blood sample is 34 to 50 seconds, depending on the number of platelet counting cycles necessary. Only one sample may be introduced into the instrument at a time.

When agglutination of the red blood cells is present (e.g., cold agglutinin), the RBC will be invalidly low and the MCV invalidly high. In this situation, the only useful parameters determined by the instrument are the WBC, hemoglobin, and platelet count.

COULTER COUNTER Models S Plus II, III, IV, V, VI, and STKR

Coulter Corporation has modified the basic COULTER COUNTER® Model S Plus and enlarged the instrument's capabilities. The basic operating unit shows only minor changes. One major addition is the data terminal.

The *COULTER COUNTER Model S Plus II* tests blood samples at the rate of 90 per hour and uses a reagent system modified slightly from the one used in the Model S Plus. This has resulted in the reporting of lymphocyte number and percentage, and the RDW is calculated as a true C.V. (coefficient of variation). This model is capable of determining and reporting the absolute number and percentage of lymphocytes per μL of blood. A data terminal may also be utilized with this model, which provides quality control capabilities (including $\bar{X}_B$ analysis), the ability to flag abnormal results, and white blood cell, red blood cell, and platelet histograms. A matrix printer plotter is capable of printing all information displayed by the data terminal.

The COULTER COUNTER Model S Plus III is able to test over 115 samples per hour.

The *COULTER COUNTER Model S Plus IV*, in addition to the modifications made in the S Plus II, uses a 100 μL patient sample in place of the 1.0 mL of blood that was previously required. The manually diluted microsample used in previous models is therefore no longer needed. The number of parameters tested has increased to 16 and includes WBC, RBC, hemoglobin, hematocrit, MCV, MCH,

MCHC, RDW, MPV (mean platelet volume), and a WBC differential (percentage and absolute number of granulocytes, lymphocytes, and mononuclear cells, plus eosinophils less than 700/μL and basophils less than 200/μL). Red cell, white cell, and platelet histograms are displayed on the CRT screen along with the numerical results for each patient sample. A hard copy (printed) report of these results may be obtained from the matrix printer plotter. An MPV nomogram (using the MPV and platelet count) is generated by the data terminal and may be obtained on each patient sample for which a platelet count and MPV are resulted. Up to 138 samples per hour may be analyzed. There is an optional bar code reader wand for use in matching results with the patient requisition or online data. This mechanism is also available on the Coulters S Plus V, VI, and STKR.

The *COULTER COUNTER Model S Plus V* performs all of the testing and reporting as described above for the S Plus IV. A major change is in the addition of an automated cap piercer used in aspirating the patient sample. The capped tube of well-mixed whole blood is placed into a window in the front of the diluter unit door. When the instrument is in the ready stage, it senses the tube and automatically pierces the cap, removing 100 μL of blood for analysis, and proceeds with testing. The tube of blood travels down a small exit ramp to be removed by the operator. There is also a secondary aspirator, which may be used to aspirate hand held specimens that have their caps removed.

The *COULTER COUNTER Model S Plus VI* performs testing and reporting as described for the S Plus V above. This model uses an additional unit, the autosampler, which contains two rotating wheel-shaped sample trays each capable of holding 32 patient tubes. Specimens for premixing are placed on the right side of the unit, where they are rotated and mixed prior to testing. The sample tray may then be removed and placed on the front of the unit for testing, where a premix cycle may be used to ensure complete mixing. When the specimens have been mixed, the sampler wheel stops briefly, and the first sample is automatically aspirated by means of a special cap piercer. Sample analysis is begun, and when the instrument is ready to aspirate the next sample, the sampler wheel stops at the next blood sample long enough to aspirate the specimen. To make this a true walk-away system this model has a continuous-feed fanfold printer. STAT samples may be tested at any time, and there are audible and visual signals given when all of the specimens on the wheel have been tested. Like the Model S Plus V there is a secondary aspirator for hand-held uncapped specimens, which uses 125 μL of whole blood. The automatic sampling mode uses 750 μL of whole blood.

The *COULTER COUNTER Model S Plus STKR* (pronounced "stacker") shows a variety of additional capabilities over the previously described S Plus VI. This model is capable of accepting and mixing up to 144 patient samples at one time in preparation for automatic identification, aspiration (using a cap piercer), and sample analysis. A bar code label is placed on each specimen tube and up to 12 samples are placed into an S Plus STKR cassette. Up to 12 cassettes may be placed in the right side of the STKR, where they are mixed by a back and forward motion. The first cassette is transported to the center of the diluter unit. Tube and cassette/position bar codes are read at the time of aspiration, that is, when the sample is removed from the tube by a cap piercing aspirator. Sample analysis is begun, the next specimen is moved to the test station, and when the instrument is ready, the bar code is read and the sample is aspirated. (The instrument may be operated with or without the tube bar code.) Cassettes are automatically stored on the left side of the instrument when testing is complete. There is a secondary aspirator for hand-held uncapped specimens, which uses 100 μL of whole blood. The automatic sampling mode uses 200 μL of blood and requires a minimum of 1.0 mL of whole blood in the tube. STAT samples may be tested at any time during auto-processing. Throughput for this model is 138 samples per hour. The printer is capable of automatic reporting and can read the bar code labels, which enables it to print results on labeled forms in any sequence. There is a keypad and display on the printer that allows for manual operation when desired.

Data Terminal. The data terminal receives information from the analyzer unit and sends it to the printer and the matrix printer plotter. It determines the MCV, RDW, platelet count,

MPV, and white cell percentages and absolute counts, and provides a quality control program. Extended data terminal capabilities are available, which allow for additional storage of up to 3900 numerical patient reports or up to 550 complete reports (numerical results and histograms) on the Coulters S Plus Jr., IV, V, VI, STKR, and JT Series. These same instruments will flag abnormal results: values exceeding pre-set laboratory limits, results exceeding delta checks, abnormal WBC differential results, abnormal volume distribution histograms, and abnormal MPV nomograms. The basic program used in the data terminal is made up of seven parts, each of which is termed a *menu*:

1. The *Sample analysis menu* is used during sample testing, displays specimen results, and contains information about the $\bar{X}_B$ program.
2. The *Data entry menu* allows the operator to enter information into the data terminal.
3. The *Start-up menu* is used primarily in setting up the instrument each day.
4. The *Control data menu* allows the operator to select the control file, enter and delete control values, and review control data.
5. The *Special tests menu* allows the operator to perform checks on the functioning of the different units of the instrument.
6. The *Prime menu* allows specimens to be tested on the instrument without the results being included in the $\bar{X}_B$ analysis.
7. The *Calibration menu* provides a quality control program for automatic calibration calculations.

All information displayed on the data terminal may be printed on the matrix printer plotter by depressing the plot key on the data terminal.

Interpretive Report. All Coulter Model S Pluses (Jr., IV, V, VI, STKR, JT Series) report a complete white cell histogram with an accompanying interpretive report that "flags" the abnormal test result for further review. The interpretive report is based on testing limits that may be set by each individual laboratory. When preset thresholds are exceeded, the instrument can report definitive flags for lymphocytosis, lymphopenia, granulocytosis, granulopenia, anisocytosis, microcytosis, macrocytosis, hypochromia, large platelets, and

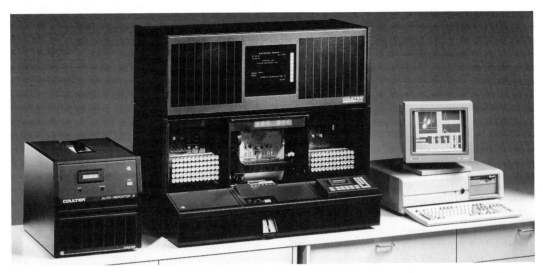

FIG. 7–21. Coulter STKS. (Courtesy of Coulter Corp., Hialeah, FL.)

small platelets. A second part of the interpretive report indicates suspect cell types: eosinophilia >700/μL, basophilia >200/μL, atypical lymphocytes, immature granulocytes, blasts, NRBCs, platelet clumps, and red cell and platelet abnormal distributions. The third portion of this report gives the message "Review Nomogram" when the MPV is smaller or larger than expected for a given platelet count.

Coulter STKS

The COULTER STKS (pronounced stack-S) is an automated hematology analyzer and white blood cell differential counter. The STKS reports the following parameters: CBC, red blood cell indices, RDW, platelet count, MPV (mean platelet volume), PDW (platelet distribution width, a measure of variation in platelet size), and the absolute number and percentage of lymphocytes, monocytes, neutrophils, eosinophils, and basophils. Components of the STKS (Fig. 7–21) are the power supply (1), the diluter unit (2), the analyzer (3), and the data management system (4). Optional units are the graphic printer (5) and the auto-reporter ticket printer (not shown).

The *power supply* provides electronic power, which regulates voltages to the STKS's computer circuitry, and pneumatic power, which supplies pressure and vacuum to the diluter.

The *diluter unit* aspirates, dilutes, mixes, lyses, and transports the blood samples. It also houses the *triple transducer module* and *laser unit* used for the WBC differential determination. The *analyzer* controls the operation of the diluter, and counts, measures, and computes results. The *data management system* (*DMS*) receives information from the analyzer and displays, stores, and transmits results to the peripheral printers and host computer.

Instrument Start UP. The *main power circuit breaker* on the power supply is used to turn on power to the analyzer and diluter. A 30 minute warmup is required when the power is first turned on. The pneumatic system is activated by pressing the *prime apert key* on the diluter. A start up cycle is initiated by pressing the *start up key* on the analyzer. During the start up cycle, cleaning reagent in the hydraulic lines is replaced by diluent. A background count is performed, measurements of hemoglobin-blank and sample voltages are taken, and a series of electronic checks are performed.

Sample Aspiration. Sample processing in the primary mode begins by loading bar coded specimens into a sample *cassette*. Up to 12 cassettes of 12 samples each may be loaded onto the STKS at one time. Sample tubes must contain a minimum of 1.0 mL of blood in a 5 mL tube. The sample volume aspirated is 250 μL. A bar code label identifies the cassette and each position in it. This permits the operator to trace a sample back to a specific cassette and position. Filled cassettes are placed in the *loading bay* on the right side of the diluter unit. The *start/cont key* on the diluter keypad is pressed to begin sample analysis. The *right lift platform* beneath the stacked cassettes in the loading area rises, and the bottom cassette is placed on the *transport platform*. The platform lowers the first cassette, and moves it onto the *rocker bed*, which moves the cassette back and forth for sample mixing. The cassette continues to move to the left on the rocker bed until it reaches the *tube sensor* at the *sensing station*. When the sample tube is detected, the *stripper plate* locks onto the tube. After a minimum of 14 rocks, the rocker bed locks in a 45° forward position.

When the first tube reaches the *sampling station*, the specimen tube is locked into position while the *cap piercing needle* rotates upward. The *tube ram* pushes the specimen tube out of the cassette and toward the needle, causing the needle to pierce the tube cap. The *bar code reader* scans both the cassette and specimen tube labels at this time.

After the cap is pierced, a pump draws 250 μL of sample through the needle into the *blood sampling valve (BSV)*. Two *blood detectors* monitor passage of the sample through the BSV. The tube ram is withdrawn and the sample tube is repositioned in the cassette. The cap piercing needle rotates into the *rinse trough*, where it is washed with diluent.

Sample Dilution. The BSV consists of fixed front and rear sections and a center section that rotates. The center section separates the sample into two segments. Isoton III (10 mL) passes through the BSV, picking up the 1.6 μL segment of blood, and goes to the RBC bath. This dilution, 1:6250, is used for the RBC and platelet counts, the MCV, and MPV. A second aliquot of Isoton III (6 mL) is delivered through the BSV, where it picks up the second segment of blood (28 μL) and carries it to the WBC bath. This dilution is used for the white blood cell count and hemoglobin. As the diluted sample is entering the WBC bath, 1 mL of Lyse S III Diff reagent enters the bath to lyse the red blood cells and convert the hemoglobin to cyanmethemoglobin. The final dilution in the WBC bath is

1:251. While the Lyse S III Diff reagent is dispensed, the hemoglobin blank pump transfers 5 mL of diluent into the hemoglobin cuvet for the hemoglobin blank reading.

As the samples are being delivered to the RBC and WBC baths, the *diff segmenting module* segments 31 μL of sample for the white blood cell differential. This sample and 1.07 mL of Erythrolyse II reagent are delivered to the *mixing chamber*. The Erythrolyse II reagent rapidly lyses the red blood cells and reduces the resultant cellular debris to an insignificant level, while leaving the white blood cells unaltered. During sample mixing, 0.2 mL of Stabilyse (a white cell preservative) is added to the dilution. This reagent neutralizes the hemolytic action of the Erythrolyse II reagent and permits the WBC size, surface, and cytoplasmic characteristics to remain intact.

Sample Testing. The STKS determines the RBC, WBC, and platelet counts using the Coulter aperture impedance method described previously. Pulses from the red cell bath representing cells 36 fL and greater are classified as red blood cells. Pulses from the white cell bath representing cells greater than 35 fL are classified as white blood cells. For the WBC count, RBC count, MCV, RDW, platelet count, and MPV, the analyzer unit votes on data from each aperture to verify that at least two apertures have produced data within an established statistical range of each other. Data that do not meet this criteria are voted out and not included in the final count. The analyzer corrects the counts for coincidence (presence of more than one cell within the aperture boundaries at the same time). A steady stream of diluent flows behind the RBC apertures during the count period to prevent cells from re-entering the aperture's sensing zone and being counted as platelets.

The RBC histogram is developed by the analyzer through a process of editing out pulses caused by cells that did not pass through the center of the aperture. After editing, pulse information is digitized (converted to a number that corresponds to the size of the cell). The digital information is then analyzed according to volume in a size distribution histogram.

Pulses detected in the RBC bath that represent cells from 2 to 20 fL are classified as platelets. The platelet pulse information is digitized and further analyzed according to size to construct the platelet size distribution histogram. The histogram is further analyzed by a fitting process, and the analyzer then votes on the platelet count, MPV, and PDW.

The analyzer's computer derives the MCV and RDW from the red cell histogram. The MPV and platelet count are derived from the platelet histogram. The hematocrit, MCH, and MCHC are computed.

At the conclusion of the WBC count cycle, the dilution is drained from the WBC bath into the hemoglobin cuvet where the hemoglobin is measured spectrophotometrically at 525 nm. At the end of this sequence, the center section of the BSV rotates back to the aspirate position.

The five part differential is performed in the flow cell of the *triple transducer module* located in the diluter unit. The diluted sample is injected into the center of a sheath stream, and the flow cell aperture current is activated. The sample is guided through the center of the flow cell aperture by a surrounding sheath of Isoton III diluent. This process is called hydrodynamic focusing. A stream of diluent on the exit side of the flow cell aperture prevents cells from re-entering the aperture. Approximately 8,000 cells are analyzed in a typical sample using a high frequency electromagnetic probe and a helium-neon laser for making conductivity, light scatter, and volume measurements.

Data Management System (DMS). Data from cell counts, size distribution histograms, and the WBC scatter plot are sent to the DMS, which will display test results and plots, in addition to flagging messages based on computer set limits for abnormal cell distributions or populations and operator set limits for the numeric results. Up to 1,000 sets of results may be stored by the DMS. There are 15 quality control files, each capable of storing 100 runs per file. The DMS main menu selections are as follows:

1. *Sample analysis*, which permits the operator to run samples, make data base inquiries, prepare worklists, and access $\bar{X}_B$ analysis.
2. *Controls*, in which the operator may run, review, and print quality control numerical and/or graphed data.

3. *Start-up*, in which the start-up cycle is initiated.
4. *Special functions*, which allows the operator to run reproducibility and carry-over checks, set definitive flag limits, set host computer communication, and perform instrument calibration.

Cell Classification Report. Sample results are routinely displayed on the DMS screen: WBC scatterplot (DF1 plot), RBC and platelet histograms, numeric results for the CBC, RBC indices, RDW, platelet count, MPV, five cell differential, and any abnormal flagging codes or messages. This report may also be printed by the graphic printer. The following messages may appear on the final printed report: (1) *Condition* messages indicate whether the WBC, RBC, and platelet populations are normal or abnormal; (2) *Suspect* messages will indicate abnormal cell distributions or populations, including the presence of blasts, immature granulocytes/bands, variant lymphs, NRBCs, dimorphic RBC population, micro RBCs/RBC fragments, RBC agglutination, platelet clumps, and giant platelets. These messages are computer-set and do not require operator set limits. (3) *Definitive* messages are based on operator-set numeric limits, and include increased and decreased levels for all parameters tested, in addition to anemia and poikilocytosis. Results that generate an abnormal message should be confirmed by manual review of a stained blood smear.

Discussion. The STKS may be operated in the secondary mode, which allows the operator to manually introduce a sample to the aspirator tip and requires 150 µL of sample (250 µL is required in the primary mode). The STKS will test a maximum of 100 samples per hour.

Technicon H™ Systems

The Technicon H™ system instruments perform a CBC, RBC indices, an RDW, a platelet count, and a white cell differential count. Six white cell types are identified: neutrophil, eosinophil, basophil, monocyte, lymphocyte, and large unstained cell. A lobularity index (left shift indicator) is also reported. Testing may be performed as only a CBC and platelet

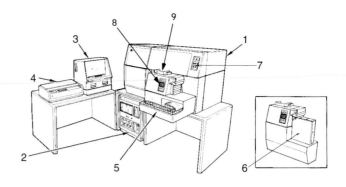

FIG. 7–22. Technicon H-2 Hematology System. (Courtesy of Technicon Instruments Corp., Tarrytown, NY.)

count, or may include the differential, as the operator chooses. The Technicon H-2 system (Fig. 7–22) is a second generation instrument that adds several design changes and improvements to the technology developed in the H-1. The Technicon H-1 is able to test 60 samples per hour, whereas the H-2 has a throughput of 100 samples per hour for testing of all parameters. Sample aspiration may be performed in either a manual open or automated closed tube mode on the H-2 (all sample aspiration is performed manually on the H-1).

There are four modules that make up both the H-1 and H-2 instruments. The *analytical module* (1) aspirates, dilutes, processes, and tests each sample. The electrical outputs from each test channel are sent to the *electronics module* (2), where they are converted to test results. In addition, this unit controls the system operation and performs all data processing and management functions. The *VDT/keypad ticket printer module* (3) prints numerical test results and morphology on inserted report forms. This unit also contains the video display terminal with associated keyboard for operator communication with the instrument. The optional *screen printer* (4) is used to obtain printouts of the contents of the video display screen (except for message lines). The Technicon H-2 uses an additional *automated closed tube (act) sampler* (a continuous linear automated sampling system [*class act*] (5) or a *cassette sampler* [*cassette act*] (6)) for automated closed tube specimen aspiration.

System On/Off

The instrument is turned on by depressing the *sys on* switch (*module status panel* [7]). As long as power is supplied to the system the

indicator light will remain lit. The *sys off* switch is pressed to turn the unit off. If the instrument will not be used for a period of time the *standby* switch may be activated. (The unit will also go into the standby mode automatically after 1 hour of non-use.) The *ready* light, when lit, indicates that a sample may be aspirated into the unit. While a sample is being tested, the *in process* light is lit. A hydraulic or mechanical problem will be indicated by the *error* light.

Sample Aspiration

The operator chooses the mode of analysis using the *mode selector valve*, mounted above the sample aspiration probe. It is set in the open position for manual aspiration and in the closed position for automated closed sampling. Open sampling aspiration requires 125 μL of whole blood, closed sampling, 145 μL.

Manual Aspiration. Prior to sample aspiration in the manual mode, select the test(s) to be performed by pressing the *CBC* or *CBC/diff* switch. The corresponding indicator will light up. Sample identification for the open mode is performed manually via keypad entry or via the optional *hand-held bar code reader*. During the test cycle the *pwr on* indicator will light. If the laser power has been halted because of a problem (power failure), the *pwr intrpt* indicator lights. To turn this light off, press the *intrpt reset* switch. The *ready to sample* green indicator light should be lit (to indicate the unit is ready to aspirate a sample). The well-mixed whole blood sample is placed under the *sample probe* and the *push to aspirate* switch depressed to begin the testing cycle.

Automated Sampling. Closed tube sampling is

performed by one of two automated closed tube (act) sampler configurations: the continuous linear automated sampling system (class act) or the cassette (cassette act) sampler. Each of these sampler systems can accommodate five different sizes of blood collection tubes as well as control and calibrator vials: 10 mm × 47 or 64 mm (2 or 3 mL), 13 mm × 75 or 100 mm (5 or 7 mL), 16 mm × 75 mm (7 mL), and 16 mm × 55 (5 mL, controls). A bar code label is placed on each sample tube. Specimen identification is performed by an automatic bar code reader positioned before the *sample aspiration station*. The bar code number contains the sample ID, test selection (CBC or CBC/diff), and sample type (patient sample, control, or calibrator) information. Each collection tube is placed in an *adapter* designed for the tube size. The adapter (with tube) is then placed into a *link*. The appropriate links (each containing a sample) are snapped together to form the *belt*, which makes up the *resident chain* of the sampling system. (The class act sampler resident chain is composed of 120 links and fits onto the instrument as shown in Figure 7–22 [5]). Approximately 45 of these links are accessible to the operator at any one time. The remaining links are inside, behind the *sampler covers*. The cassette act sampler chain consists of 50 sample links. The loaded cassette is positioned onto the instrument for patient sample processing (Fig. 7–22 [6]). Movement of the sampler chain for both the class and cassette systems is initiated or stopped by pressing the *run/stop key* on the *sampler unit status panel* (8). The chain of samples on both the class and cassette units moves through the sampler transport system until the first sample in the chain reaches the *mixing, identification, and aspiration station* (9), where these functions are then carried out.

The sample is drawn through the *sample shear valve* (Fig. 7–23) by a vacuum. During aspiration, the sample travels in and out of the rear portion of the sample shear valve four times, before passing through a *conductivity detector*, located after the sample shear valve, which notes the presence of the sample and causes the aspiration process to stop. The sample is divided into four separate segments within the rear section of the sample shear

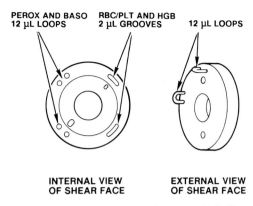

FIG. 7–23. Sample sheer valve, Technicon H-2. (Courtesy of Technicon Instruments Corp., Tarrytown, NY.)

valve: 2 µL (RBC/plt.), 12 µL (baso/lob.), 12 µL (WBC, diff.), and 2 µL (hgb.).

Sample Dilution

Dilution of the sample is performed by the combined action of the sample shear valve, *reagent shear valve*, and *diluent syringes*. Following aspiration of the sample, the back section of the sample shear valve rotates to its second position. The sample probe is rinsed inside and out, and dried. The four outer *reagent syringe drives* dispense Perox Dil 1 (WBC), Hgb Dil (hgb.), RBC Dil (RBC/plt.), and Baso Dil (baso/lob.), respectively, through separate pathways in the *reagent shear valve*. The reagents travel through the sample shear valve, where they each pick up the measured blood segment, and go to the appropriate reaction chamber (hemoglobin, RBC/plt., peroxidase, basophil/lobularity). While this is occurring, the two center reagent syringes fill with Perox Dil 2 and Perox Dil 3, respectively. These reagents are dispensed directly from the reagent shear valve into the peroxidase (WBC) reaction chamber. At the same time, the four outer reagent syringes fill with reagent for the next sample. Specimen dilutions are mixed in the appropriate reaction chambers.

Hemoglobin Measurement

The blood sample is diluted 1:250 with cyanmethemoglobin reagent (Hgb Dil) and mixed in the *hemoglobin reaction vessel*, which also

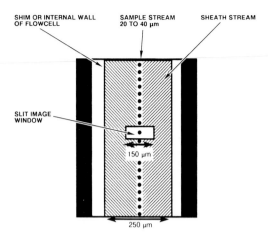

SHIM OR INTERNAL WALL
OF FLOWCELL

SAMPLE STREAM
20 TO 40 μm

SHEATH STREAM

SLIT IMAGE
WINDOW

150 μm

250 μm

FIG. 7–24. Sheath stream flowcell, Technicon H-2. (Courtesy of Technicon Instruments Corp., Tarrytown, NY.)

serves as a cuvet. It is located between a *546 nm light source* and a *photodetector*. When the hemoglobin reading has been made, the sample dilution leaves the reaction chamber and travels to the *waste chamber*. The reaction chamber is rinsed and a reading is taken of the rinse solution, to be used as the hemoglobin blank.

RBC/Platelet Count

The whole blood is diluted 1:625 with RBC/Plt Dil fluid and mixed in the *RBC/plt reaction vessel*. In this reagent the red cells absorb fluid until they are spherical in shape (their total volume is unchanged). The diluting fluid also lightly fixes (preserves) the red cells and platelets. A diaphragm pump pushes RBC/Baso Sheath fluid toward the *flow cell*. The sheath fluid is then pulled through the flow cell by a *sheath syringe* to ensure consistent flow of the fluid. The sheath fluid, traveling through the flow cell, completely covers all of the inner surfaces and leaves only a very narrow, open central channel for the diluted sample to pass through. The diluted specimen is pulled through this central channel in the middle of the flow cell by the *RBC/baso sample syringe* in a very thin stream (20 to 40 μm in diameter), which allows only one cell at a time to pass in front of the *laser beam* (Fig. 7–24). The constant pressure of the sheath stream, the constant velocity of both the sample and sheath streams, and the uniform internal diameter of the flow cell (250 μm) combine to provide a sample flow that is without turbulence or hydraulic fluctuation. This process is known as *laminar flow*. A laser is located on one side of the flow cell. As a cell or particle passes in front of this beam it is counted by a light scatter detector using two different gain settings, one for red cells and the second for platelets. The red cells, because they have been sphered, will not fold over, and will be round in shape (sickled red cells may be the only exception). This enables the instrument to make a more accurate determination of the MCV. The volume of the red blood cells and platelets is measured by comparing the low angle and high angle light scatter created by each particle as it passes in front of the laser beam. The concentration of the hemoglobin in each red blood cell is also determined by scatter transformation from the laser. All of these informational signals are then converted into histogram plots, one for the RBC, one for hemoglobin concentration, and one for platelets.

WBC and Differential (Peroxidase Dilution)

The blood specimen is initially diluted 1:22 with Perox Dil 1 fluid and mixed in the *peroxidase reaction vessel*. During the first 20 seconds, the chamber is heated to 72° C which, with the reagent, causes lysis of the red blood cells and platelets. In addition, the white cells are dehydrated and fixed. For the next 13 seconds Perox Dil 2 and Perox Dil 3 (primary ingredient is 4-chloro-l-naphthol) fluids are added to the original dilution in the chamber, bringing about the following reaction in those white cells containing peroxidase (neutrophils, eosinophils, and monocytes):

H_2O_2 + 4-chloro-l-naphthol cellular

peroxidase → a dark precipitate

The lymphocytes, basophils, and large unstained cells contain no peroxidase and therefore do not stain. The white cell dilution, like the RBC/plt dilution, is surrounded by a layer of sheath fluid and passed through a flow cell for testing. This channel uses a *tungsten-based optical system* in place of the laser beam used for the red cells. A diaphragm pump pushes the Perox Sheath fluid toward the flow cell.

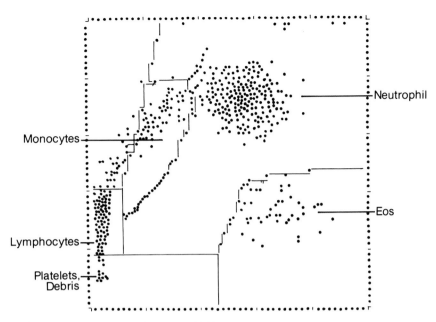

FIG. 7–25. WBC/peroxidase cytogram, Technicon H-1™.

The fluid is pulled through the cell by the sheath sample syringe. The sheath fluid leaves a narrow opening through the flow cell. The *perox sample syringe* pulls the diluted sample through the flow cell. The tungsten lamp is located on one side of the flow cell. As the cell passes through the beam of light, the stain intensity (absorbance) is measured, and the cell size determined (by use of forward light scatter). The individual impulses are counted to determine the white blood count. Peroxidase is contained in eosinophils, neutrophils, and monocytes in known amounts. The instrument uses this information, together with the cell size, to classify each of the cells. In this channel, the basophils are classified with the lymphocytes. A scattergram is constructed, plotting absorption vs. light scatter (Fig. 7–25).

Basophil/Lobularity Index

The whole blood sample is diluted with Baso/Lob Dil fluid and mixed in the *baso reaction vessel*. This fluid contains an acid that lyses the red blood cells and platelets, and ruptures the cytoplasm of all of the white cells (except basophils), thus freeing each cell nucleus. The baso/lob. dilution uses the same flow cell and laser beam as the RBC/plt. dilution, but uses

it at a different time during the test cycle. As in the RBC/plt. dilution, the same diaphragm pump and syringes move the sheath fluid and diluted sample through the flow cell. As each cell or nucleus pass in front of the laser beam, the light is scattered. Absorption and low and high angle light scatter are measured. The basophils are counted. A ratio of the signals is used to determine the degree of lobularity of the nuclei. This information is used to indicate the degree of left shift present. A scattergram is constructed, plotting high angle scatter versus low angle scatter (Fig. 7–26).

When the diluted samples leave the reaction vessels, each chamber is washed with rinse fluid. The diluted samples and the rinse solutions from the flow cells and hemoglobin cuvet travel to the waste chamber and, at the end of the cycle, exit the unit.

Test Reporting

A hematology report form may be placed in the VDT/ticket printer module at any time during the sample cycle. The numerical results will automatically print out at the end of each test. If the optional screen printer is attached to the system and programmed to print sample results, numerical results, histograms, and cytograms will automatically be

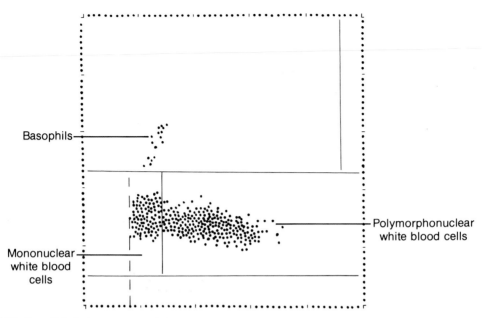

FIG. 7–26. Baso/lobularity cytogram, Technicon H-1™.

printed for each test sample. Several report formats are available from the H-2. These reports contain all numerical data. In addition, a variety of graphic plots may be selected in combination with the morphology flags, or the operator may choose to report the RBC cytogram (a cytogram plot of RBC volume vs. cellular hemoglobin concentration) instead of the morphology flags.

Result Flags

The flagging system may be divided into four categories: RBC size, RBC color, WBC, and other. The RBC size flags are for aniso, micro, and macro. These are determined by instrument analysis of the RDW and the red cell volume histogram. Flags for RBC color (hemoglobin concentration) are var (variation), hypo (hypochromia), and hyper (hyperchromia). These flags are determined by analysis of the HDW (hemoglobin distribution width [S.D. of the hemoglobin concentration histogram]) and the hemoglobin concentration histogram (distribution of hemoglobin in the RBC population). The WBC flags include left shift, atyp (atypical), and blasts. The left shift (unsegmented neutrophils) flag is derived from monitoring the

value for the LI (lobularity index) and analysis of the separation of mononuclear and polymorphonuclear populations in the baso/lobularity cytogram. The atyp flag is determined by evaluation of the values for the percent of LUCs (large unstained cells) obtained from the peroxidase channel and the percentage of blasts obtained from the baso/lobularity channel. The blast flag is determined by analysis of the same values used for atyp determination but meets different criteria to trigger the blast flag. Flags included in the "other" category are as follows: (1) NF H (no fit high) indicates that the WBC count in the peroxidase channel is too high for routine analysis; (2) NF L (no fit low) indicates that too few cells are present for analysis in the peroxidase channel (WBC <1,000/µL); (3) NF P (no fit peroxidase) indicates that >25% of the cells in the peroxidase channel cannot be classified; (4) Plt indicates a platelet count of <50,000/µL; (5) WBC indicates a white blood cell count of <1,000/µL or greater than 40,000/µL; (6) RBC indicates that the hemoglobin value is <7.0 g/dL; (7) ++ indicates that there are too few cells or too much noise in the baso/lobularity channel for reliable analysis; (8) IG (immature granulocytes) is determined by analysis of the promyelocyte, myelocyte, and metamyelocyte percentage of neutrophils and eosinophils obtained from the peroxidase channel, and the percentage of polymorphonuclear cells obtained from the baso/lobularity channel; (9) N indicates the possible presence of NRBC and/or other abnormal cell types. This flag is triggered when the separation between noise and the lymphocyte population on the peroxidase cytogram is less distinct than normal. It is also triggered when the sum of the neutrophil and eosinophil counts obtained from the peroxidase channel does not equal the polymorphonuclear cell count obtained from the baso/lobularity channel within specified limits.

In addition to morphology flags, asterisk errors may appear to alert the operator to certain questionable results due to sample abnormality or instrument malfunction. These errors may be triggered if data do not meet certain internal comparison requirements or if excessive noise is detected in an analysis channel. Error messages are displayed in the upper left corner of the CRT and alert the operator to various instrument malfunctions.

Video Display Functions

The top line on the video display screen is divided into three sections for messages: the *system message* area (left) alerts the operator to situations that require the operator's attention; *next sample* area (middle) indicates the next type of sample to be processed; and *system status* area (right) displays the status of the instrument. At the bottom of the screen, the last line is divided into five parts (F1 through F5). The display screen indicates the function for each of these, depending on the current video display. The line above the bottom line is divided into three sections: (1) *prompt* field (left) displays messages for operating the system, (2) *data entry* field (middle) displays operator-entered data, and (3) *entry error* field (right) displays errors of data entry by the operator.

The main portion of the video display screen enables the operator to view the list of system checks when the instrument is turned on, review test results as they are determined, troubleshoot problems, perform some maintenance procedures, store and review quality control data, calibrate, and set sample and control ranges. When the instrument is turned on a *List of System Checks* will be displayed, with an indication of Passed or Ready next to each if there are no problems. If there is a failure, it will be noted and the instrument will stop. During sample processing the *patient report* will be displayed on the screen. There are several different formats from which the operator may choose. If any sample results are flagged (marked by an asterisk), the operator may change the display to the *Asterisk Analysis Screen*, which will indicate the flagged problem.

The *main menu* is composed of five files:

1. *QC file* (F1) for input and review of control data, input of control limits, calibration, and calculation of control means and S.D.s.
2. *System setup* (F2) is divided into menu A and menu B. Menu A is used for starting up the instrument, setting desired options, and flagging ranges. Through menu B, the date and test units may be set, and laboratory computer interface settings may be changed.
3. *System status* (F3) is used for setting various aspects of the moving average Q.C. program, and for setting the test generator and printer automatically on or off, and contains settings for a laboratory computer.
4. *Hydraulics* (F4) function is used to perform maintenance procedures on the instrument.
5. The *utilities* (F5) function enables the operator to check various aspects of the instrument for troubleshooting problems.

Discussion

1. The batch size for the moving average may be set, within limits, by the individual laboratory. The parameters to be included may also be varied.
2. The Q.C. function will hold up to eight different controls plus a ninth control of whole blood.
3. Whole blood specimens are stable for testing for 24 hours when stored at room temperature (except for the MCV, which is stable for 8 hours, and the lobularity index [LI], which is stable for 6 hours). Refrigerated samples are stable for 54 hours (except for the MPV and LI, which are stable for less than 24 hours).

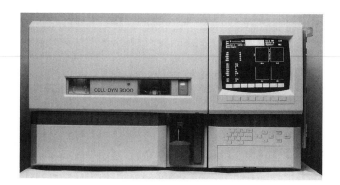

FIG. 7-27. Cell-Dyn 3000, Abbott Diagnostics. (Courtesy of Abbott Diagnostics, Mountain View, CA.)

4. The presence of a very high white count (>50,000/μL), or lipemia, will give falsely elevated hemoglobin readings.

5. Red cell agglutination may give an erroneous MCV and red cell count.

6. In the RBC dilution, sickled red cells may not become spherical and will give a falsely elevated RDW.

7. In patients with an elevated blood urea nitrogen (above 300 mg/dL) there may be incomplete lysis of the red cells in the WBC (peroxidase) dilution.

8. Differential results may be affected in patients showing a deficiency in peroxidase.

9. In some abnormal disorders (such as leukemia), some white cells, other than basophils, may be resistant to lysis in the baso/lob. dilution, which will cause a falsely elevated basophil count.

Cell-Dyn 3000/3000 SL

The Cell-Dyn 3000 is a 22 parameter automated hematology analyzer manufactured by Abbott Diagnostics. The instrument performs a complete blood count, RBC indices, RDW (RBC distribution width, a measure of anisocytosis), platelet count, MPV* (mean platelet volume), PDW* (platelet distribution width), PCT* (platelet hematocrit), and five part white blood cell differential (neutrophil, lymph, mono, eo., baso.).

The components of the Cell-Dyn 3000 (Fig. 7-27) are the analyzer module (1) and the data station module (2).

The *analyzer module* aspirates, dilutes, and

---

* Nonreportable test parameters.

counts the sample. The upper area of the analyzer houses the *helium neon laser* and *flow cytometer* used to differentiate white blood cells. Vacuum and pressure pumps, regulators, power supply, and electronics are also contained in this unit and control the operation of the analyzer itself.

The *data station module* contains the *video display screen, system computer,* and *keyboards* (6). The data station's video display and keyboards allow the operator access to seven operating menus, selectable from the main screen: The *setup menu* is used to insert or revise system operation settings. The *run menu* is used for testing patient samples and controls. In the *data menu* results from stored data may be accessed for reviewing and/or printing. Using the *QC logs menu* stored Q.C. data from any of the 21 Q.C. files may be reviewed and/or printed. The *calibration menu* is used to review or perform instrument calibration. The *diagnostics menu* is used for troubleshooting instrument problems. A *special protocols menu* is used when performing daily shutdown and cleaning procedures. The data station will store numerical results for the most recent 10,000 cycles, with complete graphic data available for the previous 2,000 cycles. Test results may be automatically transmitted from the data station module to a standard *graphics printer* to obtain a hardcopy printout of results and may also be directly sent to a host computer.

Sample Aspiration and Dilution

Blood samples may be aspirated in the closed sampler/cap piercer mode or the open sampler mode, or via the optional sample loader

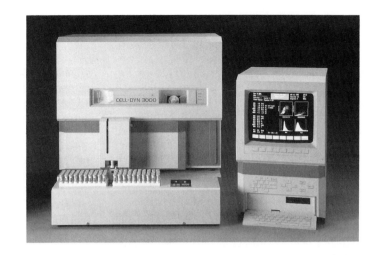

FIG. 7–28. Cell-Dyn 3000 SL, Abbott Diagnostics. (Courtesy of Abbott Diagnostics, Mountain View, CA.)

module (Cell-Dyn 3000 SL). The operator selects the aspiration mode on the data station using the run screen. (1) For *closed mode* aspiration, each sample is placed in the *closed sampler module* (3) by the operator. The *touch plate* is pressed to begin sample aspiration (270 µL). The closed sampler module contains a *holder* to accept the tube, a *tube retainer* to properly position the tube in the holder, and a *needle* that pierces the tube cap, vents vacuum or pressure within the tube, and then aspirates the sample into the *specimen shear valve*. (2) In the *open sampling mode*, the operator removes the specimen cap and holds the tube under the *open sample probe* (5). The *touch plate* is pressed to begin sample aspiration (175 µL). (3) The Cell-Dyn 3000 SL (sample loader) is equipped with a *sample loader* (Fig. 7–28). This unit attaches to the front of the analyzer module and is able to hold up to 100 sample tubes for testing. Specimen tubes are automatically forwarded to the testing area and mixed by high-speed counterrotation. While the tube is being mixed, a *laser scanner* reads the tube's bar code identification. The specimen is then aspirated (350 µL) in the same manner as used in the closed sampler non-automated method. Sample identification in the non-automated closed and open modes is performed by the operator using keyboard entry or by an optional hand-held bar code wand.

As the blood sample is aspirated into the instrument by the *sample aspiration pump* it enters the *specimen sheer valve*. This three piece valve isolates individual segments of whole blood in the center section as the front and rear sections rotate. The *RBC diluent dispense syringe* forces Isotonic Diluent through the specimen sheer valve, where it picks up a 0.64 µL segment of whole blood and sends it to the *RBC/plt transducer bath*. The final 1:12,500 dilution is used to count and size the red blood cells and platelets. In like manner, the *WBC sheath reagent syringe* forces Sheath Reagent through the specimen sheer valve to pick up a 32 µL segment of whole blood, which is transported to the *WBC mixing chamber*. This 1:51 dilution is used to count the white blood cells and to perform the five part white blood cell differential. The Sheath Reagent maintains the cellular integrity of the white blood cells (does not alter, fix, or stain the cells). Hemoglobin Reagent and Isotonic Diluent dilute a 12 µL segment (measured in the specimen sheer valve) of whole blood (1:250) for the hemoglobin determination. These reagents are dispensed by the *hemoglobin reagent dispense syringe* and the *hemoglobin diluent dispense syringe*, respectively, and transported through the specimen sheer valve to the *hemoglobin mixing chamber*.

Specimen Testing

Three channels are used for sample analysis. (1) The *impedance channel* for RBC and platelet testing, (2) the *laser channel* for the WBC and differential determinations, and (3) the *hemoglobin channel* for measurement of the hemoglobin concentration.

RBC and Platelet Count Measurements. The RBC and platelet counts are performed using electrical impedance. This method is based on the measurement of changes in electrical current produced by particles suspended in an isotonic diluent, as they pass through a sensing orifice. As particles pass through the orifice (60 μm by 70 μm), changes in the electrical current between electrodes (located on each side of the orifice) are produced. These changes in current are recorded as electrical pulses. The number and size of the pulses produced by the particles is directly proportional to the number and size of the particles (red blood cells or platelets). A red cell that does not pass through the orifice in a straight line will cause an alteration in the size of the pulse. These particles are included in the RBC count, but are not included in the RBC size determination. This exclusion (from the size determination) is called the *red cell editing ratio*. Occasionally, two or more particles will pass the sensing zone (through the orifice) simultaneously, causing the loss of one or more pulses. Because this loss of pulses, referred to as *coincidence passage loss*, is statistically predictable, the final red blood cell and platelet counts are automatically corrected for it.

A process called *volumetric metering* controls the volume of diluted specimen (100 μL) measured during each RBC/plt counting cycle. A *metering tube* (glass column) contains two optical detectors set 100 μm apart. The tube is used to determine the count time for the RBC and platelet measurements. Hemoglobin Reagent fills the metering tube at a constant rate. As the top of the reagent (the meniscus) passes the (optical path of the) first (start) detector on the metering tube, a voltage change occurs, which begins the counting cycle. When the top of the reagent (meniscus) reaches the top optical (or stop) detector, the resultant voltage change causes the counting cycle to end.

The RBC and platelet count and size data are used to create the RBC and platelet size distribution curves (histograms) (size [X-axis] vs. count [Y-axis]). The RDW (CV method [previously described under Coulter Counter section]) and MCV are determined from the RBC size distribution data. The hematocrit, MCH, and MCHC are calculated from RBC, MCV and hemoglobin values. Platelet parameters (the MPV, PDW, and PCT) are similarly derived from the platelet count and size distribution data.

WBC Measurements. The WBC dilution is transferred from the WBC mixing chamber to the *optical transducer sample feed nozzle* by the *WBC peristaltic pump*. The dilution is dispensed through this nozzle at a controlled low velocity into a high velocity stream of Sheath Reagent by the *WBC metering syringe*. This process, called *hydrodynamic focusing*, narrows the stream of diluted sample to a diameter of 25 to 30 μm, which causes the cells to pass single file through the sensing region of the *flow cell*.

A high resolution flow cytometer is used to count and classify (differentiate) the white blood cells. In addition to the traditional forward (0°) and side (90°) light scatter analysis used to characterize lymphocytes, monocytes and granulocytes, a *multi-angle polarized scatter separation (M.A.P.S.S.™)* is used to classify the white blood cells. This technology uses two additional scatter analyses: narrow angle (10°) (for basophil analysis) and 90° depolarized light (for eosinophil analysis). Various combinations of these four light scatter measurements are used to classify the white blood cells (as neutrophils, lymphocytes, monocytes, eosinophils, and basophils) and to provide morphologic flagging. Each cell is characterized by the four specific angles of light scatter. The light source is a polarized helium-neon laser with a wavelength of 632.8 nm. The laser is positioned so that the plane of polarization is vertical. As light passes from the laser to the flow cell, it is shaped and focused to provide a wide beam of uniform intensity, which is focused onto the center of the flow cell. White blood cells passing through the flow cell scatter the light in all directions. Two photodetectors measure low angle scatter (0° and 10°). These are plotted on the X and Y axis of a scatterplot and are relative indicators of cell size (0°) and complexity (structure) (10°). Lymphocyte, monocyte, basophil, and neutrophil-eosinophil populations are obtained from these light scatter measurements. Two photomultipliers detect polarized and depolarized (90°) light scatter. Eosinophils are separated from other cells by computerized analysis of this scatter. A second plot of polarized (X axis) versus depolarized (Y axis) 90° scatter is made. In this plot the eosinophils fall above the other cell types because their granules depolarize more light than the granules of other cells. Because monocytes and lymphocytes contain few if any granules, they are positioned to the left of the neutrophils on the same scatterplot.

The accumulated data from the four angles of light scatter are analyzed to determine the five white blood cell subpopulations. The white blood cell count and percentages of each cell type are determined from the test data. Two WBC histograms are constructed, plotting cell count and size data. WBC 1 histogram displays lymphocyte, basophil, and monocyte data. WBC 2 histogram displays mononuclear and polymorphonuclear data. These histograms are accessible on the data station display screen.

Hemoglobin Measurement. The hemoglobin concentration of the sample is determined by the hemiglobincyanide (cyanmethemoglobin) method. A zero (reagent blank) reference is obtained spectrophotometrically during each cycle when the hemoglobin flow cell is rinsed with hemoglobin reagent. Five separate readings are made on the test dilution (at 540 nm) for the final hemoglobin determination.

Interpretive Report. An interpretive report is displayed by the data station module, and a printed copy may be obtained. There are seven areas of displayed information: (1) specimen identification, (2) date and time of specimen run, (3) white blood cell count and differential results (expressed as absolute numbers and as percentages), (4) scatterplots (WBC1 and WBC2) and histograms (RBC and platelet), (5) red cell parameters, (6) platelet results, and (7) alert messages (flags). Alert messages will appear on the interpretive report if analysis of the test data indicates an abnormality. Flags are determined by computer software and are not operator-adjustable. There are five categories: (1) *Diff alert* indicates an abnormality of the 0° versus 10° scatterplot, (2) *Morphology alert* suggests the possible presence of bands, immature granulocytes, blasts, or variant lymphocytes (Fig. 7–29), (3) A *WBC count alert* will occur if the white blood cell count is suspect, (4) the *RBC alert* indicates possible abnormal red blood cell morphology as indicated by analysis of

the RDW, MCV, and/or MCH results, and (5) The *platelet alert* suggests interference with the separation of particles at the lower and/or upper floating size thresholds of the platelet distribution curve. The presence of any alert message is an indication to the operator that further review of the results is required.

Discussion

After a sample is aspirated in the open sampler mode, the sample probe is retracted and rinsed (inside and out) with Isotonic Diluent prior to being extended for the next sample. When the closed sample mode is selected the open mode sampler probe retracts. Isotonic diluent is also used to rinse the closed sampler needle.

Status and indicator lights on the front of the analyzer inform the operator of "ready," "busy," or "fault" status of the instrument. When a fault exists, an informative message will appear on the data station's run screen (such as "diluent empty").

Specimen testing may be performed at the rate of 100 samples per hour.

BLOOD SMEAR PREPARATION AND STAINING

Miniprep® Automatic Blood Smearing Instrument

The Geometric Data Miniprep® automatic smear maker (Fig. 7–30) prepares wedge smears of consistently good quality. The instrument is portable, light in weight, and is small enough to be carried to an outpatient clinic or to the patient's bedside.

Principles of Operation

A slide is firmly seated in each *tray* with the labeled end at the front of the tray. Using a nonheparinized microhematocrit tube (or capillary pipet), a small drop of blood is placed over the *target area* (black dot on front of the tray). (The size of the drop is critical to good smear preparation.) The lever is pressed down with a smooth, gentle stroke and released as soon as it reaches the bottom position. As the lever is pressed down, the spreaders move forward until reaching the

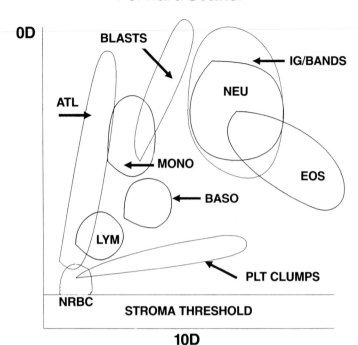

Forward Scatter

FIG. 7–29. Population locations, Cell-Dyn 3000, Abbott Diagnostics. (Courtesy of Abbott Diagnostics, Mountain View, CA.)

target area, where the *spreader blades* come in contact with the drop of blood. They hesitate momentarily to allow the blood to spread along the edge of the respective blades and then return to their original position, pulling the blood along each slide. The prepared smears are removed from the tray and allowed to air dry.

Discussion

1. The thickness of the smear may be changed by adjusting the *smear control knob* to alter the speed with which the blood is pulled across the slide. For thin smears (to increase speed), turn the knob clockwise (to the right), and for thicker smears (to decrease speed), turn the knob counterclockwise (to the left).
2. The width of the smear may be changed using the *pause control adjuster* (located underneath the instrument). This is accomplished by varying the amount of time the spreader is in contact with the drop of blood before the smear is pulled. To increase this time (increase the width of the

smear), turn the screw clockwise. To decrease, turn the screw counterclockwise. This adjustment is factory-set and generally does not need to be changed. The pause time should be exactly 1 second.
3. Spreader blades must be replaced if they become chipped. To replace a spreader blade, remove the protective backing from the tape on the spreader. Lift the *spreader holder* and place the blade in the slot, making certain the polished (spreading) edge

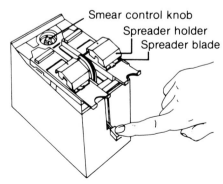

FIG. 7–30. Miniprep® automatic smear maker.

faces upward. Carefully place the blade in the center of the slot (sticky side against the lid).

4. A blood smear that is too long indicates too large a drop of blood, a very low hematocrit, and/or too thin a blood smear; specimen carryover to the next sample may be increased. Short smears indicate a very high hematocrit, a thick smear, and/ or too little blood. If most of the blood remains in the target area, the drop of blood was placed too far back on the slide. If the smear is streaked or uneven, the spreader blades may be dirty or damaged, or the slide may be dirty.

5. If one smear is prepared on each patient, only one tray should be used. Place a slide on the unused tray. It is not necessary to place a blade in this spreader holder.

6. Reticulocyte smears may also be prepared on this instrument. The smear control knob may need to be adjusted for these smears.

7. There may be carry-over of cells from one smear to the next in the amount of 0.5% or less. The spreader blades must be kept clean and washed periodically, especially when an excessive amount of blood has been placed on a slide. Clean the spreaders with 0.85% sodium chloride (w/v).

Hemaspinner Automatic Blood Cell Spinner

The Geometric Data Hemaspinner (Fig. 7–31) is used to prepare a monolayer film of whole blood on a glass slide.

Principles of Operation

The *power light* on the front panel, when lit, indicates that the instrument is on. For smear preparation, a clean glass slide is inserted into the grooves of the *platen*, and three to four drops of blood are placed on the middle of the slide (a drop the size of a quarter). The top of the instrument is closed immediately and held down firmly. The *spin light* will go on as soon as the platen (with slide) begins spinning. During the spin cycle, a beam of light (*spin light*) from the *light source* (located beneath the *catch basin*) passes up through the slide onto the *optical sensor* (located in the lid). When the cells have separated to the proper

degree the light hitting the optical sensor attains a specific intensity that signals the platen to stop spinning. (In this manner, spreading of the blood is generally consistent from one smear to the next, irrespective of the hematocrit.) While spinning, excess blood thrown from the slide is collected in the catch basin. At the conclusion of spinning, the spin light shuts off, indicating that the lid may be raised and the slide removed. The smear is ready for staining as soon as it is dry.

The *mode switch* contains settings that allow the instrument to be run in the automatic mode, as described above, or in the manual mode, where the spin time may be set by the operator using the *spin setting knob*. The optical sensing system is checked using the test mode setting.

Discussion

1. To obtain consistently well prepared smears, it is necessary to keep the Hemaspinner clean at all times. After every 25 to 30 slides, or whenever the glass shield covering the optical sensor is splashed with blood, the catch basin should be removed and washed and the optical system cleaned.

2. The Hemaspinner contains an aerosol removal system. During the spinning process, a positive airflow is created which travels through a duct in the back of the spin chamber and into a submicron filter.

3. The lid gasket should be changed at least once every 3 months, any time it appears to be damaged, or when improper sealing occurs.

Hemastainer Automatic Slide Stainer

The Geometric Data Hemastainer (Fig. 7–32) is an automated slide stainer that may also be operated manually if a mechanical breakdown occurs.

Principles of Operation

Staining solutions are prepared fresh each day, or every 4 to 8 hours during operation, depending on the stain used. *Station #1* contains methanol (500 mL) for fixing the

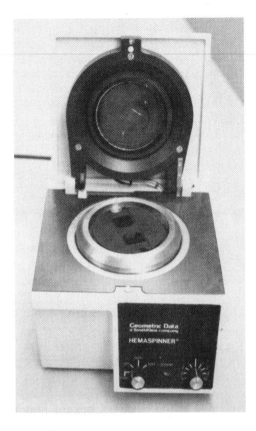

FIG. 7–31. Hemaspinner.

smears. Wright (or Wright-Giemsa) stain (500 mL) is placed in *station #2*, while a stain-buffer mixture (80 mL Wright or Wright-Giemsa stain plus 420 mL phosphate buffer) is in *station #3*, where the major staining occurs. Deionized water (1 L) is placed in the pump tank (*station #4*) for rinsing the slides. The final rinse cycle takes place at *station #5*, which contains phosphate buffer (500 mL). Warm air circulates in *station #6*.

The *power switch* on the instrument is set in the on position and sample slides are placed in the *staining basket* (capable of holding up to 50 slides), with the thickest end of the smear up (a small portion at the top of the slide will not be immersed in the solutions). The stain basket is attached to the *basket hanger* over station # 1 and the screw tightened. For automated staining the *right/left switch* is set on left, the *swing switch* to on, and the *pump switch* to auto. The covers are removed from all solutions and the staining process begun by setting the *auto/manual switch* to auto. The staining basket descends into the first solution (methanol at station #1), where it will remain for 10 to 15 seconds. The basket then moves up out of the methanol and over to station #2 (stain) for 2 minutes. It then travels to the stain-buffer mixture, where it remains for 5 minutes. It rinses in deionized water, which is circulated between station #4 and the *pump tank* by the *recirculating pump assembly* (in the pump tank) through *water rinse hoses* for 20 seconds. It then moves to the buffer solution (station #5) for 1 minute. When rinsing is complete a buzzer sounds and the stain basket is moved

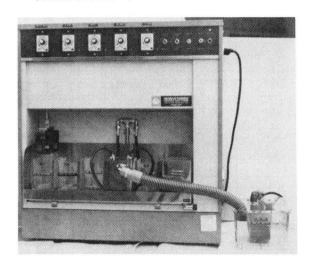

FIG. 7–32. Hemastainer automatic slide stainer.

to *station #6*, where forced warm air is circulated for drying. The slides should remain in this area for a minimum of 3 minutes, at which time the operator must set the auto/manual switch to manual in order to stop the cycle. The basket lifts out of the drying station and moves automatically to the left, where it will stop and remain over station #1 until the next staining cycle is started. The hanger screw is loosened and the stain basket, containing the dry stained smears, is removed from the instrument.

For manual operation the stain reagents and rinse remain the same. The deionized water rinse (station #4) is eliminated. Slides are placed in the staining rack and the rack is manually placed in station #1 for 2 to 3 seconds. Methanol is drained from the rack and then placed in station #2 for 2 minutes, after which the excess stain is drained from the rack and it is placed in the stain-buffer mixture for 5 minutes. During this process the staining rack is not agitated. To rinse the smears, the rack is dipped about 20 times (1 minute) in the phosphate buffer (station #5), and the smears are allowed to air dry.

There is one *station timer* for each station (except the drying area), which is used for setting the time intervals at each station in the automatic staining mode. Fixing, staining, rinsing, and drying takes approximately 12 minutes from start to finish. The fixing (station #1) and stain (station #3) solutions should be covered when the stainer is not in use.

Discussion

1. If the purple stain is too intense (nuclei very dark purple), dilute the Wright's stain in station #2 with methanol.

Hema-Tek® 1000 Slide Stainer

The Hema-Tek® 1000 slide stainer (Miles, Inc., Diagnostics Division) provides an automated method for Wright (or Wright-Giemsa) staining blood films. (See Fig. 7–33.)

Principles of Operation

When the *stain-pak* (stain, buffer, and rinse solutions) is first opened, each bottle is vented by making a small hole in the container at the top. A *cannula* (long, pointed needle) is inserted into each solution and the tip pushed all the way to the bottom of the stain-pak. A *pump tube set* (tubing) is installed to transport the solutions from the stain-pak. The #1 tubing is attached to the stain cannula, #2 to the buffer cannula, and #3 to the rinse cannula. The tubing is installed through its respective *solution pump* and attached to the appropriate fitting on the back of the *circuit board* (on which the operating level and stain lights are located). *Under platen tubing* (three lines) is installed from the back of the circuit board to the appropriate spout under the platen and carries the solutions to the staining area (*platen*). The *circular level* beneath the lid of the instrument is set so that the bubble is centered. This is accomplished by adjusting the *levelers* located at the bottom front at each end of the stainer.

The instrument is turned on using the *operating lever*. The *on light* should then be lit. The solution lines are filled by placing the operating lever in the *prime* position until all three solutions emerge through the openings on the platen. When there is a sufficient volume of solution in the stain-pak the *stain light* will be lit. When the amount of reagent is insufficient to stain 20 slides this light will turn off.

Prior to staining, the platen is cleaned by flooding with methanol and wiping dry (from right to left) with soft gauze. To begin the staining process, up to 25 slides are placed vertically, on their side with the smear facing left, into opposing grooves of the *conveyor spirals*. As the spirals turn, the slide is moved along toward the staining portion of the platen. When the first slide reaches the platen the conveyor spirals allow the slide to advance to a face-down position. The platen is constructed so that there is a very small space between the underside of the slide and the top of the platen. As the slide moves along this platform, the edge of the slide triggers the *stain sensing switch* (located above the back edge of the platen, underneath the *circuit board cover*) when the slide is over the stain outlet hole in the platen. This activates the stain pump sequence and a pre-set volume of stain fills the capillary space between the slide and the platen. The slide, with the stain moves along at a specific speed to the *buffer sensing switch*. During this time the smear is

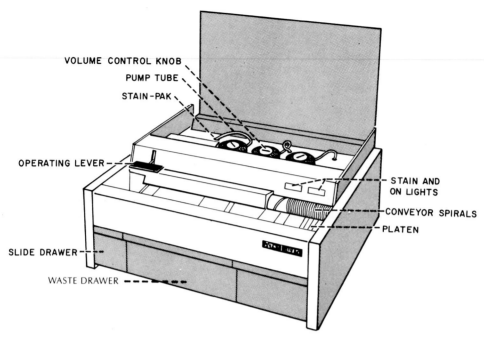

FIG. 7–33. Hema-Tek® 1000 Slide Stainer.

fixed. Buffer emerges from the outlet hole in the platen and, by means of the grooves in the platen, mixes with the stain already under the slide. The smear (with the stain and buffer mixture) moves along the platen, during which time staining of the smear occurs. When the slide reaches the end of the platen, the stain-buffer mixture is drained into the *waste drawer* if an outside waste line is not used. The slide comes in contact with the *rinse sensing switch*, which turns on. The slide is rinsed, dried by a stream of air, and allowed to drop into the *slide drawer*, which will hold up to 100 slides.

Discussion

At least once per hour, the stain tubing should be rinsed well in methanol. Prior to performing this procedure, remove the buffer and rinse cannulas from their respective containers.

The pump tubing sets should be changed after the use of three stain paks. The under-platen tubing may be changed every 10 stain paks, except for the stain tubing, which may need to be changed every four stain paks depending on how often methanol is used to clean the stain lines.

If the sensing switches become bent or out of position, refer to the operator's manual for the repositioning procedure.

Three *volume control knobs* are located on the solution pumps for altering the volumes delivered to each slide. The amount of solution delivered is increased by turning the control knob clockwise, and decreased by turning the knob counterclockwise.

Hema-Tek® 2000 Slide Stainer

The Hema-Tek® 2000 slide stainer (Fig. 7–34) (Miles, Inc., Diagnostics Division) uses the same principles of operation as the Hema-Tek® 1000. The major difference between the two instruments is the improved staining system made possible by new pumps and volume controls, which allow the operator to electronically adjust the stain, buffer, and rinse reagents. The platen mixing grooves have also been newly designed.

Guidelines for Obtaining Optimal Staining

For well-stained blood smears, proper stain: buffer ratio (1:2 to 1:3), a clean platen, and proper functioning of the sensing switches

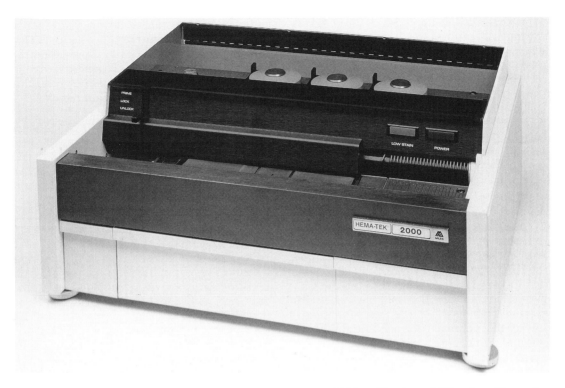

FIG. 7–34. Hema-Tek 2000 Slide Stainer, Miles, Inc., Diagnostics Division. (Courtesy of Miles, Inc., Diagnostics Division.)

are of utmost importance. Very small changes in the stain:buffer ratio will result in lighter or darker staining. If staining is not acceptable, the following procedure may be used to check the system.

All tubing should be replaced: pump tubing and underplaten tubing. The platen is cleaned using methanol and a soft material. The area should be wiped in the same direction the slide travels (from right to left). The platen grooves are carefully cleaned using methanol and cotton tipped applicators. The leveling bulb is centered to ensure that the stainer is level. Each solution bottle in the stain pak is checked to make certain it is properly vented.

The sensing switches are checked to ensure they are turning on at the proper time. Stain should emerge from the platen when the slide has moved half-way across the stain orifice. Buffer should be released when about 1/8 inch of the slide has moved across the buffer orifice.

When the stain and buffer volume control knobs are at the 0 setting (mid-way between

−2 and +2) the stain:buffer ratio is approximately 1:2.5. To check proper reagent amounts, prime instrument and run a minimum of five blank slides. The stain knob should be adjusted so that the stain *just fills* the area between the slide and platen (with no overflow). (Increase amounts by turning knob clockwise, decrease by turning knob counterclockwise.) Ignore any small air holes that occur in the area *after* filling. When at least two slides have filled properly, check the buffer volume. As the slide moves across the buffer outlet and the mixing grooves, it should appear *underfilled* because of the increased area under the slide (mixing grooves are recessed on the platen). The buffer should appear to pulse out from the orifice onto the platen. Too much buffer will reduce this pulsing action, and complete flooding of the second groove indicates too much stain or buffer. When the slide reaches the smooth area of the platen, the stain-buffer mixture should just fill the capillary space under the slide.

The rinse solution contains a small amount of methyl alcohol for quick drying. Excess rinsing will cause some fading of the stain, whereas inadequate rinsing may leave stain precipitate on the slide. Approximately 1 mL of rinse solution (0 setting on the volume control) is needed to adequately wash the slides. Stained smears should be checked to determine the correct rinse setting.

Once the stain, buffer, and rinse volumes have been set to give well stained smears, the stain:buffer ratio should be determined. (This may be used as a reference for troubleshooting future problems.) Disconnect the underplaten tubing from the spouts on the platen. Prime all lines (catch reagents from the lines in a beaker). Place the stain and buffer lines into separate 10 mL graduated cylinders, and the rinse line into a 25 mL graduated cylinder. Process 10 clean slides through the stainer (all reagents will empty into their respective cylinders). At the end of staining, record the volumes of each solution. The stain:buffer ratio is calculated as

$$1: \frac{\text{buffer volume}}{\text{stain volume}}$$

The amount of each reagent per slide is obtained by dividing the total volume in each graduated cylinder by 10. The rinse volume should be approximately 1.0 mL.

Each two increments (e.g., 0 to +2) on the stain and buffer volume control knobs will change the volume by approximately 0.01 mL/slide, whereas the same setting will change the rinse volume by 0.05 mL/slide.

Once set, the stain:buffer ratio should not need to be changed very frequently if the instrument is kept clean and well cared for. The above procedure is also applicable to the Hema-Tek 1000® using the volume control knobs on the pumps.

RETICULOCYTE TESTING

Sysmex R-1000

The Sysmex R-1000 is an automated reticulocyte analyzer manufactured by TOA Medical Electronics Co., Ltd. This instrument uses flow cytometry to determine the reticulocyte count (percentage and absolute number). In addition, the technology used by the R-1000 allows for the determination of three stages of reticulocyte maturity: the low fluorescence ratio (LFR), middle fluorescence ratio (MFR), and high fluorescence ratio (HFR). The reaction phase of the count cycle produces cells that are fluorescently labeled. The intensity of the fluorescence is a function of the cell's nucleic acid content. The greater the fluorescence, the greater a cell's RNA/DNA content. The greater the RNA/DNA content, the less mature the cell. Reticulocytes classified in the LFR group show the least amount of RNA/DNA and are the most mature reticulocytes, the MFR cells are of intermediate RNA content and maturity, and the HFR cells have the greatest RNA/DNA content and are the least mature reticulocytes. The LFR, MFR, and HFR values may be used as an addition to the reticulocyte count to monitor a patient's erythropoietic activity (red blood cell production). A decreased reticulocyte count (near 100% LFR value) represents aplasia (lack of red cell production), whereas a rise in the reticulocyte count (with an increase in the percentage of HFR cells) indicates a return of erythropoietic activity (regeneration of red blood cells).

The R-1000 (Fig. 7–35) consists of the *main unit* (1) with a built-in *data processing unit* (*DPU*), a *laser power unit* (2), and a *pneumatic unit* (3). Optional components of the R-1000 are the *autosampler* (4) with a *bar code reader*, *graphic printer* (5), and *data printer* (6).

The main unit has three subsystems: (1) the *hydraulic system*, which aspirates and dilutes the sample, mixes the diluted specimen with dye, and forms the sheath flow, (2) the *optical system*, which contains the *argon laser*, and (3) the *electronic system*, which converts optical data for analysis and output to the DPU and printers. The DPU displays results for the latest sample analyzed and informs the operator of instrument analysis status via one of 19 status messages such as Ready, Not Ready, Autorinsing, and QC Ready. The R-1000 has a self monitoring capability that alerts the operator to abnormalities in the instrument by displaying an error message on the *DPU screen*. The DPU enables the operator to enter sample identification numbers, and allows data to be processed, stored, and transmitted to external printers or a host computer. Up to 500 sample results may be retained in Stored Data. The QC program has four files,

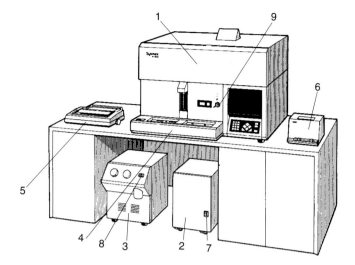

FIG. 7-35. Sysmex R-1000. (Courtesy of TOA Medical Electronics Corp., Ltd.)

each capable of storing up to 60 data points, which may be retrieved as individually run values or in chart form.

The *laser Power Unit* supplies the main unit with power for the *argon laser* (Light Amplification by Stimulated Emission of Radiation) *light source*.

The *pneumatic unit* provides the vacuum and pressures necessary for the operation of the main unit's hydraulic system.

The *sampler unit* eliminates the need for hand aspiration of samples and allows specimens to be automatically mixed, aspirated, and analyzed, and allows results to be stored in the DPU. It accommodates up to five racks of 10 samples each. A pen type *bar code reader* is available for use with the sampler unit.

The *data printer* functions as a ticket printer, and the *graphic printer* provides a hard copy printout of numerical and scattergram results.

Aspiration of Sample

Rocker switches (7, 8) are pressed to turn on the laser and pneumatic units, and the main unit is powered on by turning the *key switch* (9). The R-1000 will automatically perform a series of self-check tests, a laser warm-up and stabilization, an autorinse, and a background count. To aspirate samples in the automode the opened specimen tubes are placed in the sample rack on the right side of the sampler unit. ID and rack position numbers are entered into the DPU. The *sampler switch* on the

sampler unit is pressed and the rack is automatically forwarded to the *measurement line*, where it is moved to the left, one sample tube distance at a time. The *blood volume sensor* checks for an adequate amount of blood (sample height must be greater than, or equal to, 5 mm to be detected by the sensor). The volume of blood must be between 0.5 mL and 4.0 mL depending on the diameter of the test tube. If adequate sample is present, the *mixer paddle* is lowered into the first tube, where it rotates to mix the sample. (If sample volume is insufficient, testing will not be performed on the specimen.) After the first sample is mixed, the rack moves one position to the left. The *sample aspiration pipet* and mixer are lowered into tubes #1 and #2 where they are aspirated and mixed respectively.

Manual mode analysis is performed by first entering the sample ID number into the DPU. The sample aspiration pipet is inserted into the tube of well-mixed whole blood. The *start switch* is pressed and the *aspiration light* above the switch lights. When an audible triple beep is heard and the aspiration light goes out, the tube is removed.

Dilution of Sample

The specimen is drawn up through the *sample rotor valve* (SRV), which consists of left and right fixed sections and a center rotating piece. The SRV operates in four sequences: (1) the *whole blood sample aspiration syringe* aspirates 100 μL of whole blood through the

SRV; (2) the center section of the SRV rotates clockwise, and the 10 μL of whole blood sample in the center section is lined up with the diluent ports of the left and right sections of the SRV; (3) the *diluent syringe* forces the 10 μL blood sample and 1.95 mL of Retsearch diluent through the SRV to the *reactor chamber*, which is housed in the *reactor block*; (4) the center section of the *SRV* rotates counterclockwise to its initial position and the *sample aspiration line* is rinsed with sheath reagent by action of the whole blood aspiration syringe. The *rinse cup* is supplied with sheath reagent to automatically rinse the aspirator pipet and mixer paddle.

Reticulocyte Staining

The *dye syringe* adds 40 μL of Retsearch dye to the reactor chamber containing the diluted sample. (Retsearch dye contains auramine-O, a nucleic acid specific dye that binds to RNA.) The sample, now at a final dilution of 1:200, is mixed, incubated at 35°C, and allowed to react in the temperature controlled reactor chamber for 25 seconds. The reaction of cells with dye results in fluorescently labeled cells (auramine-O is bound to RNA and DNA present in the blood cells).

Reticulocyte Counting

The *sheath flow syringe* injects the diluted, fluorescently labeled sample into the *sheath flow line*, where it is then forced through the *sample tube* by the *sample sheath syringe*. It enters the center of the *flow cell* from the *sample tube* through the *sample nozzle* mounted in front of the flow cell. As the sample passes through the flow cell, it is hydrodynamically focused (surrounded by a sheath of particle-free fluid and directed, one cell at a time, through the center of the flow cell). The cells are analyzed by *flow cytometry*, which combines the use of hydrodynamic focusing and optical light scatter characteristics to identify and count cells (Fig. 7–36). (After the sample passes through the flow cell it is directed by the sheath reagent into the catcher tube. [This channelling of cells into the catcher tube eliminates recirculation of cells through the sheath flow cell.]) As each cell passes through the flow cell it is illuminated by an argon laser (light source) at a wavelength of 488 nm. The cell scatters the light in all directions, and the fluorescent tags on the cell (auramine-O bound nucleic acids) become energized (excited). Each cell scatters the light at an angle proportional to its volume and structural features. Forward light scatter (180° from the light source) is an indicator of cell size, whereas side fluorescence (90° from the light source) is a measure of the RNA/DNA content. *Collector lenses* focus the forward scatter and side fluorescence. Forward scatter passes to a *photodiode* (detector), which converts the optical light scatter signals to electrical signals. Side fluorescence is directed through a *wavelength selection filter*, which detects light from the energized fluorescent molecules in each cell. A *photomultiplier* (detector) converts the optical side fluorescence signals to electrical signals. The electrical signals from both forward scatter data and side fluorescence data are passed into the main unit's *microprocessor*, where these signals are converted into digitized information. The DPU screen displays this information on a scattergram plotting fluorescence (X axis) against forward scatter (Y axis). The scattergram is divided into three major areas (RBC, reticulocytes, platelets) by two floating discriminators (Fig. 7–37). A discriminator line is placed between the RBC/reticulocytes and the platelets at the area of lowest (particle) density. A second discriminator line is located between the RBC and reticulocytes. (These are floating discriminators and will be placed differently for each specimen, depending on areas of lowest particle density, which is determined by particle volume, counts, and degree of fluorescence.) The reticulocyte percentage (Ret %) is then determined from this scattergram. The absolute reticulocyte count (Ret #) is calculated from the red blood cell count and the reticulocyte percentage (RBC × Ret %). The reticulocyte area is further subdivided by invisible discriminators into the three equal sections previously described (LFR, MFR, HFR), based on the degree of fluorescence. There is also a fourth and a fifth area of fluorescence beyond the HFR, which is not displayed on the scattergram. The fourth area is termed the Upper Particle Plateau (UPP) and is to the right of the HFR region, where the cells of higher fluorescence are contained (stress reticulocytes, nucleated RBC, and RBC containing Howell-Jolly bodies). The fifth

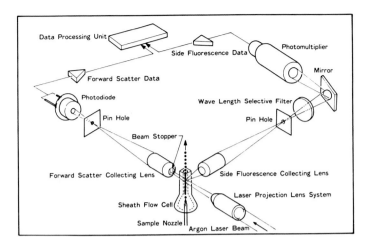

FIG. 7–36. Optical light scatter of the R-1000, (Courtesy of TOA Medical Electronics Corp., Ltd.)

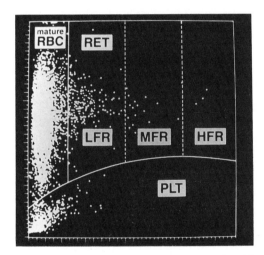

FIG. 7–37. Forward scatter intensity vs intensity of fluorescence, Sysmex R-1000. (Courtesy of TOA Medical Electronics Corp., Ltd.)

area, to the right of the UPP section, contains all WBC (highly fluorescent). Results (Ret % and #, LFR, MFR, and HFR) print on the graphic and/or data printers.

Discussion

The R-1000 analyzes a diluted sample volume of 2.78 μL. Approximately 32,000 of the total cells counted during the 7 second counting cycle are displayed on the scattergram.

K. Wanatabe (R-1000 Automated Reticulocyte Analyzer, Reports on the Clinical Utility) gives normal ranges for the reticulocyte counts as:

Ret % = 0.8–2.2%
Ret # = 31.5–108.8 × 10^6 μL
LFR % = 85.7–97.3%
MFR % = 3.6–14.7%
HFR % = 0.1–1.4%

Stress reticulocytes contain greater amounts of RNA than normal reticulocytes. These cells, because of their resultant higher fluorescence, will fall to the right of the HFR region and will therefore not be counted in the reticulocyte percentage or number. This is advantageous because it is usually not desirable to include these cells in a reticulocyte count (because of the fact that they are present in the blood for several days). In the manual count, when these cells are present, a "corrected" reticulocyte count (Reticulocyte Production Index %) is calculated. Elimination of these cells from the reticulocyte count is a more accurate reflection of true erythropoietic activity.

Iron containing granules (siderocytes, Pappenheimer bodies) have no affinity for the fluorescent dye used in this test. Their presence will therefore not affect results.

Basophilic stippling (aggregates of RNA) will stain with the auramine-O as they do with the manual reticulocyte dyes. These cells will therefore be counted in both procedures.

Howell-Jolly bodies will stain with auramine-O. However, they bind much larger amounts of the dye than reticulocytes and will fall in the region beyond the HFR area and will not be counted in this procedure. They are generally not as easily discernible in the manual procedure.

Platelets contain RNA and are differentiated in this procedure by their size (forward light scatter). However, clumped or giant platelets may be counted as reticulocytes. Therefore, when the discrimination between platelets and reticulocytes becomes indistinct, the instrument will show a platelet discrimination error. It may then be advisable to perform a manual reticulocyte count. Because of the wide range of error in the manual count, however, the R-1000 may still reflect a more accurate count.

In the presence of cold agglutinins (clumping of red blood cells), there may be an increase in fluorescence because of the additive effects of the clumped red cells. This will cause the red cells to fall in the reticulocyte region of the scattergram. In these instances, manual counts may be performed, or the blood sample may be warmed prior to testing. Given the poor precision of manual reticulocyte counts this latter procedure may be preferred.

Reporting the absolute reticulocyte count is advantageous over reporting the reticulocyte percentage in that the count does not depend on the red blood count and does not have to be "corrected" for anemia.

A red blood cell count and a platelet count may also be obtained from this instrument (without histograms).

This instrument is also available with automatic bar code reading and sampling from the tube.

The newly released R-3000 reticulocyte analyzer automatically mixes, aspirates (via closed tube sampling), and performs reticulocyte counts on specimens as small as 100 μL. It also has bar code reading capabilities and is similar in function to the R-1000. Additional improvements include more compact instrumentation, more sensitive optics, and increased data processing functions.

ERYTHROCYTE SEDIMENTATION TESTING

Automated ESR System

The Automated ESR System by Vega Biomedical (Lincoln, RI and Brea, CA) is a fully automated instrument for measurement of the erythrocyte sedimentation rate (ESR). The blood specimen (1 mL) is collected in a special vacutainer tube containing liquid sodium citrate. This tube is compatible with the standard Vacutainer system. The filled, stoppered tube is placed in the Ves-Matic analyzer where it is automatically mixed, allowed to sediment, and read at the appropriate time. Results are reported to be comparable with the standard Westergren ESR procedure. Testing takes 22 minutes.

Three models of the Ves-Matic analyzer are available: The *Mini-Ves* tests four samples at one time and reports results on a display; the *Ves-Matic 20* (Fig. 7–38) processes up to 20 samples simultaneously and prints results; the *Ves-Matic 60* holds up to 60 samples at one time, may be interfaced with a host computer (both the 20 and 60 models), can be equipped with a bar code reader for sample identification, and will print final test results.

Principles of Operation (Ves-Matic 20)

The instrument is turned on by pressing the *power switch* located on the back of the unit, at which time a system check is performed. The date is entered by the operator using the *TM* and up and down *arrow* keys. The display reads "Ves-Matic Jr., Select Function." The *cover* of the Ves-Matic is opened and the specimens to be tested are removed from their collection holders and placed in the numbered slots on the *sample holder plate*. The instrument cover is replaced and the *F1* key is pressed followed by the *Run* key. (If an ESR corresponding to a 2 hour sedimentation rate is desired the *F2* key is pressed instead of the F1 key.) The display will indicate the F key pressed and an option to set the temperature mode on or off. (When the temperature is set in the on mode the Ves-Matic automatically makes the appropriate corrections to give ESR results as if the test had been performed at 18°C.) The testing time of 20 (minutes) (equivalent to a 1 hour ESR) or 40 (equivalent to a 2 hour ESR) is also displayed. The cycle number, function (F1 or F2), temperature setting (on or off), and date are then printed for that run of specimens.

The testing cycle is begun when the sample holder plate makes a 90° change in position, so that the sample tubes are almost horizontal. The plate containing the specimens begins a series of 360° rotations for the next 2

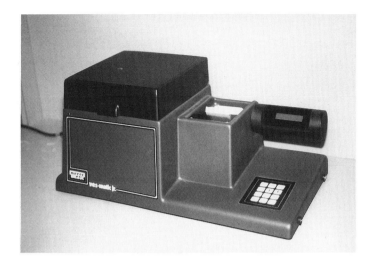

FIG. 7-38. Ves-Matic 20.

minutes in order to adequately mix the samples. At the end of the mixing period, the sample holder plate returns to its original position. A *movable carriage assembly* lifts the *optical reading assembly* into place to measure the level of blood in each tube. A photo-optical system is used to detect the opacity (nontransparency) of the blood. Improperly filled tubes (overfilled or underfilled) unsuitable for testing will also be detected at this time. The sample holder plate containing the tubes remains in place for the next 20 minutes, and the blood is allowed to sediment. At the end of this period a second reading is taken on each tube. (If F2 was pressed, a third reading will be taken 20 minutes after the second reading. This corresponds to the Westergren second hour ESR reading.)

As soon as the final reading is taken, the Ves-Matic analyzes the data and prints the ESR results. The printed report contains the sample plate holder number with the corresponding ESR result. If any tubes were improperly filled "****" will print in place of the result. Any sample plate holder spaces that did not contain a sample will be indicated by "Sample Absent" printed next to the holder number. Specimens with a hematocrit of 10% or lower cannot be tested using this system.

Discussion

The *keyboard* contains 12 keys for operator use: (1) Print, (2) Run, (3) Feed, used to advance the printer paper, (4) Test, used to perform a sensor test of the optical reading assembly, (5) TM, used to enter the date, (6) and for scanning data on the display, entering the date, and transforming results for temperature correction, (7) Reset, which will reset the instrument in case of error situations, (8) F1 and F2, which when pressed prior to Run determine the 20 or 40 minute test mode, (9) Stop, which will halt instrument function when pressed, and (10) Disp, which activates the display.

During the 20 (or 40) minute sedimenting period the tubes are held in the sample holder plate in a nonvertical position.

The sedimentation of the blood takes place in three stages: an initial delay, a period of linear sedimentation, and a level period.

The optical system should be checked daily using a standard cuvet supplied with the instrument.

Specimens should be tested as soon as possible after they are obtained, following the same guidelines used for the Western ESR procedures.

Coulter Zetafuge™

The zeta sedimentation ratio (ZSR) is a measurement similar to the erythrocyte sedimentation rate and is determined by use of the Coulter Zetafuge™ (Fig. 7–39).

Normally, red blood cells are negatively charged and repel each other. In the presence of an increased concentration of fibrinogen and/or gamma globulin, the net negative charge of the erythrocytes decreases, thus permitting an increase in rouleaux formation

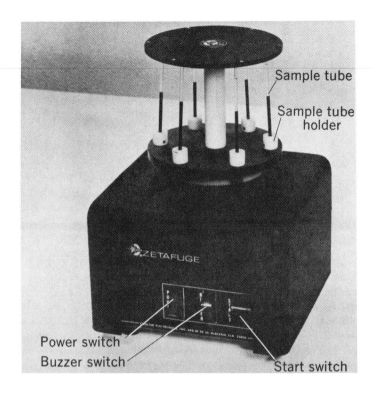

FIG. 7–39. Coulter Zetafuge. (Courtesy of Coulter Electronics, Inc., Hialeah, Florida.)

and a more rapid erythrocyte sedimentation rate.

Principles of Operation

A capillary *tube* (75 mm long with an inner diameter of 2.0 mm) is ¾ filled with well-mixed EDTA anticoagulated whole blood (approximately 0.2 mL). Each tube is closed at one end with a sealing clay to a depth of approximately 5 mm. The tubes are immediately placed into the *sample tube holder* in a vertical position so that the instrument is balanced. The *power switch* is pushed to the on position and the *buzzer switch* is also turned on. Both switches should light up indicating the on position. The *start switch* is then depressed to begin the spin cycle. The Zetafuge will revolve at a constant low speed for 45 seconds. During this time, the centrifugal force applied to the tube forces the red blood cells to migrate across the diameter of the tube to the outer wall, where rouleaux formation is accelerated. At the conclusion of the first 45 seconds, the Zetafuge stops and automatically rotates the capillary tube 180°. The Zetafuge restarts, and spins the tube for

a second 45-second period. The rouleaux formation (now on the inner wall) partially disperses, moves across the diameter of the tube, and reforms on the outer wall. The Zetafuge stops and rotates the tubes 180° a second and third time, thus allowing four 45-second centrifuge periods. Each time the rouleaux formation moves across the diameter of the tube, it sediments downward because of the force of gravity on the erythrocyte mass. At the conclusion of the 3 minute spin cycle the buzzer will sound. The operator switches the buzzer off, and immediately removes the sample tubes. The percentage of space occupied by the fallen red blood cells is measured. A mark may be made on each tube to indicate the level of sedimented red blood cells (Fig. 7–40) (the level to be read is termed the *knee* of the curve), or the tubes may be read immediately using a microhematocrit tube reader. The hematocrit (PCV) is determined for each sample and the ZSR ratio calculated:

$$\text{ZSR \%} = \frac{\text{Hematocrit \%}}{\text{Zetacrit \%}} \times 100$$

The ZSR, therefore, measures how close the red blood cells approach one another under

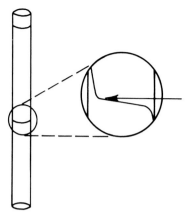

FIG. 7–40. Sedimented level of red blood cells.

a specific standardized stress. The packing of the red cells depends on their net negative charge, which in turn depends primarily on the concentration of fibrinogen and γ (gamma) globulin.

The ZSR takes approximately 4 minutes to perform and is unaffected by anemia. The normal range for the ZSR is 40 to 51% and is the same for both males and females. Values of 51 to 54% are considered to be borderline; 55 to 59%, mildly elevated; 60 to 64%, moderately elevated; and greater than 65%, markedly elevated.

Discussion

1. At least once/day, check that the mechanism which rotates the tubes 180° is operating satisfactorily. During a complete spin cycle of the instrument, observe the *speed indicator* (not shown) on one of the sample tube holders. This indicator should be pointed alternately in and out during the four-spin cycles.

COAGULATION TESTING

Fibrosystem® (Fibrometer®)

The FibroSystem® (BBL Microbiology Systems, Division of Becton Dickinson and Co.) is a semiautomated, electromechanical instrument for performing coagulation procedures. It consists of the *Fibrometer® coagulation timer* (Fig. 7–41), the *thermal prep block* (incubator) (Fig. 7–42), and an *automatic pipet*

(Fig. 7–43). The main unit is the Fibrometer, which contains a *timer*, several *warming wells*, and a clot detector (*probe arm* with *electrodes*). The thermal prep block plugs into the Fibrometer and contains additional *warming wells* for the *coagulation test cups* and several deeper incubation wells for heating larger amounts of reagent or plasma. The automatic pipet attaches to the Fibrometer, and when in the on position starts the timer when the *plunger* is depressed (expelling the contents of the pipet). It will dispense 0.1 or 0.2 mL aliquots, depending on the setting of the plunger. Most coagulation procedures that use a clot as their end point may be performed on this system.

Principles of Operation

The *pipet switch* is placed in the off position and the plunger completely depressed and turned to align the single notch (0.1 mL) or double notch (0.2 mL) with the *alignment indicator* on the pipet for the appropriate volume to be pipetted. The test reagent (or specimen/control plasma) is added to a disposable coagulation cup and placed in a warming well to heat to 37°C. When ready for testing the cup is placed in the *reactor well*. The pipet switch is placed in the on position. As soon as the sample (or reagent) is pipetted into the cup, the timing mechanism of the Fibrometer is activated (via the automatic pipet). (If the automated pipet is not used, the *timer bar* on the Fibrometer is depressed simultaneously as the sample (or reagent) is added to the cup in the reactor well. Within 0.5 to 1.8 seconds of instrument activation, the probe arm drops down, placing the electrodes into the reaction mixture. During testing, the *probe foot* (Figs. 7–44 and 7–45) rests on a segmented *cam* in the bottom of the Fibrometer. This cam is constantly rotating when the Fibrometer is activated. As it rotates, it moves the probe foot up and down in an elliptical pattern, causing the moving electrode to sweep through, up, and out of the mixture every 0.5 seconds. Because of the design of the cam, when the moving electrode is in the down position (Fig. 7–44) (immersed in the sample mixture), the probe foot is resting on the insulated portion of the cam and there is no electric current passing to the probe. When the cam rotates, and the probe foot comes in contact with the electrically active portion of

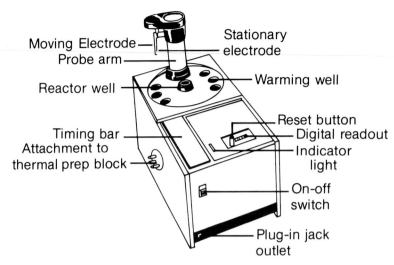

FIG. 7–41. Fibrometer®.

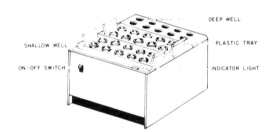

FIG. 7–42. Thermal prep block.

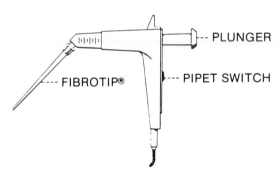

FIG. 7–43. Automatic pipet.

the cam (Fig. 7–45), the electric current is passed through the probe foot to the moving electrode. At the same time, due to the shape of the cam, the probe foot is forced upward, causing the moving electrode to move up and out of the sample mixture. When a clot forms, it is caught by the small hook on the moving electrode. As the moving electrode moves out of the liquid to the up position, the electric current passes from the cam to the moving electrode and simultaneously to the attached clot, through the clot, and into the liquid in which the clot is partially immersed. The electric current passes to the stationary electrode and the circuit is complete, stopping the timing mechanism. The clotting time is then recorded and the *reset button* depressed to reset the timer to 000.0. The probe arm is lifted up to its resting position, the probes carefully cleaned with a lint-free cloth, and the coagulation cup discarded. The instrument is ready for further testing. Duplicate testing should be used on this instrument.

Discussion

1. When the moving electrode is in the up position, during testing, it should be 1.27 mm above the liquid level in the cup. The level of the liquid in the disposable cup is critical. If the liquid level is too high (or the electrodes too long), the moving electrode will not leave the liquid when it is in its up position, the electric circuit will automatically be complete within the first 2 to 3 seconds of starting and the timer will stop. (The electric current will pass from the activated moving electrode, through the mixture, to the stationary electrode.) Conversely, if the liquid level is too low (or the electrodes too

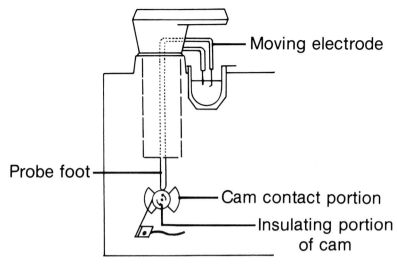

FIG. 7–44. Probe arm position during sample testing (Fibrometer).

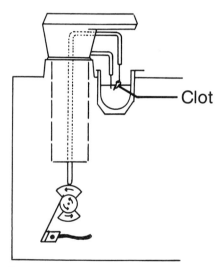

FIG. 7–45. Probe arm position during sample testing (Fibrometer).

short), when the clot forms, it will not be detected. In this instance, the electric circuit is broken because the clot does not remain in contact with the mixture when attached to the moving electrode in its up position (carrying an electric charge).

2. The electrodes must be kept free of lint and debris to eliminate falsely shortened results. They may be cleaned using distilled water or a solution of 1% phosphoric acid followed by a through rinsing with distilled water (the use of acids may pit the electrodes). It is advisable to remove the probe and dip the electrodes into the acid solution. Rinse with distilled water and wipe dry with lint-free material.

3. The disposable plastic *FibroTip* should only be used one time. However, when pipetting the same reagent, the tip may be reused, but should be tightened periodically so that it does not come loose from the pipet.

4. If the timing mechanism is started inadvertently, turn the *on-off switch* on the Fibrometer to off. Turn the unit back on, replace the probe arm in its resting position, and reset the digital readout.

5. Two probe arms are available: one for testing a final volume of 0.3 mL, and an alternate for testing 0.4 mL volumes.

6. When using the automatic pipet, develop the habit of moving the pipet switch to off as soon as the timing mechanism has been activated.

7. After the plunger on the automatic pipet is depressed, a small amount of solution will remain in the FibroTip. This is acceptable and has been allowed for in the calibration of the pipet.

8. The stationary and moving electrodes must be in a position parallel to one another. If they become bent, they should be realigned very carefully.

9. If the Fibrometer does not appear to be detecting a clot, fill a coagulation cup with 0.5 mL of reagent. Press the timer bar. Due to excess liquid in the cup, the Fibrometer should stop within 0.5 second of when the probe unit drops to the down position. If it does not, check the cam (beneath the probe) for dirt. This area may be cleaned with a cotton-tipped applicator immersed in 70% isopropyl alcohol. A shortened moving electrode may also cause this problem. This electrode may be lengthened a short amount by carefully pushing the probe foot up slightly. (See operator's manual.)

10. If the Fibrometer stops within 0.5 to 3.0 seconds after the probe drops down, the moving electrode may be too long. Place 0.3 mL of reagent into a coagulation cup. Press the timer bar. If the moving electrode is too long the Fibrometer will stop as soon as the probe drops down. The probe may be shortened by carefully pulling down on the probe foot (see operator's manual).

Coag-A-Mate XC

The Coag-A-Mate XC is a semi-automated coagulation instrument that automatically pipets reagent and detects clot formation via a change in optical density. The PT, APTT, thrombin time, fibrinogen, and factor assays may be performed on the instrument in addition to almost any coagulation test that has the formation of a clot as the end point. The XC will also calculate and store factor assay and fibrinogen curves, report results in percentage of activity (factor assays), in mg/dL (fibrinogen), and in a ratio of clotting time to normal for the PT and APTT, in addition to reporting results in seconds (Fig. 7–46).

Principles of Testing (Factor VIII Assay)

The factor VIII assay is outlined below because this procedure best exemplifies the flexibility and operation of the XC.

Instrument Preparation. The instrument is turned on by pressing the *on/off switch*. The XC will automatically proceed through a systems check. The *display* and the *printer* will indicate "System Self Check." When this test is complete, "Coag-A-Mate XC—Unit Warming, Proceed with Calibrations" is displayed and the mode is automatically set for PTs. The printer displays "Coag-A-Mate XC, Version xxxx." The instrument is allowed to reach 37.5°C (the *Ready NO key* is lit until the proper temperature is reached, at which time the *Ready YES key* will light up). When the instrument is at the proper temperature the display and the printer indicate, "Warm-up Complete." The XC automatically runs the analog channel test and returns to the PT mode. The *APTT key* on the *touch entry panel* is pressed. Two sets of reagent tubing are installed: The delivery tip of the long tubing is inserted into the hole on the *reagent incubation arm* and pushed down until the tip extends $1/16$ of an inch below the arm. The tubing is gently seated into the groove on the incubation arm, working it toward the base of the arm. It must not be stretched. The area of tubing between the two collars (which will be placed in the pump) is very lightly lubricated. The tubing is seated around the *pump*, by sliding it into the slot on either side of the stator, and making certain the tubing is properly positioned in the appropriate notch. To place the back collar snugly against the stator, the appropriate prime key (1 or 2) is pressed. The second reagent tubing is installed in the same manner. A vial of APTT reagent with stir bar is placed in storage well 1 (left), and the pick up tip of the reagent tubing placed into the reagent vial. In like manner, the vial of calcium chloride is placed in the second storage well on the right and the reagent tubing placed in the vial.

Sample Preparation. The reference plasma dilutions for the factor assay are prepared as described for the manual procedure. Factor deficient plasma (0.1 mL) is pipetted into wells #1 through 10. The reference plasma dilutions (0.1 mL) are added to the appropriate wells. The first and last cuvet numbers (1 and 10) are entered by pressing *first test key*, #1, Enter, *Last Test key*, #1, 0, and Enter. The reagent tubing is primed by lifting the incubation arm, holding a suitable container $1/2$ inch below the delivery tip, and pressing the *prime 1 key* until the APTT reagent flows continuously from the delivery tip. This procedure is repeated for the calcium chloride reagent line using the *prime 2 key*. The filled *test*

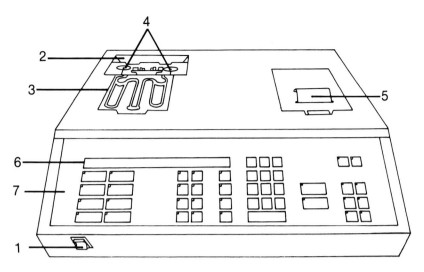

FIG. 7–46. Coag-A-Mate XC.

tray is placed on the *incubation test plate*, matching the notch in the tray with the notch in the hub. The reagent incubation arm is lowered and seated firmly in place.

Testing of Standard Curve. The *start key* is pressed to begin the test cycle. The printer will type out the first and last test cuvet numbers, plate temperature, test mode, and the preset instrument parameters. The samples will be incubated on the test plate for 1 minute prior to the addition of APTT reagent. During this time the display counts down from 60 seconds indicating, "Cuvette Warming . . . Seconds Left=xx." After the incubation period the display shows "Test in Progress," during which time the APTT reagent is added to all cuvets and the display reads "Activation, Seconds left=xxx." At the conclusion of the activation period, calcium chloride is added to the cuvets, timing is begun, and the display reads "Test in Progress." During testing the only panel key able to be activated is the *cancel key* (stops testing). Once all reagents have been added, each cuvet is monitored for clot formation (change in optical density). A single light source is divided into 12 channels, each of which passes through the sample to its own corresponding sensor. Thus, all samples are tested simultaneously. As each sample clots, the change in optical density is detected, and this information is stored until all test samples have clotted.

Preparation of Standard Curve. At the end of the test cycle the instrument gives an audible beep, and test results are displayed and printed. The printout also contains the date and time. The reagent incubation arm is raised and the test tray removed and discarded. Duplicate results are averaged for each reference plasma dilution. The *factor assay key* is pressed. The display prompts, "Factor ____ Enter File (1–12)." Using the numeric keypad the number 8 (or whatever number is required by the laboratory's numbering system) is pressed followed by Enter. "APTT Factor File 8" is displayed. The *std curve key* is pressed and then the *calib. key*. The display prompts, "Enter number of Standards (3–10) ____." The appropriate number (5) is entered and the Enter key pressed. The display prompts, "1% Activity=____." The percentage concentration (to 1 decimal point) of the highest standard (dilution #1) is entered and the Enter key pressed. The display shows "1% Activity=xxx" and prompts "Time = ____." The average time for that standard is entered and the Enter key pressed. The display continues to prompt for the remaining standards (percentage concentration and clotting times). After all information has been entered, the display prompts "Calibration Printout (Y/N)?". If the *YES key* is pressed the percentage concentrations and clotting times are printed along with the Coefficient of Determination (an indicator of the best fit line).

This number should be equal to or >0.985. (If it is not the standard curve is repeated.)

Patient/Control Testing. Dilutions of the patient and control plasmas are prepared and tested as described for the standard curve. However, when testing the patient and control plasmas the APTT, Std. Curve, and Factor Assay keypads are activated (pressed) in order to obtain results in percentage activity along with seconds. At the conclusion of testing, the clotting times in seconds and percentage activity are printed for each test sample. The Coefficient of Determination, calibration curve points, and clotting times are also printed on the header of each report.

Test Conclusion. When testing is complete, the reagent is removed from the reagent lines by pressing the YES and *Deprime 1 keys,* and YES and *Deprime 2 keys.* The reagent lines are flushed with distilled water and air by pressing the YES, Prime 1, and Prime 2 keys, alternating air and water for the duration of the cycle. The tubing is removed from the pumps if no further testing is to be performed.

Discussion

1. A result of "***.*" indicates that an end point has not been detected because of incomplete clotting, clot formation during the blank time, or insufficient change in optical density during testing that prevented the instrument from detecting the clot.
2. Additional keys on the Touch Entry Panel not used in the above procedure have a variety of functions. Selection of procedures is done by pressing *PT, APTT, TT* (thrombin time), and *Fibrinogen* keys. *Two Stage FA* key is used in the two stage factor VIII assay. The *Ratio* key is used with the PT or APTT for reporting results in a ratio of patient result to normal. *Pump 1 and 2 vol.* keys, when pressed, display the calibration volumes of the pumps, and the *Blank Time* key indicates the length of that time period. *Max Time* key, when pressed, will display the maximum time period for which the specimens will be monitored for clot formation. The *Act. Time* indicates

the amount of time between the addition of the first and second reagent to the test samples. The date and time may be displayed by pressing the *Date/Time* key. Pump volumes and blank, maximum, and activation times are changed using the *Modify* key. Printer paper may be advanced by activation of the *Paper Feed* key. The *Recall* key is used to reprint results from the most recent testing run (provided the instrument has not been turned off) and to obtain a printout of the instrument parameters.

3. This instrument is very flexible. Total cuvet volumes for testing may vary from as little as 0.3 mL to as much as 0.5 mL. The pump volumes may be set at 50 to 300 μL, the blank time from 1.0 to 20.0 seconds, maximum time from 50 to 300 seconds, and the activation time from 0 to 999.9 seconds. These parameters may be set temporarily for one run of testing or may be permanently set.
4. In order to obtain the parameter settings for an individual test, press the test key (e.g., PT) and the Recall key. To obtain a printout of a factor assay curve, press the test key, Std. Curve key, and the Recall key.

Coag-A-Mate XM

The Coag-A-Mate XM (extended manual) (Fig. 7–47) is manufactured by Organon Teknika Corp. It is a manually operated photo-optical coagulation instrument with data management capabilities. The XM may be used for determination of the PT (with a semiquantitative fibrinogen), APTT, thrombin time, fibrinogen, and factor assays.

Instrument Description

The XM has two *clot detection stations,* each of which contain two *read (test) stations,* thus permitting the performance of two tests in duplicate, simultaneously. A *dual test tray* (containing two cuvets) is used to hold the test mixtures. Contained in the *incubation test plate* are four *reagent storage compartments* (the inner two of which are equipped with magnetic stir bar capabilities) and six *warming*

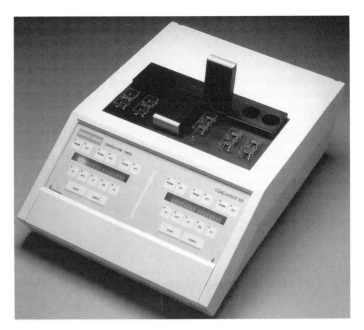

FIG. 7–47. Coag-A-Mate XM. (Courtesy of Organon Teknika Corp.)

stations (allow for timed incubation of test plasmas or reagents). The incubation test plate temperature is operator controllable. Two *display areas* serve as a means for operator interaction with the instrument and will exhibit test results. A data management system allows for (1) the conversion of clotting times (in seconds) to other report units (mg/dL, percentage activity, INR [PT], and ratio), (2) retention of information for fibrinogen, factor activity, and dose-response curves, (3) identification of specimens by assigned number, and (4) automatic assessment of duplicate testing reproducibility. Output ports (back of unit) provide the option to interface the XM with a data management system or printer. Instrument *programming keys* allow the operator to communicate with the instrument: (1) *warm* keys allow the operator to time the warming cycle in the warming or testing well, and the *act*(ivate) keys allow timing of the activation time for APTT samples in the same areas, (2) test keys allow for test selection, (3) *start* and *cancel* keys begin and terminate testing, (4) programming keys (*permanent modify, modify, step, audio, temperature*) provide a means for customizing the instrument to each laboratory's procedures, (5) *enter*, (6) *clear* key permits entries to be changed from the keyboard, and (7) *numerical* keys.

Principles of Operation—Fibrinogen

The test station cover is placed in the closed position and any test trays removed to avoid blockage of the optical light paths. The XM is turned on using the *power switch* located on the rear of the instrument. The displays will exhibit COAG-A-MATE XM along with a program revision letter and number. During the 10 minute warmup period, the instrument automatically performs a series of memory and optical self checks. The display prompts the operator to enter the date and time using the numeric keypad (the enter key is pressed after each entry). The display will then read UNIT WARMING. When the instrument has reached the operating temperature of 37°C, the display indicates WARM-UP COMPLETE and proceeds to check the voltage output of the optical channels at each read station. After the optical self check, the instrument is ready for use. It automatically defaults to the PT test mode, and displays the pre-programmed standard parameters for the PT (blank time, activation time, maximum time [B = X, A = X, M = X]). The fibrinogen test mode is selected by pressing the appropriate key (FIB) for test station 1 or 2 (or both) depending on which clot detection stations are to be used. The standard parameters for the fibrinogen will be displayed (B = 1.0, A = 0.0, M = 60, if the default settings are used). Thrombin reagent is prepared according to manufacturer's instructions and the reagent maintained at room temperature. The patient or control plasma is diluted according to the manual procedure. A dual test tray is placed in either a warm or read (test) station and 0.2 mL of the diluted plasma added to each of the two cuvets. The warm key is pressed to begin a 1 minute warming cycle. The display will read WARMING. At the completion of 1 minute, the display will flash and a tone will sound. The warm key is pressed to shut off the audible tone. The test tray is placed in the read station, and the cover closed. The display reads START TEST. The start key is pressed. The display reads ADD REAGENT. Thrombin reagent (0.1 mL) is added through one of the ports in the read station cover. (The pipet tip must be wiped clean *prior to* adding the reagent [placing pipet tip in the read station cover port].) A tone sounds to acknowledge that reagent has been added to one side of the test tray and the LED displays TEST IN PROGRESS. Thrombin is immediately added to the second cuvet through the appropriate port in the read station cover. A second tone sounds to acknowledge addition of this reagent. The clotting reaction is begun with the addition of the thrombin. The first period of time after reagent addition is called the blank time, which allows for mixing of the plasma and reagent, and for the disappearance of any bubbles. During this time the instrument does not respond to any optical changes in the test mixture. At the end of the blank time the instrument monitors the test mixture in the cuvet for fibrin (clot) formation. A beam of light is transmitted through the cuvet onto a photodetector. This light is increasingly scattered as fibrin is formed, and the amount of light reaching the photodetector decreases. The clot formation is measured by the rate of change of light transmission through the reaction mixture and must exceed a preset threshold in order for a clot to be detected. (If a clot is not detected by the instrument within the maximum period of time, testing is stopped.) A tone will sound when testing is complete. The result, in seconds, will be displayed for each sample: TIME:XXX.X YYY.Y (X and Y = clotting time for each plasma sample). The step key is pressed. The average of the two clotting times for the specimen are displayed if they are within acceptable preset ranges. The step key is pressed a second time to obtain the fibrinogen reading in mg/dL for each of the clotting times. (Results are obtained from the fibrinogen curve in instrument memory previously entered by each laboratory.) The average fibrinogen reading for the two results is obtained by pressing the step key a third time. Results are manually recorded as they are displayed. If the XM is interfaced with a printer, results will be printed as they are displayed.

Discussion

1. Each time a key is selected, a tone will sound to indicate that a function has been initiated. Tones will also sound at the completion of warming, upon addition of reagent, and at completion of a test.
2. The message TURBID REACTION may be displayed if a lipemic sample is tested or if the sample/reagent mixture is below the limit of detection by the optical system, or the message CALIBRATE OPTICS may be displayed if the sample/reagent mixture is beyond the optical system detection limit.
3. The final reagent in each reaction mixture must be added within 30 seconds of starting the test procedure.
4. If no reagent addition is detected, "***.*" will be displayed, whereas ">>>.>" indicates no clot detection.
5. If duplicate samples exceed preset limits for precision (CV limit or 10%), DUP PREC ERROR will be displayed.
6. REAGENT TEMP ERROR will be displayed and a tone will sound when the reagent temperature exceeds $\pm$ 0.5°C of the preprogrammed temperature.
7. The step key is used to scan through options when programming and to scan through test results when in a testing mode.
8. The read stations are provided with accessory covers for fibrinogen assays for prevention of contamination with thrombin reagent.
9. The read station covers must remain closed during testing.

10. Parameters changed using the modify option will be held in memory until the instrument is turned off, at which time these changes will default to those settings entered using the permanent modify key.
11. The audio key may be used to turn the tone that sounds at the end of the warming cycle on or off.
12. A diagnostics mode is available to assist the operator in troubleshooting and is entered by pressing any key when turning the unit on.
13. The XM allows a throughput of 200 PT tests per hour and 50 APTT tests per hour.
14. A semiquantitative fibrinogen test may be performed simultaneously with the prothrombin time. This is accomplished by the instrument monitoring the test mixture during the prothrombin time until the clot is fully formed. The change in the voltage reading between the end of the blank time and that of the fully formed clot is directly proportional to the amount of fibrinogen present in the test plasma. This difference is compared to known values in the instrument memory (previously calibrated/standardized by the performance of prothrombin times with known and varying concentrations [50 to 750 mg/dL] of fibrinogen).

Coag-A-Mate 2001

The Coag-A-Mate 2001 (Fig. 7–48) is able to perform up to 12 PTs or 12 APTTs simultaneously.

Principles of Operation

The Coag-A-Mate 2001 is turned on by means of the *on/off switch* and is ready for testing when the *temperature indicator* reads 37°C (±1°C). By use of the *mode switch*, either PT or APTT is selected, depending on which test is to be run. The *reagent dispenser pumps* are set by the operator to deliver the correct reagent volumes. The rear panel of the instrument contains a *PT cycle switch* to select sequential testing or simultaneous testing. Also located in this area is the *APTT activation time switch* for setting the activation time at 180,

240, or 300 seconds. The appropriate test reagents are placed in the *reagent storage wells*, and the tip of the *tubing assemblies* are placed into the reagent vials. The tubing is placed in the *reagent incubation arm*, and the tubing nozzles (through which the reagent is dispensed to the test samples) are put into place in the incubation arm. *Prime #1* and *prime #2 switches* are depressed to activate the left and right *dispenser pumps*, respectively, to prime the tubing with reagent. Plasma samples are manually pipetted (0.1 mL) into the *circular test tray*, which is placed onto the *incubation test plate* (beneath the *light shield* containing the incubation arm). The *first sample* and *last sample switches* are set to tell the instrument where to begin and end testing. The light shield is kept closed during testing. The test cycle is begun by depressing the *start switch*, at which point the electronic timing mechanism is activated. Reagents are automatically added to the samples. A single *light source* within the instrument is divided into 12 channels. This light passes through each sample onto its corresponding sensor. As each plasma sample clots the change in optical density is detected by the sensor and the clotting time registered by the instrument. The *station number display* will indicate the sample number and the clotting time on the *time-seconds display*. If maximum time has occurred before clotting, UU.U will be displayed, and the test should be repeated by another method. When all testing is complete, the *cycle-button/light* will be lit, and the *print module* will print out the sample results with the corresponding cuvet number. Those samples which did not clot will be indicated by --.– on the printer tape. The circular test tray is removed, and the instrument is ready for further testing.

Coag-A-Mate Dual Channel Analyzer

The Coag-A-Mate dual channel automated coagulation analyzer (Fig. 7–49) detects clot formation by means of a photocell sensing circuit that reads the optical density change when a clot is formed. This instrument automatically pipets all reagents necessary for testing and is capable of performing the PT, APTT, and factor assays. The PT and APTT may also be performed simultaneously.

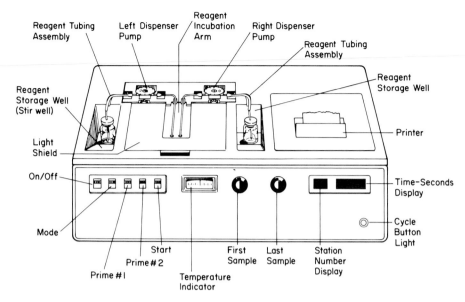

FIG. 7–48. Coag-A-Mate 2001.

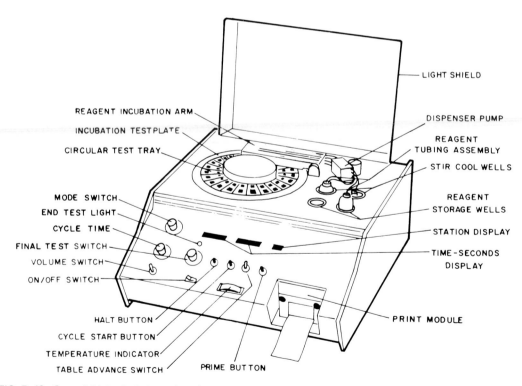

FIG. 7–49. Coag-A-Mate dual channel analyzer.

Principles of Operation
(Simultaneous PT and APTT Testing)

The instrument is turned on by means of the *on/off switch* and is ready for testing when the red *decimal point temperature indicator* in the *time seconds display* illuminates. To perform PTs and APTTS simultaneously the *mode switch* is appropriately set (PT/APTT). This automatically determines the length of the delay period (time elapse between reagent addition and when the instrument monitors an optical density change in case bubbles are formed when reagent is added), which is 8 seconds for PTs and 20 seconds for APTTs. The *cycle time switch* is set to 110 for a 4 minute APTT activation or 150 for a 5 minute activation time. The *volume switch* is set at 0.1. Vials of thromboplastin (PT) reagent (with stir bar) and partial thromboplastin (APTT) reagent (with stir bar) are placed in *stir cool wells* and a vial of calcium chloride is placed in the *reagent storage well*. The vials are capped with a three hole stopper and the appropriate *reagent tubing assemblies* are placed in each vial. The *reagent incubation arm* (warms reagents to 37°C) is lifted and an appropriate dish is placed under the reagent delivery tips while pressing the *prime button* to activate the *dispenser pumps* in order to fill the tubing with reagent. Plasma and control specimens to be tested are pipetted (0.1 mL) into the *circular test tray* (inner [PT] and outer [APTT] wells) beginning with cuvet #1 and ending no higher than cuvet #22 (#23 and #24 collect excess reagent). When all specimens to be tested have been pipetted into the test tray, it is placed on the *incubation test plate* (the blue area cools the samples and the red area warms the samples to 37°C prior to testing), matching the notch in the test tray with the notch in the hub. The reagent incubation arm is carefully lowered into place. The *final test switch* is set to indicate the last cuvet containing a sample to be tested. The *light shield* is closed. Testing is begun by pressing the *cycle button*. The first plasma samples (one in the inner cuvet and one in the outer cuvet) enter the first of two *incubation stations* where the samples are heated to 37°C. At the first station, 0.1 mL of partial thromboplastin reagent is added to the outer cuvet for the APTT. At the end of the preset cycle time (110 or 150 seconds), the test tray advances one

station. When the first pair of samples (inner and outer cuvet) reach the *test station*, 0.2 mL of thromboplastin (two reagent lines each delivering 0.1 mL) is added to the inner cuvet (PT) and the timer is started. At the same time, 0.1 mL of calcium chloride is added to the outer cuvet (APTT) and a second timer is started. During testing the *time seconds display* shows the elapsed time for each sample being tested while the *station display* indicates the cuvet number currently in the test station. When fibrin formation occurs, the photoelectric cell detects the sudden change in optical density, and the timing mechanism is automatically stopped. The clotting time is printed out by the *printer module* to the closest tenth of a second. When both test samples have clotted, the test tray is ready to rotate to the next two test samples. The time elapse between clot formation and the beginning of the next two tests depends on the cycle time mode that has been selected by the operator. If a clot does not form within the 110 (or 150 seconds, 000.0 is printed on the tape. At the completion of the final test the *end test light* comes on and an audible beep is given.

The testing cycle may be stopped at any time by pressing the *halt button*. The *cycle start button* is used to reactivate the test cycle when it has been stopped.

Discussion

1. Erratic results may be due to one of several causes: (a) reagents, (b) improper sample collection, (c) dirty, twisted, or improperly seated reagent tubing, (d) jerky pump operation (pump tubing may need lubrication), (e) delivery tip dirty or in wrong position, or (f) mode switch in wrong position.

2. Reagent should not remain in the reagent tubing for more than 30 minutes after testing has been completed. Remove the reagent and clean the tubing by alternately drawing distilled water and air through the lines using the prime button. Remove the tubing assembly from the pump if the instrument is not to be used right away.

3. Depending on usage, the rotor should be removed from the pump and cleaned with isopropanol on a scheduled basis. The reaction temperatures and reagent delivery

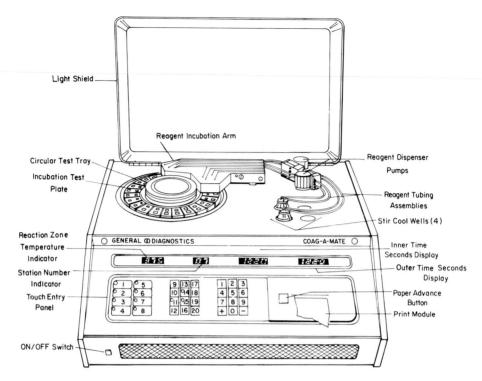

FIG. 7–50. Coag-A-Mate ·X2.

volume should also be checked routinely. See operations manual.

Coag-A-Mate·X2

The Coag-A-Mate·X2 coagulation instrument (Fig. 7–50) detects clot formation by means of a photocell sensing circuit that reads the optical density change when a clot is formed. The instrument is capable of performing the majority of coagulation procedures and automatically pipets all necessary reagents for testing. It will perform two tests simultaneously: two different tests or two like tests in duplicate, or four like tests performed singularly.

Principles of Testing (Simultaneous Performance of the PT and APTT)

Instrument Preparation. The *rocker switch* is pressed to turn the instrument on. NOT READY is displayed, indicating the instrument temperature has not reached 37°C (±0.5°C). When the proper temperature has

been attained, READY will be displayed. (The instrument cannot be used for testing as long as NOT READY is displayed.) The *PT/APTT* key (3) on the *touch entry panel* is pressed (the light on the key will illuminate). The date is entered by pressing *date* key (16), a two digit number for the month, the day, and the year, and pressing *Enter* (20) after each entry. One vial each of thromboplastin, activated partial thromboplastin, and 0.025 M calcium chloride are placed in the *stir cool wells*. A clean magnetic stir bar is placed in the PT and APTT reagent vials (as recommended by manufacturer). A cap with an appropriate opening for the reagent line is placed on each vial. The *reagent lines* are installed as described in Table 7–1. The delivery tip of each reagent tubing is placed in the appropriate hole on the *reagent incubation arm*, and pushed down until it extends 1/16 inch below the opening. Without stretching the tubing, it is firmly pressed into the appropriate groove of the incubation arm, working from the delivery tip to the base of the arm. The tubing is lightly lubricated between the collars. Using both hands, the two collars on the piece of tubing are held

TABLE 7–1. PLACEMENT OF REAGENT TUBING FOR THE COAG-A-MATE X2 (FOR PT AND APTT TESTING)

INCUBATION ARM SLOT	TUBING	REAGENT	PUMP #	PUMP SLOT #
D and E	Red collar (2)	Thromboplastin	2	6 and 7
F	Clear collar	Calcium chloride	2	8
B	Blue collar	Partial thromboplastin	1	3

and stretched around the front of the *pump rotor.* The tubing is slid into the slot on either side of the stator and positioned in the appropriate notch. Both collars must fit firmly on either side of the pump area. The appropriate prime (1 or 2) button may be pressed to ensure proper seating of the tubing around the pump. The pick up tips of the reagent tubing are installed in the appropriate reagent vials, making certain they are inserted to the bottom of each vial. The reagent lines are filled by priming the pumps: The reagent incubation arm is lifted to a 45° angle, a small dish held under lines D, E, and F, and the *prime 2* button (10) on the touch entry panel depressed until all three reagents are expelled from the lines in a steady stream. Line B is primed in a similar manner using the *prime 1* button (9).

Sample Preparation. Patient and control plasmas (0.1 mL) are pipetted into the appropriate cuvets in the *circular test tray.* Plasma samples for the APTT are placed in the cuvet in the outer channel of the test plate, while PT test samples are placed in the inner channel of cuvets. The tray is placed on the *incubation test plate* (maintains samples at a cool temperature prior to testing), matching the notch in the tray with the notch in the hub. The reagent incubation arm is lowered to its bottom position (horizontal). The *light shield* is lowered, making certain all tubing is completely under the shield. The light shield must be closed at all times while the instrument is testing (the busy light displayed). The station number, as indicated on the *station number indicator,* must correspond to the cuvet number containing the first sample to be tested. If a different number appears in the station number window, the *index* key (19) must be

depressed until the station number corresponds to the first sample cuvet number. The end test station (last cuvet containing a test sample) is set by pressing *end test* (13), entering the two digit number of the last cuvet, and pressing enter.

Sample Testing. Testing is begun by pressing the *start* key (17). As soon as the instrument is activated, the test plate revolves, carrying the first four test samples into the heating zone, where they are warmed to 37°C for a preset time period prior to and during testing. A printout is given at this time with the following information: End test station, reaction zone temperature, sensitivity, pumps #1 and #2 volumes, blank time (PT and APTT), and minimum and maximum times. If two reagents are required for a test (e.g., APTT), the first reagent is added to each cuvet at a set time interval prior to its arrival at the test station. When the first four samples arrive at the test station, the correct amount of reagent is automatically pipetted into each of the four cuvets, and the timing mechanisms are started. When fibrin formation occurs, the photoelectric cell detects the sudden change in optical density, and the timing mechanism is automatically stopped. During testing, the control panel will show the following: Busy light illuminated, the station number display will shift back and forth between the two cuvet numbers currently at the test stations, the *inner time seconds display* will shift back and forth showing the time elapsed or clotting times of the PTs being tested or just completed, and the *outer time seconds display* shows the same information for the APTTs. As each set of plasmas clot, the test results are printed on the printer tape. After a preset period of time the test tray rotates to the next four nm. The ability of the optical system to monitor multiple cuvets (15 reaction wells) at different wavelengths allows the MDA the flexibility of performing clotting, chromogenic, and immunoassays simultaneously. The optics module contains five detector arrays. The light that passes through the 15 reaction wells is divided into 35 wavelengths with a diffraction grating and passes through a rotating shutter, which interrupts each of the 15 beams so that only one beam falls onto a detector at the time. The arrays are scanned electronically in sync with the shutter so that the signals from all of the 15 wells are acquired five times per second. Because the MDA tracks each specimen by the timing of the lead screw (to which the cuvet is attached), it is able to relate the information from the detectors to the test performed in each individual reaction well. (That is, it knows which test is performed in each reaction well and therefore uses the light signal information accordingly. It therefore automatically monitors each reaction mixture at the correct wavelength and analyzes the data appropriately.)

When testing has been completed, the used cuvets are automatically transported to the closed *cuvet waste receptacles*.

Discussion

Tests can be ordered individually or as user defined test panels (such as mixing studies or intrinsic or extrinsic factor panels).

The pipet probes are rinsed between all samples and reagents to eliminate carryover. All sample and reagent aspirations are controlled by positive displacement syringe pumps, which eliminates the need for tubing changes and calibration.

Sample throughput is 180 tests per hour in any combination of clotting, chromogenic, and/or immunoassay.

Lyophilized reagents (and controls) may be reconstituted using the positive displacement syringe pumps.

Self-monitoring is performed on temperatures, sample/reagent delivery volumes, waste levels, and all moving mechanisms.

Results are available immediately at completion of an assay and may be accessed on the PC monitor, an optional printer, or the host computer.

The monitoring of patient samples will detect hemolysis and increased bilirubin, correct for lipemia, and detect microclots.

STAT samples can be introduced into a test cycle at any time by placing the specimen tube in the rack just prior to the bar code reader.

All reagent delivery arms contain fluid sensors allowing the probe tip to make contact with a minimum amount of reagent/diluent/plasma, which also reduces carryover. Fluids are added to the reaction well in a manner to obtain maximum mixing. When necessary, reagents are heated in the reagent arm during transfer to the test cuvet.

Test cuvets are maintained at 15°C by the temperature of the transport track. The track near and at the test station is 37°C so that all testing is carried out at this temperature.

Specimen tubes are maintained at a decreased temperature in the MDA and may be left in the instrument until testing is complete, or they may be removed following aspiration of the sample.

MLA Electra 750

The MLA Electra 750 (Fig. 7–52) is a semi-automated blood coagulation timer. Clot formation is timed automatically and is detected by means of a photocell which reads the optical density change when the clot is formed. The unit contains a heating block which maintains the reagents and plasma samples at 37°C prior to and during testing. Pipetting of the reagents and plasma samples is performed manually, utilizing disposable tipped pipets included with the instrument. An improved sensitivity and optical range allow the instrument to detect the clot on samples that may be chylous or icteric. There are five mode switches located on the front of the instrument. All routine coagulation testing may be performed on the MLA 750 in addition to the thrombin time, fibrinogen assay, factor assay, and saline dilutions.

MLA Electra® 800

The MLA Electra® 800 (Fig. 7–53) is an automated multitest coagulation timer that uses a photo-optical clot detection system. Four

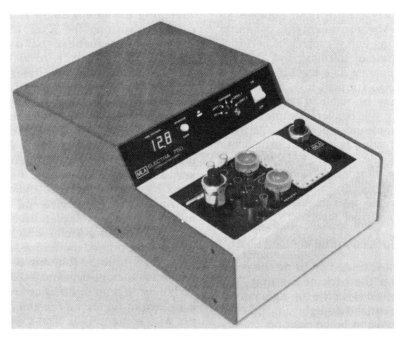

FIG. 7–52. MLA Electra 750. (Courtesy of Medical Laboratory Automation, Mount Vernon, New York.)

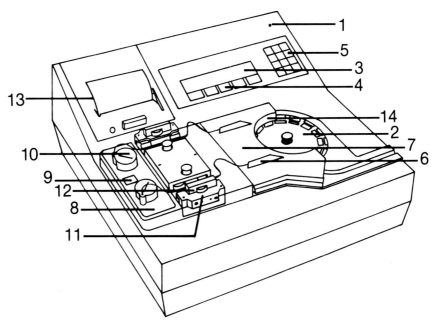

FIG. 7–53. MLA Electra 800.

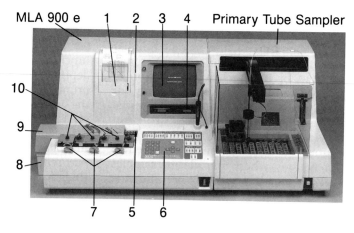

MLA 900 e   1   2   3   4   Primary Tube Sampler

10
9
8
7   5   6

FIG. 7–54. MLA Electra 1000C (including the MLA Electra 900C). (Courtesy of Medical Laboratory Automation, Inc.)

which also contain magnetic stirring capabilities. Three peristaltic *pumps* deliver reagent to the test cuvet, and can be programmed to dispense volumes from 25 μL to 500 μL. The *heater trough cover* serves as protection for the reagent heaters and reagent nozzles in position over the testing area. The cover also helps to maintain the temperature at $37°C \pm 0.2°C$. The *cuvet transport* (5) *system* consists of a 100 position linear transport belt onto which a maximum of 40 individual test cuvets (samples) may be loaded at any one time. The *cuvet disposal bin* (8) collects the used cuvets after testing. The thermal *printer* (1) supplies a hardcopy printout of results, temperature status, error messages, and standard curves. A *paper advance button* allows the operator to easily detach the printout from the instrument. A series of output ports located on the back of the MLA provides the means to interface the MLA with a host computer, and to add an external printer, an auxillary keyboard, and a bar code scanner.

Principles of Operation

To begin testing on the MLA 900/900C the operator places the program disk in drive A and the data disk in drive B. The MLA is powered up by pressing the on/off switch at the right front of the unit. The power on indicator will light, the computer will load programming, and after several minutes the cuvet transport belt will move and the monitor will display the Main Menu. The test mode is selected from the display by pressing the number on the keypad that corresponds to the appropriate test.

The reagent reservoir cup assemblies are chosen according to the test selection: the blue cup is used for delivery of 0.1 mL of heated reagent, red delivers 0.2 mL heated reagent, and yellow delivers 0.1 mL of unheated reagent. The reagent cups are placed into the refrigerated reservoir wells for the appropriate pump. The associated tubing is placed into the pump slot, with the pump lever in the open position. The first and second tubing connectors are slid into position at the first and second pump posts, respectively, and the pump lever is closed. The heat exchangers are positioned in the heater trough, depending on the procedures to be run. Reagents are placed in the appropriate reagent cups and stir bars added as necessary.

The specimens are manually pipetted into test cuvets. Both single-well (single testing) and double-well (duplicate testing) cuvets are available and may be used in the same run. The MLA automatically detects the cuvet type and will test singly or in duplicate, as indicated by the cuvet.

Reagents are primed by selecting "Pumps" from the Main Menu: The heat exchanger is removed from the heater trough and held over the open reagent cup, at a slight angle, with the nozzle pointing toward the side of the cup. To begin priming, the number corresponding to the pump to be primed is pressed, followed by the Enter key. When reagent flows smoothly from the nozzle and the reagent in the exchanger is bubble-free, priming is stopped by pressing any key. The reagent cup is covered, the heat exchanger is replaced in the heating trough by sliding it down and forward into position, and the nozzle is centered in the nozzle guide. To ensure proper sample/reagent mixing the priming process is repeated for all pumps to be used. The Esc(ape) key or "Quit" is pressed to return to the Main Menu.

The sample cuvets are loaded onto the cuvet transport belt. A clamp mechanism on the belt holds the cuvets in position during transport and testing.

At the start of a working shift or when changing test modes, it is recommended that a Confidence test be run. Select "Run" from the Main Menu, and "1-Confidence Test" from the Run Menu. The Confidence test is a two phase system self-check that includes an optical check of the 550 nm filter (clotting tests), the 405 nm filter (chromogenic assays), and the neutral density filter. A digitized clot image (numerical data) is also sent through the system to provide an additional check on the clotting and chromogenic test modes. The monitor display returns to the Run Menu upon completion of the Confidence test. Testing is initiated by selecting "Run Test" from the Run Menu or it will begin automatically 10 seconds after the Run Menu is displayed on the monitor.

The cuvets are moved to the testing station on the transport belt where reagents are automatically added to the samples and the reaction monitored by a photo-optical detection system. When testing starts, the monitor will display the Test Run screen, with test sequence numbers, test mode, location of samples in the transport belt, and the results of each test as it is completed.

During clotting assays, four optical channels simultaneously measure the endpoint of four test mixtures. Light (at 550 nm) passing through the sample is monitored by a photodetector. As clotting progresses, the amount of light detected decreases and causes a change in the electrical signal output from the detector. This signal is processed by the MLA's computer to determine the clotting time of the sample.

For chromogenic assays, the MLA measures the rate of optical density change. Light (at 450 nm) passes through the sample and is monitored by a photodetector. The reaction between the reagent and the analyte releases the chromophore paranitroaniline. This colored reaction product absorbs light and causes a change in optical density of the sample. This optical density change causes a corresponding change in the amount of light falling on the detector. The signal output from the detector describes this change as the change in absorbance during a defined period of time. The MLA takes a series of O.D. readings and determines the linearity of the data and the change in absorbance (delta ABS) per minute. This absorbance change is compared to the reference calibration curve programmed into the instrument by the laboratory. The final test result is determined from this curve and is reported in the appropriate units.

After testing is complete for each group of four samples, the transport belt moves the cuvets and drops them into the disposal bin.

Discussion

A patient list may be created to identify patient samples and test modes.

Because the MLA is a continuous loading device, additional test cuvets may be added to the transport belt, and patients to the patient list, while a run is in progress.

The MLA can be programmed to automatically deprime the pumps at the end of testing.

Programs are available to set specific test parameters, to create, alter, and recall standard curves from memory, to run instrument diagnostic checks, and to set report formats.

The maximum test rate for PTs is 360 per hour, and for APTTs, 136 per hour.

The monitor will display information above and below the menu to assist the operator. Status lines, above the menu, describe the present condition of the instrument, and prompt lines displayed below the menu options define the choices available in each menu selection. Additional help screens, called pop-ups, are also available to assist the operator.

MLA Electra 1000C

The MLA Electra 1000C (Medical Laboratory Automation, Inc.) is a computerized coagulation system consisting of two units, an MLA Electra 900C and an automatic primary tube sampler for automated pipetting of patient plasmas. This unit accepts up to 10 racks of 10 tubes each and will automatically pipet (and dilute) samples into cuvets. (See Fig. 7–54.)

Autosampler Operation

In preparation for running the autosampler, the operator loads the *cuvet hopper* (5) with up to 350 single-well, clear cuvets. The *sampler power on/off switch* and the *power switch* on the MLA 900C are set in the on position. A *diluent bottle* (6) and *rinse container* (7) are filled and placed under the cover on the right side of the unit. Centrifuged specimens (with caps removed) are placed into *sample rack* A (14) and the rack is placed into the *rack holder* (13) at the top of the *keypad* (12) on the MLA 900C. Sample ID numbers may be entered manually into the computer via the patient list function or, if the tubes are barcoded, the ID numbers may be entered by scanning with the *bar code wand* (2). A beep will sound after each ID number, confirming that the scanner has read the bar code information. When all sample numbers have been entered for the specimens in the rack, the barcode wand is used to scan the location bar code on the sample rack (below each tube) (working from left to right) in the same order the sample IDs were entered. Test selection is made using the bar codes located on the keypad. When the first rack (A) is completed, successive racks (B, C, D, etc.) may be scanned and tests selected.

Sample racks are next loaded onto the *sampler* (10), rack A to the far left, followed in order by racks B, C, D, etc. The test cycle is started from the Run Test Menu. A *blade* inside the cuvet hopper rotates to pick up and move cuvets to the exit ramp where the *carrier system* transports them from the exit ramp to either the *dilution station* (for assays that require a dilution step) or to the *conveyor plate* for addition of the plasma specimen. The *sample probe* (4), connected by teflon tubing to the *syringe pump*, is mounted on the *sampler arm* and controlled by the XYZ assembly. It aspirates the appropriate samples, diluents, and/or factor deficient plasmas and dispenses these into the cuvets. Three motors control the X (left to right), Y (forward to back), and Z (up and down) movement of the arm. The conveyor plate then moves to the *shuttle mechanism* (3), which loads the cuvets (four at a time) onto the *transport belt* (11) of the MLA 900C. The cuvets are moved to the *cuvet reader* (test station) where the final reagents are added and test results read. At the conclusion of testing the cuvets are moved, via the transport belt, into the disposal bin.

Discussion

When the sampler is in operation, the *sampler rack door* must be closed. In addition, the *sample rack shield* prevents the operator from reaching into the area when the probe arm is in motion.

A *pause switch* (8) allows the operator to temporarily halt pipetting in order to add a cuvet to the hopper or to replenish diluent supplies.

Racks are labeled A through K. There is no I rack. Rack K is designated as a "stats only" rack.

The *plasma reagent rack assembly* (9) is a refrigerated (8°C) area for up to 12 controls, reference plasmas, and/or factor deficient plasmas.

A *diluent pump* delivers diluent from the diluent bottle to the diluent cup for preparation of prediluted samples or calibration reference plasmas.

The *wash station* (1) provides a receptacle for rinsing the probe's internal teflon liner and external surface with distilled water following each aspiration.

KoaguLab* 40-A Automated Coagulation System

KoaguLab 40-A (Fig. 7–55) is manufactured by Ortho Diagnostic Systems Inc. and is a microprocessor-controlled coagulation analyzer. It automatically pipets sample aliquots, adds the appropriate reagents to each sample cuvet, and measures the clotting times using two photo-optical detectors. Results are displayed and printed on a paper tape (except for fibrinogen results, which are not displayed, but are printed). The PT, APTT, factor assay, thrombin time, and fibrinogen may be performed on the KoaguLab 40-A. In addition, the instrument is able to perform the PT and APTT simultaneously. All testing is performed in duplicate if the samples are pipetted by the instrument.

The KoaguLab 40-A is composed of the *control module* (2) and the *sample handling module* (1). The control module contains the *display panel* (12), which exhibits test results, current test station, temperature warning lights, and

---

* Trademark of Ortho Diagnostic Systems

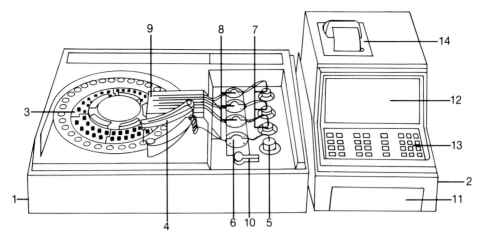

FIG. 7–55. KoaguLab 40-A Automated Coagulation System.

instrument messages. The *keyboard* (13) contains keys used to operate the instrument and is divided into five areas: (1) test selection keys, (2) operational keys (Run, Stop, Stat, Random Test), (3) special function keys (Print, Print Adv., Incub/End Pt., Man. Mode, Time/Date, Pump Calib., Temp. check, and Service Access), (4) quality control keys for selecting, reviewing, deleting, and clearing results, and (5) numeric keys. The *switch panel* (11) is located on the front bottom of the unit behind a door and contains switches for temperature adjustment, sample container size, beeper on/off, prime/deprime of pumps, and standby/operational mode selection.

Principles of Operation

Uncapped, centrifuged blood samples are placed directly into the *sample carousel* (3). Alternatively, the plasma may be poured into 2 mL sample cups and placed on the carousel. Reagent vials are placed in the appropriate *reagent wells* (7). The reagent lines in the *reagent arm* (9) and the *sample arm* (4) are primed (using the *reagent* [8] and *sampler* [6] *pumps* respectively). The *sample container switch* is set and the instrument is started. At the beginning of a run, the sample carousel moves forward until position 1 is adjacent to the sample arm, which moves out of the wash well (5) and positions itself over the sample. An air bubble is aspirated into the tip to leave a space between the distilled water and the sample to be aspirated. The sample arm moves down into the sample to a set depth and aspirates the sample. (For the PT or APTT it aspirates 0.6 mL of plasma.) The sample arm moves out of the sample, dispenses approximately 0.1 mL of sample back into the sample container, moves across to the cuvet tray, lowers the tip to the cuvet, and dispenses 0.1 mL of sample into two adjacent cuvets for duplicate testing. The sample arm moves back and is lowered into the wash well where the sample is flushed from the tip and washed with 1.3 mL of distilled water. (In the PT/APTT combination mode, samples are placed in every other position in the sample carousel. The sample arm picks up 0.8 mL of sample, dispenses 0.1 mL back into the sample tube, moves across to the cuvets and dispenses 0.1 mL of plasma into two adjacent cuvets. The samples arm then moves back to its position over the wash well, the carousel moves forward one position, the sample arm moves over the cuvet tray, and 0.1 mL of the same plasma is added to the next two adjacent cuvets.)

The cuvet tray advances one position at a time at a preset rate for the tests being performed. When the samples reach the incubation plate, they are heated to 37.5°C. Reagents are added to the cuvets as they reach the test station (or, for the APTT, the activated partial thromboplastin reagent is added when it reaches one of the stations in the incubation plate, dependent on the activation time desired). The *photo-optical detection system* is located in the test station. A timer is started

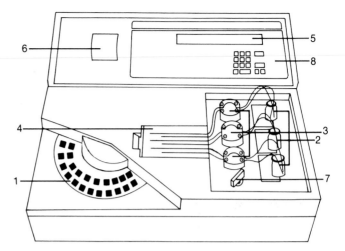

FIG. 7–56. Koagulab 16-S Coagulation System.

when the reagent is added. Elapsed time is displayed on the appropriate channel display. As clotting occurs the mixture becomes cloudy. When this change in optical density is detected, the timing mechanism is automatically stopped, the channel display indicates the clotting time, and the *printer* (14) produces a hard copy of the results. At a preset time, the carousel moves forward one position and the previously described timing process is repeated for the next sample until all testing is complete.

The *pump engage/release lever* (10) is released by the operator when testing and rinsing are complete in order to remove pressure from the tubing.

Discussion

The quality control program allows the operator to store data for ten different populations, and will calculate a T value, number of specimens, the mean, 1 S.D., the C.V., the range (± 2 S.D.), and the sum of X and X^2. Twenty-five sets of duplicate controls are entered for each file and transferred to CUM population as a group.

KoaguLab* 16-S Coagulation System

KoaguLab 16-S (Fig. 7–56) (Ortho Diagnostic Systems) is an automated coagulation analyzer that performs the PT, APTT, PT/APTT

* Trademark of Ortho Diagnostic Systems

combination, thrombin time, fibrinogen, and factor assays. Specimens may be tested in duplicate or singly, and the plasma samples are pipetted into the sample cuvets by the operator. PT results may be reported in percentage activity, as a ratio (to the population range), and as an International Normalized Ratio (INR). The APTT results may be reported as a ratio, using the normal average clotting time.

Principles of Operation

Plasma samples are pipetted into a *cuvet tray* and placed on the *sample carousel* (1) (maintained at room temperature). The reagents are placed in the *reagent wells* (2) and the tubing is primed (filled with reagent) by activating the *reagent pumps* (3). The tubing passes through the *reagent arm* (4) where the reagents are warmed to 37.5°C (± 0.5°C). The instrument is started by using the *enter* key. The carousel indexes forward and the first set of samples move under the reagent arm and onto the *incubation plate* (located under the carousel) where they are warmed to 37.5°C (± 0.5°C). There are four positions on the incubation plate in addition to the *test station*. The carousel moves the cuvet tray forward to the test station at a preset rate. (In the APTT test, the APTT reagent is added to the sample cuvet at a preset time before arriving at the test station.) When the first plasma sample reaches the test station, reagent is added to each of two sample cuvets and the timing mechanism for each is started.

Clot detection system. The clot detection system consists of an ultra-high intensity light-emitting diode (LED) and a photodetector for each channel. When reagent is added to the plasma sample in the test station, a blank time is initiated. During this period, the intensity of the LED is continuously adjusted by a feedback circuit to compensate for variability in the plasma sample (e.g., lipemia). If the amount of light reaching the photo detector is not within an acceptable range, a message, 'Channel Check,' is printed with the final test result. At the completion of the blank time the intensity of the LED is locked in and the photo detector continues to take measurements every 0.2 or 0.5 second (depending on the test being performed) until the maximum end point is reached. These readings (absorbance and time) represent the strength, rate, and time of the clot reaction and are plotted (absorbance vs. time). The shape of the curve is examined and the clotting time determined. The final result is accepted and printed, appended with a message (to indicate atypical parameters), or the data is rejected and "No Data" is reported.

The results are displayed on the *message display* (5) and printed on paper tape by the *printer* (6). After a preset time the carousel moves forward to the next sample and the above procedure is repeated until all testing is complete. The *pump engage/release lever* (7) is released by the operator when testing and rinsing are complete in order to remove pressure from the tubing.

Discussion

Using the KoaguLab 16-S, the operator selects the desired test(s) to be performed from the *Operational Menu*. The *Utility Menu* contains a service mode and is used to set the pump calibration, incubation times, maximum end points, duplicate or single testing, starting position in the cuvet tray, patient identification number, precision flags, a reprint of the previous run, and different reporting formats.

The *keypad* (8) contains 15 keys for operator interaction with the instrument. The numeric keys, *0 to 9*, allow the operator to enter information into the instrument. The *prime button* is used for priming, depriming, and rinsing the reagent tubing. The *clear button* is used to remove a number not yet entered into the

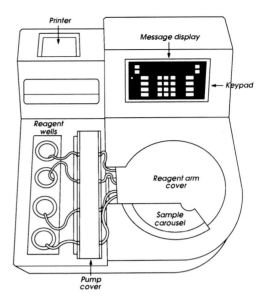

FIG. 7–57. KoaguLab 60-S. (Courtesy of Ortho Diagnostic Systems, Inc.)

instrument, allows the operator to return to the utility menu from the service mode, and allows the operator to move back and forth between the operational menu and the utility menu. The *arrow keys* allow the operator to move up and down through the displayed menu. The *enter key* is used to enter information into the instrument, begin testing, and add samples during the cycle.

Ortho KoaguLab 60-S

The KoaguLab 60-S (Ortho Diagnostic Systems, Inc.) (Fig. 7–57) is a microprocessor-controlled coagulation instrument capable of performing the PT, APTT, fibrinogen, thrombin time, and factor assays in a variety of combinations. The only limitation is that fibrinogen assays and thrombin times cannot be performed in the same run. All other test combinations are possible, from one test procedure to four different tests in the same batch.

A *message display* (two rows, 60 columns wide) and *keypad* allows for operator interaction with the system. Four *soft keys*, one located at each corner of the display, are used for menu selection. There are four *reagent wells* that hold vials and are cooled to 17°C ±3°C. Magnetic stirrers may be used in wells

1, 2, and 4. The four *peristaltic reagent pumps* deliver reagent from the reagent vials to the plasma mixtures. The *reagent arm* containing the reagent lines, along with the *reagent arm cover*, preheat the reagents to 37.5°C ± 0.6°C, and keep stray light from entering the test area. The *sample carousel*, capable of holding up to five *cuvette trays* of 12 wells each, is numbered from 1 to 60 so that a maximum of 60 plasmas may be tested in each run. A thermal *printer* provides a hardcopy record of numerical and graphic patient and control results, assay curves from the instrument memory, and a copy of instrument settings.

Principles of Operations

The KoaguLab 60-S is turned on using the power switch, and the instrument is allowed to warm-up for 15 minutes before testing. Reagent vials are placed in the reagent wells and the reagent intake tubes inserted into the appropriate vials. The reagent tubing is placed in the reagent arm and the delivery tips positioned directly over the center of the cuvette. A tip protector is mounted on the underside of the arm to prevent damage to the tip.

The first test selected in the instrument will determine the test settings for the entire run, but all tests must have the same maximum end point (amount of time instrument monitors a sample for clot formation). The coagulation menu is selected by pressing the appropriate soft key. The start position (in the sample carousel) is then selected by pressing the corresponding soft key. The appropriate number is entered to denote the first test cuvette, followed by pressing Enter. The first test procedure is selected by pressing the corresponding soft key. (The arrow key may be used to scroll through the test menu if necessary.) After selecting the first test the operator is prompted for the number of samples to be tested for that procedure. This number is entered and the Enter key pressed. The instrument will print the cuvette positions for the selected test. The next procedure is chosen as outlined above and the number of samples to be tested is entered as prompted by the display. Two additional procedures may be selected, if desired, using the same method just described. When all test selections have been made, a summary of the test run is printed out containing the cuvette number for each procedure.

Plasma samples are manually pipetted into the appropriate cuvettes in the tray(s) using the printed summary (from above). The Run key is pressed. The display reads Load, Prime, Press Run to Start Else Clear. An empty priming tray is placed under the reagent arm during the priming cycle to catch overflow reagent. The pumps are primed (tubing filled with reagent) by pressing the Prime key.

The cuvette trays are placed onto the sample carousel. Run is pressed to initiate the test cycle. The display reads Samples Incubating. The cuvette tray sensor will scan for the presence of the tray. The sample plate maintains the plasmas at 17°C prior to testing. The carousel advances at a preset rate to the incubation plate area where the cuvettes and their contents are warmed to 37.5°C. Reagent is added to four cuvette wells at a time.

The last area in the incubation plate is the test area in which there are four test stations. A light source is broken up into four channels, each containing an electro-optical detector. As clotting occurs, the turbidity of the reaction mixture increases and causes a decrease in the amount of light reaching the detector. This voltage change is measured by the detector and determines the clotting time for the sample.

Results are displayed and printed by the instrument. If duplicate testing was selected, the individual results as well as the average clotting time will be printed. If duplicate samples do not agree within preset limits, a warning is printed. If desired, a graph of the clotting curve may be printed (O.D. vs. time). At the completion of the test cycle, data can be reprinted or sent to a host computer.

Display Program

There are three Main Menu selections on the message display:

1. The *Coagulation menu* is used for test selection, to enter specimen ID numbers, and to program, edit, or run an assay using a standard curve stored in instrument memory.
2. The *Utility menu* allows the operator to calibrate pumps, set assay parameters and conditions, set report formats, and obtain clot graph data.

3. The *Service menu* is used to troubleshoot instrument problems and to set the output configuration for a host computer.

Discussion

An optional bar code wand is available for entering sample ID numbers. Sample testing may be performed singly or in duplicate, and testing may be carried out using full sample and reagent volumes or half volumes.

A variety of messages may be displayed to alert the operator to certain conditions prior to, during, or after a run. These messages are to prevent operator errors or to alert the operator to problems in the system.

Throughput will vary depending on how the operator programs the unit for incubation time and maximum end points. Duplicate PT testing set at a 30 second maximum end point will yield a throughput of 180 duplicate results per hour. Duplicate APTTs with a 3 minute incubation and 60 second maximum end point will have a throughput of 90+ duplicate results per hour.

There are two methods for programming test selection:

1. Using the *auto-random* method the PT and APTT may be performed in the same run in addition to the fibrinogen or the thrombin time. One test (PT/APTT, or the thrombin time or fibrinogen assay) is selected as the Tab On test and the other the Tab Off test. The instrument will detect the presence or absence of the tabs (torn off by the operator). This will determine which test the instrument performs on each cuvette.
2. When using the *auto-manual* procedure, test selection and cuvette assignments are made by the operator via the display and keyboard (as described above).

Samples with clotting times longer than the maximum end point (amount of time the KoaguLab 60-S will monitor a sample for clot formation) will print out as 000.0 seconds with the message "No Data." The message "Specimen Warning" or "Data Fit Warning" may print out to indicate that a sample does not meet the clot detection specifications of the KoaguLab 60-S.

The quality control program provides storage of data for four control levels per test method. A sample ID function and an operator-selected control ID number are used for identification of Q.C. specimens. Summary statistics (mean, S.D., and C.V.) are stored, and a Levey-Jennings plot of the 30 most recent data points may be printed at any time.

A PT or APTT ratio (test value/mean of the normal clotting time), percentage activity (PT), and the INR (PT) may be automatically calculated by the instrument, if desired.

ACL 3000

The ACL (Automated Coagulation Laboratory) 3000 (Fig. 7–58) is manufactured by Instrumentation Laboratory, Lexington, MA. It is an automatic microcomputer-controlled centrifugal analyzer capable of performing the PT, APTT, fibrinogen, thrombin time (TT), factor assays, protein C, and chromogenic assays (antithrombin III, α-2-antiplasmin, plasminogen, and heparin).

The ACL contains two measuring systems. *Nephelometry* is used to detect the end point for clot detection; *photometry*, measuring absorbance (optical density), is used for reading the chromogenic assays. In the clotting test a beam of light (from the LED) passes through the sample mixture. The finely dispersed particles in the sample scatter this light, which is measured by a photodetector positioned at right angles (90°) to the light path (nephelometric analysis).

Instrument Components

Disposable rotors contain 20 reaction cuvettes in which testing takes place. Each cuvette contains two wells with a dividing ridge to temporarily separate sample and reagent.

A *sample tray* (1) contains 20 positions and is loaded with the centrifuged specimen tube or sample cups (0.5 or 2.0 mL for controls and/or calibration plasmas). Two tray types are available, depending on the sample volume of the specimen tubes (5.0 or 3.5 mL).

There are three *reagent reservoirs* (2), two of which are cooled to approximately 15°C and hold reagent-filled cups, which may be mixed by magnetic stir bars. The third reservoir is maintained at room temperature. A fourth compartment contains a combination waste/rinse cup.

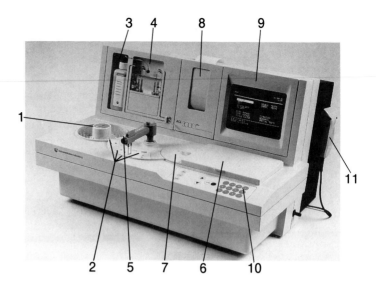

FIG. 7–58. ACL 3000. (Courtesy of Instrumentation Laboratory, Lexington, MA.)

The *sampling/dispensing system* consists of a bottle of silicone emulsion that is used for rinsing the sample and reagent pipets and also serves as the optical reference for the clotting channel. The *piston block* (4) contains two cylinders for use in the pipetting of sample and reagents and pipet rinsing.

The *arm assembly* (5) contains two needles, one for sample aspiration and one for reagent pipetting. The arm is capable of movement from side to side and up and down. *Fluidic sensors* are also present for detection of the plasma and/or reagent level. These sensors function during the incubation phase of the testing cycle to detect the presence of reference emulsion, specimens in the sample tray, and reagents in the reservoirs.

The *measuring chamber* is located under the cover on the top of the right side of the instrument. It consists of a temperature controlled (36 to 39°C) *rotor preheater* (6) on which up to 10 cuvette rotors may be stored, and the *optical measuring system and rotor holder* (7) (controlled at a temperature of 38.5°C ± 0.5°C) on which the cuvette rotor is placed for testing. There are two optical pathways: the nephelometric channel for clotting assays and the chromogenic path. The light source for clotting assays is an LED (light emitting diode) of 660 nm. The photodetector for this system is positioned below the rotor holder and measures the light scatter at right angles (90°) to the light path. The light source for chromogenic assays is a halogen lamp, and a 405 nm interference filter is used. The optical detector for this system is mounted directly above (180°) the rotor holder in the cover of the measuring chamber.

Microprocessors are responsible for controlling all functions of the instrument: mechanical movement of the arm assembly and spinning of the rotor, aspiration of samples and reagents, data accumulation and processing, and interfacing with input and output devices.

A *thermal printer* (8) is built into the ACL. It is capable of both graphic and numeric output.

The *video display unit* (9) informs the operator of instrument status (upper part of screen), displays menus, results, and graphs, and provides information on how to proceed through the steps of a testing sequence (central section of screen); it also displays general operational instructions (lower portion of display).

An 18 character membrane style *keyboard* (10) is used to enter the various operating modes of the instrument. The *stop* key, when used in conjunction with the *enter* key, will abort a testing cycle. The *PRT* (print) key activates the thermal printer. The *PROG* (special program menu) key will display a list of secondary programs that allow the operator to verify or modify certain functions and settings according to the laboratory's individual needs. The *cursor* and *enter* keys are used to make and confirm menu selections, respectively. *Numeric* keys are available for data input.

A standard *interface port* is provided for output of data to a host computer or PC (personal computer).

A hand-held *bar code scanner* (11) allows for the identification of patient samples with input of this information into the system.

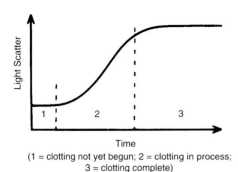

FIG. 7–59. Normal clotting curve, ACL 3000.

An *internal cooling system* maintains the instrument temperature. The cooling system has two alarms, one that warns the operator but allows testing to continue and one that shuts off the instrument.

Principles of Testing

A testing cycle begins with the pipetting of patient samples and reagents into a disposable plastic rotor containing 20 reaction cuvets. All pipetting is performed by the arm assembly (using a microprocessor controlled positive displacement system). Up to 18 plasma samples may be tested in each run. One cuvet is filled with the reference solution for establishing the baseline light scatter and a second cuvet is used for a calibration or control plasma. When all samples and reagents have been pipetted, the rotor spins at a speed of 1200 RPM. The centrifugal action forces the sample and reagent to move together to the outer well of each cuvette. The rotor stops abruptly, resulting in a homogeneous sample/reagent mixture. The rotor spins again for a specified period (usually 110 seconds), making approximately 20 revolutions per second. During this time a fixed beam of light passes through each cuvette. A measurement of light scatter is made every two revolutions (or 10 readings/second). Up to 1,100 readings for each reaction are collected by the microcomputer during this period. These readings are measured in relation to the optical reference solution initially placed in the rotor cuvette. The microcomputer plots a curve, graphing light scatter versus time for each sample (Fig. 7–59). Because each clot formed will be slightly different, an "offset" must be determined for each plasma

sample. This offset is determined during the initial reading of light scatter before the reaction starts. The curve is therefore "zeroed" (aligned with the X-axis [i.e., similar to reading a patient blank in spectrophotometry]) by averaging the first 10 readings (during the first second of centrifugation). The graph also contains two preset thresholds (Fig. 7–60). If the curve does not reach the first (lower) threshold, NO COAG is displayed. If the higher (second) threshold is not reached, COAG ERROR is displayed. This will occur in the presence of a low fibrinogen. The "S" shaped curve plotted for each sample determines the clotting time, which is defined as the amount of time it takes for the clot curve to reach a preset threshold. The fibrinogen concentration is determined from the PT curve. The last 10 readings (when the clot is well stabilized) of the PT curve are compared to the baseline of the same curve. The difference in light scatter is directly proportional to the fibrinogen concentration. This difference is compared to a standard curve in the instrument for determination of the clottable fibrinogen concentration. In this procedure, every plasma is examined for a total of 169 seconds (in the extended mode) irrespective of the clotting time.

When chromogenic assays are performed, because of the reagents used, a colored product is formed. A halogen lamp is used as the light source at a wavelength of 405 nm. The change in optical density is plotted against time and then compared with the appropriate

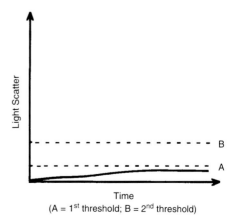

FIG. 7–60. Abnormal clotting curve (no clot formation), ACL 3000.

2. There are four color-coded *channel operation switches*, one for each channel. The first time the button is depressed, a 100% baseline value is read and stored. The second depression of the switch determines the 0% baseline, sets 0% on the printer paper, and begins the paper transport. Depressing the switch a third time terminates printing for that particular channel. When all channel switches have been depressed for the third time, the percentage aggregation and slope for each channel is printed out.

3. The *mode switch* has two settings: (1) When the green light is on, the instrument is ready for testing. If the switch is then depressed, the orange light comes on. (2) The orange light indicates the stir speed position, and the display will indicate the stir speed in each channel. The stir speed may be changed, using the appropriate *stir speed control* (make certain the test wells are empty). (All stir speeds used should be in the range of 600 to 1500 RPM. If speeds lower or higher are used an error message will be displayed.)

4. The *temperature indicator* will light when the incubation block reaches 37°C (8 to 10 minutes after the instrument is turned on).

5. The *micro-volume switch* is utilized when micro sample volumes (with microcuvettes) are used. This switch deactivates the magnetic stir bar detector and allows use of the micro stir bar.

6. The *memory switch* is used to initiate the instrument's memory recall. The aggregation patterns generated in each channel will remain in memory until another sample is tested in that channel. The patterns are stored in the unfiltered form but may be recalled as filtered or unfiltered.

7. *Display* will give information concerning the instrument operation, test status, stir speeds, and temperature when the instrument is on.

8. Each channel has its own color-coded *filter switch*. When this switch is activated, the oscillations (a function of the size of the platelet aggregate) generated during platelet aggregation are filtered out.

9. The platelet aggregation patterns are printed out on the *printer paper*, which may be manually advanced by depressing the *paper advance switch*.

10. There are four *incubation wells* maintained at 37°C for each of the four channels.

11. There is one *test well* for each of the four channels, in which platelet aggregation is tested and monitored.

See the Coagulation chapter of this book for the platelet aggregation test procedure.

Bio/Data Platelet Aggregation Profiler PAP-4C

The Bio/Data platelet aggregation profiler model PAP-4C is the same instrument as the model PAP-4 with the added feature of a program for chromogenic assays (antithrombin III, plasminogen, protein C, factor VIII, Factor Xa, heparin assays, and others).

The *chromogenic assay program* has four testing modes, a data storage mode and an exit mode. When installing a curve, channels 1, 2, and 3 are used for testing the reference standards for the curve, and if desired, a control or patient plasma may be tested in channel 4 at the same time.

1. The *% Act Curve 0–100%* mode is programmed to accept a three point curve (0%, 50%, and 100%) and reports results in percentage activity. It is recommended that indirect test methods be used in this mode—methods in which the change in optical density (absorbance) increases as the concentration of the analyte decreases.

2. The *% Act Curve 25–125%* also accepts a three point curve, but with concentrations of 25%, 75%, and 125%. Results are reported in percentage activity and direct test methods are used: as the absorbance increases, the concentration of the analyte increases.

3. The *IU Curve 0.1–0.7 IU* mode reports results in international units and is used for the heparin assay. It accepts concentrations of 0.1, 0.4, and 0.7 for the reference curve.

4. In the *Sample Test Mode* up to four separate patient samples may be run simultaneously. If a standard curve is present in working memory, all results from this test mode will automatically be plotted on the

curve and reported in the units of that curve.

5. The *Access Stored Data* mode allows up to eight standard curves to be stored in memory and allows curves to be reviewed, recalled (to working memory), or deleted (from memory). When a curve is recalled to working memory from this mode, all subsequent results are determined from the recalled curve. Curves stored in memory will remain when the instrument is turned off.

6. The *Exit Chromo* mode is used to exit from the chromogenic testing modes. The instrument returns to the aggregation mode and the 620 nm filter is restored.

The chromogenic test procedure uses reagents similar to those used in the manual methods. The final reagent used to halt the reaction, however, is not used, and instead of an absorbance reading being taken of the final color change, the *rate* of absorbance change is measured. When this reaction is graphed (O.D. vs. time) the slope of the resultant line is proportional to the enzyme concentration. The optical density is read at a wavelength of 405 nm and the instrument monitors the rate of O.D. change until adequate color develops. This time period will vary between procedures from 10 seconds to as long as 2 minutes.

Discussion

Magnetic stirring improves the reproducibility of the results by assuring a homogeneous mixture, especially important in fast reactions.

The printout of test results includes the standard curve with sample results automatically calculated.

Microsample adapters afford the use of greatly reduced sample and reagent volumes.

A chromogenic program template provides instructions for access into the chromogenic assay mode. The template fits over the channel switches. Space is provided on the template to record the locations and types of curves stored in memory.

BIBLIOGRAPHY

Ackerman, G.A.: Substituted naphthol AS phosphate derivatives for the localization of leukocyte alkaline
phosphate activity, Lab. Invest., *11*, 563, 1962.

American Diagnostica: DVVtest™, pkg. insert, Greenwich, CT, 1991.

American Optical Corporation: *Reference Manual Series 10
Microstar Advanced Laboratory Microscopes*, Buffalo, NY,
Scientific Instrument Division, 1974.

Applied Technology Associates, Inc.: Profile-Coulter
STKS hematology system, Lifshitz, M.S., and Di-
Cresce, R., editors, The Instrument Report, Chicago,
3, 1991.

Ash, L.R., and Orihel, T.C.: *Parasites: A Guide to Laboratory
Procedures and Identification*, ASCP Press, Chicago,
1987.

Babior, B.M., and Stossel, T.P.: *Hematology, A Pathophysi-
ological Approach*, Churchill Livingstone, New York,
1986.

Baxter Healthcare Corp.: Dade® adsorbed plasma and
serum reagents, pkg. insert, Dade Division, Miami,
FL, 1988.

Baxter Healthcare Corp.: Data-Fi euglobulin lysis reagents, pkg. insert, Dade Division, Miami, FL, 1989.

Baxter Healthcare Corp.: Data-Fi protamine sulfate reagents, pkg. insert, Dade Division, Miami, FL, 1985.

Becton, Dickinson and Company: *Laboratory Procedures Using the Unopette Brand System*, Rutherford, NJ, Becton,
Dickinson and Company, 1977.

Berenbaum, M.C.: The use of bovine albumin in the
preparation of marrow and blood films, J. Clin. Pathol., *9*, 381, 1956.

Betke, K., Marti, H.R., and Schlict, I.: Estimation of small
percentages of foetal haemoglobin, Nature, *184*,
1877, 1959.

Beutler, E.: A series of new screening procedures for
pyruvate kinase deficiency, glucose-6-phosphate dehydrogenase deficiency, and glutathione reductase
deficiency, Blood, *28*, 553, 1966.

Beutler, E., Dern, R.J., and Alving, A.S.: The hemolytic
effect of primaquine. VI. An in vitro test for sensitivity
of erythrocytes to primaquine, J. Lab. & Clin. Med.,
45, 40, 1955.

Biggs, R., and Douglas, A.S.: The thromboplastin generation test, J. Clin. Path., *6*, 23, 1953.

Bio/Data Corp.: vW factor assay™ for the quantitation of
von Willebrand factor, pkg. insert, Hatboro, PA, Bio/
Data Corp., 1986.

Bio/Data Corp.: *Operating Instructions and Methods Manual,
Platelet Aggregation Profiler® Model PAP-4*, Hatboro, PA,
Bio/Data Corp., 1985.

Bio/Data Corp.: *Operating Instructions and Methods Manual
Supplement. Platelet Aggregation Profiler Model PAP-4C
with Chromogenic Program*, Bio/Data Corp., Horsham,
PA, 1989.

Bithell, T.C.: Platelets and Megakaryocytes, in *Fundamentals of Clinical Hematology*, by Thorup, O.A., ed.,
W.B. Saunders Co., Philadelphia, 1987.

Boggs, D.R., and Winkelstein: *White Cell Manual*, F.A.
Davis Co., Philadelphia, 1983.

Bowie, E.J.W., and Owen, C.A.: The value of measuring
platelet "adhesiveness" in the diagnosis of bleeding
disorders, Am. J. Clin. Pathol., *60*, 302, 1973.

Brecher, G., and Cronkite, E.P.: Morphology and enumeration of human blood platelets, J. Appl. Physiol.,
3, 365, 1950.

Breen, F.A., Jr., and Tullis, J.L.: Ethanol gelation: A rapid
screening test for intravascular coagulation, Ann. Intern. Med., *69*, 1197, 1968.

Briere, R.O., Golias, T., and Batsakis, J.G.: Rapid qualitative and quantitative hemoglobin fractionation.
Cellulose acetate electrophoresis, Am. J. Clin. Pathol.,
44, 695, 1965.

Broden, P.: Hydrodynamic focusing in cell counting and
sizing, unpublished, Japan, TOA Medical Electronics
Co., Ltd., 1984.

Broden, P., and Culp, N.: *Sysmex NE Series Interpretive Flagging Definitions*, TOA Medical Electronics (USA) Inc.,
McGaw Park, IL, 1990.

Bruce, A.W.: *Basic Quality Assurance and Quality Control in
the Clinical Laboratory*, Little Brown, Boston, 1984.

Buchanan, G.R., and Holtkamp, C.A.: A comparative
study of variables affecting the bleeding time using
two disposable devices, Am. J. Clin. Pathol., *91*, 45,
1989.

Bull, B.S., and Brailsford, D.: The Zeta sedimentation ratio, Blood, Oct., 1972.

Burnett, R.W.: Accurate estimation of standard deviations for quantitative methods used in clinical chemistry, Clin. Chem., *21*, 1935, 1975.

Callahan, J.B., Jones-Green, C., and Magerko, D.J.: Coag-A-Mate XM: A new coagulation instrument for moderate-to-low volume applications, Interface, 1988.

Carr, J.M., Emery, S., Stone, B.F., and Tulin, L.: Babesiosis, diagnostic pitfalls, Am. J. Clin. Pathol., *95*, 774, 1991.

Carrell, R.W., and Kay, R.: A simple method for the detection of unstable haemoglobins, Br. J. Haematol., *23*, 615, 1972.

Cartwright, G.E.: *Diagnostic Laboratory Hematology*, New York, Grune & Stratton, Inc., 1963.

Cembrowski, G.S., and Carey, R.N.: *Laboratory Quality Management*. QC QA, Am. Soc. Clin. Pathol., Chicago, 1989.

Centers for Disease Control: Recommendations for prevention of HIV Transmission in Health-care Settings, MMWR, *36* (2S), 1987.

Chakrabarti, M., Bielawiec, J.F., Evans, J.F, and Fearnley, G.R.: Methodological study and a recommended technique for determining the euglobulin lysis time, J. Clin. Path., *21*, 698, 1968.

Claus, A.: Rapid physiological coagulation method for the determination of fibrinogen, Acta Haematol., *17*, 237, 1957.

Cocchi, P., Mori, S., and Becattini, A.: N.B.T. tests in premature infants, Lancet, *2*, 1426, 1969.

Colfs, B., and Vekeyden, J.: A rapid method for the determination of serum haptoglobin, Clin. Chem. Acta, *12*, 470, 1965.

Comp, P.C.: Laboratory evaluation of protein S status, Semin. Thromb. Hemost., *16*, 177, 1990.

Coulter Corporation: Evaluation of the Coulter Counter Model S-Plus IV differential in normal and hospitalized subjects, Hematology Analyzer, *6–4*, Hialeah, FL, Coulter Corporation, 1985.

Coulter Corporation: *Coulter Counter Model S-Plus IV with Data Terminal Product Reference Manual*, Hialeah, FL, Coulter Corporation, 1983.

Coulter Corporation: *Coulter S-Plus IV*, Hialeah, FL, Coulter Corporation, 1983.

Coulter Corporation: *Coulter S-Plus V*, Hialeah, FL, Coulter Corporation, 1983.

Coulter Corporation: *Coulter S-Plus VI*, Hialeah, FL, Coulter Corporation, 1984.

Coulter Corporation: *Instruction Manual for Coulter Zetafuge*, Hialeah, FL, Coulter Corporation, 1973.

Coulter Corporation: *STKR*, Hialeah, FL, Coulter Corporation, 1985.

Coulter Corporation: The advantage of Coulter pulse editing, Hematology Analyzer, Hialeah, FL, Coulter Corporation, *6–5*, 1985.

Coulter Corporation: *Coulter STKS Operator's Guide*, Coulter Corporation, Hialeah, FL, 1991.

Coulter Corporation: *Coulter STKS Service and Maintenance Manual*, Coulter Corporation, Hialeah, FL, 1991.

Coulter Corporation: *Coulter STKS Reference Manual*, Coulter Corporation, Hialeah, FL, 1991.

Dacie, J.V., and Lewis, S.M.: *Practical Hematology*, 6th ed., New York, Churchill Livingstone, Inc., 1991.

Daland, G.A., and Castle, W.B.: A simple and rapid method for demonstrating sickling of the red blood cells: The use of reducing agents. J. Lab. Clin. Med., *33*, 1082, 1948.

Davis, G.L.: Technical aspects of enzyme immunosorbent assays, Clin. Lab. Sci., *4*, 338, 1991.

Deacon-Smith, R.: The ascorbate cyanide test and the detection of females heterozygous for glucose-6-phosphate dehydrogenase deficiency, Med. Lab. Sciences, *39*, 139, 1982.

DeCresca, R.: The Technicon H-1: A discrete, fully automated complete blood count and differential analyzer, Lab., Med., *17*, 17, 1986.

Dharan, M.: *Total Quality Control in the Clinical Laboratory*, C.V. Mosby Co., St. Louis, 1977.

Diagnostica Stago: Asserachrom® Protein S Enzyme Immunoassay of Protein S, pkg. insert, Diagnostica Stago, Seine, France, 1991.

Diagnostica Stago: Asserachrom® vWF Enzyme immunoassay of vonWillebrand factor, pkg. insert, Diagnostica Stago, Seine, France, 1992.

Diagnostica Stago: F.S. test, pkg. insert, Diagnostica Stago, Seine, France, 1989.

Diagnostica Stago: Staclot® Protein C, pkg. insert, Diagnostica Stago, Seine, France, 1990.

Diagnostica Stago: Staclot® Protein S Clotting Assay of Protein S, pkg. insert, Diagnostica Stago, Seine, France, 1991.

Division of Host Factors, Center for Infectious Diseases, CDC: *Laboratory Methods for Detecting Hemoglobinopathies*, Atlanta, GA, Center for Disease control, 1984.

Dow, P.A., Petteway, M.B., and Alperin, J.B.: Simplified method for G-6-PD screening using blood collected on filter paper, Am. J. Clin. Pathol., *6*, 333, 1974.

Duke, W.W.: The pathogenesis of purpura haemorrhagica with especial reference to the part played by the blood platelets, Arch. Inter. Med., *10*, 445, 1912.

Efremov, CD., Huisman, T.H.J., and Wrightstone, R.N.: Microchromatography of hemoglobins. II. A rapid method for the determination of hemoglobin A_2, J. Lab. Clin. Med., *83*, 657, 1974.

Engelkirk, P.G., and Koester, S.K.: Proposed functions of eosinophils, J. Med. Tech., *3:3*, 181, 1986.

Erslev, A.J., and Gabuzda, T.G.: *Pathophysiology of Blood*, Philadelphia, W.B. Saunders Co., 1985.

Evelyn, K.A., and Malloy, H.T.: Microdetermination of oxyhemoglobin, methemoglobin, and sulfhemoglobin in a single sample of blood, J. Biol. Chem., *126*, 655, 1938.

Exner, T., Papadopoulos, G., and Koults, J.: Use of a simplified dilute Russell's viper venom time (DRVVT) confirms heterogeneity among "Lupus Anticoagulants," Blood Coag. Fibrinol., *1*, 259, 1990.

Fahey, J.L., Barth, W.F., and Solomon, A.: Serum hyperviscosity syndrome, JAMA, *192*, 464, 1965.

Feffer, S.E., Carmosino, L.S., Lin, J.H., and Fox, R.S.: In-vitro detection of heparin-induced humoral antiplatelet activity, South. Med. J., *79*, 315, 1986.

Funk, C., Gmür, J., Herold, R., and Straub, P.W.: Reptilase®-R—A new reagent in blood coagulation, Br. J. Haem., *21*, 43, 1971.

Gardlund, B.: The lupus inhibitor in thromboembolic disease and intrauterine death in the absence of systemic lupus, Acta Med. Scand., *215*, 293, 1984.

Garza, D., and Becan-McBride, K.: *Phlebotomy Handbook*, Appleton & Lange, Norwalk, CT, 1989.

Golde, D.W.: Overview of myeloid growth factors, Semin. Hematol., *27*, 1, 1990.

Graham, R.C., Lundholm, U., and Karnovsky, M.J.: Cytochemical demonstration of peroxidase activity with 3-amino-9-ethylcarbazole, J. Histochem. Cytochem., *13*, 150, 1965.

Green, M.: Centrifugal analysis as applied to coagulation testing, Cl. Hemostasis Rev., *5*, 11, 1991.

Ham, T.H.: Studies on destruction of red blood cells. Chronic hemolytic anemia with paroxysmal nocturnal hemoglobinuria, Arch. Intern. Med., *64*, 1271, 1939.

Harmening, D.M.: *Clinical Hematology and Fundamentals of Hemostasis*, F.A. Davis Co., Philadelphia, 1992.

Harrison, R.L., and Birotte, R.: The thrombin clotting time, Am. J. Clin. Pathol., *89*, 81, 1988.

Hartmann, R.C., Jenkins, D.E., Jr., and Arnold, A.B.: Diagnostic specificity of sucrose hemolysis test for paroxysmal nocturnal hemoglobinuria, Blood, *35*, 462, 1970.

Hattersley, P.G., and Hayse, D.: The effect of increased contact activation time on the activated partial thromboplastin time, Am. J. Clin Path., *66*, 479, 1976.

Hayash, M., and Okamoto, K.: The Sysmex total Hematology System, Sysmex J., *13*, 354, 1990.

Helena Laboratories: Beta-Thal Hemoglobin A₂ Quik Column™ Procedure, pkg. insert, Beaumont, TX, Helena Laboratories, 1984.

Helena Laboratories: Hemoglobin Electrophoresis Procedure, pkg. insert, Beaumont, TX, Helena Laboratories, 1985.

Helena Laboratories: Titan IV citrate hemoglobin electrophoresis procedure, pkg. insert, Beaumont, TX, Helena Laboratories, 1983.

Helena Laboratories: *ProtoFluor®-Z Hematofluorometer Operator's Manual*, Beaumont, TX, 1990.

Helena Laboratories: ProtoFluor® reagent system, pkg. insert, Beaumont, TX, 1987.

Helena Laboratories: Ristocetin Cofactor Assay, pkg. insert, Helena Laboratories, Beaumont, TX, 1985.

Henry, J.B., ed.: *Clinical Diagnosis and Management by Laboratory Methods*, Philadelphia, W.B. Saunders Co., 1991.

Hermelin, L.I.: Heparin-induced thrombocytopenia. Diagnosis and confirmation, Am. Clin. Prod. Rev., 1984.

Hicks, R., Schenken, J.R., and Steinrauf, M.A., eds.: *Laboratory Instrumentation*, Hagerstown, Harper & Row, 1980.

Hillman, R.S., and Finch, C.A.: *Red Cell Manual*, Philadelphia, F.A. Davis Co., 1985.

Hoffman, R., Benz, E.J. Jr., Shattil, S.J., et al.: *Hematology, Basic Principles and Practice*, Churchill Livingstone, New York, 1991

Howanitz, J.H., and Howanitz, P.J.: *Laboratory Medicine, Test Selection and Interpretation*, Churchill Livingstone, New York, 1991.

Hyun, B.H., Gulati, G.L., and Ashton, J.K.: Hematopoiesis and Blood Cell Morphology, In *Laboratory Medicine*, Howanitz, J.H., and Howanitz, P.J., eds., Churchill Livingstone, New York, 1991.

Instrumentation Laboratory: *ACL 3000 Coagulation System Operator's Manual*, Instrumentation Laboratory, Milan, Italy, 1991.

International Committee for Standardization in Hematology (Expert Panel on Rheology), Guidelines on selection of laboratory tests for monitoring the acute phase response, J. Clin. Pathol., *41*, 1203, 1988.

International Technidyne Corp.: Surgicutt, pkg. insert, International Technidyne Corp., Edison, NJ, 1988.

International Technidyne Corp.: Surgicutt Jr., pkg. insert, International Technidyne Corp., Edison, NJ.

International Technidyne Corp.: Surgicutt Newborn, pkg. insert, International Technidyne Corp., Edison, NJ, 1989.

International Technidyne Corp., Tenderfoot™, pkg. insert, Edison, NJ.

International Technidyne Corp.: Tenderlett™, pkg. insert, International Technidyne Corp., Edison, NJ, 1991.

Jacob, H.S., and Jandl, J.H.: A simple visual screening test for glucose-6-phosphate dehydrogenase deficiency employing ascorbate and cyanide, N. Engl. J. Med., *274*, 1162, 1966.

Janckila, A.J., Li, C., Lam, K., and Yam, L.T.: The cytochemistry of tartrate-resistant acid phosphatase, Am. J. Clin. Pathol., *70*, 45, 1978.

Jandl, J.H.: *Blood, Textbook of Hematology*, Little Brown, Boston, 1987.

Jandl, J.H.: *Blood: Pathophysiology*, Blackwell Scientific Publications, Boston, 1991.

Jones, J.A., Broszeit, H.K., LeCrone, C.N., and Detter, J.C.: An improved method for detection of red cell hemoglobin H inclusions, Am. J. Med. Tech., *47*, 94, 1981.

Kabi Diagnostics: Coatest® Protein C Assay, pkg. insert, Kabi Diagnostics, Sweden, 1988.

Kaplow, L.S.: Substitute for benzidine in myeloperoxidase stains, Am. J. Clin. Pathol., *63*, 451, 1975.

Kasper, C.K.: *Progress in Clinical Biological Research*, Alan R. Liss, New York, 87–98, 1984.

Kasper, C.K., and Ewing, N.P.: Acquired inhibitors of plasma coagulation factors, J. Med. Tech., *3*, 431, 1986.

Katayama, I., and Yang, J.P.S.: Reassessment of a cytochemical test for differential diagnosis of leukemic reticuloendotheliosis, Am. J. Clin. Pathol., *68*, 268, 1977.

Kisner, H.J.: Technicon H-2 hematology system, Clin. Lab. Mgmt. Rev., May/June, 190, 1991.

Knowles, D.M.: Lymphoid cell markers. Their distribution and usefulness in the immunophenotypic analysis of lymphoid neoplasms, Am. J. Surg. Path., *9(3)*, 85, 1985.

Kocoshis, T.A., Triplett, D.A.: CAP survey results for factor VIII assays (1977–1978), Am. J. Clin. Path., *72*, 346, 1979.

Koepke, J.A.: *Practical Laboratory Hematology*, Churchill Livingstone, New York, 1991.

Labbe, R.F., and Rettmer, R.L.: Zinc protoporphyrin: A product of iron-deficient erythropoiesis, Semin. Hematol., *26*, 40, 1989.

Lamberg, S.L., and Rothstein, R.: *Laboratory Manual of Hematology and Urinalysis*, Westport, CT, Avi Publishing Co., Inc., 1978.

Lampasso, J.A.: Error in hematocrit values produced by excessive ethylenediaminetetracetate, Techn. Bull. Regist. Med. Techn., *35*, 109, 1965.

Lampasso, J.A.: Changes in hematologic values induced by storage of ethylenediaminetetracetate human blood for varying periods of time, Techn. Bull. Regist. Med. Techn., *38*, 37, 1968.

Largo, R., Heller, V., and Straub, P.W.: Detection of soluble intermediates of the fibrinogen-fibrin conversion using erythrocytes coated with fibrin monomers, Blood, *47*, 991, 1976.

Lathem, W., and Worley, W.E.: The distribution of extracorpuscular hemoglobin in circulating plasma, J. Clin. Invest., *38*, 474, 1959.

Lee, R.I., and White, P.D.: A clinical study of the coagulation time of whole blood, Am. J. Med. Sci., *145*, 495, 1913.

Lenahan, J., and Smith, K. (eds.): Clotters Corner, Durham, NC, Organon Teknika Corp., 1986.

Lenahan, J.G., and Smith, K.: *Hemostasis*, Durham, N.C., Organon Teknika Corp., 1985.

Lilli, R.D., and Fullmer, H.M.: *Histopathologic Technic and Practical Histochemistry*, New York, McGraw-Hill Book Co., 1976.

Losowsky, M.S., Hall, R., and Goldie, W.: Congenital deficiency of fibrin-stabilizing factor, Lancet, *2*, 156, 1965.

MacGregor, R.G.S., Richards, W., and Loh, G.L.: The differential leucocyte count, J. Pathol. Bacteriol., *51*, 337, 1940.

Magath, T.B., and Winkle, V.: Technic for demonstrating 'L.E.' (lupus erythematosus) cells in blood, Am. J. Clin. Pathol., *22*, 586, 1952.

Maronde, G.R., et al.: A quality control system utilizing duplicate patient specimens, Am. J. Med. Tech., *40–4*, 165, 1974.

McBride, J.H.: Amino acids and proteins, in *Laboratory Medicine Test Selection and Interpretation*, by Howanitz, J.H. and Howanitz, P.J., eds., Churchill Livingstone, New York, p. 171, 1991.

McGlasson, D.L.: Specimen processing requirements for detection of lupus anticoagulant, Clin. Lab. Sci., *3*, 18, 1990.

McKenzie, S.B.: *Textbook of Hematology*, Philadelphia, Lea & Febiger, 1988.

McLucas, E., and Harrison, R.L.: The lupus anticoagulant, J. Med. Tech., *3*, 440, 1986.

McManus, J.F.A.: Histological demonstration of mucin after periodic acid, Nature, *158*, 202, 1946.

Medical Laboratory Automation, Inc.: *Operator's Manual, MLA 750*, Pleasantville, NY, Medical Laboratory Automation, Inc., 1981.

Medical Laboratory Automation, Inc.: *Operator's Manual, MLA Electra 800*, Pleasantville, NY, Medical Laboratory Automation, Inc., 1985.

Medical Laboratory Automation, Inc.: *Electra 900C Operator's Manual*, Medical Laboratory Automation, Inc., Pleasantville, NY, 1990.

Medical Laboratory Automation, Inc.: *Electra 1000C Automatic Coagulation Timer*, Medical Laboratory Automation, Inc., Pleasantville, NY, 1992.

Mielke, C.H., et al: The standardized normal Ivy bleeding time and its prolongation by aspirin, Blood, *34*, 204, 1969.

Miles Inc.: *Hema-Tek® Slide Stainer Operating Manual*, Miles Inc., Diagnostics Division, Elkhart, IN, 1986.

Miles Inc.: *Hema-Tek 2000 Operating Manual*, Miles, Inc., Diagnostics Division, Elkhart, IN, 1990.

Nalbandian, R.M., et al.: Dithionite tube test—a rapid, inexpensive technique for the detection of hemoglobin S and non-S sickling hemoglobin, Clin. Chem., *17*, 1028, 1971.

Nalbandian, R.M., et al.: Automated dithionite test for rapid, inexpensive detection of hemoglobin S and non-sickling hemoglobinopathies, Clin. Chem., *17*, 1033, 1971.

National Committee for Clinical Laboratory Standards: *Reference Procedure for the Human Erythrocyte Sedimentation Rate (E.S.R.) Test*, Code #H2-T2, NCCLS, Villanova, PA, 1983.

National Committee for Clinical Laboratory Standards: *Procedures for the Collection of Diagnostic Blood Specimens by Venipuncture*, Code #H3-A2, NCCLS, Villanova, PA, 1984.

National Committee for Clinical Laboratory Standards: *Procedures for the Collection of Diagnostic Specimens by Skin Puncture*, Code #H4-A2, NCCLS, Villanova, PA, 1986.

National Committee for Clinical Laboratory Standards: *Procedure for Determining Packed Cell Volume by the Microhematocrit Method*, Code #H7-A, NCCLS, Villanova, PA, 1985.

National Committee for Clinical Laboratory Standards: *Solubility Test for Confirming the Presence of Sickling Hemoglobins*, Code #H10-A, NCCLS, Villanova, PA, 1986.

National Committee for Clinical Laboratory Standards: *Screening Red Blood Cell Glucose-6-Phosphate Dehydrogenase Activity*, Code #H12-A, NCCLS, Villanova, PA, 1984.

National Committee for Clinical Laboratory Standards: *Proposed Guidelines for the Quantitative Measurement of Fetal Hemoglobin by the Alkali Denaturation Method*, Code #H13-P, NCCLS, Villanova, PA, 1982.

National Committee for Clinical Laboratory Standards: *Reference Procedure for the Quantitative Determination of Hemoglobin in Blood*, Code #H15-A, NCCLS, Villanova, PA, 1984.

National Committee for Clinical Laboratory Standards: *Method for Reticulocyte Counting, Proposed Standard*, Code #H16-P, NCCLS, Villanova, PA, 1985.

National Committee for Clinical Laboratory Standards: *Leukocyte Differential Counting*, Code #H20-T, NCCLS, Villanova, PA, 1984.

National Committee for Clinical Laboratory Standards: *Guidelines for the Standardized Collection, Transport and Preparation of Blood Specimens for Coagulation Testing and Performance of Coagulation Assays*, Code #H21-A, NCCLS, Villanova, PA, 1986.

National Committee for Clinical Laboratory Standards: *Citrate Agar Electrophoresis for Confirming Identification of Variant Hemoglobins*, (H23-T), NCCLS, Villanova, PA, 1988.

National Committee for Clinical Laboratory Standards: *Additives to Blood Collection Devices: Heparin*, Code H24-T, NCCLS, Villanova, PA, 1988.

National Committee for Clinical Laboratory Standards: *Proposed Guidelines for a Standardized Procedure for the Determination of Fibrinogen in Biological Samples*, Code #H30-P, NCCLS, Villanova, PA, 1982.

National Committee for Clinical Laboratory Standards: *Romanowsky Blood Stains*, Code #H32-P, NCCLS, Villanova, PA, 1986.

National Committee for Clinical Laboratory Standards: *Determination of Factor VIII Coagulant Activity (VIII:C), Proposed Guideline*, Code #H34-P, NCCLS, Villanova, PA, 1986.

National Committee for Clinical Laboratory Standards: *Additives to Blood Collection Devices: EDTA*, Code H35-P, NCCLS, Villanova, PA, 1989.

National Committee for Clinical Laboratory Standards: *Proposed Guidelines for Citrate Agar Electrophoresis for Confirming Identification of Mutant Hemoglobins*, NCCLS, Villanova, PA, 1981.

National Committee for Clinical Laboratory Standards: *Use of Blood Film Examination for Parasites*, Code M15-P, NCCLS, Villanova, PA, 1990.

Okamura, K., Kato, H., Matsuda, N., and Takahashi, H.: An improved nitroblue tetrazonium test and its correlation with toxic neutrophils, *62*, 27, 1974.

Organon Teknika Corp.: Automated APTT, pkg. insert, Organon Teknika Corp., Durham, NC, 1990.

Organon Teknika Corp.: Chromostrate™ Antithrombin III Assay, pkg. insert, Durham, NC, Organon Teknika Corp., 1987.

Organon Teknika Corp.: Chromostrate™ Heparin Anti-Xa Assay, pkg. insert, Organon Teknika Corp., Durham, NC, 1988.

Organon Teknika Corp.: Chromostrate™ Plasminogen Assay, pkg. insert, Durham, NC, Organon Teknika Corp., 1987.

Organon Teknika Corp.: *Coag-A-Mate 2001 Operator's Manual*, Durham, NC, Organon Teknika Corp., 1979.

Organon Teknika Corp.: *Coag-A-Mate Dual Channel Operator's Manual*, Durham, NC, Organon Teknika Corp., 1974.

Organon Teknika Corp.: *Coag-A-Mate·X2 Operations Manual*, Durham, NC, Organon Teknika Corp., 1981.

Organon Teknika Corp.: *Coag-A-Mate XM Operator Manual*, Organon Teknika Corp., Durham, NC, 1990.

Organon Teknika Corp.: Fibrinosticon, latex agglutination immunoassay, pkg. insert, Organon Teknika Corp., Durham, NC, 1990.

Organon Teknika Corp.: *Fibriquik*, pkg. insert, Durham, NC, Organon Teknika Corp., 1983.

Organon Teknika Corp.: International Normalized Ratio (INR), pkg. insert, Organon Teknika Corp., Durham, NC, 1989.

Organon Teknika Corp.: *MDA Coagulation Instrumentation Manual*, Organon Teknika Corp., Durham, NC, 1991.

Organon Teknika Corp.: Simplate Bleeding Time Device, pkg. insert, Durham, NC, Organon Teknika Corp., 1985.

Organon Teknika Corp.: Thromboquick™ thrombin reagent, pkg. insert, Organon Teknika Corp., Durham, NC, 1990.

Ortho Diagnostic Systems, Inc.: *KoaguLab* 16-S Coagulation System*, Raritan, NJ, Ortho Diagnostic Systems, Inc., 1985.

Ortho Diagnostic Systems, Inc.: *KoaguLab* 40-A Automated Coagulation System*, Raritan, NJ, Ortho Diagnostic Systems, Inc., 1984.

Ortho Diagnostic Systems, Inc.: *KoaguLab 60-S Coagulation System Operator's Manual*, Ortho Diagnostic Systems, Inc., Raritan, NJ, 1990.

Pappas, A.A., Palmer, S.K., Meece, D., and Fink, L.M.: Rapid preparation of plasma for coagulation testing, Arch. Pathol. Lab. Med., *115*, 816, 1991.

Park, B.H., Fikring, S.M., and Smithwick, E.M.: Infection and nitroblue-tetrazolium reduction by neutrophils, Lancet, *2*, 532, 1968.

Parpart, A.K., et al.: The osmotic resistance (fragility) of human red cells, J. Clin. Invest., *26*, 636, 1947.

Pearson, R.W., Houwen, B., and Mast, B.: Sysmex Sulfolyser, TOA Medical Electronics (USA), Inc., Los Alamitos, CA, 1991.

Pendergraph, G.E.: *Handbook of Phlebotomy*, Philadelphia, Lea & Febiger, 1984.

Pimental, E.: Colony stimulating factors, Ann. Clin. Lab. Sci., *20*, 36, 1990.

Powers, L.W.: *Diagnostic Hematology: Clinical and Technical Principles*, C.V. Mosby Co., St. Louis, 1989.

Proctor, R.R., and Rapaport, S.I.: The partial thromboplastin time with kaolin, Am. J. Clin. Path., *36*, 212, 1961.

Quick, A.J.: *Bleeding Problems in Clinical Medicine*, Philadelphia, W.B. Saunders Co., 1970.

Quick, A.J.: Salicylates and bleeding: The aspirin tolerance test, Am. J. Med. Sci., *252*, 265, 1966.

Randolph, T.G.: Differentiation and enumeration of eosinophils in the counting chamber with a glycol stain, J. Lab. Clin. Med., *34*, 1696, 1949.

Ratnoff, O.D., and Forbes, C.D., editors: *Disorders of Hemostasis*, Orlando, FL, Grune & Stratton, Inc., 1990.

Raven, J.L., and Tooze, J.A.: α-thalassaemia in Britain, Br. Med. J., *4*, 486, 1973.

Richardson-Jones, A.: An automated hematology instrument for comprehensive WBC, RBC, and platelet analysis, Am. Clin. Lab., Jan./Feb., 1991.

Salzman, E.W.: Measurement of platelet adhesiveness. A simple in-vitro technique demonstrating an abnormality in von Willebrand's disease, J. Lab. Clin. Med., *62*, 724, 1963.

Schneiderman, L.J., Junga, I.G., and Fawley, D.E.: Effect of phosphate and non-phosphate buffers on thermolability of unstable haemoglobins, Nature, *225*, 1041, 1970.

Selwyn, J.G., and Dacie, J.V.: Autohemolysis and other changes resulting from the incubation in vitro of red cells from patients with congenital hemolytic anemia, Blood, *9*, 414, 1954.

Sheehan, H.L., and Storey, G.W.: An improved method of staining leukocyte granules with sudan black B, J. Path. Bact., *59*, 336, 1947.

Shephard, M.K., Weatherall, D.J., and Conley, C.L.: Semiquantitative estimation of the distribution of fetal hemoglobin in red cell populations, Bull. J. Hopkins Hosp., *110*, 293, 1962.

Sigma Diagnostics: Alkaline Phosphatase, pkg. insert, St. Louis, Sigma Chemical Co., 1988.

Sigma Diagnostics: Atroxin® (Bothrops atrox venom). Determination of Plasma Clotting Time, pkg. insert, St. Louis, Sigma Chemical Co., 1989.

Sigma Diagnostics: Fetal hemoglobin, pkg. insert, St. Louis, MO, 1988.

Sigma Chemical Co.: Glutathione Reductase Deficiency in Blood, pkg. insert, St. Louis, Sigma Chemical Co., 1986.

Sigma Diagnostics: Glucose-6-Phosphate Dehydrogenase (G-6-PDH) Deficiency, pkg. insert, St. Louis, Sigma Chemical Co., 1989.

Sigma Diagnostics: Pyruvate Kinase Deficiency, Qualitative, Visual Fluorescence Determination in Red Cells, pkg. insert, St. Louis, Sigma Chemical Co., 1987.

Sigma Chemical Co.: Nitroblue tetrazolium (NBT) reduction, histochemical demonstration in neutrophils, pkg. insert, St. Louis, Sigma Chemical Co., 1985.

Simmons, A.: *Hematology, A Combined Theoretical and Technical Approach*, W.B. Saunders Co., Philadelphia, 1989.

Simson, E., Ross, D.W., and Kocher, W.D.: *Atlas of Automated Cytochemical Hematology*, Technicon Instruments Corp., Tarrytown, NY, 1988.

Singer, K., Chernoff, A.I., and Singer, L.: Studies on abnormal hemoglobins. 1. Their demonstration in sickle cell anemia and other hematologic disorders by means of alkali denaturation, Blood, *6*, 413, 1951.

Sirchia, G., Soldano, F., and Mercurial, F.: The action of two sulfhydryl compounds on normal human red cells. Relationship to red cells of paroxysmal nocturnal hemoglobinuria, Blood, *25*, 502, 1965.

Smith, J.W., Melvin, D.M., Orihel, T.C., et al.: *Atlas of Diagnostic Medical Parasitology, Blood and Tissue Parasites*, American Society of Clinical Pathologists Press, Chicago, 1976.

Spinco Division, Beckman Instruments Inc.: *Preliminary Instruction Manual for Model R-101 Microzone Electrophoresis Cell*, Palo Alto, CA, Spinco Division, Beckman Instruments Incorporated, 1963.

Straight, D.L.: The physiologic inhibitors of blood coagulation and fibrinolysis, J. Med. Tech., *3*, 443, 1986.

Sun, T., Li, C., and Yam, L.T.: *Atlas of Cytochemistry and Immunochemistry of Hematologic Neoplasms*, Am. Soc. Clin. Pathol. Press, Chicago, 1985.

Sundberg, R.D., and Broman, H.: The application of the Prussian blue stain to previously stained films of blood and bone marrow, Blood, *10*, 160, 1955.

Technicon Instruments Corp.: *Technicon H-1™ System Operator's Guide*, Tarrytown, NY, Technicon Instruments Corp., 1985.

Technicon Instruments Corp.: *Technicon H-1™ System Course Guide*, Tarrytown, NY, Technicon Instruments Corp., 1985.

Technicon Instruments Corp.: *H-2 System Manuals: Unit 2, Operation; Unit 4, Troubleshooting; Unit 5, Reference Manual*, Technicon Instruments Corp., Tarrytown, NY, 1990.

Thorup, O.A., ed.: *Fundamentals of Clinical Hematology*, W.B. Saunders Co., Philadelphia, 1987.

TOA Medical Electronics Co., Ltd.: *Sysmex, E-Series Training Manual Part 1*, Japan, TOA Medical Electronics Co., Ltd., 1985.

TOA Medical Electronics Co., Ltd.: *E-500 Operator's Manual*, Japan, TOA Medical Electronics Co., Ltd., 1985.

TOA Medical Electronics (USA) Inc.: *NE-8000 Activity Guide/Training Manual*, Baxter Scientific Products Division, McGaw Park, IL, 1989.

TOA Medical Electronics (USA) Inc.: *NE-8000 Operator's Manual*, Baxter Scientific Products Division, McGaw Park, IL, 1988.

TOA Medical Electronics Co., Ltd.: *Sysmex R-1000 Operator's Manual*, TOA Medical Electronics Co., Ltd., Japan.

TOA Medical Electronics Co., Ltd.: *Sysmex H-Series, product brochure*, Kobe, Japan, 1991.

Tocantins, L.M.: Technical methods for the study of blood platelets, Arch. Path., *23*, 850, 1937.

Triplett, D.A.: *Laboratory Evaluation of Coagulation*, Chicago, Am. Soc. Clin. Path. Press, 1982.

Triplett, D.A., Brandt, J.T., Kaczor, D., and Schaeffer, J.: Laboratory diagnosis of lupus inhibitors: A comparison of the tissue thromboplastin inhibition procedure with a new platelet neutralization procedure, Am. J. Clin. Path., *79*, 678, 1983.

Triplett, D.A., Harms, C.S.: *Procedures for the Coagulation Laboratory*, Chicago, Am. Soc. Clin. Path. Press, 1981.

Turgeon, M.L.: *Clinical Hematology*: Little Brown, Boston, 1988.

Unipath Corp. (Abbott Diagnostics): Cell-Dyn 3000 laser

differential scatterplot interpretation, Unipath Corp., Mountain View, CA, 1989.

Unipath Corp. (Abbott Diagnostics): *Cell-Dyn 3000 Operator's Manual*, Unipath Corp., Mountain View, CA, 1990.

U.S. Dept. of HEW, Public Health Service, CDC, Bureau of Laboratories, Hematology Division, HEW Pub. #(CDC)78–8266: *Basic Laboratory Methods of Hemoglobinopathy Detection*, Atlanta, GA, U.S. Dept. of HEW, 1978.

U.S. Department of Health and Human Services/Public Health Service, *Laboratory Methods for Detecting Hemoglobinopathies*, Center for Disease Control, Atlanta, 1984.

Walters, J., and Fritsma, G.: Technical analysis of the R-1000 reticulocyte analyzer and comparison to manual reticulocyte counts, Hematology Monograph, Baxter Healthcare Corp., Scientific Products Division, July, 1990.

Walton, J.R.: Uniform grading of hematologic abnormalities, Am. J. Med. Technol., *39*, 517, 1973.

Wanatabe, K.: R-1000 automated reticulocyte analyzer. Reports on the clinical utility, TOA Medical Electronics Co., Ltd., Japan.

Warner, B.A., and Reardon, D.M.: A field evaluation of the Coulter STKS, Am. J. Clin. Pathol., *95*, 207, 1991.

Wellcome Diagnostics: Thrombo-Wellcotest. Rapid latex test for detection of fibrinogen degradation products,

pkg. insert, Dartford, England, The Wellcome Foundation Ltd., 1986.

Wellcome Research Laboratories: Russell Viper Venom, pkg. insert, Beckenham, England, Wellcome Research Laboratories, 1977.

Westgard, J.O., and Groth, T.: A multi-rule Shewhart chart for quality control in clinical chemistry, *27*, 493, 1981.

Wiernik, P., Canellos, G.P., Kyle, R.A., and Schiffer, C.A.: *Neoplastic Diseases of the Blood*, New York, Churchill Livingstone, Inc., 1991.

Williams, N., and Levine, R.F.: The origin, development and regulation of megakaryocytes, Br. J. Haematol., *52*, 173, 1982.

Williams, W., Beutler, E., Erslev, A.J., and Lichtman, M.A.: *Hematology*, New York, McGraw-Hill Book Co., 1990.

Yam, L.T., Li, C.Y., and Crosby, W.H.: Cytochemical identification of monocytes and granulocytes, Am. J. Clin. Path., *55*, 283, 1971.

Zinkham, W.H., and Conley, C.L.: Some factors influencing the formation of L.E. cells. A method for enhancing L.E. cell production, Bullet. Johns Hopkins Hosp., *98*, 102, 1956.

Zuck, T.F., Bergin, J.J, Raymond, J.M., and Dwyre, W.R.: Implications of depressed antithrombin-III activity associated with oral contraceptives, Surg. Gynecol. Obstet., *133*, 609, 1971.

INDEX

Page numbers in *italics* indicate illustrations; numbers followed by ''t'' indicate tables.